BASIC TECHNIQUES
FOR THE MEDICAL
LABORATORY

BASIC TECHNIQUES FOR THE MEDICAL LABORATORY

Jean Jorgenson Linné, B.S., M.T. (ASCP)

Karen Munson Ringsrud, B.S., M.T. (ASCP)

DEPARTMENT OF LABORATORY MEDICINE AND PATHOLOGY
UNIVERSITY OF MINNESOTA

Second Edition

McGraw-Hill Book Company • New York • St. Louis • San Francisco • Auckland
Bogotá • Düsseldorf • Johannesburg • London • Madrid • Mexico • Montreal • New Delhi
Panama • Paris • São Paulo • Singapore • Sydney • Tokyo • Toronto

BASIC TECHNIQUES FOR THE MEDICAL LABORATORY

4 5 6 7 8 9 0 DODO 7 8 3 2 1

This book was set in Press Roman by Hemisphere Publishing Corporation.
The editor was Stuart D. Boynton; the designer was Hermann Strohbach;
the production supervisor was Milton J. Heiberg.

Library of Congress Cataloging in Publication Data

Linné, Jean Jorgenson.
    Basic techniques for the medical laboratory.

    First ed. (c1970) published under title: Basic
laboratory techniques for the medical laboratory technician.
    Bibliography: p.
    1. Diagnosis, Laboratory–Laboratory manuals.
I. Ringsrud, Karen Munson, joint author. II. Title.
[DNLM: 1. Technology, Medical. QY25.3 L578b]
RB37.L67 1979   616.07'5   78-12209
ISBN 0-07-037948-3

TO

David and Peter — our husbands

David, Erik, and Jonathan — our children

CONTENTS

CHAPTER FOUR
COAGULATION AND HEMOSTASIS 271

CHAPTER FIVE
URINALYSIS 287

CHAPTER SIX
EXAMINATION OF MISCELLANEOUS EXTRAVASCULAR FLUIDS 379

CHAPTER SEVEN
EXAMINATION OF THE FECES 391

PREFACE TO THE SECOND EDITION

The first edition of this text, "Basic Laboratory Techniques for the Medical Laboratory Technician," has met with favorable response. Because of this success, and in order to update and to generally improve and enhance the material covered in the first edition, this second edition was written. The goals of the book remain the same as those for the first edition.

Significant advances in laboratory medicine have demanded the rather extensive revision seen in the second edition. Much of the information contained in the first edition remains unchanged, but a significant amount of information has been added, including new chapters covering serology, hemostasis and coagulation, examination of extravascular fluid, and examination of the feces. One chapter on basic metabolic rate and electrocardiography tests has been deleted.

It is anticipated that this basic general information will be applicable to persons at various levels of clinical laboratory training. As in the first edition, the clinical laboratory specialties of hematology, urinalysis, and chemistry are stressed, and these chapters have been expanded considerably.

The reader will notice that a change in the title of the textbook has also been made. The new title, "Basic Techniques for the Medical Laboratory," is less cumbersome and conveys the general intent of the second edition.

Several new illustrations have been added to enhance the written word. Photomicrograph reproductions of various blood cells and urinary sediment structures have also been included to visually describe these common microscopic findings.

Since publication of the first edition of this text, the authors have been involved in the teaching of basic laboratory techniques to medical students at the University of Minnesota under the direction of Dr. G. Mary Bradley. We want to thank Dr. Bradley for her inspiration, practical knowledge, and clinical expertise, which we hope has been conveyed in this revision.

In the preparation of this second edition, the authors were assisted once again by many interested persons in the Department of Laboratory Medicine and Pathology at the University of Minnesota. We extend another word of thanks to Dr. Ellis S. Benson, professor and head of the Department of Laboratory Medicine and Pathology, for his continued support. In addition to those persons mentioned in the preface to the first edition, we wish to thank Dr. G. Mary Bradley, Sandra Carter, Marilyn Cavanaugh, Helen Hallgren, Mary Damron, Dolores Harvey, Grace Mary Ederer, Patricia Johnson, and Karen Viskochil.

A special thanks to Ruth Hovde and Verna Rausch who originated the medical laboratory assistant course at the University of Minnesota. Without their foresight, this textbook would never have been written.

Several new illustrations have been added, thanks to the fine artwork of Mr. Martin Finch and Mrs. Linda Richter. We want to thank Drs. Robert McKenna and Richard Brunning for their advice in preparing several of the photomicrographs of blood cells and the urinary sediment. A very special thanks to Peter Ringsrud for the many days he spent in the darkroom processing these photomicrographs in addition to his photography, which is included in the text. Thanks also to Drs. Patrick Ward and G. Mary Bradley and to the University of Minnesota Medical School for permission to use several photomicrographs of the urinary sediment from slide collections of the Department of Laboratory Medicine and Pathology.

We also wish to thank Dorothy Lekson and her fellow instructors in the medical laboratory assistant course at the St. Paul Technical Vocational Institute for their helpful cooperation and suggestions during the writing of this second edition.

Revising a textbook requires a great deal of time. The authors wish to thank their families—husbands and children—for their patience and support throughout the revision process, which was a time of personal disruption. Erik and Peter Ringsrud and Jonathan, David, and David Linné were a continual source of encouragement and survival.

Jean Jorgenson Linné
Karen Munson Ringsrud

PREFACE TO THE FIRST EDITION

In the modern medical laboratory a wide variety of analyses ranging from simple to complex are utilized by the physician and are essential to him in the management of his patients. Laboratory personnel, to qualify for such work, require specific training and education. Usually the laboratory is under the direction of a medical doctor, the pathologist, who is a physician specializing in pathology, the study of disease. Under the direction of the pathologist is the medical technologist, who is educated to perform the complex laboratory procedures, to engage in teaching activities, and to handle supervisory and administrative duties. To assist the medical technologist, the medical laboratory technician is specifically trained for routine tasks.

Although the laboratory technician has proper understanding of basic fundamentals and techniques so as to be flexible in the use of his training and skills, he is not qualified to make technical and administrative decisions.

It takes a special type of person to work in a clinical laboratory. He must understand the need for accuracy, be conscientious, and above all, want to be of service to the patient.

The materials for this textbook have been developed from the lectures given students in the medical laboratory assistant program at the University of Minnesota. It is intended to provide the student technician with basic information in the departments of the clinical laboratory where technicians will work; these departments include chemistry, hematology, urinalysis, blood banking, microbiology, electrocardiography, and basal metabolism. In addition to these chapters, a discussion of basic laboratory fundamentals is included.

The authors gratefully acknowledge the contributions of Ruth Hovde, Verna Rausch, Margaret Ohlen Hanson, Elizabeth Lundgren, Ruth Brown Anderson, Marilyn Scovil Cavanaugh, and Mary Lou Kuefner Carlson, people who formerly were associated with the instruction and the administration of the medical laboratory assistant program from which the material for this book evolved.

The authors express their appreciation to Mary Damron, Barbara Merritt, Grace Mary Ederer, Patricia Hanauer Bordewich, Donna Blazevic, Sandra Benson, and Margaret Halsted for their assistance in reviewing the various sections of the book during its preparation, and to Mr. Martin Finch for his assistance in the preparation of the illustrations.

The authors thank Dr. Ellis S. Benson, Professor and head of the Department of Laboratory Medicine, for his encouragement and support of this project.

Jean Jorgenson Linné
Karen Munson Ringsrud

ONE
FUNDAMENTALS OF THE CLINICAL LABORATORY

The aim of this chapter is to give general information that applies to most laboratory work. The use of certain laboratory equipment (the microscope, the photometer, glassware, and the centrifuge, for example) is discussed, as well as laboratory calculations, units of measurement, quality control programs, laboratory safety, the proper preparation of reagents, and the cleaning of laboratory glassware. Certain general techniques are also discussed, such as weighing, pipetting, and titration. The proper collection of laboratory specimens, including the procedure for collecting blood, is covered. A knowledge of these subjects is basic information for those who engage in the major areas of laboratory work covered in the chapters that follow.

SAFETY IN THE LABORATORY

The importance of laboratory safety and correct first-aid procedures cannot be overemphasized to anyone working in the medical laboratory. Students as well as laboratory personnel should be constantly reminded of safety precautions. Most accidents do not just happen—they are caused by carelessness. For this reason, safety should be foremost in the mind of anyone involved in doing laboratory work of any kind.

Most laboratory accidents are preventable by the exercise of good technique and by the use of common sense. There are many potential hazards in the laboratory, but they can be controlled by taking simple precautions. In every medical institution, the administration supplies the laboratory with safety devices for equipment and personal use, but it is up to the individual to make use of them. Safety is personal, and its practice must be a matter of individual desire and accomplishment. Real appreciation for safety requires a built-in concern for the other person, for an unsafe act may harm the bystander without harming the person who performs the act.

To ensure that workers have safe and healthful working conditions, the United States government created a system of safeguards and regulations under the Occupational Safety and Health Act of 1970.[1] This system touches almost every person working in the United States today. It is especially relevant to discuss the meaning of the act in any presentation concerning safety in the clinical laboratory. In this setting there are special problems with respect to potential safety hazards, and diseases or accidents associated with preventable causes cannot be tolerated in the busy laboratory today.

The Occupational Safety and Health regulations apply to all businesses with one or more employees and are administered by the U.S. Department of Labor through the Occupational Safety and Health Administration (OSHA). The program deals with many aspects of safety and health protection, including compliance arrangements, inspection procedures, penalties for noncompliance, complaint procedures, duties and responsibilities for administration and operation of the system, and how the many standards are set. Responsibility for compliance is placed on both the administration of the institution and the employee. The maximum fine for noncompliance with the OSHA regulations is $1000 per day.

A person who understands the potential hazards in a laboratory and knows the basic safety precautions can prevent accidents. The Occupational Safety and Health Act requires a safety program in every clinical laboratory. Identification of potential hazards is a most important part of any such program. In each department in the laboratory, the type of hazard is slightly different. However, many hazards are commonly found throughout the laboratory.

One safeguard that can be taken is to see that all containers are properly labeled. Labeling may be the simplest, single important step in the proper handling of hazardous substances. Because many hazards of the clinical laboratory are unique, a special term, *biohazard*, was devised. This word is posted throughout the laboratory to denote infectious materials or agents that present a risk or even a potential risk to the health of humans or animals in the laboratory. The potential risk can be either through direct infection or through the environment. Biological infections are frequently caused by accidental aspiration of infectious material orally through a pipet, accidental inoculation with contaminated needles or syringes, animal bites, sprays from syringes, and

centrifuge accidents. Some other sources of laboratory infections are cuts or scratches from contaminated glassware, cuts from instruments used during animal surgery or autopsy, and spilling or spattering of pathogenic samples on the work desks or floors. People working in laboratories on animal research or other research involving biologically hazardous materials are most susceptible to the problems of biohazards. The symbol shown in Fig. 1-1 is used to denote the presence of biohazards. A label for a container should include a date and the chemical contents of the container. When the contents of one container are transferred to another container, this information should also be transferred to the new container. Proper labeling of containers is discussed further under Quantitative Transfer in this chapter.

The fact that clinical laboratories present many potential hazards simply because of the nature of the work done there cannot be overemphasized; open flames, electrical equipment, glassware, chemicals of varying reactivity, flammable solvents, biohazards, and toxic fumes are but a few. One serious hazard in laboratory work is the

Fig. 1-1. Biohazard symbol.

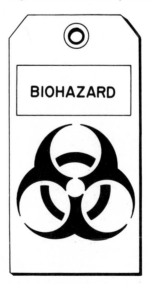

potential for fire and explosion when flammable solvents such as ether and acetone are used. These materials should always be stored in special safety cans or other appropriate storage devices. Even with proper storage of these materials, there is always some release of flammable vapors in a working laboratory. A good ventilation system in the room and vent sites for the storage area will help to eliminate some of the potential hazard. When using flammable materials, proper precautions must be taken; for instance, flammable liquids should be poured from one container to another slowly, they should never be used when there is an open flame in the room, and they should be kept in closed containers when they are not being used.

Other sources of injury in the laboratory are poisonous, volatile, caustic, or corrosive reagents such as strong acids or bases. Chemicals and reagents can present different types of hazards. Some are dangerous when inhaled (sulfuric acid), some are corrosive to the skin (phenol), some are caustic (acetic acid), some are volatile (many solvents), and some combine these hazards. Acids and bases should be stored separately in well-ventilated storage units. When not in use, all chemicals and reagents should be returned to their storage units. Bottles of particularly volatile substances should not be left open for extended periods. Some chemicals that must be handled with care and some potential hazards in their use are:

Sulfuric acid: At a concentration above 65% may cause blindness; may produce burns on the skin; if taken orally may cause severe burns, depending on the concentration.

Nitric acid: Gives off yellow fumes that are extremely toxic and damaging to tissues; overexposure to vapor can cause death, loss of eyesight, extreme irritation, smarting, itching, and yellow discoloration of the skin; if taken orally can cause extreme burns, may perforate the stomach wall, can cause death.

Acetic acid: Severely caustic; continuous exposure to vapor can lead to chronic bronchitis.

Hydrochloric acid: Inhalation of vapors should be avoided; any on the skin should be washed away immediately to prevent a burn.

Sodium hydroxide: Extremely hazardous in contact with the skin, eyes, and mucous membranes (mouth), causing caustic burns; dangerous even at very low concentrations; any contact necessitates immediate care.

Phenol (a disinfectant): Can cause caustic burns or contact dermatitis even in dilute solutions; wash off skin with water or alcohol.

Carbon tetrachloride: Damaging to the liver even at an exposure level where there is no discernible odor.

Trichloroacetic acid: Very severely caustic; respiratory tract irritant.

Ethers: Cause depression of central nervous system.

When using any potentially hazardous solution or chemical, protective equipment for the eyes, face, head, and extremities, as well as protective clothing or barriers, should be used. Volatile or fuming solutions should be used under a fume hood. In case of accidental contact with a hazardous solution or a contaminated substance, quick action is essential. The laboratory should have a safety shower where quick, all-over decontamination can take place immediately. Another safety device that is essential in all laboratories is a face or eye washer that streams aerated water directly onto the face and eyes to prevent burns and loss of eyesight. Any action of this sort must be undertaken immediately, so these safety devices must be present in the laboratory area.

In case of fire hazards, various types of fire-extinguishing agents must be available and their use must be understood. Fire in clothing should be smothered with a fire blanket or heavy toweling or the flame should be beaten out; it should not be flooded with water. Everyone in the laboratory should know the correct use of the fire alarm.

It is a generally accepted rule that all pipetting must be done by mechanical means and not by using mouth suction. For pipetting use either mechanical suction or aspirator bulbs. This procedure safeguards against burning the mouth with caustic reagents and against contamination by pathogenic organisms in samples. All specimens of human origin that are used in the laboratory (blood, urine, spinal fluid, stools, etc.) should be considered potentially infectious. Hepatitis B virus is a serious biohazard found in the laboratory.

One well-known virus, which causes type B viral hepatitis, can be transmitted through the blood of a patient with that virus. In hospitals where renal transplants are done, this problem is especially serious. Those most heavily exposed to blood from renal patients—for example, through accidental inoculation, ingestion of blood, or inhalation of blood aerosols while doing laboratory work on these samples—run the greatest risk of infection. Laboratories must exert every effort to make this risk factor as low as possible. This can start with prevention of contamination while the specimens are collected and delivered to the laboratory (see under Collection, Preservation, and Preparation of Laboratory Specimens). A large percentage of the specimens sent to the laboratory contain blood, and their safe collection and transportation must take top priority in any discussion of safety in the laboratory. Disposal of contaminated needles and blades used in collecting the specimens must also be done properly. For example, they may be discarded in a special wax-lined, heavy cardboard box, coded with red stripes.[2] When these specially labeled and coded boxes are full, they can be taped shut, marked *contaminated*, and autoclaved before being incinerated.

To further eliminate the risk of transmitting type B hepatitis virus, those working in the laboratory with blood specimens must take precautions. Washing the hands frequently is one of the most important ways of preventing contamination. At least one sink in the laboratory should be equipped with a foot pedal for operating the faucets, and it should also have a foot pedal dispenser with an antiseptic solution for the hands. Wearing disposable rubber gloves and a special protective laboratory coat while handling blood, serum, or any biological specimen from a patient is another preventive measure. Such coats are worn only in the laboratory and never leave the laboratory except when they are specially bagged for the laundry.

More recently, attention has been drawn to chemical agents that are carcinogenic. A carcinogen is any agent that can produce cancer. Many carcinogens are not noticed in a normal inspection for hazards in the laboratory. OSHA has published a list of carcinogenic agents, which should be found in a prominent location in all laboratories.[3] Where chemical carcinogens are being used, several extra precautions must be taken: protective clothing should be worn; protective equipment such as a face mask or a respirator should be worn; a shower should be taken immediately after exposure to a carcinogen; there should be no eating, drinking, or smoking in the area; no oral pipetting should be done; and all personnel should wash their hands after completing procedures involving the use of any carcinogen. If proper techniques are used, safeguards against most of the carcinogens found in the clinical laboratory are provided.

Biohazards are generally treated with great respect in the clinical laboratory. The effects of pathogenic substances on the body are well documented. The presence of pathogenic organisms is not limited to the culture plates in the microbiology laboratory. Aerosols can be found in all areas of the laboratory where human specimens are used. Substances can become airborne when the cork is popped off a blood-collecting container, a serum sample is poured from one tube to another, or a serum tube is centrifuged. Another step that should be taken to lessen the hazard from aerosols is to exercise caution in handling pipets and other equipment used to transfer human specimens, especially pathogenic materials. These materials should be discarded properly and carefully.

The preferred method for decontamination and disinfection of toxic or infectious materials is autoclaving. Autoclaving depends on humidity, temperature, and time. Under pressure, steam becomes hotter than boiling water and kills bacteria much more quickly. Autoclaves must be used with caution.

To clean up the work area, a strong bleach solution can be used for any spills of biological materials. Desk tops can be cleaned daily with a dilute solution of bleach. Any contaminated laboratory ware that must be reused cannot be cleaned with bleach because it corrodes stainless steel containers and coagulates proteins. A strong detergent solution such as 3% phenolic detergent can be used before autoclaving. Contaminated pipets should be placed in long horizontal covered trays deep enough to minimize the chance of spilling when they are transported to the autoclave.

Shocks from the various pieces of electrical apparatus in the clinical laboratory are a common source of injury if one is not aware of the potential hazard. This may be one of the most serious hazards in the laboratory. The important thing to understand with respect to danger to the human body is the effect of an electrical current. Current flows when there is a difference in potential between two points, and this knowledge is used in determining the approach to safety in the use of electrical equipment. Grounding of all electrical equipment is essential. If there is no path to ground, such a path might be established through the human in contact with the apparatus, resulting in serious injury. Attempts to repair or inspect a disabled electrical device should be left to someone who is trained to do it.

The use of many kinds of glassware is basic to anyone working in the clinical laboratory. Caution must be used to prevent unnecessary or accidental breakage. Some types of glassware can be repaired, but most glassware used today is discarded when it is broken. Any broken or cracked glassware should be discarded in a special container for broken glass, and not thrown into the regular waste containers. Common sense should be used in storing glassware, with heavy pieces placed on the lower shelves and tall pieces placed behind smaller pieces. Shelves should be placed at reasonable heights; glassware should not be stored out of reach. Broken or cracked glassware is the cause of many lacerations, and care should be taken to avoid this laboratory hazard.

General rules for safety in the clinical laboratory

1. Know where the fire extinguishers are located, the different types for specific types of fires, and how to use them properly.
2. Pipet *all* solutions by using mechanical suction or an aspirator bulb. Never use mouth suction.
3. Handle all flammable solvents and fuming reagents under a fume hood. Store in a well-ventilated cabinet.
4. Use an explosion-proof refrigerator to store ether. Never use ether near an open flame, as it is highly flammable.
5. Do not use *any* flammable substance near an open flame.
6. Wear gloves when handling infectious substances or toxic substances such as bromine or cyanide.
7. Mercury is poisonous. Clean up spilled mercury immediately.
8. If glass tubing is to be cut, hold the tubing with a towel to prevent cuts of the hands. This precaution also applies to putting a piece of glass tubing through a rubber stopper.
9. Use extreme caution when handling laboratory glassware. Broken glass is probably the greatest source of injury in the laboratory. Immediately discard cracked or broken glassware in a separate container, not with other waste.
10. If strong acids or bases are spilled, wipe them up immediately, using copious amounts

of water and great care. Keep sodium bicarbonate on hand to assist in neutralizing acid spillage.

11. Plainly label all laboratory bottles, specimens, and other materials. When a reagent bottle is no longer being used, store it away in its proper place.

12. Put away safely or cover any equipment that is not being used.

13. Replace covers, tops, or corks on all reagent bottles as soon as they are no longer being used. Never use a reagent from a bottle that is not properly labeled.

14. If water is spilled on the floor, wipe it up immediately. Serious injuries can result from falls caused by slipping on a wet floor.

15. Never taste any chemical. Smell chemicals only when necessary and then only by fanning the vapor of the chemical toward the nose.

16. When handling blades or needles, use extreme caution to avoid cuts and infections. Dispose of all blades and needles properly.

17. Always pour acid into water for dilution. Never pour water into acid. Pour strong acids or bases slowly down the side of the receiving vessel to prevent splashing.

18. Use caution when pipetting any specimen from a patient. Handle blood, serum, plasma, cerebrospinal fluid, urine, or any other patient specimen with care, as it may be contaminated. Severe infections and illnesses can result from handling such specimens carelessly.

19. Wash hands frequently while working in the laboratory, especially after handling patient specimens or reagents. *Always* wash hands before leaving the laboratory.

20. Wear safety goggles when preparing reagents with strong chemicals (such as the dichromate acid cleaning solution used to clean laboratory glassware, or aqua regia, another cleaning solution). Some states (e.g., Minnesota) have enacted laws that require students, teachers, and visitors in educational institutions who are participating in or observing activities in eye-protection areas (areas where work is performed that is potentially hazardous to the eyes) to wear devices to protect their eyes.

21. In case of severe fire or burns, know where the safety shower is located and how to operate it.

22. Know the location of a fire blanket, which is used to smother flames in case of fire.

23. Most hospitals and teaching institutions have some type of warning signal and a procedure to follow in the event of a fire. This procedure should be understood thoroughly by anyone working in that institution, whether as a student or an employee. Such institutions also have disaster plans, with which every worker must be thoroughly familiar.

24. When using burners and other heating devices, keep them far enough away from the working area that there is no possibility that anything will catch fire.

25. Never lean over an open flame. Extinguish flames when they are no longer being used.

26. Learn the procedure used in the laboratory for discarding hazardous substances such as strong acids and bases.

27. Never pour volatile liquids down a sink.

28. To free a frozen glass stopper, run hot water over it, tap it lightly with a towel wrapped around it, or grasp it with a rubber glove or tourniquet.

29. Wear gloves when cleaning glassware in case there is broken glass in the sink or soaking bucket.

30. If blood or another body specimen comes in contact with the mouth, spit it out immediately into the sink, rinse with mouthfuls of tap water, never swallowing but discarding each mouthful of rinse water. The most important thing is to spit out the blood or other specimen immediately without swallowing it.

31. Handle all hot objects with tongs, not hands.

Extremely hot objects are to be handled with asbestos gloves.

32. If contaminated materials such as human specimens or bacterial agents are spilled on the work area, discard the contaminated material properly and wipe off the work area with phenol, bleach solution, or another laboratory disinfectant.

33. Cover all centrifuges to avoid flying broken glass. Do not open centrifuges before they have stopped. Do not stop the centrifuge head by hand.

34. Be familiar with the Occupational Safety and Health rules and regulations and be ready for an inspection by OSHA.

Every clinical laboratory should have at its disposal a safety reference library. This library should be available at all times to all technical personnel, students, and employees. It should include books and manuals that will be helpful in preventing unsafe conditions and that provide a guide to safe procedures to be employed in the event of an accident in the laboratory. The following list includes some of the more valuable references for a safety library:

1. U.S. Department of Labor, Occupational Safety and Health Administration, "Guide for Applying Safety and Health Standards," 29 CFR 1910, Government Printing Office, Washington, D.C., 1972.

2. U.S. Department of Labor, Occupational Safety and Health Administration, Occupational Safety and Health Standards, *Fed. Regist.*, vol. 29, no. 125, part II, 1974.

3. "Laboratories in Health-Related Institutions," National Fire Protection Association, Boston, 1973.

4. Norman V. Steere (ed.), "Handbook of Laboratory Safety," 2d ed., Chemical Rubber Company, Cleveland, 1971.

5. "A Laboratory Safety Guide," California Association of Public Health Laboratory Directors, April 1976.

6. National Institutes of Health, "Biohazards Safety Guide," Government Printing Office, Washington, D.C., 1974.

Basic first-aid procedures

Since there are so many potential hazards in a clinical laboratory, it is easy to understand why a basic knowledge of first aid should be an integral part of any educational program in laboratory medicine. The first emphasis should be on removal of the accident victim from further injury; the next involves definitive action or first aid to the victim. By definition, first aid is "the immediate care given to a person who has been injured or suddenly taken ill." Any person who attempts to perform first aid before professional treatment by a physician can be arranged should remember that such assistance is only a stopgap—an emergency treatment to be followed until the physician arrives. Stop bleeding, prevent shock, then treat the wound—in that order.

A rule to remember in dealing with emergencies in the laboratory is to keep calm. This is not always easy to do, but it is very important to the well-being of the victim. Keep crowds of people away and give the victim plenty of fresh air.

Because so many of the possible injuries are of such an extreme nature and because in the event of such an injury immediate care is most critical, application of the proper first-aid procedures must be thoroughly understood by every person in the medical laboratory. A few of the more common emergencies and the appropriate first-aid procedures are listed below. These should be learned by every student or person working in the laboratory.

1. *Alkali or acid burns on the skin or in the mouth.* Rinse thoroughly with large amounts of running tap water. If the burns are serious, consult a physician.

2. *Alkali or acid burns in the eye.* Wash out thoroughly with running water for a minimum of 15 minutes. Help the victim by holding the

eyelid open so that the water can make contact with the eye. An eye fountain is recommended for this purpose, but any running water will suffice. Use of an eyecup is discouraged. A physician should be notified immediately, while the eye is being washed.

3. *Heat burns.* Apply cold running water (or ice in water) to relieve the pain and to stop further tissue damage. Use a wet dressing of 2 tablespoons of sodium bicarbonate in 1 qt of warm water. Bandage securely but not tightly. If it is a third-degree burn (the skin is burned off), do not use any ointments or grease, and consult a physician immediately.

4. *Minor cuts.* Wash carefully and thoroughly with soap and water. Remove all foreign material, such as glass, that projects from the wound, but do not gouge for embedded material. Removal is best accomplished by careful washing. Apply a clean bandage if necessary.

5. *Serious cuts.* Direct pressure should be applied to the cut area to control the bleeding, using the hand over a clean compress covering the wound. Call for a physician immediately.

In cases of serious laboratory accidents, such as burns, medical assistance should be summoned while first aid is being administered. For general accidents, competent medical help should be sought as soon as possible after the first-aid treatment has been completed. In cases of chemical burns, especially where the eyes are involved, speed in treatment is most essential. Remember that first aid is useful not only in your working environment, but at home and in your community. It deserves your earnest attention and study.

LABORATORY UNITS OF MEASUREMENT
(THE INTERNATIONAL SYSTEM OF UNITS)

The ability to measure accurately is the keystone of the scientific method. Therefore, a student in any scientific course must have a working knowledge of the systems and units of measurement. Until the Metric Conversion Act was signed in 1975, students of laboratory medicine and other scientific fields in the United States, unlike the general population, had to learn two systems of measurement: the metric system and the English system. Now, at last, everyone is becoming conversant with the more convenient and rational metric system, which is based on a decimal system of divisions and multiples of tens. In the clinical laboratory we must become familiar with a further standardization of measurement called the SI system (International System of units). The SI system was established in 1960 by international agreement and is now the standard international language of measurement. In this book the term metric system generally refers to the SI system; however, outdated terms that remain in common usage are described. Since the English system is still in common everyday use, English equivalents are also given in our discussion of units. The International Bureau of Weights and Measures, near Paris, is responsible for maintaining the standards on which this system of measurement is based.

In the SI system the basic units of measurement are the metre (meter), kilogram, second, mole, ampere, kelvin, and candela. These seven basic units of the SI system and accepted symbols are listed in Table 1-1.

All units in the SI system can be qualified by standard prefixes that serve to convert values to more convenient forms, depending on the size of the object being measured. These prefixes are listed in Table 1-2.

Various rules should be kept in mind when combining these prefixes with their basic units and using the SI system; some of these rules follow.[4,5] An *s* should not be added to form the

Table 1-1. Units of the SI system

Measurement	Unit name	Symbol
Length	Metre[a]	m
Mass	Kilogram	kg
Time	Second	s
Amount of substance	Mole	mol
Electric current	Ampere	A
Temperature	Kelvin[b]	K
Luminous intensity	Candela	cd

[a]The spelling *meter* is more commonly used in the United States and is used in this book.

[b]Although the basic unit of temperature is the kelvin, the degree Celsius is regarded as an acceptable unit, since kelvins may be impractical in many instances. Celsius is more commonly used in the clinical laboratory.

plural of the abbreviation for a unit or for a prefix with a unit. For example, 25 millimeters should be abbreviated as 25 mm, not 25 mms. Do not use periods after abbreviations (use mm, not mm.). Do not use compound prefixes; instead, use the closest accepted prefix. For example, 24×10^{-9} gram (g) should be expressed as 24 nanograms (24 ng) rather than 24 millimicrograms (25 mμg). Commas should not be used as spacers in recording large numbers since they are used in place of decimal points in some countries. Instead, groups of three digits

should be separated by spaces. When recording temperature on the Kelvin scale, omit the degree sign. Therefore, 295 kelvins should be recorded as 295 K, not 295°K. However, the symbol for degree Celsius is °C, and 22 degrees Celsius should be recorded as 22°C. Multiples and submultiples should be used in steps of 10^3 or 10^{-3}. Only one solidus or slash (/) should be used when indicating *per* or a denominator: use meters per second squared (m/s^2), not meters per second per second (m/s/s), or millimoles per liter-hour (mmol/L · hour), not millimoles per liter per hour (mmol/L/hour). Finally, although the preferred SI spellings are *metre* and *litre*, the spellings *meter* and *liter* remain in common usage in the United States and are used in this book.

The basic units of measurement that you will be most concerned with in the clinical laboratory are length, mass, and volume. These are now further described.

Length

The standard unit for the measurement of length or distance is the meter (m). The meter is standardized as 1 650 763.73 wavelengths of a certain orange light in the spectrum of krypton-

Table 1-2. Prefixes of the SI system

Prefix name	Symbol	Power of 10	Decimal
Tetra	T	10^{12}	1 000 000 000 000
Giga	G	10^9	1 000 000 000
Mega	M	10^6	1 000 000
Kilo	k	10^3	1 000
Hecto	h	10^2	100
Deca	da	10^1	10
Deci	d	10^{-1}	0.1
Centi	c	10^{-2}	0.01
Milli	m	10^{-3}	0.001
Micro	μ	10^{-6}	0.000 001
Nano	n	10^{-9}	0.000 000 001
Pico	p	10^{-12}	0.000 000 000 001
Femto	f	10^{-15}	0.000 000 000 000 001
Atto	a	10^{-18}	0.000 000 000 000 000 001

86. One meter equals 39.37 inches (in), slightly more than a yard in the English system. There are 2.54 centimeters (cm) in 1 in.

Further common divisions and multiples of the meter, using the system of prefixes previously discussed, follow. One-tenth of a meter is a decimeter (dm), one-hundredth of a meter is a centimeter (cm), and one-thousandth of a meter is a millimeter (mm). One thousand meters equals 1 kilometer (km). The following examples show equivalent measurements of length:

$$25 \text{ mm} = 0.025 \text{ m}$$

$$10 \text{ cm} = 100 \text{ mm}$$

$$1 \text{ m} = 100 \text{ cm}$$

$$0.1 \text{ m} = 100 \text{ mm}$$

Other units of length that were in common usage in the "metric system" but are no longer recommended in the SI system are the angstrom and the micron. The angstrom (Å) is equal to 10^{-10} m or 10^{-1} nanometer (nm). This unit is permitted but not encouraged. The micron (μ), which is equal to 10^{-6} m, is replaced by the micrometer (μm).

Mass (and weight)

Mass denotes the quantity of matter, while weight takes into account the force of gravity and should not be used in the same sense as mass. However, they are commonly used interchangeably and may be so used in this book. The standard unit for the measurement of mass in the SI system is the kilogram (kg). This is the basis for all other mass measurements in the system. The standard kilogram is determined by the mass of a block of platinum-iridium kept at the International Bureau of Weights and Measures. One kilogram weighs approximately 2.2 pounds (lb) in the English system. Conversely, 1 lb equals approximately 0.5 kg.

The kilogram is further divided into thousandths, called grams (g). One thousand grams equals 1 kg. The gram is used much more often than the kilogram in the clinical laboratory. The gram is divided into thousandths, called milligrams (mg). Grams and milligrams are units commonly used in weighing substances in the clinical laboratory. One-millionth of a gram, a microgram (μg), may also be encountered. Some examples of weight measurement equivalents follow:

$$10 \text{ mg} = 0.01 \text{ g}$$

$$0.055 \text{ g} = 55 \text{ mg}$$

$$25 \text{ g} = 25\ 000 \text{ mg}$$

$$1.5 \text{ kg} = 1500 \text{ g}$$

Units that were once used to describe mass and that may still be encountered are the gamma and parts per million. The term gamma (γ) should not be used; instead, use microgram (μg). The term parts per million (ppm) should be replaced by micrograms per gram (μg/g).

Volume

In the clinical laboratory the unit of volume is the liter (L). You may have noticed that it was not included in the list of basic units of the SI system. The liter is a derived unit. The standard unit of volume in the SI system is the cubic meter (m^3). However, this unit is quite large and the cubic decimeter (dm^3) is a more convenient size for use in the clinical laboratory. Thus in 1964 the Conférence Générale des Poids et Mésures (CGMP) accepted the litre (liter) as a special name for the cubic decimeter. Previously, the standard liter was the volume occupied by 1 kg of pure water at $4°C$ (the temperature at which a volume of water weighs the most) and at normal atmospheric pressure. On this basis, 1 L equals 1000.027 cubic centimeters (cm^3), and the units milliliters and cubic centimeters were used interchangeably, although there is a slight difference between them.[6] One liter is slightly more than 1 quart (qt) in the English system (1 L = 1.06 qt).

The liter is further divided into thousandths, called milliliters (ml); millionths, called microliters (μl); and billionths, called nanoliters (nl). Some examples of volume equivalents are:

$$500 \text{ ml} = 0.5 \text{ L}$$

$$0.25 \text{ L} = 250 \text{ ml}$$

$$2 \text{ L} = 2000 \text{ ml}$$

Since the liter is derived from the meter (1 L equals 1 dm^3), it follows that 1 cm^3 is equal to 1 ml and that 1 millimeter cubed (mm^3) is equal to 1 μl. The older abbreviation for cubic centimeter cc is replaced by cm^3. Although this is a common means of expressing volume in the clinical laboratory, milliliter (ml) is preferred.

Amount of substance

The standard unit of measurement for the amount of a (chemical) substance in the SI system is the mole (mol). The mole is defined as the quantity of a chemical equal to that present in 0.0120 kg of pure carbon-12. A mole of a chemical substance is the *relative atomic* or *molecular mass unit* of that substance. Formerly, the terms atomic and molecular weight were used to describe the mole. These will be further defined and discussed under Expressions of Solution Concentration.

Temperature

Three scales are commonly used to measure temperature, namely, the Kelvin, Celsius, and Fahrenheit scales. The Celsius scale is sometimes referred to as the centigrade scale, which is an old-fashioned term.

The basic unit of temperature in the SI system is the kelvin (K). However, as mentioned previously, the degree Celsius is regarded as an acceptable unit, since the kelvin may be impractical in many instances. The Celsius scale is the one used most often in the clinical laboratory. The Kelvin and Celsius scales are closely related, and conversion between them is simple since the units (degrees) are equal in magnitude. The difference between the Kelvin and Celsius scales is the zero point. The zero point on the Kelvin scale is the theoretical temperature of no further heat loss, which is absolute zero. The zero point on the Celsius scale is the freezing point of pure water. Remember, however, that the magnitude of the degree is equal on both scales. Therefore, since water freezes at 273 kelvins (273 K), it follows that 0 degrees Celsius ($0°C$) equals 273 kelvins (273 K) and that 0 kelvin (0 K) equals minus 273 degrees Celsius ($-273°C$). Thus, to convert from kelvins to degrees Celsius add 273; to convert from degrees Celsius to kelvins subtract 273.

$$K = °C + 273$$

$$°C = K - 273$$

Since the Celsius scale was devised so that $100°C$ is the boiling point of pure water, the boiling point on the Kelvin scale is 373 K.

Converting from Celsius to Fahrenheit is not as simple, since the degree is not equal in magnitude on these two scales. The Fahrenheit scale was originally devised with the zero point at the lowest temperature attainable from a mixture of table salt and ice, while the body temperature of a small animal was used to set $100°F$. Thus, on the Fahrenheit scale the freezing point of pure water is 32°, while the temperature at which pure water boils is 212°. It is rare that readings on one of these scales must be converted to the other, as almost without exception readings taken and used in the clinical laboratory will be on the Celsius scale.

Examples of comparative readings of the three scales with common reference points are given in Table 1-3.

It is possible, however, to convert from one

Table 1-3. Common reference points on the three temperature scales

	Kelvin	Degrees Celsius	Degrees Fahrenheit
Boiling point of water	373	100	212
Body temperature	310	37	98.6
Room temperature	293	20	68
Freezing point of water	273	0	32
Absolute zero (coldest possible temperature)	0	−273	−459.4

scale to the other, and a student or technician in the clinical laboratory should be able to do this if the need arises. The basic conversion formulas are:

1.
$$1°C = \tfrac{9}{5}°F$$
$$1°F = \tfrac{5}{9}°C$$

2. To convert Fahrenheit to Celsius:
   Method A: Add 40, multiply by $\tfrac{5}{9}$, and subtract 40 from the result.
   Method B: $°C = \tfrac{5}{9}(°F - 32)$.
3. To convert Celsius to Fahrenheit:
   Method A: Add 40, multiply by $\tfrac{9}{5}$, and subtract 40 from the result.
   Method B: $°F = \tfrac{9}{5}°C + 32$.

LABORATORY CALCULATIONS

A sound background in basic mathematics (including algebra), an understanding of the units in which quantities are expressed, and a knowledge of the methods of analysis are all necessary in performing laboratory calculations. There are no simple formulas for solving all such problems, but certain fundamentals are a part of many of the problems encountered in a clinical laboratory.

Proportions

The use of proportions involves a commonsense approach to problem solving. Proportions are devices used to determine a quantity from a given ratio. A ratio is an amount of something compared to an amount of something else; for instance, 5 g of something dissolved in 100 ml of something else can be expressed by the ratio 5/100, 5:100, or 5 ÷ 100, or by the decimal 0.05. Proportion is a means of saying that two ratios are equal. Thus, the ratio 5:100 is equal or proportional to the ratio 1/20. This proportion can be expressed as 5:100 = 1:20. In the laboratory, proportions and ratios are useful when it is necessary to make more (or less) of the same

thing. However, ratios and proportions can be used only when the concentration (or any other kind of relationship) does not change.

Example

A formula calls for 5 g of sodium chloride (NaCl) in 1000 ml of solution. If only 500 ml of solution is needed, how much NaCl is required?

$$\frac{5 \text{ g}}{1000 \text{ ml}} = \frac{x \text{ g}}{500 \text{ ml}}$$

$$x = \frac{5 \text{ g} \times 500 \text{ ml}}{1000 \text{ ml}}$$

$$x = 2.5 \text{ g of NaCl}$$

In setting up ratio and proportion problems, the two ratios being compared must be written in the same order and they must be in the same units.

Relating concentrations

To relate different concentrations of solutions that contain the same amount of substance (or solute) a basic relationship is used. The volume of one solution (V_1) times the concentration of that solution (C_1) equals the volume of the second solution (V_2) times the concentration of the second solution (C_2), or $V_1 \times C_1 = V_2 \times C_2$. If any three of the values are known, the fourth may be determined. This relationship shows that when a solution is diluted, the volume is increased as the concentration is decreased. However, the total amount of substance (or solute) remains unchanged. Several applications of this relationship are used in the clinical laboratory, two of them being in titrations (see under Titration) and in the preparation of weaker solutions from stronger solutions.

Example

A sodium hydroxide (NaOH) solution is available that has a concentration of 10 g of NaOH per deciliter (dl) of solution (1 dl = 100 ml). To calculate the volume of the 10 g/dl NaOH solution required to prepare 1000 ml of 2 g/dl NaOH:

$$V_1 \times C_1 = V_2 \times C_2$$

$$x \text{ ml} \times 10 \text{ g/dl} = 1000 \text{ ml} \times 2 \text{ g/dl}$$

$$x = \frac{2 \text{ g/dl} \times 1000 \text{ ml}}{10 \text{ g/dl}} = 200 \text{ ml}$$

Notice that this relationship is not a direct proportion; instead, it is an inverse proportion. As in proportion problems, it is important to remember that the concentrations and volumes on both sides of the equation must be expressed in the same units.

Dilution problems and dilution factors

It is often necessary to dilute specimens being analyzed or to make weaker solutions from stronger solutions in various laboratory procedures. It is therefore necessary to be capable of working with various dilution problems and dilution factors. In these problems one must often

be able to determine the concentration of material in each solution, the actual amount of material in each solution, and the total volume of each solution. Some such problems follow.

Dilution factors

In most laboratory determinations, a small sample is taken for analysis, and the final result is expressed as concentration per some convenient standard volume.

Example

In a certain procedure, 0.5 ml of blood is diluted to a total of 10 ml with various reagents. 1 ml of this dilution is then analyzed for a particular chemical substance. The final result is to be expressed in terms of the concentration of that substance per 100 ml of blood. A *dilution factor* by which all determination answers are multiplied to give the concentration per 100 ml of sample (blood) may be determined as follows.

First determine the volume of blood that is actually analyzed in the procedure. By use of a simple proportion, it is evident that 0.5 ml of blood diluted to 10 ml is equivalent to 1 ml of blood diluted to 20 ml.

$$\frac{0.5 \text{ ml of blood}}{10 \text{ ml of solution}} = \frac{1 \text{ ml of blood}}{x \text{ ml of solution}}$$

$$x = \frac{1 \text{ ml} \times 10 \text{ ml}}{0.5 \text{ ml}} = 20 \text{ ml}$$

In other words, there is a 1:20 dilution of blood in this procedure—that is, 1 ml of blood diluted to a total volume of 20 ml with the desired diluent (usually saline or deionized water) or reagents. This is the same as 1 ml of blood plus 19 ml of diluent.

The concentration of specimen (blood) in each milliliter of solution may be determined, by the use of another simple proportion, to be 0.05 ml of blood per milliliter of solution.

$$\frac{1 \text{ ml of blood}}{20 \text{ ml of solution}} = \frac{x \text{ ml of blood}}{1 \text{ ml of solution}}$$

$$x = \frac{1 \text{ ml} \times 1 \text{ ml}}{20 \text{ ml}} = 0.05 \text{ ml}$$

Since 1 ml of the 1:20 dilution of blood (often stated as 1 ml of filtrate) is analyzed in the remaining steps of the procedure, 0.05 ml of blood is actually analyzed (1 ml of the dilution used $\times$ 0.05 ml/ml = 0.05 ml of blood analyzed).

To relate the concentration of the substance measured in the procedure to the concentration in 100 ml of blood (the units in which the result is to be expressed) another proportion may be used.

$$\frac{100 \text{ ml (volume of blood desired)}}{0.05 \text{ ml (volume of blood used)}}$$

$$= \frac{\text{concentration desired}}{\text{concentration used or determined}}$$

Concentration desired

$$= \frac{100 \text{ ml} \times \text{concentration determined}}{0.05 \text{ ml}}$$

Concentration desired = 2000 $\times$ value determined

In other words, the concentration of the substance being measured in the volume of blood actually tested (0.05 ml) must be multiplied by 2000 in order to report the concentration per 100 ml of blood.

The preceding material may be summarized by the following statement and equations. In reporting results obtained from laboratory determinations, one must first determine the amount of specimen actually analyzed in the procedure and then calculate the factor that will express the concentration in the desired terms of measurement. Thus, in the previous example the following equations may be used:

$$\frac{0.5 \text{ ml (volume of blood used)}}{10 \text{ ml (volume of total dilution)}}$$

$$= \frac{x \text{ ml (volume of blood analyzed)}}{1 \text{ ml (volume of dilution used)}}$$

$x = 0.05$ ml (volume of blood actually analyzed)

$$\frac{100 \text{ ml (volume of blood required for expression of result)}}{0.05 \text{ ml (volume of blood actually analyzed)}}$$

$$= 2000 \text{ (dilution factor)}$$

Other dilution problems

When the concentration of a particular substance in a specimen is too great to be accurately determined, or when there is less specimen available for analysis than the procedure requires, it may be necessary to dilute the original specimen, or to further dilute the initial dilution (or filtrate). Such dilutions are usually expressed as a ratio, such as 1:2, 1:5, or 1:10, or as a fraction, $\frac{1}{2}$, $\frac{1}{5}$, or $\frac{1}{10}$. These ratios or fractions refer to 1 unit of the original specimen diluted to a final volume of 2, 5, or 10 units, respectively. A dilution therefore refers to the volume of concentrate in the total volume of final solution. A dilution is an expression of concentration; it indicates the relative amount of substance in solution. Dilutions can be made singly or in series.

To calculate the concentration of a single dilution, multiply the original concentration by the dilution expressed as a fraction.

Example (calculation of the concentration of a single dilution)

A specimen contains 500 mg of substance per deciliter of blood. A 1:5 dilution of this specimen is prepared by volumetrically measuring 1 ml of the specimen and adding 4 ml of diluent (usually distilled water or saline). The concentration of substance in the dilution is

$$500 \text{ mg/dl} \times \tfrac{1}{5} = 100 \text{ mg/dl}$$

Notice that the concentration of the final solution (or dilution) is expressed in the same units as that of the original solution.

To obtain a dilution factor that can be applied to the determination answer in order to express it as a concentration per standard volume, proceed as follows. Rather than multiply by the dilution expressed as a fraction, multiply the determination value by the reciprocal of the dilution fraction. In the case of a 1:5 dilution, the dilution factor that would be applied to values obtained in the procedure would be 5, since the original specimen was five times more concentrated than the diluted specimen tested in the procedure.

Example (use of dilution factors)

A 1:5 dilution of a specimen is prepared and an aliquot (one of a number of equal parts) of the dilution is analyzed for a particular substance. The concentration of the substance in the aliquot is multiplied by 5 to determine its concentration in the original specimen. If the concentration of the dilution is 100 mg/dl, the concentration of the original specimen is

100 mg/dl $\times$ 5 (the dilution factor)

$$= 500 \text{ mg/dl in blood}$$

As mentioned previously, dilutions can be made singly or in series, where the original solution is further diluted. A general rule for calculating the concentrations of solutions obtained by dilution in series is to multiply the original concentration by the first dilution (expressed as a fraction), this by the second dilution, and so on until the desired concentration is known.

Example (calculation of the concentration after a series of dilutions)

A working solution is prepared from a stock solution. In so doing, a stock solution with a concentration of 100 mg/dl is diluted 1:10 by volumetrically adding 1 ml of it to 9 ml of diluent. The diluted solution (intermediate solution) is further diluted 1:100 by volumetrically

measuring 1 ml of intermediate solution and diluting to the mark in a 100-ml volumetric flask. The concentration of the final or working solution is

$$100 \text{ mg/dl} \times \frac{1}{10} \times \frac{1}{100} = 0.1 \text{ mg/dl}$$

Serial dilutions

Several laboratory procedures, especially serological ones, make use of a dilution series where all dilutions, including or following the first one, are the same. Such dilutions are referred to as *serial* dilutions. A complete dilution series usually contains 5 or 10 tubes, although any single dilution may be made directly from undiluted specimen or substance. In calculating the dilution or concentration of substance or serum in each tube of the dilution series, the rules previously discussed apply.

Example

A five-tube twofold dilution may be prepared as follows (see Fig. 1-2). A serum specimen is diluted 1:2 with buffer. A series of five tubes are prepared where each succeeding tube is rediluted 1:2. This is accomplished by placing 1 ml of diluent into each of 4 tubes (tubes 2-5). Tube 1 contains 1 ml of undiluted serum. Tube 2 contains 1 ml of undiluted serum plus 1 ml of diluent, resulting in a 1:2 dilution of serum. A 1-ml portion of the 1:2 dilution of serum is placed in tube 3, resulting in a 1:4 dilution of serum ($\frac{1}{2} \times \frac{1}{2} = \frac{1}{4}$). A 1-ml portion of the 1:4 dilution from tube 3 is placed in tube 4, resulting in a 1:8 dilution ($\frac{1}{4} \times \frac{1}{2} = \frac{1}{8}$). Finally, 1 ml of the 1:8 dilution from tube 4 is added to tube 5, resulting in a 1:16 dilution ($\frac{1}{8} \times \frac{1}{2} = \frac{1}{16}$). 1 ml of the final dilution is discarded so that the volumes in all the tubes are equal. Notice that each tube is diluted twice as much as the previous tube and that the final volume in each tube is the same. The undiluted serum may also be given a dilution value, namely 1:1.

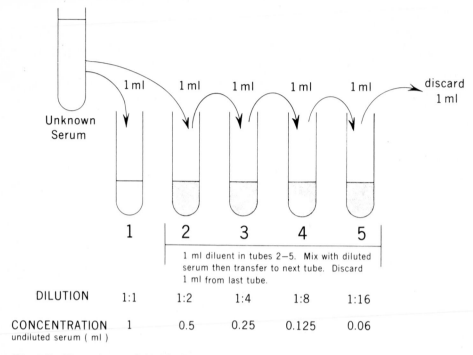

Fig. 1-2. Five-tube twofold dilution.

The concentration of serum in terms of milliliters in each tube is calculated by multiplying the previous concentration (ml) by the succeeding dilution. In this example tube 1 contains 1 ml of serum, tube 2 contains 1 ml $\times \frac{1}{2} = 0.5$ ml of serum, and tubes 3–5 contain 0.25, 0.125, and 0.06 ml of serum, respectively.

Other serial dilutions might be 5-fold or 10-fold, where each succeeding tube is diluted 5 or 10 times. A 5-fold series would begin with 1 ml of serum in 4 ml of diluent and a total volume of 5 ml in each tube, while a 10-fold series would begin with 1 ml of serum in 9 ml of diluent and a total volume of 10 ml in each tube. Other systems might begin with a 1:2 dilution and then dilute five succeeding tubes 1:10. The dilutions in such a series would be 1:2, 1:20 ($\frac{1}{2} \times \frac{1}{10} = \frac{1}{20}$), 1:200 ($\frac{1}{20} \times \frac{1}{10} = \frac{1}{200}$), 1:2000, 1:20 000, and 1:200 000.

Significant figures

Using more digits than are necessary to calculate and report the results of a laboratory determination has several disadvantages. It is important that the number used contain only the digits necessary for the precision of the determination. Using more digits than necessary is misleading in that it ascribes more accuracy to the determination than is actually the case. There is also the danger of overlooking a decimal point and making an error in judging the magnitude of the answer. Digits in a number that are needed to express the precision of the measurement from which the number is derived are known as *significant figures*. A significant figure is one that is known to be reasonably reliable. Judgment must be exercised in determining how many figures should be used. Some rules to assist in making such decisions are:

1. Use the known accuracy of the method to determine the number of digits that are significant in the answer, and, as a general rule, retain one more figure than this.

Example

A urea nitrogen result was reported as 11.2 mg/dl. This would indicate that the result is accurate to the nearest tenth and that the exact value lies between 11.15 and 11.25. In reality, the accuracy of most urea nitrogen methods is ±10%, so that the result reported as 11.2 mg/dl could actually vary from 10 to 12 mg/dl and should be reported as 11 mg/dl. In addition, if the decimal point were omitted or overlooked, the result could be taken as 112 mg/dl.

2. Take the accuracy of the least accurate measurement, or the measurement with the least number of significant figures, as the accuracy of the final result. In doing so, certain things must be done in the addition and subtraction or multiplication and division of numerals.

Example (addition or subtraction)

In order to add

$$206.1$$
$$7.56$$
$$\underline{0.8764}$$

rewrite it as

$$206.1$$
$$7.6$$
$$\underline{0.9}$$

In this example, the least accurate figure is accurate to one decimal place; this is therefore the determining factor. In determining the least accurate figure, the following rule was utilized: in a column of addition or subtraction, in which the decimal points are placed one above the other, the number of significant figures in the final answer is determined by the first digit encountered going from left to right that terminates any one numeral.

Example (multiplication or division)

In the multiplication of

$$32\,500 \times 0.001\,25$$

the result should be reported as 40.6. In this example, the final product should be reported to three significant figures since each factor in the problem has three significant figures. This was determined by utilizing the following general rule: the number of significant figures in the final product or quotient should not exceed the least number of significant figures in any one factor.

3. The following general rule may be used in rounding off decimal values to the proper place. When the figure next to the last one to be retained is less than 5, the last figure should be left unchanged. When the figure next to the last one to be retained is greater than 5, the last figure is increased by 1. If the additional digit is 5, the last digit reported is changed to the nearest even number.

Examples

2.314 63 g is rounded off to 2.3146 g.
5.346 59 g is rounded off to 5.3466 g.
23.5 mg is rounded off to 24 mg.
24.5 mg is rounded off to 24 mg.

EXPRESSIONS OF SOLUTION CONCENTRATION

Concentrations of solutions of reagents may be expressed in one of three general ways: by *proper name*, by *physical units*, or by *chemical units*.

Proper name

There are very few instances where a solution is described by proper name as far as its concentration is concerned. Under Urinalysis, the use of Benedict's solution is discussed. This solution is prepared with specific amounts of ingredients according to a series of instructions or directions. When Benedict's solution is needed, one knows exactly what is meant and which chemicals in specific amounts are used in its preparation. Another example of a reagent described by proper name is Wright's stain, which is used in the hematology laboratory.

Physical units

Physical units are commonly used to express concentration. The units used are either of *mass* or of *volume*. One way of expressing concentration is by *mass per unit volume* (or *M/V*). When mass per unit volume is used, the amount of solute (the substance that goes into solution) per volume of solution is expressed. Mass per unit volume is used most often when a solid chemical is diluted in a liquid. The usual way to express mass per unit volume is as grams per liter (g/L) or milligrams per milliliter (mg/ml). If a concentration for a certain solution is given as 10 g/L, it means that there are 10 g of solute for every liter of solution. If a solution with a concentration of 10 mg/ml is desired and 100 ml of this solution is to be prepared, the use of a proportion formula can be applied.

Example

$$\frac{10 \text{ mg}}{1 \text{ ml}} = \frac{x \text{ mg}}{100 \text{ ml}}$$

$$x = 1000 \text{ mg, or } 1 \text{ g}$$

One gram of the desired solute is weighed and diluted to 100 ml (see under Reagent Preparation).

In working with *standard solutions* it will be seen that their concentrations, almost without exception, are expressed as milligrams per milliliter.

Another way of expressing concentration in physical units is by *volume per unit volume* (*V/V*). Volume per unit volume is used to express concentration when a liquid chemical is diluted with another liquid; the concentration is expressed as the number of milliliters of liquid chemical per unit volume of solution. The usual way to express volume per unit volume is as milliliters per milliliter (ml/ml) or milliliters per liter (ml/L). The number of milliliters of liquid chemical in 1 ml or 1 L of solution utilizes the volume per unit volume expression of concentration. If 10 ml of alcohol is diluted to 100 ml with water, the concentration is expressed as 10 ml/100 ml, or 10 ml/dl, or 0.1 ml/ml, or 100 ml/L. If a solution with a concentration of 0.5 ml/ml is desired and 1 L is to be prepared, a proportion can again be used to solve the problem.

Example

$$\frac{0.5 \text{ ml}}{1 \text{ ml}} = \frac{x \text{ ml}}{1000 \text{ ml}}$$

$$x = 500 \text{ ml}$$

Thus 500 ml of the liquid chemical is measured accurately and diluted to 1000 ml (1 L).

To express concentration in milliliters per liter, one needs to know how many milliliters of liquid chemical there are in 1 L of the solution.

Any chemical (liquid or solid) can be made into a solution by diluting it with a solvent. The usual solvent is deionized or distilled water (see under Kinds of Water Used in the Clinical Laboratory). If the desired chemical is a liquid, the amount needed is measured in milliliters or liters (on occasion liquids are weighed, but the usual method is to measure their volume); if the desired chemical is a solid, the amount needed is weighed in grams or milligrams.

A third way of expressing concentration in

physical units is by *mass per unit mass* (*M/M*). This expression is not commonly used. Not many reagents are prepared by using only solid chemicals and no liquid solvent. When the desired chemical is a solid and it is mixed with, or diluted with, another solid, the expression of concentration is mass per unit mass. The usual ways to express mass per unit mass is as milligrams per milligram (mg/mg), grams per gram (g/g), or grams per kilogram (g/kg). The number of milligrams or grams of one solid in the total number of milligrams or grams of the dry mixture is the mass per unit mass.

An example of a chemical reagent using this expression of concentration is Rothera's reagent, which is used in the detection of acetone in the urine. Rothera's reagent is prepared by mixing two dry chemicals together in specific amounts.

A now outdated expression of concentration in physical units is the *percent solution* (%). In the SI system the preferred units are kilograms (or fractions thereof) per liter (mass/volume) or milliliters per liter (volume/volume). A description of the old percent solution follows, as this expression of concentration is still used for biological samples. Percent is defined as *parts per hundred parts* (the part can be any particular unit). Unless otherwise stated, a percent solution usually means grams or milliliters of solute per 100 ml of solution (g/100 ml or ml/100 ml). Recall that 100 ml is equal to 1 deciliter (dl). Percent solutions can be prepared by using either liquid or solid chemicals. Percent solutions can be expressed either as mass per unit volume percent (*M/V%*) or volume per unit volume percent (*V/V%*), depending on the state of the solute (chemical) used—that is, whether it is a solid or a liquid. When a solid chemical is dissolved in a liquid, percent means *grams of solid in 100 ml of solution*. If 10 g of NaCl is diluted to 100 ml with deionized water, the concentration is expressed as 10% (10 g/dl). If 2.5 g is diluted to 100 ml, the concentration is 2.5% (2.5 g/dl). The following is an example of concentration expressed in percent.

Example

Ten grams of NaOH is diluted to 200 ml with water. What is the concentration in percent? A proportion can be set up to solve this problem.

$$\frac{10 \text{ g}}{200 \text{ ml}} = \frac{x \text{ g}}{100 \text{ ml}}$$

$$x = 5\% \text{ solution (preferably 5 g/dl)}$$

Remember that the percent expression is based on how much solute is present in *100 ml (or 1 dl)* of the solution.

When specifically stated, some concentrations of solutions are expressed as the milligrams of solute in 100 ml of solution (mg%). When this is used, *mg%* is always stated. If 25 mg of a chemical is diluted to 100 ml, the concentration in milligrams percent would be expressed as 25 mg% (preferably 25 mg/dl).

If a liquid chemical is used to prepare a percent solution, the concentration is expressed as volume per unit volume percent, or milliliters of solute per 100 ml of solution. If 10 ml of hydrochloric acid (HCl) is diluted to 100 ml with water, the concentration is 10% (preferably 10 ml/dl). If 10 ml of the same acid is diluted to 1 L (1000 ml), the concentration is 1% (preferably 1 ml/dl).

Chemical units

The third main way to express concentration is by using *chemical units*. In the following discussion of the use of chemical units, the terms *molarity* and *normality* of a solution will be explained.

Molarity

The molarity of a solution is defined as the gram molecular mass of a compound per liter of solution. Another way to define molarity is as the number of moles per liter (mol/L) of solution. A *mole* is the molecular mass of a compound in grams (one mole equals one gram molecular mass). The number of moles of a compound equals the number of grams divided by the gram molecular mass of that compound. One gram molecular mass equals the sum of all atomic weights in a molecule of the compound, expressed in grams.

To determine the gram molecular mass of a compound, the correct formula must be known. When this formula is known, the sum of all the atomic masses in the compound can be found by consulting a periodic table of the elements or a chart with the atomic masses of the elements.

Examples

1. Sodium chloride has one sodium ion and one chloride ion; the formula is written NaCl. The gram molecular mass is derived by finding the sum of the atomic weights:

$$Na = 23$$

$$Cl = 35.5$$

$$\text{Gram molecular mass} = 58.5$$

If the gram molecular mass of sodium chloride is 58.5 g, a 1 molar (*M*) solution of sodium chloride would contain 58.5 g of NaCl per liter of solution, because molarity equals moles per liter, and 1 mol of NaCl equals 58.5 g.

2. For barium sulfate ($BaSO_4$), the gram molecular mass equals 233 (the formula indicates that there are one barium, one sulfate, and four oxygen ions).

$$1\,Ba = 137 \times 1 = 137$$

$$1\,S = 32 \times 1 = 32$$

$$4\,O = 16 \times 4 = \underline{64}$$

$$233$$

Since the gram molecular mass is 233, a 1 *M*

solution of barium sulfate would contain 233 g of $BaSO_4$ per liter of solution.

The quantities of solutions needed will not always be in units of whole liters, and often concentrations using fractions or multiples of a 1 *M* concentration will be desired. Parts of a molar solution are expressed as decimals. If a 1 *M* solution of sodium chloride contains 58.5 g of NaCl per liter of solution, a 0.5 *M* solution would contain one-half of 58.5 g, or 29 g/L, and a 3 *M* solution would contain 3 × 58.5 g, or 175.5 g/L.

Example

What is the molarity of a solution containing 10 g of NaCl per liter? Molarity equals the number of moles per liter, and the number of moles equal the grams divided by the gram molecular mass.

Step 1: Find the gram molecular mass of NaCl. It is 58.5 g (Na = 23 and Cl = 35.5).
Step 2: Find the moles per liter.

$$\frac{10\ \text{g/L}}{x} = \frac{58.5\ \text{g/L}}{1\ \text{mol}}$$

$$x = \frac{10\ \text{g/L} \times 1\ \text{mol}}{58.5\ \text{g/L}} = 0.171\ \text{mol of NaCl}$$

Step 3: Knowing that the number of moles per liter of solution equals the molarity, the solution in the example is therefore 0.171 *M*.

Equations might prove useful to some in working with molarity solutions. However, all of these equations can be derived by applying a common-sense proportion approach to molarity problems, as described in Laboratory Calculations. Some of these equations are listed below.

1. Molarity $= \dfrac{\text{moles of solute}}{\text{liters of solution}}$

2. Molarity

$$= \frac{\text{grams of solute}}{\text{gram molecular mass}} \times \frac{1}{\text{liters of solution}}$$

3. Moles of solute = molarity × liters of solution
4. Grams of solute = molarity × gram molecular mass × liters of solution

Note: These equations are all on the basis of 1 L of solution; if something other than 1 L is used, refer back to the 1-L basis (500 ml = 0.5 L, or 2000 ml = 2 L, for example).

Molarity does not provide a basis for direct comparison of strength for all solutions. An example of this is that 1 L of 1 M NaOH will exactly neutralize 1 L of 1 M HCl, but it will neutralize only 0.5 L of 1 M sulfuric acid (H_2SO_4). It is therefore more convenient to choose a unit of concentration that *will* provide a basis for direct comparison of strengths of solutions. Such a unit is referred to as an *equivalent* (or equivalent weight or mass), and this term is used in describing the next unit of concentration to be discussed—*normality*.

Normality

The *equivalent* (equiv) is the mass in grams that will liberate, combine with, or replace one gram atom (g atom) of hydrogen ion (H^+). By using equivalents, the numbers of units of all substances involved in a reaction are made numerically equal.

Examples

Reaction 1:

1 equiv of NaOH + 1 equiv of HCl →

1 equiv of H_2O + 1 equiv of NaCl

Reaction 2:

1 equiv of NaOH + 1 equiv of H_2SO_4 →

1 equiv of H_2O + 1 equiv of Na_2SO_4

The balanced equation for this reaction is

$$2NaOH + 1H_2SO_4 \rightarrow 2H_2O + 1Na_2SO_4$$

This same reaction expressed using moles is

1 mol of NaOH + 0.5 mol of H_2SO_4 →

1 mol of H_2O + 0.5 mol of $NaSO_4$

One equivalent of any acid will neutralize one equivalent of any base.

In discussing molarity, the term moles per liter (mol/L) is used; in units of normality, the terms equivalents per liter (equiv/L), milliequivalents per milliliter (meq/ml), and milliequivalents per liter (meq/L) are used. The normality of a solution is defined as the number of gram equivalents (or equivalent weights) per liter of solution, or the number of milliequivalents per milliliter of solution. The *equivalent weight* (or mass) is the weight in grams that will liberate, combine with, or replace one gram atom of hydrogen. The equivalent weight may be found by dividing the gram molecular mass by the total combining power, or valence, of the positive ion (ions) of the substance. The SI system prefers the use of molarity (mol/L) to express the amount of substance in chemical units. A disadvantage of the concept of normality is that a particular solution may have more than one normality depending on the reaction in which it is used, while it will always have the same molarity since there is only one molecular mass for any substance.

Examples (equivalent weights)

Hydrochloric acid has one atom of H^+ and one atom of Cl^-; therefore, the gram equivalent weight equals the molecular mass.

Hydrogen sulfide (H_2S) has two atoms of H^+ and only one atom of S^{2-}, *or* one atom of H^+ and $\frac{1}{2}$ atom of S^{2-}; therefore, the equivalent weight equals one-half the molecular mass or

$$\frac{\text{Molecular mass}}{\text{Total positive valence}} = \frac{34}{2} = 17$$

NaCl has one atom of Cl^- and one atom of Na^+ (Na^+ replaces H^+); therefore, the gram equivalent weight equals the gram molecular mass.

A liter of a 1 normal (N) solution of H_2SO_4 contains the same number of equivalents as 1 L of $1\,N$ HCl, or $1\,N$ NaOH, or $1\,N$ barium hydroxide $[Ba(OH)_2]$. Again, equations might prove useful in working with normality solutions; some of these are

$$Normality = \frac{\text{equivalents of solute}}{\text{liters of solution}}$$

$$Normality = \frac{\text{grams of solute}}{\text{GMM/combining power (valence)}}$$
$$\times \frac{1}{\text{liters of solution}}$$

where GMM means gram molecular mass

$$Normality = \frac{\text{moles}}{\text{combining power}} \times \frac{1}{\text{liters of solution}}$$

$$Normality = \frac{\text{grams of solute}}{\text{equivalent weight}} \times \frac{1}{\text{liters of solution}}$$

$$Normality = \frac{\text{equivalents}}{\text{liters}}$$

$$Normality = \frac{\text{milliequivalents}}{\text{milliliters}}$$

Once again, all of these equations can be derived by applying a commonsense proportion approach to problem solving, as described in Laboratory Calculations.

Interconversion of molarity and normality

On occasion, it is necessary to convert an expression of concentration in molarity to one in normality and vice versa. Two simple formulas are available for this purpose:

Molarity
$$= \frac{\text{normality}}{\text{total positive combining power (valence)}}$$

Normality
$$= \text{molarity} \times \text{total positive combining power}$$

To prepare 1 L of a $2\,N$ NaCl solution, first calculate the gram molecular mass, using the known formula for the compound: $Na = 23$, $Cl = 35.5$, the gram molecular mass thus being 58.5 g. In working with normality problems, the gram equivalent weight is used; therefore, the next step is to calculate this. The gram equivalent weight equals the gram molecular mass divided by the valence, or 58.5 g divided by 1; the gram equivalent weight is therefore 58.5 g. For 1 L of a $1\,N$ solution of this compound, 58.5 g would be weighed; for 1 L of a $2\,N$ solution, $58.5\,g \times 2$, or 117 g, of NaCl is needed per liter.

An example of another such problem follows.

Example

Prepare 200 ml of a $0.5\,N$ calcium chloride ($CaCl_2$) solution.

Step 1: Calculate the gram molecular mass.

$$Ca = 40 \times 1 = \quad 40$$
$$Cl = 35.5 \times 2 = \quad \underline{71}$$
$$111\,g = \text{gram molecular mass}$$

Step 2: Calculate the gram equivalent mass.

$$\text{Equivalent weight} = \frac{\text{GMM}}{\text{valence}} = \frac{111}{2} = 55.5\,g$$

Step 3: Solve for normality. A $1\,N$ solution would contain 55.5 g/L. A $0.5\,N$ solution would contain only half as much chemical per liter of solution, or 27.8 g. A proportion could be set up to solve this:

$$\frac{55.5\,g/L}{1\,N\,\text{solution}} = \frac{x\,g/L}{0.5\,N\,\text{solution}}$$

$$x = 27.8\,g$$

However, only 200 ml of this solution is needed. Therefore another proportion could be set up for this:

$$\frac{27.8 \text{ g}}{1000 \text{ ml}} = \frac{x \text{ g}}{200 \text{ ml}}$$

$$x = 5.6 \text{ g}$$

Step 4: Actual preparation of solution. 5.6 g of $CaCl_2$ is weighed and diluted to 200 ml volumetrically (see under Reagent Preparation).

KINDS OF WATER USED IN THE CLINICAL LABORATORY

For use in the clinical laboratory, all water should be free from substances that could interfere with the tests being performed. It is important that anyone involved in doing clinical laboratory procedures understand the reasons for the special emphasis placed on the kinds of water used and the difficulties involved in obtaining and maintaining pure water. Water used in the clinical laboratory is generally distilled water or deionized water. Either may be used satisfactorily in most laboratory procedures. The term deionized water used in this text may be used interchangeably with distilled water unless otherwise stated.

Many minerals are found in natural water. Among those commonly found in water are iron, magnesium, and calcium. Water from which these minerals and others have been removed by distillation is known as *distilled water.* In the process of distillation, water is boiled, and the resulting steam is cooled; condensed steam is distilled water. Distilled water is often used in the laboratory.

Another kind of water used is known as *deionized water.* In the process of deionization, water is passed through a resin column containing positively (+) and negatively (−) charged particles. These particles combine with ions present in the water to remove them. Therefore, only substances that can ionize will be removed in the process of deionization. Organic substances and other substances that do not ionize are not removed. Both deionized and distilled water are used widely in the clinical laboratory.

However, distilled or deionized water is not necessarily pure water. There may be contamination by dissolved gases, by nonvolatile substances

carried over by steam in the distillation process, or by dissolved substances from storage containers. For example, in tests for nitrogen compounds (such as urea nitrogen, a common clinical chemistry determination) it is important to use ammonia-free (nitrogen-free) water. This may be specially purchased by the laboratory for such determinations or prepared in the laboratory by a specific method, double distillation, to remove the contaminating ammonia.

Water of higher purity is also produced by special distillation units in which the water is first deionized and then distilled; this eliminates the need for double distillation. Other systems may first distill the water, then deionize it. The presence of ionizable contaminants in distilled or deionized water is most easily determined by measuring the conductance, or electrical resistance, of the water. This is the basis for having *purity meters* or conductivity warning lights on distillation and deionization apparatus. Water of the highest purity will vary with the actual method of preparation and may be referred to as nitrogen-free water, double distilled water, or conductivity water, depending on the actual method used. However, a measure of conductance does not consider the presence of nonionized substances (organic contaminants) such as dissolved gases. Especially important in the clinical laboratory is dissolved carbon dioxide. Water free of such dissolved gases may be obtained by boiling it immediately before use and is often referred to as gas-free, or carbon dioxide-free, water. Such water may be necessary for the preparation of strongly alkaline solutions. As mentioned previously, another contaminant of water may be the presence of substances dissolved from the storage container. Thus laboratory water should be stored in borosilicate (Pyrex or Kimax) glass or plastic bottles to prevent contamination and should be tightly stoppered to prevent the absorption of gases.

Rarely is tap water used in the clinical laboratory, the exception being for the initial washing of glassware. Whenever water is needed in any procedure or reagents are to be made and diluted with water, care should be taken to use the type of water best suited to the test or reagent. Plain tap water is not used in any procedures or in making reagents.

LABORATORY GLASSWARE

Most clinical laboratories still use glassware for the greater part of the analytical work done, even with the advent of modern plasticware and stainless steel. Glassware is used in all departments of the laboratory, and special types of glass apparatus have been devised for special uses. These special types of glassware will be discussed where applicable. The chemistry department probably has the greatest variety and amount of glassware. Certain types of glass can be attacked by reagents to such an extent that the determinations done in them are not valid. It is therefore important to use the correct type of glass for the determinations being done. Clinical laboratory glassware can be divided into five types: glass with high thermal resistance, high-silica glass, glass with a high resistance to alkali, low-actinic glass, and standard flint glass.

High thermal resistant glass is usually a borosilicate glass with a low alkali content. This type of glassware is resistant to heat, corrosion, and thermal shock and should be used whenever heating or sterilization by heat is employed. Borosilicate glass, known by the commercial name of Pyrex or Kimax, is used widely in the laboratory because of its high qualities of resistance. Laboratory apparatus such as beakers, flasks, and pipets are usually made from borosilicate glass. Exax brand glassware is a lower-grade borosilicate glass and may be used when a high-quality borosilicate glass is not necessary. If the various pieces of glassware found in the laboratory are examined, it will be seen that one or more of these brand names will be found on many different kinds of glassware. It is essential to choose glassware that has a reliable composition and that will be resistant to laboratory chemicals and conditions. In borosilicate glassware, mechanical strength and thermal and chemical resistance are well balanced. Two other brands of high thermal resistant glass are Corex and Vycor. Corex glassware is made from a special alumina-silicate glass that is six times stronger than borosilicate glass. Vycor glassware can withstand drastic thermal and chemical treatment.

High-silica glass has a silica content of more than 96%, which makes it comparable to fused quartz in its heat resistance, chemical stability, and electrical characteristics. High-silica glass is made from borosilicate glass by removing almost all the elements except silica. This type of glassware is used for high-precision analytical work and can also be used for optical reflectors and mirrors. It is not used for the type of glassware generally found in the laboratory.

Glass with high resistance to alkali was developed particularly for use with strong alkaline solutions. It is boron-free. It is often referred to as *soft glass*, as its thermal resistance is much less than that of borosilicate glass and it must be heated and cooled very carefully. Its use should be limited to times when solutions of or digestions with strong alkalis are made.

Low-actinic glassware contains materials that usually impart an amber or red color to the glass and reduce the amount of light transmitted through to the substance in the glassware. It is used for substances that are particularly sensitive to light, such as bilirubin.

Standard flint glass, or soda-lime glass, is composed of a mixture of the oxides of silicon, calcium, and sodium. It is the most inexpensive glass and is readily made into a variety of types of glassware. This type of glass is much less resistant to high temperatures and sudden changes of temperature, and its resistance to chemical attack is only fair. Glassware made from soda-lime glass can release alkali into solutions and can therefore cause considerable errors in certain laboratory determinations. For instance, pipets made from soda-lime glass may release alkali into the pipetted liquid.

In recent years the widespread introduction of relatively inexpensive disposable glassware has greatly reduced the need to clean glassware. This disposable glassware is made to be used and discarded, and no cleaning is necessary either before or after use, in most cases. Disposable glass and plastic is used to manufacture test tubes of all sizes, pipets, slides, Petri dishes for microbiology, and specimen containers, to mention but a few. Considering the recent awareness of the need to conserve resources and raw materials, however, the technician should be instructed in the use of reusable glassware and the cleaning processes that are necessary with it.

There are two main categories into which most laboratory glassware can be separated: (1) *containers and receivers*, and (2) *volumetric* apparatus. Examples of containers and receivers are beakers, test tubes, Erlenmeyer flasks, and reagent bottles. Examples of volumetric glassware are volumetric flasks, pipets, graduated cylinders, and burets.

Containers and receivers

This category of laboratory glassware includes many of the most frequently used and most common pieces of glassware known to the student. Containers and receivers must be made of good-quality glass. They are not calibrated to hold a particular or exact volume, but rather are available for various volumes, depending on the use desired. Beakers, Erlenmeyer flasks, test tubes, and reagent bottles are made in many different sizes (Fig. 1-3). This glassware, like the volumetric glassware described in the next section, has certain information indicated directly on the vessel. The volume and the brand name, or trademark, are two pieces of information found on items such as beakers and test tubes. Containers and receivers are not as expensive as volumetric glassware, because the process of exact volume calibration is not necessary.

Beakers

Beakers are available in many sizes and in several forms. The most common form used in the clinical laboratory is known as the *Griffin low form*. Beakers should be made of glass that is resistant to the many chemicals used in them and also resistant to heat.

Erlenmeyer flasks

Erlenmeyer flasks are used commonly in the laboratory for preparing reagents, for titration procedures, and for preparing blood filtrates. They, too, come in various sizes and must be made from a resistant form of glass.

Test tubes

Test tubes come in many sizes, depending on the use for which they are intended. Test tubes without lips are the most satisfactory, because there is less chance of chipping and eventual breakage. Disposable test tubes are used for many laboratory purposes. Since chemical reactions occur in test tubes used in the chemistry laboratory, test tubes intended for such use should be made of borosilicate glass, which is resistant to thermal shock.

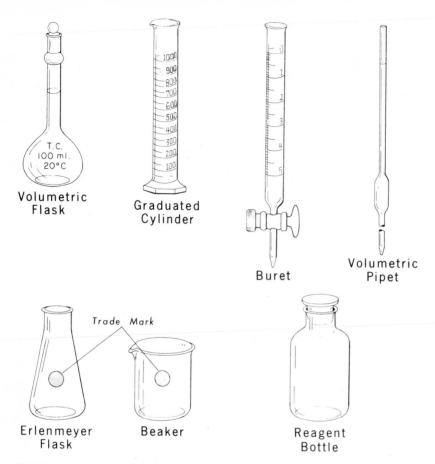

Fig. 1-3. Laboratory glassware.

Reagent bottles

All reagents should be stored in a reagent bottle of some type. These can be made of glass or some other material; some of the more commonly purchased ones now are made of polyethylene. Reagent bottles come in various sizes; the size used should meet the needs for the particular situation.

Photometry cuvettes

The special tubes used for photometry are called cuvettes or absorption cells. They may be round, square, or rectangular and may be made of glass, silica (quartz), or plastic. For most routine use in the clinical laboratory, a round cuvette made of good-quality glass is used. The amount of light transmitted by the cuvette varies significantly with the material used to make it. To be able to use cuvettes interchangeably, they must be of uniform inside diameters so that the absorbance of a solution will be within a specified tolerance when measured in different cuvettes. To ensure this uniformity, the cuvettes must be calibrated (see under Calibration of Cuvettes for the Photometer).

Volumetric glassware

Volumetric glassware must go through a rigorous process of volume calibration to ensure the accuracy of the measurements required for laboratory determinations. In very precise work it is never safe to assume that the volume contained or delivered by any piece of equipment is exactly that indicated on the equipment. The calibration process is lengthy and time-consuming; therefore the cost of volumetric glassware is relatively high compared with the cost of noncalibrated glassware (beakers, test tubes, etc.).

Volumetric flasks

Volumetric flasks are flasks with a round bulb at the bottom. This tapers to a long neck, on which the calibration mark is found. The specifications set up by the National Bureau of Standards apply to all volumetric glassware and therefore to volumetric flasks (Fig. 1-3).[7] Volumetric flasks are calibrated to contain a specific amount or volume of liquid, and therefore the letters T.C. are inscribed somewhere on the neck of the flask. There are many different sizes of volumetric flasks, for the different volumes of liquid that are used. The following are some of the sizes in which volumetric flasks can be purchased: 10, 25, 50, 100, and 500 ml, and 1 and 2 L.

Volumetric flasks have been calibrated individually to contain the specified volume. For each size of volumetric flask there are certain allowable limits within which its volume must lie. This is called the *tolerance* of the flask. All volumetric glassware has a specific tolerance, the capacity tolerance, which is dependent on the size of the glassware. For example, a 100-ml volumetric flask has a tolerance of ±0.08 ml. Conditions are controlled during the calibration of a 100-ml volumetric flask to guarantee these limits. A tolerance of ±0.08 indicates that the allowable limits for the volume of a 100-ml volumetric flask are from 99.92 to 100.08 ml. A tolerance of ±0.05 ml for a 50-ml volumetric flask indicates allowable limits ranging from 49.95 to 50.05 ml for the volume of the flask. Volumetric flasks are used in the preparation of specific volumes of reagents or laboratory solutions. They should be used with reagents or solutions at room temperature. Solutions diluted in volumetric flasks should be repeatedly mixed during the dilution so that the contents are homogeneous before they are made up to volume. In this way, errors due to the expansion or contraction of liquids during mixing are made negligible. An important factor in the use of any volumetric apparatus is an accurate reading of the meniscus level. For more information on reading a meniscus, see under General Considerations in Pipetting.

Graduated measuring cylinders

A graduated measuring cylinder is a long cylindrical piece of glassware with calibrated markings on it. Graduated cylinders are used to measure volumes of liquids when a high degree of accuracy is not essential. They can be made from plastic or polyethylene as well as from glass (Fig. 1-3). Graduated cylinders come in various sizes according to the volumes they measure: 10, 25, 50, 100, 500, and 1000 ml. A 100-ml graduated cylinder can measure 100 ml or a fraction thereof, depending on the calibration, or graduation, marks on it. Most graduated cylinders are calibrated to deliver. This will be indicated directly on the glassware by the inscription T.D. The letters T.D. can be found on many kinds of volumetric glassware, especially on the numerous kinds of pipets used in the laboratory (see under Pipets).

Graduated cylinders can be used to measure a specified volume of a liquid, such as water, in the preparation of laboratory reagents. The calibration marks on the cylinder indicate its capacity at different points. If 450 ml of water is to be measured, the most satisfactory cylinder to use would be one with a capacity of 500 ml. Graduated cylinders are not calibrated as accurately as volumetric flasks. Therefore, the capacity tolerance for graduated cylinders allows a greater variation in volume. The capacity tolerance is greater for the larger graduated cylinders. A 100-ml graduated cylinder (T.D.) has a tolerance of ±0.40 ml, meaning that the allowable limits are from 99.60 to 100.40 ml.

Pipets

Pipets are another type of volumetric glassware used extensively in the laboratory. Many types of pipets are available. It is important, however, to use only pipets manufactured by reputable companies. Care and discretion should be used in selecting pipets for clinical laboratory use, since their accuracy is one of the determining factors in the accuracy of the procedures carried out. A pipet is a cylindrical glass tube used in measuring fluids. It is calibrated to deliver, or transfer, a specified volume from one vessel to another (Fig. 1-3).

Each pipet has at least one calibration or graduation mark on it, as does all volumetric glassware. A pipet is filled by using mechanical suction or an aspirator bulb. Mouth suction is never used. Strong acids, bases, solvents, or human specimens are much too potent or contaminated to risk pipetting them by mouth. Caustic liquids and some solvents are very dangerous; some destroy tissue immediately on contact. Some solvents have harmful vapors (see under Safety in the Laboratory).

For most general laboratory use, there are two main types of pipets, the volumetric (or transfer) pipet and the graduated (or measuring) pipet. They are classified according to whether they contain or deliver a specified amount. For this reason, they may be called *to-contain* or *to-deliver* pipets. A to-contain pipet is identified by inscribed letters T.C. and a to-deliver one by the letters T.D. The T.D. pipet is filled properly and allowed to drain completely into a receiving vessel. Portions of nonviscous samples, such as filtrates, serum, and standard solutions, are accu-

rately measured by allowing the volumetric pipet to drain while it is held in the vertical position and by using only the force of gravity (see under General Pipetting Procedure). For most volumetric glassware the temperature of calibration is usually 20°C, and this is inscribed on the pipet (see under Calibration of Volumetric Glassware).

The opening (orifice) at the delivery tip of the pipet is of a certain size to give a specified length of time for drainage when the pipet is held vertically. A pipet must be held vertically to ensure proper drainage. It will not drain as fast when held at a 45° angle. The actual procedure is discussed further under Pipetting (see Pipetting Technique).

Volumetric pipets

A pipet that has been calibrated to deliver a fixed volume of liquid by drainage is known as a *volumetric* pipet, or *transfer* pipet. These pipets consist of a cylindrical bulb joined at both ends to narrow glass tubing. A calibration mark is etched around the upper suction tube, and the lower delivery tube is drawn out to a fine tip.[8] Some important considerations concerning volumetric pipets are that the calibration mark should not be too close to the top of the suction tube, the bulb should merge gradually into the lower delivery tube, and the delivery tip should have a gradual taper. To reduce drainage errors, the orifice should be of such a size that the flow out of the pipet is not too rapid. These pipets should be made from a good-quality glass, such as Kimax or Pyrex (Fig. 1-4).

Volumetric pipets are suitable for all accurate measurements of volumes of 1 ml or more. They are calibrated to deliver the amount inscribed on them. This volume is measured from the calibration mark to the tip. A 5-ml volumetric pipet will deliver a single measured volume of 5 ml, and a 2-ml volumetric pipet will deliver 2 ml. The tolerance of volumetric pipets increases with the capacity of the pipet. A 10-ml volumetric pipet will have a greater tolerance than a 2-ml

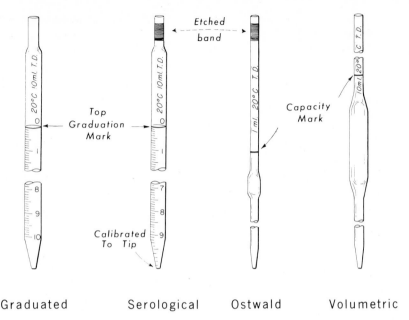

Graduated   Serological   Ostwald   Volumetric

Fig. 1-4. Types of pipets.

one. The tolerance for a 5-ml volumetric pipet is ±0.01 ml. When volumes of liquids are to be delivered with great accuracy, a volumetric pipet is used. Volumetric pipets are used to measure standard solutions, unknown blood and plasma filtrates, serum, plasma, urine, spinal fluid, and some reagents.

Measurements with volumetric pipets are done individually, and the volumes can only be whole milliliters (e.g., 1, 2, 5, and 10 ml). To transfer 1 ml of a standard solution into a test tube volumetrically, a 1-ml volumetric pipet is used. To transfer 5 ml of the same solution, a 5-ml volumetric pipet is used. After a volumetric pipet drains, a drop remains inside the delivery tip. This drop is *not* to be blown out: the specific volume the pipet is calibrated to deliver is dependent on the fact that the drop is left in the tip of the pipet. Information inscribed on the pipet includes the temperature of calibration (usually 20°C), capacity, manufacturer, and usage (T.D.). The technique involved in using volumetric pipets correctly is very important, and a

certain amount of skill is required (see under Pipetting Technique).

Graduated pipets

Another way to deliver a particular amount of liquid is to deliver that amount of liquid contained between two calibration marks on a cylindrical tube, or pipet. Such a pipet is called a *graduated*, or *measuring*, pipet. It has several graduation, or calibration, marks (Fig. 1-4). Many measurements in the laboratory do not require the precision of the volumetric pipet. Graduated pipets are used when great accuracy is not required. This does not mean that these pipets may be used with less care than the volumetric pipets. Graduated pipets are used primarily in measuring reagents, but they are not calibrated with sufficient tolerance to use in measuring standard or control solutions, unknown specimens, or filtrates.

A graduated pipet is a straight piece of glass tubing with a tapered end and graduation marks on the stem separating it into parts. Depending on the size used, graduated pipets can be used to measure parts of a milliliter or many milliliters. These pipets come in various sizes or capacities, including 0.1, 0.2, 1, 2, 5, 10, and 25 ml. If 4 ml of deionized water is to be measured into a test tube, a 5-ml graduated pipet would be the best choice. Since graduated pipets require draining between two marks, they introduce one more source of error, compared with the volumetric pipets with only one calibration mark. This makes measurements with the graduated pipet less precise. Because of this relatively poor precision, the graduated pipet is used where speed is more important than precision. It is used for measurements of reagents and is generally not considered accurate enough for measuring samples and standard solutions.

Two types of pipets are calibrated for delivery (Fig. 1-4). One (called a Mohr pipet) is calibrated between two marks on the stem, and the other (a serological pipet) has graduation marks down to the delivery tip. The serological pipet has a larger orifice and therefore drains faster than the Mohr pipet (see under Serological Pipets).

The volume of the space between the last calibration mark and the delivery tip is not known in the Mohr pipet. In graduated pipets, this space cannot be used for measuring fluids. Graduated pipets are calibrated in much the same manner as volumetric pipets; however, they are not constructed with as strict specifications and they have larger capacity tolerances. The allowable tolerance for a 5-ml graduated pipet is ±0.02 ml.

To-contain pipets (micropipets)

The to-contain pipet, when used properly, is one of the more precise pipets used in the clinical laboratory. This type of pipet is calibrated to *contain* a specified amount of liquid. If a pipet contains only 0.1 ml, and 0.1 ml of blood is needed for a chemistry determination, then none of the blood can be left inside the pipet. The entire contents of the pipet must be emptied. If this pipet is *rinsed well* with a diluting solution, then all the blood or similar specimen will be removed from it. The correct way to use a to-contain pipet is to rinse it with a suitable diluent. Thus, a to-contain pipet cannot be used properly unless the receiving vessel contains a diluent; that is, a to-contain pipet should not be used to deliver a specimen into an empty receiving vessel. Since all the liquid in a to-contain pipet is rinsed out and used, there is only one graduation mark.

To-contain pipets are used when micro amounts of blood or specimen are needed, and they are also called *micropipets* in many areas of the laboratory. Many procedures require only a small amount of blood, and a micropipet is used for this measurement. Because even a minute volume remaining in the pipet can cause a significant error in micro work, most micropipets are calibrated to contain (T.C.) the stated volume rather than to deliver it. They are generally available in small sizes, such as 20, 50, 100, and 200 μl. A common micropipet used is the Sahli hemoglobin pipet, calibrated to contain 0.02 ml or 20 μl.

A special disposable micropipet used in the hematology laboratory is a self-filling pipet accompanied by a polyethylene reagent reservoir (see under Hematology). This unit is called a Unopette (Becton, Dickinson & Co., Rutherford, N.J.) and is used by many laboratories. A glass capillary pipet is fitted in a plastic holder and fills automatically with blood by means of capillary action. The plastic reagent bottle (called the reservoir) is squeezed slightly while the pipet is inserted. On release of pressure, the sample is drawn into the diluent in the reservoir. Intermittent squeezing fills and empties the pipet to rinse out the contents of the pipet. This type of unit has been adapted for several chemical and hematological determinations.

Ostwald pipets

A special type of pipet designed for use in measuring viscous fluids such as blood or serum is known as the *Ostwald* pipet (or the *Ostwald-Folin* pipet). When blood is to be measured in the chemistry laboratory, the Ostwald pipet is used. This pipet is similar in appearance to the volumetric pipet, except that the bulb is closer to the delivery tip (Fig. 1-4). Ostwald pipets are usually calibrated to be blown out, and therefore an etched ring or band will be seen near the suction hole. To minimize the effects of viscosity, the Ostwald pipet is designed with a large oval bulb and a short delivery tip.

Ostwald pipets come in several sizes; the most common ones are 0.5, 1, and 2 ml. When using an Ostwald pipet to measure blood, the blood should be allowed to drain as slowly as possible so that no residual film is left on the sides of the pipet. Contrary to the usual practice of reading the bottom of the meniscus for liquids being measured by pipet, when blood is pipetted in the Ostwald pipet, the top of the meniscus is read (blood is not transparent and the bottom of the meniscus cannot be seen clearly).

Serological pipets

Another pipet used in the laboratory, but not often in the chemistry laboratory, is called a *serological* pipet. It is much like the graduated pipet in appearance (Fig. 1-4). The orifice, or tip opening, is larger in the serological pipet than in other pipets. The rate of fall of liquid is much too fast for great accuracy or precision. For use in chemistry it would be necessary to retard the flow of liquid from the delivery tip of the serological pipet. The serological pipet is graduated to the end of the delivery tip and has an etched band on the suction piece. It is therefore designed to be blown out. The serological pipet is less precise than any of the pipets discussed above. It is designed for use in serology, where relative values are sought. It is best not to use the serological pipet for chemistry.

Stopcock pipets

The *stopcock* pipet is designed for delivering blood into a Van Slyke machine, which is used for the determination and analysis of gases such as oxygen and carbon dioxide. The stopcock pipet can be used to deliver anything that is not to be exposed to the air. It resembles a small volumetric pipet with a stopcock attached near the delivery tip; this is used for better control of the delivery of the sample into the machine. Stopcock pipets have two calibration marks, one on either side of the bulb.

Automatic pipets

Automatic and semiautomatic versions of pipets are useful in many areas of laboratory work. Use of automatic pipetting devices eliminates pipet cleaning and reduces the error resulting from the variation in pipetting techniques. Several different types are available, and each must be carefully calibrated before it is used. The problems encountered with automatic pipetting devices depend to a large degree on the nature of the solution being pipetted. Some reagents cause more bubbles than others, and some are more viscous. Each of these tendencies can cause problems with the measurement and delivery of samples and solutions.

Automatic pipetting devices permit measuring out a whole series of equal volumes. They provide very efficient delivery of equal volumes of specimens followed by equivalent volumes of diluent. These automatic devices can be operated either manually or by a motor. Since proper care and calibration are essential for accurate sampling, it is important to read and follow the manufacturer's instructions.

Burets

The fourth category of volumetric glassware consists of burets. A buret is a long cylindrical piece of glassware with graduation divisions on it and a stopcock closing at one end (Fig. 1-3). The stopcock on the delivery tip of the buret serves to control the flow of liquid. A buret is used to deliver measured quantities of fluids or solutions. Like all other volumetric glassware, burets are carefully calibrated according to the specifications set up by the National Bureau of Standards.

Burets also have a specific capacity tolerance depending on their size. Smaller burets are more accurate than larger ones (as they have smaller tolerances). Burets with a maximum capacity of 2.0 ml or less are called *microburets.* They are usually calibrated with 0.01-ml or smaller divisions. Some common capacities for burets are 5, 10, and 25 ml. The capacity tolerances for burets are similar to those for graduated pipets, which burets resemble very closely. For a 5-ml buret, the tolerance is ±0.02 ml. This means that the allowable limits for the volume of this particular buret range from 4.98 to 5.02 ml. The chief difference between the buret and the graduated pipet is that the buret has a stopcock. The stopcock is made from either glass or Teflon. A glass stopcock requires the use of a lubricant, but a Teflon stopcock does not. Burets are used in titration, a means of quantitative measurement (see under Titration for more information on the use of the buret).

Calibration of volumetric glassware

Calibration is the means by which glassware or other apparatus used in quantitative measurements is checked to determine its exact volume. To calibrate is to divide the glassware or mark it with graduations (or other indexes of quantity) for the purpose of measurement. Calibration marks will be seen on every piece of volumetric glassware used in the laboratory. Specifications for the calibration of glassware are set up by the National Bureau of Standards.[9]

Each piece of volumetric glassware must be checked and must comply with these specifications before it can be accurately used in the clinical laboratory. Pipets, burets, volumetric flasks, and other volumetric glassware are supposed to hold, deliver, or contain a specific amount of liquid. This specified amount, or volume, is known as the *units of capacity* and is indicated by the manufacturer directly on each piece of glassware.

Volumetric glassware is usually calibrated by weight, using distilled water. Water is commonly used as the liquid for calibration because it is readily available and because it is similar in viscosity and speed of drainage to the solutions and reagents ordinarily used in the clinical laboratory. The units of capacity determined will therefore be the volume of water contained in, or delivered by, the glassware at a particular temperature. The manufacturer knows what the weights of various amounts of distilled water are at specific temperatures. This information is used in the calibration of volumetric glassware. If a manufacturer wants a volumetric flask to contain 100 ml, a sensitive balance such as an analytical balance is used. Weights corresponding to what 100 ml of distilled water weighs at a specific temperature are placed on one side of the balance. The flask to be calibrated is placed on the other side of the balance, and distilled water is gradually added to it until equilibrium is achieved. The manufacturer then makes a permanent calibration mark on the neck of the flask at the bottom of the water meniscus level. This flask is then calibrated to contain 100 ml. Other sizes and types of volumetric glassware are similarly calibrated.

The volume of a particular piece of glassware varies with the *temperature.* For this reason it is necessary to specify the temperature at which the glassware was calibrated. Glass will swell or shrink with changes in temperature, and the volume of the glassware will therefore vary with changes in temperature. Most volumetric glassware for routine clinical use is calibrated at 20°C. This means that the calibration process and checking took place at a controlled temperature of 20°C. On all volumetric glassware the inscription 20°C will be seen. Although 20°C is almost universally adopted as the standard temperature for calibration of volumetric glassware, each piece of glassware will have the temperature of calibration inscribed on it. The volume of a volumetric flask is less at a low temperature than at a higher temperature. A 50-ml volumetric flask that was calibrated at 20°C would contain less than 50 ml at 10°C.

Since the laboratory depends to such a great extent on the quality of its glassware to produce reliable results, it is necessary to be certain that the glassware is of the *very best quality.* The glass used for volumetric glassware must meet certain standards of quality. It must be transparent and free from striations and other surface irregularities. It should have no defects that would distort the appearance of the liquid surface or portion of the calibration line seen through the glass.

The *design and workmanship* for volumetric glassware is also specified by the National Bureau of Standards. The shape of the glassware must permit complete emptying and thorough cleaning, and it must stand solidly on a level surface.

Plasticware

The clinical laboratory has benefited greatly from the introduction of plasticware. In many cases, plasticware designed for laboratory usage has replaced glassware. Beakers, bottles, funnels, centrifuge tubes, graduated cylinders, tubing, and pipets manufactured from polyethylene or polypropylene have unusual impact and tensile strength and are resistant to corrosion. When possible, plasticware should be used in place of glassware. It is unbreakable, which is its greatest advantage. The disadvantages of plasticware are that there is some leaching of surface-bound constituents into solutions, some permeability to water vapor, some evaporation through breathing of the plastic, and some absorption of dyes, stains, or proteins. Because evaporation is a significant factor in using plasticware, small volumes of reagent should never be stored in oversized plastic bottles for long periods of time.

Cleaning laboratory glassware

Among the many factors that ensure accurate results in laboratory determinations is the use of *clean*, unbroken glassware. There is no point in exercising care in obtaining specimens, handling the specimens, and making the laboratory determination if the glassware used is not extremely clean.

There are various methods of cleaning glassware, the one chosen depending on its use. In all cases, glassware for the clinical laboratory must be physically clean, in most cases it must be chemically clean, and in some cases it must be bacteriologically clean, or sterile.

Glassware that cannot be cleaned immediately after use should be rinsed with tap water and left to soak in a basin or pail of water to which a small amount of detergent has been added. Never allow dirty glassware to dry out. Once dried out on the surface, it is difficult to remove most soil by ordinary means. For this reason it is important to have a soaking bucket available in the working area. Glassware that is new is often slightly alkaline and should be soaked for several hours in a dilute hydrochloric acid or nitric acid solution (about 1 ml/dl is satisfactory). This glassware should then be washed in the regular manner.

Glassware that is contaminated, as by use in the microbiology laboratory, must be sterilized before it is washed. This can be done by boiling, autoclaving, or some similar procedure.

General cleaning methods involve the use of a

soap, detergent, or cleaning powder. In most laboratories, detergents are used. If the dirty glassware has been soaking in a solution of the detergent water, the cleaning job will be much easier.

General cleaning procedure

There are various specific methods of cleaning laboratory glassware. Most glassware (with the exception of pipets) can be cleaned in the following way.

1. Put the specified amount of detergent into a dishpan or washing bucket containing moderately hot water. Allow the detergent to dissolve thoroughly.

2. Rinse glassware (or other items that can be washed) in tap water before placing it in the detergent solution. Never allow dirty glassware to dry out; always place it in a soaking bucket. Glassware should be completely submerged in the bucket or pan. Fill large pieces with detergent water and set aside to soak. Soaking glassware for at least 1 hour before washing makes the washing procedure much more efficient.

3. Using a cleaning brush, thoroughly scrub the glassware, being certain to clean all parts. Brushes of various sizes should be available to fit the different-sized test tubes, flasks, funnels, and bottles. Excessive brushing and improper use of brushes may cause scratching of the glassware. Avoid the use of abrasive cleaners on glassware.

4. Rinse glassware under running tap water; allow the water to run into each piece of glassware, pour it out, and repeat several times (7–10 times is sufficient). Rinse the outside of the glassware too. It is especially important to *remove all the detergent from the glassware before use*; if detergent remains, the alkali in it may interfere with laboratory determinations.

5. After thoroughly rinsing the glassware with tap water, rinse it with distilled or deionized water about three times. Certain glassware used for microbiological studies requires even longer rinsing with deionized water. Use deionized or distilled water in the final rinsing of all laboratory glassware.

6. Glassware may be dried in a hot oven (no hotter than 100°C) or at room temperature. If a higher temperature is used, the glassware can become distorted. Always dry glassware or other equipment in an inverted position to ensure complete drainage of water as it dries. Never dry laboratory ware with a towel. Do not dry plasticware or rubber items in an oven.

7. Check the glassware for cleanliness by observing the water drainage. Chemically clean glassware will drain uniformly; dirty glassware will drain leaving water droplets adhering to the walls of the glass.

Cleaning pipets

Pipets used in the laboratory are cleaned in a special way. Immediately after use, the pipets should be placed in a special pipet container or cylinder containing water; the water should be high enough to completely cover the pipets. Pipets should be carefully placed in the container to avoid breakage. When the pipets are to be cleaned, they are removed from the cylinder and placed in another cylinder containing an acid cleaning solution. This cleaning solution is usually a combination of sulfuric acid and either potassium or sodium dichromate (called acid-dichromate solution). Acid-dichromate cleaning solution may be purchased commercially, or it may be prepared by dissolving 100 g of sodium or potassium dichromate in 100 ml of water and slowly adding, while stirring, the contents of one 9-lb bottle of technical grade sulfuric acid. For safe handling during the preparation, the container of acid solution should be placed in a pan or sink of cold water because of the great amount of heat generated on mixing the acid and water. Safety goggles should always be worn during the preparation of this solution, as should rubber gloves and a protective apron. It is an extremely potent solution, and it must be handled cautiously or serious burns will result (see under Safety in the Laboratory). The pipets are allowed to soak in the cleaning solution for 30 minutes.

The next step involves thorough rinsing of the pipets. This can be accomplished by hand, but more often it is done with the aid of an automatic pipet washer. The pipets are rinsed with tap water, utilizing the automatic pipet washer, for 1–2 hours. They are then rinsed in deionized or distilled water two or three times and dried in a hot oven. An alternative cleaning solution is a solution of detergent. However, the acid cleaning solution is recommended.

Cleaning diluting pipets

Pipets used in the hematology laboratory for dilution are also cleaned in a special way. They should always be rinsed immediately after use, preferably by being placed in a tumbler or beaker of water until they are cleaned. There are several ways to clean these pipets, but in general they are first cleaned with tap water, then with distilled water, and finally rinsed with either alcohol or acetone. Acetone assists in drying the inside of the pipet. Usually the cleaning is done with suction, using a special pipet holder that fits onto the suction apparatus. The pipets are also dried with suction. Periodically, the pipets should be cleaned with a detergent solution, rinsed well, and dried.

Cleaning photometry cuvettes

Cuvettes must be scrupulously clean and free from grease smudges or scratches. As soon as possible after use, cuvettes should be rinsed with tap water, filled with a mild detergent solution, and placed in a rubberized test tube rack. It is best not to put them into a regular dishwashing

bucket where they would rub against each other and be scratched. After standing with the detergent solution, the cuvettes are rinsed several times with tap water and two or three times with distilled or deionized water. When drying cuvettes, high temperatures and unclean air should be avoided. A low to medium oven (not above $100°C$) can be used for rapid drying. In some laboratories, there are special dishwashing machines that can adequately handle cuvettes.

Glass breakage and replacement

It is important in the clinical laboratory to check all glassware periodically to determine its condition. No broken or chipped glassware should be used. Many laboratory accidents are caused by the use of broken glassware. Serious cuts may result, and infections may set in.

Each time a laboratory procedure is carried out, the glassware used should be checked; equipment such as beakers, pipets, test tubes, and flasks should not have broken edges or cracks. To prevent breakage, glassware should be handled carefully; carrying too much glassware at one time from one place to another in the laboratory is to be avoided.

When glassware is broken, it must be replaced with another like piece. Breakage should be reported to an instructor or department head, so that replacement can be arranged. Several laboratory equipment catalogs are available from which the required items may be ordered. These catalogs are distributed by supply companies that handle laboratory equipment. They describe the quality, capacity, tolerance, and cost of the available items. To purchase equipment at the most reasonable price it is advisable to compare specific items in several different catalogs.

THE MICROSCOPE

The microscope is probably the piece of equipment that receives the most use (and, unfortunately, misuse) in the clinical laboratory. Microscopy is a basic part of the work in many areas of the laboratory—hematology, urinalysis, microbiology, and blood banking, to name a few. Because the microscope is such an important piece of equipment and is a precision instrument, it must be kept in excellent condition, optically and mechanically. It must be kept clean, and it must be kept aligned.

In simple terms, a microscope is a magnifying glass. The compound light microscope (the type used in most clinical laboratories) consists of two magnifying lenses, the objective and the ocular (or eyepiece). It is used to magnify an object to a point where it can be seen with the human eye. Here we must introduce the term *resolution*, which is basic in microscopy. Resolution tells how small and how close individual objects (dots) can be and still be recognizable. Practically, the resolving power is the limit of usable magnification. Further magnification of two dots that are no longer resolvable would be "empty magnification" and would result in a dumbbell appearance, as shown in Fig. 1-5.

In general terms, the human eye can separate (or resolve) dots that are 0.25 mm (0.25×10^{-3} m or 0.000 25 m) apart; the light microscope can separate dots that are 0.25 μm (0.25×10^{-6} m or 0.000 000 25 m) apart; and the electron microscope can separate dots that are 0.5 nm (0.5×10^{-9} m or 0.000 000 000 5 m) apart.

As mentioned above, the compound light microscope consists of two magnifying lenses, the objective and the eyepiece or ocular. The total magnification observed is the product of the magnifications of these two lenses. In other words, the magnification of the objective times the magnification of the ocular equals the total magnification. The magnitude of magnification is

inscribed on each lens as a number preceded by X—for example, X10. These magnification units are in terms of diameters; thus, X10 means that the diameter of an object is magnified to 10 times its original size. (The object itself or its area is not magnified 10 times—only the diameter of the object is magnified.)

Because of the manner in which light travels through the compound microscope, the image that is seen is upside down and reversed. The right side appears as the left, the top as the bottom, and vice versa. This should be kept in mind when moving the slide (or object) being observed.

Another term encountered in microscopy is *numerical aperture* (NA). The numerical aperture of a lens can be thought of as an index or measurement of the resolving power. As the numerical aperture increases, the resolution (or distance from each other at which objects can be distinguished) decreases. The numerical aperture can also be thought of as an index of the light-gathering power of a lens—a means of describing the amount of light entering the objective. Any particular lens has a constant numerical aperture, and this value is dependent on the radius of the lens and its focal length (the distance from the object being viewed to the lens or the objective). The numerical aperture is also inscribed on each objective lens. It follows that decreasing the amount of light passing through a lens will decrease the numerical aperture. The importance of this value will become apparent when we discuss proper light adjustments with the microscope.

The structures basic to all types of compound microscopes fall in four main categories: (1) the framework, (2) the illumination system, (3) the magnification system, and (4) the adjustment system (Fig. 1-6).

Parts of the microscope

The framework of the microscope consists of several units. The *base* is a firm, horseshoe-

Fig. 1-5. Resolution versus empty magnification.

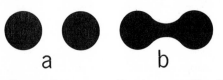

a   b

Resolution   Empty magnification

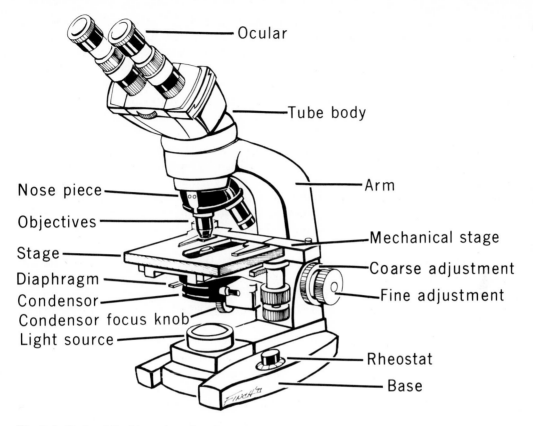

Ocular

Tube body

Arm

Nose piece

Objectives

Stage

Diaphragm

Condensor

Condensor focus knob

Light source

Mechanical stage

Coarse adjustment

Fine adjustment

Rheostat

Base

Fig. 1-6. Parts of the binocular microscope.

shaped foot on which the microscope rests. The *arm* is the structure that supports the magnifying and adjusting systems. It is also the handle by which the microscope can be carried without damaging the delicate parts. The *stage* is the horizontal platform, or shelf, on which the object being observed is placed. Most modern microscopes have a *mechanical stage*, which makes it much easier to manipulate the object being observed.

Good microscopic work cannot be accomplished without proper illumination. The illumination system is therefore an important part of the compound light microscope. Actually, there are six different illumination techniques or systems that are useful in the clinical laboratory: (1) bright-field, (2) dark-field, (3) fluorescence

(using transmitted light), (4) polarizing, (5) phase-contrast, and (6) Nomarski differential interference contrast. At this point we will describe the bright-field illumination system, which is most commonly employed in the clinical laboratory.

The illumination system begins with a *source of light*. The modern compound microscope most often has a built-in light source (or bulb). This illumination system also has a control to regulate the light intensity, ensuring both adequate illumination and comfort for the microscopist. The light source is located at the base of the microscope, and the light is directed up through the condenser system. It is important that the bulb be positioned correctly for proper alignment of the microscope. (Proper alignment means that the light path from the source of light throughout the microscope and the ocular is physically correct.) Modern microscopes are designed so that the light bulb filament will be centered if the bulb is installed properly. Many styles or types of bulbs are available, and it is important that the bulb designed for a particular microscope be used.

Some microscopes have an external rather than a built-in illumination system. These tend to be older, less commonly used microscopes. A mirror is part of the illumination system when a microscope has an external light source. It is located at the base of the microscope, approximately where the light bulb is in microscopes with built-in light sources. The mirror reflects the beam of light directed at it upward. It has two sides, one flat and the other concave. The concave side should be used for clinical microscopy work. To be certain that the mirror is at the correct angle, an ocular is removed and the light is centered while looking through the body tube.

Another part of the illumination system is the *condenser*. Modern microscopes use a substage Abbe-type condenser. The condenser directs and focuses the beam of light from the bulb or mirror onto the material under examination. The Abbe condenser is a conical lens system (actually consisting of two lenses) with the point planed off. The condenser position is adjustable; it can be raised and lowered beneath the stage by means of an adjustment knob. It must be correctly positioned to correctly focus the light on the material being viewed. When it is correctly positioned, the image field is evenly lighted. The condenser must be positioned because, being a lens, it has a fixed numerical aperture. When the microscope is properly used, the numerical aperture of the condenser should be equal to or slightly less than the numerical aperture of the objective being used. The numerical aperture of the condenser can be varied by changing its position; thus the condenser position must be adjusted with each objective used in order to maximize the light focus and the resolving power of the microscope. When the numerical aperture

of the condenser is decreased below that of the objective, contrast is gained and resolution is lost. This manipulation is often necessary in the clinical laboratory when observing wet, unstained preparations such as urinary sediment. In this case, when scanning a specimen, in order to gain contrast, the condenser is lowered (or the iris diaphragm closed), thus reducing the numerical aperture. Some microscopes are equipped with a top condenser element, which is used in place for low-power work and swings out for high power. This changes the numerical aperture of the condenser, matching it with that of the objective.

The third and last unit of the illumination system to be discussed in this section is the *iris diaphragm*. The iris diaphragm also controls the amount of light passing through the material under observation. It is located at the bottom of the Abbe condenser, under the lenses but within the condenser body. This diaphragm consists of a series of horizontally arranged interlocking plates with a central aperture. It can be opened or closed as necessary to adjust the intensity of the light by means of a lever. The size of the aperture, and consequently the amount of light permitted to pass, is regulated by the microscopist. Such regulation of the light affects the numerical aperture of the condenser; decreasing the size of the field under observation with the iris diaphragm decreases the numerical aperture of the condenser. Thus, proper illumination techniques involve a combination of proper light intensity regulation, light source position, condenser position, and field size regulation.

The magnification system contains several important parts. This system, too, plays an extremely important role in the use of the microscope. The *ocular*, or *eyepiece*, is a lens that magnifies the image formed by the objective. The usual magnification of the ocular is 10 ($\times$10); however, $\times$5 and $\times$20 oculars are also generally available. Most modern microscopes have two oculars and are called *binocular* microscopes. Some microscopes have only one ocular, and these are called *monocular* microscopes. The magnification produced by the ocular, when multiplied by the magnification produced by the objective, gives the total magnification of the object being viewed.

The *objectives* are the major part of the magnification system. There are usually three objectives on each microscope, with magnifying powers of ×10, ×45, and ×100. The objectives are mounted on the *nosepiece*, which is a pivot that enables a quick change of objectives. Objectives are also described or rated according to *focal length*, which is inscribed on the outside of the objective. Microscopes used in the clinical laboratory most commonly have 16-, 4-, and 1.8-mm objectives. The focal length is the distance from the object being examined to the center of the lens. Practically speaking, the focal length of a lens is very close in value to the *working distance*—the distance from the bottom of the objective to the material being studied. The greater the magnifying power of a lens, the smaller the focal length and hence the working distance. This becomes very important when using the microscope, as the working distance is very short for the ×45 (4-mm) and ×100 (1.8-mm) objectives. For this reason, correct focusing habits are necessary to prevent damaging the objectives against the slide on the stage. We have now described the objectives in terms of their focal length and magnifying power. The actual magnifying power will vary with different lenses; however, the actual focal length and magnifying power are inscribed directly on the outside of the objective.

Other terms that are commonly used to describe microscope objectives are low-power, high-power (also "high-dry"), and oil-immersion. The low-power objective is the 16-mm (usually ×10 magnification) one. This objective is used for the initial scanning and observation in most microscopic work. For example, blood films and urinary sediment are routinely examined by using the low-power objective first. This is also the lens employed for the initial focusing and light adjustment of the microscope. Often the term *parfocal*

is used in speaking about a microscope. It means that if one objective is in focus and a switch is made to another objective, the focus will not be lost. Thus the microscope can be focused under low power and then switched to the high-power or oil-immersion objective and it will still be in focus except for fine adjustment. The numerical aperture of the low-power objective is significantly less than that of the condenser on most microscopes (for the ×10 objective the NA is approximately 0.25; for the condenser it is approximately 0.9). Therefore, to achieve focus, the numerical apertures must be more closely matched by reducing the light to the specimen; this is done by lowering the condenser or reducing the size of the field with the iris diaphragm, or both.

The high-power or high-dry objective is the 4-mm (usually ×45) lens. This objective is used for more detailed study, as the total magnification with a ×10 eyepiece is ×450 rather than the ×100 magnification of the low-power system. The high-power objective is used to study histological sections, and to study wet preparations such as urinary sediment in more detail. The working distance of the 4-mm lens is quite short; therefore, care must be taken in focusing. The numerical aperture of the high-power lens is fairly close to (although slightly less than) that of most commonly used condensers (for most high-power objectives NA = 0.85; for the condenser NA = 0.9). Therefore, the condenser should generally be all the way up and the field slightly closed for maximum focus.

The oil-immersion (generally ×100) lens is a 1.8-mm lens. This lens has a very short focal length and working distance. In fact, the objective lens almost rests on the microscope slide when in use. The ×100 objective is also called an oil-immersion lens, since a special grade of oil, called *immersion oil*, must be placed between the objective and the slide or cover glass. Oil is used to increase the numerical aperture and thus the resolving power of the objective. Since the focal length of this lens is so small, there is a problem in getting enough light from the microscope field to the objective. Light travels through air at a greater speed than through glass, and it travels through immersion oil at the same speed as through glass. Thus, to increase the effective numerical aperture of the objective, oil is used to slow down the speed at which light travels, increasing the gathering power of the lens.[*] Since the numerical aperture of the oil-immersion objective is greater than that of the condenser in most systems (for the 0.8-mm objective $NA = 1.2$; for the condenser $NA = 0.9$), the condenser should be used all the way up and the iris diaphragm should generally be open; practically speaking, however, partial closing of the iris may be necessary. The oil-immersion lens, with a total magnification of $\times 1000$, is generally the limit of magnification with the light microscope. The oil-immersion lens is routinely used for morphological examination of blood films and microbes. The short working distance requires dry films, so wet preparations such as urinary sediment cannot be examined under an oil-immersion lens. The high-power lens is also referred to as a high-dry lens because it does not require the use of immersion oil. Other objectives that might be present on a microscope in the clinical laboratory are a lower-power $\times 5$ scanning lens or a $\times 50$ low oil-immersion lens.

The *body tube* is the part of the microscope through which the light passes to the ocular. This is the tube that actually conducts the image. The adjustment system enables the body tube to move up or down for focusing the objectives. This system usually consists of two adjustments, one coarse and the other fine. The coarse adjustment gives rapid movement over a wide range and is used to obtain an approximate focus. The

fine adjustment gives very slow movement over a limited range and is used to obtain exact focus after prior coarse adjustment.

A more detailed description of the optics of a microscope can be found in standard physics textbooks.

Care and cleaning of the microscope

The microscope is a precision instrument and must be handled with great care. When it is necessary to transport the microscope, it should always be carried with both hands; it should be carried by the arm and supported under the base with the other hand. When not in use, the microscope should be covered and put away in a microscope case, or in a desk or cupboard. It should be left with the low-power ($\times 10$) objective in place, the body tube barrel adjusted to the lowest possible position, and the condenser down.

The surface of most microscopes is finished with a black or gray enamel and metal plating that is resistant to most laboratory chemicals. It may be kept clean by washing with a neutral soap and water. To clean the metal and enamel, a gauze or soft cloth should be moistened with the cleaning agent and rubbed over the surface with a circular motion. The surface should be dried immediately with a clean, dry piece of gauze or cloth. Gauze should *never* be used to clean any of the optical parts of the microscope.

The glass surfaces of the ocular, the objectives, and the condenser are hand-ground optical lenses. These lenses must be kept meticulously clean. Optical glass is softer than ordinary glass and should never be cleaned with paper tissue or gauze. These materials will scratch the lens. To clean the lenses of the microscope, use lens paper. Before polishing with lens paper, care must be taken that nothing is present that will scratch the optical glass in the polishing process. Such potentially abrasive dirt, dust, or lint can easily be blown away before polishing. Cans of

---

[*]The speed at which light travels through a substance is measured in terms of the *refractive index*. The refractive index is calculated as the speed at which light travels through air divided by the speed at which it travels through the substance. The refractive index of air is therefore 1.00. The refractive index of glass is 1.515; immersion oil, 1.515 and water, 1.33.

compressed air are commercially available, or an air syringe can be made simply by fitting a 1-ml plastic tuberculin syringe with the tip cut off into a rubber bulb of the type used for pipetting (Fig. 1-7). Use this air syringe to blow away dust or lint that might otherwise scratch the optical glass in the polishing process.

Oil must be removed from the oil-immersion (X100) objective immediately after use by wiping with clean lens paper. If not removed, oil may seep inside the lens, or dry on the outside surface of the objective. The high-dry (X45) objective should never be used with oil; however, if this or any other objective comes into contact with oil it should be cleaned immediately. If a lens is especially dirty, it may be cleaned with a small amount of xylene or commercial lens cleaner applied to the lens paper. Xylene should be used sparingly, because it can damage the lens mounting if it is allowed to get beyond the front seal. Commercial lens cleaner has the advantage of being less harmful to the mounting medium.

Fig. 1-7. Air syringe.

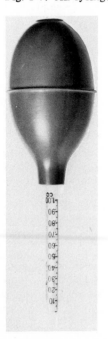

To properly clean the oil-immersion lens, lens cleaner or a small amount of xylene should be used on the lens paper. When lens cleaner or xylene is used, the lens should be dried and polished with a clean piece of lens paper. Lenses should never be touched with the fingers. Objectives must not be taken apart as even a slight alteration of the lens setting may ruin the objective. Merely clean the outer surface of the lens as described. An especially dirty objective may be removed (unscrewed) from the nosepiece, then held upside down and checked for cleanliness by using the ocular (removed from the body tube) as a magnifying glass. Dust or lint can also be removed from the rear lens of the objective by blowing it away with an air syringe. Such removal of the objective from the nosepiece is *not* a routine cleaning procedure. The final step when using the microscope should always be to wipe off all objectives with clean lens paper.

The ocular or eyepiece is especially vulnerable to dirt because of its location on the microscope and contact with the observer's eye. Mascara presents a constant cleaning problem. Dust can be removed from the lens of the ocular with an air syringe (or camel's hair brush). Air is probably easier to use and more efficient. The lens should then be polished with lens paper. At regular intervals the ocular can be taken apart and cleaned on the inside, by first blowing away dust and lint and then polishing. The ocular can be checked for additional dirt by holding it up to a light and looking through it. When one is looking into the microscope, dirt on any part of the ocular will rotate with the ocular when it is turned. The ocular should not be removed for more than a few minutes as dust can collect in the body tube and settle on the rear lens of an objective.

The light source (or mirror) and condenser should also be free of dust, lint, and dirt. First blow away the dust with an air syringe or camel's hair brush, then polish the light source and condenser with lens paper. It may be necessary to clean them further with lens paper moistened with a commercial lens cleaner or mild detergent solution before polishing them with lens paper.

The stage of the microscope should be cleaned after each use by wiping with gauze or a tissue. It may be necessary to remove oil from the stage by wiping with a piece of gauze moistened with a little xylene. After it has been cleaned thoroughly, the stage should be wiped dry.

The coarse and fine adjustments occasionally need attention, as does the mechanical stage adjustment mechanism. When there is unusual resistance to any manipulation of these knobs, force must not be used to overcome the resistance. Such force might damage the screw or rack-and-pinion mechanism. Instead, the cause of the problem must be found. A small drop of oil may be needed. It is best to call in a specialist to repair the microscope when a serious problem occurs.

Use of the microscope

When using a microscope, two conditions must first be met: (1) the microscope must be clean, and (2) it must be aligned. The cleaning procedure was described above; alignment is discussed here. When properly aligned, the microscope is adjusted in such a way that the light path through the microscope, from the light source to the eye of the observer, is correct according to the rules of physics. If a microscope is misaligned, the field of view will seem to swing—a very uncomfortable situation, often described as making the observer feel seasick. This can be corrected by properly aligning or adjusting the light path through the microscope. To check the alignment, with the low-power objective in place and the condenser up, remove the eyepiece and look down the body tube. Now close the iris field diaphragm enough to see a constricted (or partially closed) field. Center this field in the body tube by adjusting the centering screws on the condenser. (This alignment opera-

tion may be omitted by the new student; the alignment can be adjusted by the instructor or supervisor.) Looking down the microscope body tube with the eyepiece removed, one can also check for the presence of dust, lint, or dirt, which would be readily observed at this point. Besides centering the condenser, one must center the light source to give the correct light path. In microscopes that have a built-in illumination system, the light bulb filament will be correctly centered if the correct bulb is used and is installed properly. For microscopes with an external light source and mirror, use the concave side of the mirror and adjust the mirror angle and light position by centering the light while looking through the body tube with the ocular removed.

The biggest concern in learning how to use a microscope for the first time is the lighting and fine-adjustment maneuvers. One must be certain that the light source, condenser, and iris diaphragm are in correct adjustment. Light adjustment is made before any focusing is done. The light adjustment is accomplished by raising and lowering the condenser and opening and closing the diaphragm. At the start of this initial light adjustment, the condenser should be all the way up and the diaphragm all the way open, with the low-power ($\times 10$) objective in place. While looking through the ocular, the diaphragm can be closed until the field is just beginning to be closed off. Next, the condenser should be lowered until the light is even.

The object to be examined is placed on the stage and secured. Usually it is placed on a glass microscope slide. Care must be taken to avoid damaging the objectives while placing specimens on the stage. To prevent this, the barrel, or tube, of the microscope should be raised by means of the coarse-adjustment knob.

Focusing is the next technique to be mastered. With the object on the stage, and while watching from the side, the low-power ($\times 10$) objective is brought down as far as it will go, so that it almost meets the top of the specimen. The coarse adjustment is used for this procedure. The objective must not be in direct contact with the specimen. The observer must watch from the side to avoid damaging the objective. Once the objective is just at the top of the specimen, the object is slowly focused upward, using the coarse-adjustment knob and looking through the ocular while this is being done. When the object is nearly in focus, it is brought into clear focus by use of the fine-adjustment knob. Further light adjustment should now be made to ensure that the numerical aperture of the condenser corresponds to the numerical aperture of the objective, giving maximum focus and resolution. To correctly position the condenser, place the tip of a pencil on top of the light source, then move the condenser up and down until the pencil is focused in the same plane as the specimen. Next, adjust the iris diaphragm until the field is just filled with light, remove the ocular, and readjust the iris diaphragm until light from the condenser just fills the field.[10] When changing to another objective, the barrel distance need not be changed. As stated previously, most microscopes are parfocal. The only adjustment necessary should be made with the fine-adjustment knob. Fine adjustment is used continuously during microscopic examination.

If greater magnification is needed, more light is necessary. It is obtained by repositioning the condenser and iris diaphragm in the manner previously described. In general, the condenser will be raised and the iris diaphragm opened as the objective magnification increases. Additional light is provided by the use of immersion oil placed on the viewing slide when the oil-immersion lens ($\times 100$ objective) is used. The oil directs the light rays to a finer point. When the oil-immersion lens is to be used, the desired area on the slide is first found by using the $\times 10$ (low-power) objective. Once this area is located, the objective is pivoted out of position, a drop of immersion oil is placed on the slide, and the oil-immersion lens is pivoted into the oil while observing it from the side. The ocular should not

be looked through during this adjustment procedure. When the initial adjustment has been made, the fine adjustment is made while looking through the ocular. The oil remaining on the lens of the objective after the study has been completed must be cleaned off with lens paper as described above.

Types of microscopes

Until recently, bright-field illumination has, with few exceptions, been the primary type of microscope illumination system used in the routine clinical laboratory. Now other illumination systems are becoming increasingly popular as refinements in microscope design have made them more reliable and easier to use in a clinical situation. These other types of illumination systems—dark-field, transmitted light fluorescence, polarizing, phase-contrast, and Nomarski differential interference contrast—will now be briefly described. The basic principles of microscopy and rules for usage apply with all of these variations; the primary difference is the character of light delivered to the specimen and illuminating the microscope.

First we will consider *dark-field* illumination. In this system, a special substage condenser is used that causes light waves to cross *on* the specimen rather than pass in parallel waves through the specimen. Thus, when one looks through the microscope, the field in view will be black, or dark, as no light passes from the condenser to the objective. However, when an object is present on the stage, light will be deflected as it hits the object and will pass through the objective and be seen by the viewer. As a result, the object under study appears light against a dark background. Any compound microscope may be converted to a dark-field microscope by use of a special dark-field condenser in place of the usual condenser. The dark-field microscope has long been used in the routine clinical laboratory to observe spirochetes in the exudates from leptospiral or syphilitic infections. A more recent use, facilitated by newer microscope design technology, is as a low-power scanner for urinary sediment.

The transmitted light *fluorescence* microscope is a further refinement of the dark-field microscope. It is basically a dark-field microscope with wavelength selection. Certain objects have the ability to fluoresce. This means that they absorb light of certain very short (ultraviolet) wavelengths and emit light of longer (visible) wavelengths. In fluorescence microscopy with transmitted light and a compound microscope, the dark-field condenser is preceded by a special *exciter filter*, which allows only shorter-wavelength blue light to pass and cross on the specimen plane. If the specimen contains an object that fluoresces (either naturally or because of staining or labeling with certain fluorescent dyes) it will absorb the blue light and emit light of a longer yellow or green wavelength. A special barrier filter is placed in the microscope tube or eyepiece. This barrier filter will pass only the desired wavelength of emitted light for the particular fluorescent system. Thus, the fluorescence technique shows only the presence or absence of the fluorescing object. The barrier filter used must be carefully chosen so that only light of the desired wavelength will be passed through the microscope to the observer. Other objects in the specimen that do not fluoresce will not emit light of that wavelength and will not be seen. Fluorescence techniques, in particular fluorescent antibody (FA) techniques, are becoming increasingly useful in the clinical laboratory. They are used particularly in the clinical microbiology laboratory and for various immunologic studies. Different fluorescent antibody techniques may be used in the primary identification of microorganisms, or in the final identification of bacteria (such as group A streptococci), replacing older serological methods. Such techniques have the advantage of saving time, which results in earlier diagnosis for the patient, and they are often more sensitive than other techniques. They

may also be useful in the identification of organisms that cannot be cultured, such as *Treponema pallidum.*

Another increasingly popular illumination system is represented by the *polarizing* microscope. A polarizer (or polarizing filter) may be thought of as a sieve that takes ordinary light waves, which vibrate in all orientations (or directions), and allows only light waves of one orientation (say north-south or east-west) to pass through the filter. In a polarizing microscope, a polarizing filter is placed between the light source (bulb) and the specimen. A second *analyzer* (or polarizer) is placed between the objective and the eyepiece (either at some point in the microscope tube or in the eyepiece). One of the polarizers is then rotated until the two are at right angles to each other. This will be seen as the extinction of light through the microscope (one sees a dark field) since both north-south and east-west light waves are cancelled when they are at right angles to each other. However, certain objects have a property termed *birefringence*, which means that they rotate (or polarize) light. An object that polarizes bends light, and can be seen in such a system. Objects that do not bend light will not be observed in the microscope. An object that polarizes light (or is birefringent) will appear light against a dark background. The polarizing microscope is useful clinically in the study of synovial fluid and urinary sediment, and in some histological work. This technique is commonly used in geology for particle analysis, and clinically in forensic medicine. With the polarizing microscope the optical properties of an object can be determined.

A further modification of the polarizing microscope involves the addition of a first-order red plate (filter) or full-wave retardation plate placed between the two polarizing filters. With this addition the field background appears red or magenta, while the object that polarizes appears yellow or blue in relation to its orientation to the red filter and its optical properties. This is especially useful clinically for differentiating between sodium acid urate and calcium pyro-phosphate in synovial fluid. It is also becoming useful in the routine study of urinary sediment.

Another extremely useful illumination technique is *phase-contrast* microscopy. A disadvantage of bright-field illumination is that it is necessary to stain (or dye) many objects to give sufficient contrast and detail. Phase contrast facilitates the study of unstained structures, which can even be alive, since wet preparations of cells or organisms can be observed without prior dehydration and staining. As the name of the technique implies, the structures observed with this system show added contrast compared with the bright-field microscope. The phase-contrast microscope is basically a bright-field microscope with changes between the objective and the condenser. First, an annular diaphragm, which is a black ring with a black center, is put into or below the condenser. This results in a hollow cone or "doughnut" of light passing through the specimen. Next, an absorption ring is fitted into the objective. The annulus and absorption ring must be perfectly aligned or adjusted so that they are concentric and superimposed. Therefore a problem with the phase-contrast microscope is the necessity for perfect alignment. The net effect is to slow down the speed of light by one-fourth of a wavelength. This diminution of the speed of light makes the system very sensitive to differences in refractive index.

Objects with differences in refractive index, shape, and absorption characteristics show added differences in the intensity and shade of light passing through them. The end result is that one can observe unstained preparations with good resolution and detail. In the clinical laboratory, phase contrast is especially useful for counting platelets by using a direct method, and for observing structures in urinary sediment and vaginal smears.

The last illumination technique gaining in clinical use is *Nomarski differential interference contrast* illumination. This technique gives the viewer a three-dimensional image of the object under study. Like phase contrast, it is especially useful for wet preparations such as urinary sediment, showing finer details without the need for special staining techniques. The bright-field microscope is modified by the addition of a special beam-splitting (Wollaston) prism to the condenser. The two split beams are then polarized, one passes through the specimen, which alters the amplitude (or height) of the light wave, and the other (which serves as a reference) does not pass through the specimen. The two dissimilar light beams then pass separately through the objective and are recombined by a second Wollaston (beam-combining) prism. This recombination of light waves gives the three-dimensional image to the additive or subtractive effects of the light waves as they are combined.

USE OF THE CENTRIFUGE

Centrifugation is used in the separation of a solid material from a liquid. It is also used in recovering solid materials from suspensions, as in the microscopic examination of urine. The solid material or sediment packed at the bottom of the centrifuge tube is sometimes called the precipitate, and the liquid or top portion is called the supernatant. Another important use for the centrifuge is in the separation of serum or plasma

from cells in blood specimens. The suspended particles, solid material, or blood cells usually collect at the bottom of the centrifuge tube because the particles are heavier than the liquid. Occasionally the particles are lighter than the liquid and will collect on the surface of the liquid when centrifuged. Centrifugation is employed in every department of the clinical laboratory, in chemistry, urinalysis, hematology, and blood banking, among others. Proper use of the centrifuge is important for anyone engaged in laboratory work.

Centrifuges facilitate the separation of particles in suspension by the application of centrifugal force. Several types of centrifuges will usually be found in the same laboratory, each designed for special uses. There are table-model and floor-model centrifuges, some small and others very large; there are even refrigerated centrifuges for special procedures.

Directions for use of a centrifuge are most frequently given in terms of speed, or revolutions per minute (r/min). A rheostat is used to set the desired speed; the setting on the rheostat dial does not necessarily correspond directly to revolutions per minute. The setting speeds on the rheostat can also change with variations in weight load and general aging of the centrifuge.

The top speed of most conventional centrifuges is about 3000 r/min. The microhematocrit centrifuge used in many hematology laboratories for packing red blood cells attains a speed of about 10 000 r/min.

Two types of centrifuges are used in doing routine laboratory determinations. One is a conventional horizontal centrifuge and the other is an angle head centrifuge. For the horizontal-type centrifuge, the cups holding the tubes of material to be centrifuged occupy a vertical position when the centrifuge is at rest, but assume a horizontal position when the centrifuge revolves. For the angle head centrifuge, the cups are held in a rigid position at a fixed angle. This position makes the process of centrifuging more rapid than it is with the horizontal centrifuge. There is also less chance that the sediment will be disturbed when the centrifuge stops. Both types of centrifuges may be purchased as table or floor models.

The most important rule to remember in using any centrifuge is: *always balance the tubes placed in the centrifuge.* That is, in the centrifuge cup opposite the material to be centrifuged, place a container of equivalent size and shape with an equal volume of liquid of the same specific gravity as the load. For most laboratory determinations, water may be placed in the balance load.

Special centrifuge tubes should be used. These are tubes constructed to withstand the force exerted by the centrifuge. They have thicker glass walls or are made of a stronger, more resistant glass. Some of these tubes are conical, and some have round bottoms. Some are disposable and others must be washed.

Before placing the centrifuge tubes in the cups or holders, check the cups to make certain that the rubber cushions are in place. If some cushions are missing, the centrifuge will not be properly balanced. Without the cushions, the tubes are more likely to break.

Whenever a tube breaks in the centrifuge cup, it is most important that both the cup and the rubber cushion in the cup be cleaned well to prevent further breakage by glass particles left behind.

Covers specially made for the centrifuge should be used except in certain specified instances. Using the cover prevents possible danger from flying glass should tubes break in the centrifuge. Keep the centrifuge cover closed at all times, even when not using the machine. In addition to the danger from broken glass, using the centrifuge without the cover in place may cause the revolving parts of the centrifuge to vibrate, which causes excessive wear of the machine.

Do not try to stop the centrifuge with your hands. It is generally best to let the machine stop by itself. A brake may be applied if the centrifuge is equipped with one. The brake should be used with caution, as braking may cause some resuspension of the sediment. Many laboratories discourage use of the brake except where it is evident that a tube or tubes have broken in the centrifuge.

Centrifuges should be checked, cleaned, and lubricated regularly to ensure proper operation.

WEIGHING AND THE USE OF BALANCES

Many and varied pieces of laboratory apparatus are used in performing clinical determinations, and the knowledge of the proper use and handling of this equipment is an important part of any course of study dealing with laboratory work. Probably some of the most important instruments are the various types of balances used to measure weight or mass (gravimetric analysis) in preparing the reagents and standard solutions used in the laboratory. This is a method of quantitative analysis in the laboratory. Almost every procedure performed in the laboratory depends to some extent on the use of a balance. The balance considered to be the "backbone" of the clinical chemistry laboratory is the analytical balance. This balance and other types—namely the triple-beam, Cent-O-Gram, and torsion balances—will be discussed in this section. A single laboratory is likely to have all of these types, and for this reason a student in a laboratory course should understand how the various balances work. Every laboratory should have some type of analytical balance and at least one other less sensitive type of balance. These are the minimum requirements for weighing instruments.

Balances are used to weigh the chemicals used to prepare the many chemical solutions needed in the laboratory. Some solutions require more accurately weighed chemicals than others. The accuracy needed depends on what the solution is to be used for. One must decide what type of balance (or scale) is most appropriate for the precision or reproducibility required in weighing the chemicals to be used for a particular solution. The different kinds of balances are suited to particular needs. A balance that sacrifices precision for speed should not be used when precision is needed.

Analytical balance

Many different types of analytical balances are made by different companies and they have

Fig. 1-8. Manual analytical balance.

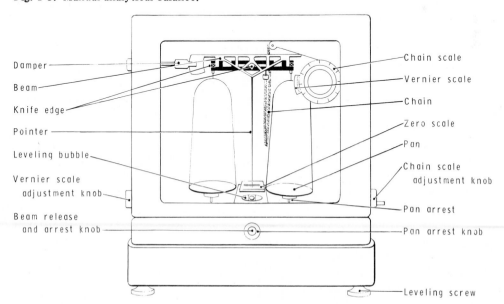

Damper

Beam

Knife edge

Pointer

Leveling bubble

Vernier scale
adjustment knob

Beam release
and arrest knob

Chain scale

Vernier scale

Chain

Zero scale

Pan

Chain scale
adjustment knob

Pan arrest

Pan arrest knob

Leveling screw

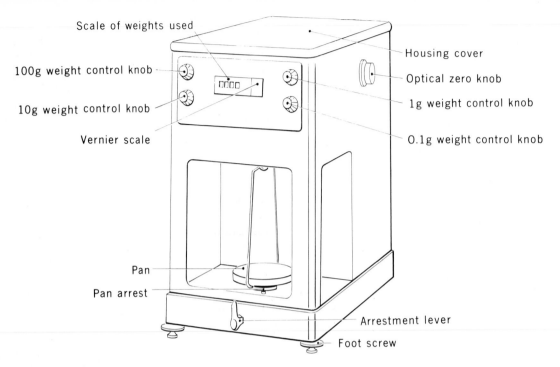

Fig. 1-9. Automatic analytical balance.

various degrees of automatic operation. In this discussion analytical balances are divided into two types: manually operated analytical (Fig. 1-8) and automatic analytical (Fig. 1-9) balances. Each company that manufactures analytical balances has its own special name for each of the various automatic analytical balances produced. All analytical balances are used to weigh very small amounts of substances with a high degree of accuracy, but just how this is accomplished differs slightly from one balance to another. Some require little or no manual operation, and some are more time-consuming and require much more manipulation on the part of the operator. Some of the fine analytical balances manufactured for use in the clinical laboratory are the Ainsworth, Voland, Gram-atic, Christian-Becker, Mettler, and Sartorius balances. Others are also available. It is important to investigate carefully several different analytical balances before deciding on one for use in a particular laboratory.

As stated previously, almost every procedure performed in the laboratory depends on the use of balances, the most important one being the analytical balance. Before any procedure is started, reagents must be prepared and standard solutions made. Standard solutions are always very accurately prepared, and the analytical balance is used to weigh the chemicals for these solutions. The analytical balance might be called the starting point of each method used in the laboratory. Its accuracy determines the accuracy of many clinical determinations. An instrument that is so sensitive and so essential must be made with great skill and treated very carefully by those using it.

The analytical balance should be cleaned and adjusted at least once a year to ensure its continued accuracy and sensitivity. Its accuracy is what makes this instrument so essential in the clinical laboratory. The accuracy to which most analytical balances used in the clinical laboratory should weigh chemicals is commonly 0.1 mg, or 0.0001 g. Whenever this accuracy is needed, the analytical balance must be used. Differences between automatic and manual analytical balances lie mainly in the manner in which the weights are added in the weighing procedure. In the manual balance the weights are actually placed on one of the balance pans by hand. In the automatic balance the weights are added by manipulating a series of dials.

It is essential that the parts of the analytical balance be thoroughly understood, so that the weighing process can be carried out to the degree of accuracy necessary. Once the correct use of an analytical balance has been mastered, one should be able to use any of the available types, as they all have the same basic parts. Each manufacturer supplies a complete manual of operating directions, as well as information on the general use and care of the balance, with each balance purchased. These directions should be followed closely.

Basic parts

1. *Glass enclosure.* The analytical balance is enclosed in glass to prevent currents of air and collection of dust from disturbing the process of weighing.

2. *Balancing screws.* Before doing any weighing on the balance, it must be properly leveled. This is done by observing the leveling bubbles, or spirit level, located near the bottom of the balance. If necessary, adjust the balancing screws located on the bottom of the balance case (usually found on each leg of the balance).

3. *Beam.* This is the structure from which the pans are suspended.

4. *Knife edges.* These support the beam at the fulcrum during weighing and give sensitivity to the balance. Knife edges are vital parts and are constructed of hard metals to give a minimum amount of friction.

5. *Pans for weighing.* In the manually operated analytical balance, there are two pans: the weights are placed on the right-hand pan and the object to be weighed is placed on the left-hand pan. In the automatic analytical balance, there is only one pan. The object to be weighed is placed on this pan. The pans are suspended from the ends of the beam.

6. *Weights.* In the manual balance, the weights are found in a separate weight box. These weights are never handled with the fingers but are removed from the box and placed on the balance pan by using ivory-tipped forceps. Mishandling of weights, either by using the fingers or by dropping, can result in an alteration of the actual and true mass of the weight. Weights come in units ranging from a 50-g to a 100-mg weight. The values of the weights are stamped directly on top of them. In the automatic analytical balance, the weights are inside the instrument and are not seen by the operator unless there is need to remove the casing for repair or adjustment. The weights are added by manipulating specific dials calibrated for the weighing process. The built-in weights are on the same end of the beam as the sample pan and are counterbalanced by a fixed weight at the opposite end; they are removed from above the pan when an object is weighed. There is always a constant load on the beam, and the projected scale has the same weight regardless of the load. The total weight of an object is registered automatically by a digital counter or in conjunction with an optical scale.

7. *Pan arrest.* This is a means of arresting the pan so that sudden movement or addition of weights or chemical will not injure the delicate knife edges. The pan arrests (usually found under the pans) can absorb any shock due to weight inequalities, so that the knife edges are not subjected to this shock. The pan must be released to swing freely during actual weighing. In the automatic analytical balance the arresting mechanism for both the pan and the beam is operated by a single lever. Partial release or full release can be obtained, depending on how the lever is moved.

8. *Damping device.* This is necessary to arrest

the swing of the beam in the shortest practical time, thus cutting down the time consumed in the weighing process.

9. *Vernier scale.* This is the small scale used to obtain precise readings to the nearest 0.1 mg. It is used in conjunction with the large reading scale to obtain the necessary readings.

10. *Reading scale.* In the manual analytical balance, this scale is actually the reading scale for the chain that is used for weighing 100 mg or less. It is used in conjunction with the vernier scale to obtain readings to the nearest 0.1 mg. In the automatic analytical balance, this is usually a lighted optical scale, giving a high magnification and sharp definition for easier reading. The total weight of the object in question is registered automatically on this viewing scale.

General rules for use of the analytical balance

Weighing errors will occur if the balance is not properly positioned. It is therefore very important that the balance be located and mounted in an optimal position. The balance must be level. This is usually accomplished by adjusting the movable screws on the legs of the balance. The firmness of support is also important. The bench or table on which the balance rests must be rigid and free from vibrations. Preferably the room in which the balance is set up should have constant temperature and humidity. Ideally, the analytical balance should be in an air-conditioned room. The temperature factor is most important. The balance should not be placed near hot objects such as radiators, flames, stills, or electric ovens. Likewise, it should not be placed near cold objects, especially not near an open window. Sunlight or illumination from high-power lamps should be avoided in choosing a good location for the analytical balance.

The analytical balance is a delicate precision instrument, which will not function properly if abused. When learning to use an analytical balance, students should make themselves responsible for knowing and adhering to the rules for the use of the particular balance with which they are provided. The following general rules apply:

1. Set up the balance where it will be free from vibration.
2. Load and unload the balance only when the pans are arrested; if the pans are not arrested, the delicate knife edges can be damaged.
3. Close the balance case before observing the reading; any air currents present would affect the weighing process.
4. Never weigh any chemical directly on the pan; a container of some type must be used for the chemical.
5. Never place a hot object on the balance pan. If an object is warm, the weight determined will be too light because of convection currents set up by the rising heated air.
6. Whenever the shape of the object to be weighed permits, handle it with tongs or forceps. Round objects such as weighing bottles may be handled with the fingers, but take care to prevent weight changes caused by moisture from the hand. Do not hold any object longer than necessary.
7. On completion of weighing, remove all objects and clean up any chemical spilled on the pans or within the balance area. Close the balance case.
8. Weighed materials should be transferred to labeled containers or made into solutions immediately.

Speed in weighing is obtained only through practice.

Procedure for weighing with a manual analytical balance

1. Sitting directly in front of the center of the balance, dust off the pans and the inside of the balance with a soft brush.

2. Check to see that the balance is level by observing the leveling bubbles. Make any necessary adjustment by means of the leveling screws on the legs of the balance.

3. To adjust the balance to a beginning reading of zero, lower the beam and release the pan arrests, making certain that the chain reading scale and the vernier scale are both set at zero. Note where the pointer comes to rest, and slowly move the chain until the pointer rests exactly at zero. Arrest the pans and raise and lock the beam. Recheck by repeating these same steps once again. The pointer should still rest exactly at zero. By use of the vernier scale adjustment knob, adjust the zero of the vernier scale to match the zero of the chain reading scale.

4. With the beam raised and locked and the pans arrested, place the weighing vessel on the left-hand pan, using tongs if possible.

5. From the box of weights provided with the balance, transfer the first weight to the right-hand pan, using the special forceps. Choose a rather large weight as the first weight: 20-g weight would be satisfactory for most purposes. Lower the beam and release the pan arrests. Note where the pointer swings in relation to the zero point. If the pointer swings to the left, the weight is heavier than the vessel. If the pointer swings to the right, the weight is lighter than the vessel. Arrest the pans, and raise and lock the beam.

6. Depending on the direction of the pointer's swing in the previous step, either add another weight from the box of weights, or remove the 20-g weight and replace it with a lighter one (10 g). Repeat this process by adding and removing weights (being certain to raise and lock the beam and arrest the pans before each change of weights) until the addition of the smallest weight in the box (100 mg) causes the pointer to swing to the left. Close the balance window.

7. At this point add weight from the chain. The chain has a total weight of 100 mg and is used when no further weights from the box can be used. With the beam locked and the pans arrested, add 50 mg from the chain by moving the chain scale adjustment knob. Lower the beam and release the pans. Observe the pointer. Again, if the pointer swings to the left the chain

weight is too light, and more weight must be added. Raise the beam and arrest the pans. Depending on the swing of the pointer, either add weight by moving the chain by 20-mg steps until the addition of 20 mg causes the pointer to swing to the left, or remove weight by 20-mg steps until the pointer swings to the right. When the chain weight has been narrowed down to within 10 mg of true balance, leave the beam lowered and the pans released, and gradually add or remove weight until balance is obtained. The weighing vessel has now been weighed, and the actual weighing of the desired chemical can commence. Record the weights used to obtain balance with the weighing vessel. To obtain the reading to the nearest 0.1 mg, the vernier scale (Fig. 1-10) must be used in conjunction with the chain scale. Raise the beam and arrest the pans.

8. To the weight of the weighing vessel add the amount of chemical to be weighed. For example, if the weighing vessel weighs 35.5646 g and the amount of chemical to be weighed is 10.5555 g, the total weight is 46.1201 g. This total weight should be on the right-hand pan. To

Fig. 1-10. Reading obtained with a vernier scale.

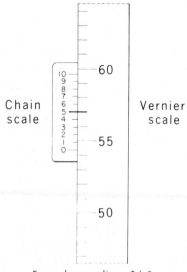

Example reading 54.5 mg

accomplish this, add the necessary weights from the box of weights and the chain scale to make up the difference.

9. Add the chemical in small amounts, using a clean spatula until balance is achieved. Before each addition of chemical raise the beam and arrest the pans. When balance is obtained, the amount of chemical has been weighed in the weighing vessel. Then transfer it quantitatively to a flask for dilution (see under Quantitative Transfer).

10. Return all weights to the box, return the chain to zero, and clean up any spilled chemical from the balance area. Leave the beam in a raised and locked position, and arrest the pans.

Procedure for weighing with an automatic analytical balance

1. Before doing any weighing, make certain that the balance is properly leveled. Observe the spirit level (leveling bubble), and adjust the leveling screws on the legs of the balance if necessary.

2. To check the zero point adjustment, fully release the balance and turn the adjustment knob clockwise as far as it will go. The optical scale zero should indicate three divisions below zero on the vernier scale. Using the same adjustment knob, adjust the optical scale zero so that it aligns exactly with the zero line on the vernier scale. Arrest the balance.

3. With the balance arrested, place the weighing vessel on the pan, using tongs if possible, so that no humidity or heat is brought into the weighing chamber by the hands. Close the balance window.

4. Weigh the vessel in the following manner: partially release the balance and turn the 100-g weight control knob clockwise. When the scale moves up, turn the knob back one step. Repeat this operation with the 10-g, 1-g, and 0.1-g knobs, in that order. Arrest the balance. After a short pause, release the balance, and allow the scale to come to rest. Read the result and arrest

the balance. With the balance arrested, unload the pan and bring all knobs back to zero.

5. Add the weight of the sample desired to the weight of the vessel just weighed to get the total to be weighed. Set the knobs (100, 10, 1, and 0.1 g) to the correct total weight needed. When the 0.1-g knob has been set at its proper reading, the balance should be placed in partial release. Slowly add the chemical to the vessel until the optical scale begins to move downward. When the optical scale starts downward, fully release the beam, and continue to add the chemical until the optical scale registers the exact position desired. To obtain the reading to the nearest 0.1 mg (the sensitivity of most analytical balances), the vernier scale must be used in much the same manner as in the manual analytical balance readings.

6. With the balance arrested, unload the pan, and bring all the knobs back to zero. Clean up any spilled chemical in the balance area.

Torsion balance

These balances are used mainly for weighing chemicals in the laboratory. They are sensitive, responsive instruments with an exceptionally long service life, during which there is no significant deterioration in performance. In normal use, they require very little maintenance. The unique attributes of the torsion balance movement, which is assembled as a single flexible structure by means of highly tensed torsion bands of watch-spring alloy, eliminate the use of knife edges, bearings, and other loose parts that would become dull, misaligned, and soiled. Having no knife edges to dull or other loose parts to be adjusted accounts for the popularity of the torsion balance. Little or no adjustment is required, and this is important in a laboratory, where the time element is so important.

The torsion balance has high sensitivity under a heavy load, permits fast weighing, and is relatively inexpensive. Care must be taken to avoid overloading these balances. Some models have a dial-controlled torque spring to eliminate the use of smaller loose weights. Other models are offered with dial-controlled built-in weights, which may further reduce the number of loose weights required. Many weighing determinations can be completed in about one-fifth the time formerly required. A sliding tare weight is provided to counterbalance the weighing vessel used. The beam is operated by a lever on the balance case. Some torsion balances are enclosed completely in glass or metal cases. Several of these balances have a damping feature, which brings the balance to equilibrium quickly. One such damping device is an oil dashpot, which is filled at the factory with silicon oil. Weighing can be done more rapidly on torsion balances with damping devices than on those lacking them.

There is usually a means by which the torsion balance can be arrested. This need only be done when the balance is to be moved to a new location or otherwise transported.

The sensitivity of the torsion balance varies with the model chosen. For most clinical laboratories, however, balances with a sensitivity of readings to the nearest 0.01 g are satisfactory. The manufacturer supplies a complete manual with directions for setting up, proper use, and care of the particular torsion balance. These directions should be followed closely.

Procedure

1. Check to be sure that the balance is level, and adjust the leveling screws if necessary.

2. Check the zero adjustment. The optical reading scale should read zero with the pan empty and clean; adjust the optical zero with the small control knob if necessary.

3. Place the weighing vessel on the pan. Turn the weight control knob until the optical reading scale reads zero.

4. Add the chemical to the vessel until the desired weight registers on the optical scale. A vernier scale is present on most models so that the weight may be read to the accuracy needed. Torsion balances used in clinical laboratories have an accuracy of either 0.1 or 0.01 g.

5. Remove the vessel with the weighed chemical from the pan. Turn the control knob to zero, and wipe up any spilled chemical immediately.

Triple-beam balance

Another common piece of laboratory apparatus used for weighing is the triple-beam or "trip" balance (Fig. 1-11). This is a less sensitive balance with accuracy to the nearest 0.1 g. Whenever reagents are to be prepared with an accuracy

Fig. 1-11. Triple-beam balance.

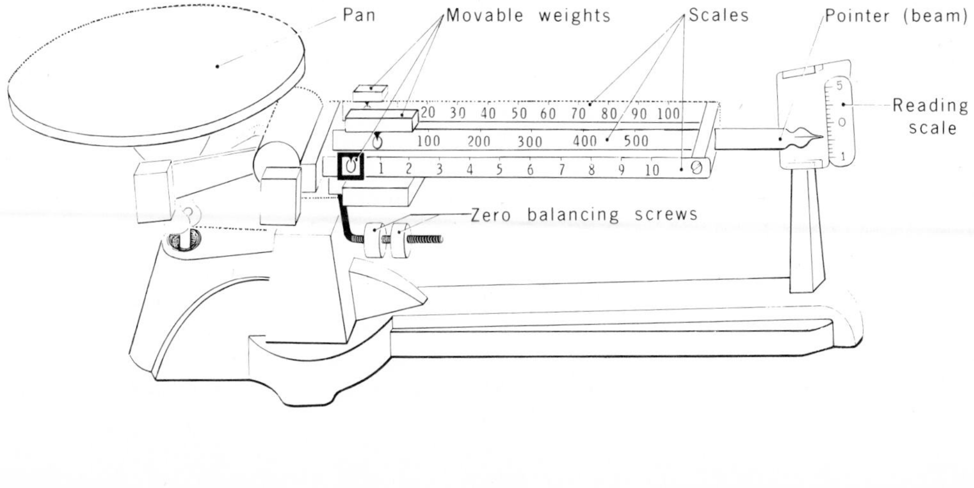

of 0.1 g or less, the triple-beam balance can be used most satisfactorily. As the words triple-beam and trip suggest, three beams are present on the balance. Each beam provides a different weighing scale. Scales reading from 0 to 100 g, 0 to 500 g, and 0 to 10 g are usually provided on the triple-beam balance. These scales are provided with movable weights. The two larger scales have weights that lock into accurately milled notches at each calibration to ensure absolute accuracy at each position.

Some models of the triple-beam balance (called the *Harvard triple-beam* balance) have two pans, and some have a single pan. The principle of the weighing process is the same whether there are two pans or only one. Two-pan balances are used when two objects must be balanced against each other, as in balancing tubes for use in the centrifuge. One-pan balances are used a great deal in the laboratory for preparing reagents and chemical solutions.

Some type of less sensitive balance such as the triple-beam or torsion balance is an essential piece of equipment for every clinical laboratory, as many reagents are prepared that do not need the accuracy of the analytical balance. When an accuracy of more than 0.1 g is not needed, the triple-beam balance can be used. It can be operated simply and rapidly and gives accurate weighings when used properly. Even a balance with less sensitivity must be used carefully and according to the directions provided with the particular model.

The triple-beam balance should be placed on a reasonably flat and level surface. The beam should be near zero balance, with all the movable weights at their zero points. A final zero balance is attained by adjusting the balancing screws. It is advisable to check the zero balance periodically, especially if the balance has been moved. If an object is to be weighed, the balance must be set at zero before the weighing is begun. If a vessel is weighed in preparation for the addition of a chemical, it is not necessary to set the balance at the exact zero reading.

Basic parts

1. *Pan.* This is where the object or weighing vessel holding the substance to be weighed is placed.

2. *Beam.* The beam is a lever supported by a knife plane bearing at the center post. The length of beam to the right of the knife plane is graduated for placement of a sliding weight and ends in a pointer. The other end of the beam is attached to the pan guide with a knife edge contact.

3. *Movable weights or poises.* These are sliding weights attached to the beam that are moved to bring the balance into equilibrium. The trip balance has three beams, and various weight increments are added as the poises are advanced toward the pointer ends of the beams.

4. *Reading scale.* This is a scale located at the end of the beam pointer that shows when the balance is in equilibrium.

5. *Balancing screws or spindle.* This is a pair of threaded weights that are used to bring the empty balance into equilibrium.

Procedure for general use

1. Place the weighing vessel on the balance pan without previously bringing the balance to zero.

2. With the weighing vessel on the pan, bring the balance to zero by adjusting the movable weights on the three scales. Record the sum of the weights required for balance.

3. To the recorded weight add the amount of chemical to be weighed. For example, if the reagent to be prepared requires 10.5 g of NaCl and the weighing vessel weighs 35.5 g, the total weight is 46.0 g. Move the movable weights on the scales to give this total weight.

4. Gradually add the chemical until the pointer of the balance rests exactly at the zero mark on the vertical reading scale. Remove the weighing vessel and return the movable weights to their zero positions. Transfer the chemical quantitatively to the flask for dilution.

5. Wipe up any spilled chemical immediately from the balance area.

A special type of triple-beam balance is known as the *Cent-O-Gram* balance. This balance also has three beams, but they are tiered on three levels, so that the readings can be obtained from a single eye level. The three beams on the Cent-O-Gram balance provide different weighing scales. The center beam is graduated to 10 g in 1-g notches. As the name implies, the sensitivity of this balance is the nearest 0.01 g. The Cent-O-Gram balance has a lever for arresting the balance when placing objects on the pan.

On any type of triple-beam balance, the balance position of an object on the pan can be determined by observing the swing of the pointer. A swing of an equal number of divisions on either side of the zero mark on the dial indicates that the scale is balanced. It is not necessary to wait for the oscillation to stop to determine the correct weight. This observation enables the weighing process to be a simple and rapid one.

REAGENT PREPARATION, CHEMICALS, AND QUANTITATIVE TRANSFER

For the various clinical laboratory determinations many types of glassware, equipment, specimens, and reagents are used. It is important to understand fully just how valuable the reagents are in the clinical laboratory, as the accuracy of the determinations depends to a great extent on the accuracy of the reagents used. A reagent is defined as any substance employed to produce a chemical reaction. In preparing reagents, instructions should be followed exactly. Often certain reagents will be purchased in a fully prepared state; in this case it is important that the reagents be obtained only from reputable chemical companies. To repeat a most important precept, *instructions must be followed*; this is a strict rule in the laboratory. One should never rely on memory in preparing a reagent, but rather follow the set of instructions or directions devised for the preparation of each reagent needed.

Instructions for preparing a reagent resemble a cake recipe in that they tell what quantities of ingredients to mix together. They tell the names of the chemicals needed, the number of grams or milligrams needed, and the total volume to which the particular reagent should be diluted. The solvent most commonly used for dilution is deionized or distilled water.

Chemical supply companies furnish ready-made reagents, which fill the needs of some laboratories. These reagents usually cost more money, and therefore in large laboratories and in teaching institutions ready-made reagents are not often used. For students it is important that the preparation of reagents be practiced, as this is one of the fundamentals of the clinical laboratory.

Reagent preparation

Preparation of reagents involves the use of a balance (the analytical, triple-beam, or torsion balance, for example) and other special volumetric measuring devices (such as volumetric flasks and graduated cylinders). The types of volumetric glassware available are discussed under Laboratory Glassware.

Since chemicals are used in the preparation of reagents and the accuracy of laboratory determinations depends on the quality of the reagents employed, it is essential that only chemicals from reliable companies be used.

Grades of chemicals

A chemical is a substance that occurs naturally or is obtained through a chemical process; it is used to produce a chemical effect or reaction. Chemicals are produced in various purities or grades. It is essential that the user of chemicals in reagent preparation understand that there are many grades of chemicals available and which grade or type should be used for which reagent.

When quantitative determinations are to be performed and accurate standard solutions prepared, it is necessary to use pure chemicals. In such cases, the more costly *reagent-grade* chemicals are necessary for accuracy. Different companies have their own descriptions for the various degrees of purity, and there is no official designation. The label on the bottle and the supplier's catalog may give important information such as the maximum limits of impurities or an actual analysis of the chemical. Recipes for reagents usually specify the grade, and in many instances state the particular brand of chemical. These directions must be followed to ensure reliable results. The following is a general description of the various grades of chemicals available for the clinical laboratory.[11]

1. *Reagent grade or analytical reagent (AR) grade.* These chemicals are of a high degree of purity and are used often in the preparation of reagents in the clinical laboratory.

2. *American Chemical Society (ACS).* The American Chemical Society has developed specifications for many reagent grade or AR chemicals, and those that meet their standards are designated by the letters ACS.

3. *Chemically pure (CP) grade.* These chemicals are sufficiently pure to be used in many analyses in the clinical laboratory. However, the designation does not reveal the limits of impurities that are tolerated, and so they may not be acceptable for research and various clinical laboratory techniques unless they have been specifically analyzed for the desired procedure. It may be necessary to use this grade when higher-purity biochemicals are not available.

4. *USP and NF grade.* These reagents meet the specifications stated in the *United States Pharmacopeia* (USP) or the *National Formulary* (NF). They are generally less pure than CP grade as the tolerances are specified so that they are not injurious to health rather than chemically pure.

5. *Purified, practical, or pure grade.* These chemicals may be used as starting materials for synthesis of other chemicals of greater purity but generally should not be used in the clinical laboratory.

6. *Technical or commercial grade.* These chemicals are used only for industrial purposes and are generally not used in the preparation of reagents for the clinical laboratory.

The purity of organic chemicals is generally inferior to that of inorganics. This is due both to the manner in which they are prepared or synthesized and to changes that occur as they stand or are stored. Because of these difficulties it may be necessary to use CP and even practical grade chemicals in some analyses.

Standards are the most highly purified types of chemicals available. The group includes *primary*, *reference*, and *certified* standards. Primary standards meet specifications set by the Committee on Analytical Reagents of the American Chemical Society. Each lot of these chemicals is assayed and the chemicals must be stable substances of definite composition. Reference standards are chemicals whose purity has been ensured by the National Bureau of Standards list of standard reference materials (SRM). Certified standards are also available. For example, the College of American Pathologists (CAP) certifies bilirubin and cyanmethemoglobin standards, and the National Committee for Clinical Laboratory Standards (NCCLS) certifies a standardized protein solution.

Chemicals used in the laboratory have various physical forms. Those using these chemicals must know the various forms and which form should be used in the preparation of a specific reagent. Some of the common forms are lumps, sticks, pellets, granules, fine granules, crystalline powder, crystals, fine crystals, powder, and liquid. There are some special forms such as chips, scales, and flakes, but these are not frequently used in reagent preparation.

It is important that chemicals kept in the

laboratory be stored properly, as described under Safety in the Laboratory. Chemicals that require refrigeration should be refrigerated immediately. Solids should be kept in a cool, dry place. Acids and bases should be stored separately and in well-ventilated storage units. Flammable solvents (such as alcohol and chloroform, to name only two) should be stored in specially constructed well-ventilated storage units with appropriate labeling in accordance with OSHA regulations. Flammable solvents such as acetone and ether should always be stored in special safety cans or other appropriate storage devices in appropriate storage units. Fuming and volatile chemicals such as solvents, strong acids, and strong bases should be opened and reagent preparation resulting in fumes should be done only under a fume hood so that the vapors will not escape into the room. Chemicals that absorb water should be weighed only after desiccation or drying in a hot oven, otherwise the weights will not be accurate.

Quantitative transfer

In preparing any solution in the clinical laboratory, it is necessary to utilize the practice known as *quantitative transfer*. It is essential that the *entire* amount of the weighed or measured substance be used in preparing the solution. In quantitative transfer, the entire amount of the measured substance is transferred from one vessel to another for dilution. The usual practice in preparing most laboratory reagents is to weigh the chemical in a beaker (or other suitable vessel, such as a disposable weighing boat) and quantitatively transfer the chemical to a volumetric flask for dilution with deionized or distilled water. The volumetric flask chosen must be of the correct size; that is, it must hold the amount of solution that is desired for the total volume of the reagent being prepared.

Procedure for quantitative transfer and dilution

1. Place a clean, dry funnel in the mouth of the volumetric flask.
2. Carefully transfer the chemical in the measuring vessel into the funnel.
3. Wash the chemical into the flask with small amounts of deionized water or the required solvent for the reagent.
4. Rinse the measuring vessel (beaker) three to five times with small portions of deionized water or the required solvent until *all* of the chemical has been transferred from the vessel into the volumetric flask (add each rinsing to the flask).
5. Rinse the funnel with deionized water or the required solvent, and remove the funnel from the volumetric flask.
6. Dissolve the chemical in the flask by shaking it. Some chemicals are more difficult to dissolve than others. On occasion, more special attention must be given to the problem of dissolving the chemical.

There are several methods by which the dissolution of solid materials can be hastened. Heating usually increases the solubility of a chemical, and heat also causes the fluid to move (the currents help in dissolving). Even mild heat, however, will decompose some chemicals, and therefore heat must be used with caution. Agitation by using a stirring rod or swirling by means of a mechanical shaker increases solubility by removing from contact with the chemical the saturated solution, which hinders further solution of the substance. Rapid addition of the solvent is another means of hastening the solution of solid materials. Some chemicals tend to cake and form aggregates as soon as the solvent is added. By adding the solvent quickly and keeping the solids in motion, aggregation may be prevented.

7. Add deionized water or the required solvent to about $\frac{1}{2}$ in below the calibration line on the flask, allow a few seconds for drainage of fluid above calibration line, and then carefully add

deionized water or the required solvent to the calibration line (the *bottom* of the meniscus must be exactly on the calibration mark).

8. Stopper the flask with a ground-glass stopper, and mix well by inverting at least 20 times.

9. Rinse a properly labeled reagent bottle with a small amount of the mixed reagent in the volumetric flask. Transfer the prepared reagent to the labeled reagent bottle for storage.

Containers for storage of reagents (usually reagent bottles) should be labeled before the material is added. A reagent should never be placed in an unlabeled bottle or container. If an unlabeled container is found, the reagent in it must be discarded. Proper labeling of reagent bottles is of the greatest importance. All labels should include the name and concentration of the reagent, the date on which the reagent was prepared, and the initials of the person who made the reagent (Fig. 1-12).

After the prepared reagent is in the reagent bottle, it must be checked by some means before it is put into actual use in any procedure. This can be done in one of several ways, depending on the reagent itself. After the reagent has been

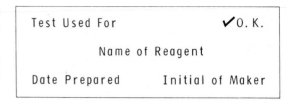

Fig. 1-12. Sample label.

checked, this is noted on the label, and the solution can then be put into active use in the laboratory.

The most common amount of solution prepared at one time is 1 L. If 1 L of reagent is needed, the measured chemical must be transferred quantitatively to a 1-L volumetric flask and diluted to the calibration mark with deionized water or the required solvent. The method of quantitative transfer requires a great deal of care and accuracy.

Using solutions of the correct concentration is of the greatest importance in attaining good results in the laboratory. Quantitative transfer, along with accurate initial measurement of the chemical, helps to ensure that the solution will be of the correct concentration.

PIPETTING

A general discussion of laboratory glassware, including types used for measuring volume, has been given in an earlier section of this chapter (see under Laboratory Glassware). The importance of knowing the correct usage of these various pieces of glassware must be thoroughly appreciated by the student. The four basic pieces of volumetric glassware—volumetric flasks, graduated measuring cylinders, burets, and pipets—are specialized types, and each has its own particular use in the laboratory.

Pipets used in volumetric measurement in the laboratory must be free from all grease and dirt. For that reason, a special cleaning solution is used for these pipets. One made from a combina-

tion of sulfuric acid and either sodium or potassium dichromate is commonly used. For a detailed description of this cleaning solution, see Cleaning Laboratory Glassware.

Since the accuracy of laboratory determinations depend to such a large extent on the equipment used and since pipetting is a principal means of volume measurement, it is imperative that any pipets used in the clinical laboratory be of the finest quality and be manufactured and calibrated by a reputable company. Care and discretion should be used in the selection of laboratory pipets.

Several types of pipets are used commonly in the laboratory. It is necessary that the student understand the uses of these different pipets and know how to handle them in a clinical determination. Practice, again, is the key to success in the use of laboratory pipets; only through practice will the student become proficient in pipetting.

As already mentioned under Volumetric Glassware, there are two categories of pipets: to-contain (T.C.) and to-deliver (T.D.). T.C. pipets are calibrated to contain a specified amount of liquid but are not necessarily calibrated to deliver that exact amount. A small amount of fluid will cling to the inside wall of the T.C. pipet, and when these pipets are used, they should be rinsed out with a diluting fluid to ensure that the entire contents of the pipet have been emptied. T.D. pipets are calibrated to deliver the amount of fluid designated on the pipet; this volume will flow out of the pipet by gravity when the pipet is held in a vertical position with its tip against the side of the receiving vessel. A small amount of fluid will remain in the tip of the pipet; this amount is to be left in the tip as the calibrated portion has been delivered into the receiving vessel. There is another category of pipet, called *blowout*. The calibration of these pipets is similar to that of T.D. pipets, except that the drop remaining in the tip of the pipet must be blown out into the receiving vessel. If a pipet is to be blown out, an etched ring will be seen near the suction opening (see under Types of Pipets).

Pipetting technique

It is important to develop a good technique for handling pipets (Fig. 1-13). It is only through practice that this is accomplished, however. With few exceptions, the same general steps apply to

Fig. 1-13. Pipetting technique.

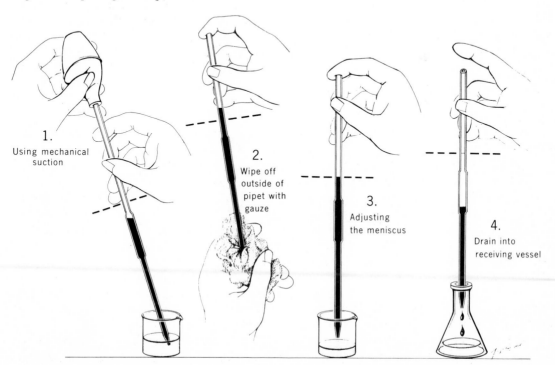

1. Using mechanical suction

2. Wipe off outside of pipet with gauze

3. Adjusting the meniscus

4. Drain into receiving vessel

pipetting with any of the pipets described under Laboratory Glassware.

1. Check the pipet to ascertain its correct size, being careful also to check for broken delivery or suction tips.

2. Hold the pipet lightly between the thumb and the last three fingers, leaving the index finger free.

3. Place the tip of the pipet well below the surface of the liquid to be pipetted.

4. Using mechanical suction or an aspirator bulb, carefully draw the liquid up into the pipet until the level of liquid is well above the calibration mark.

5. Quickly cover the suction opening at the top of the pipet with the index finger.

6. Wipe the outside of the pipet dry with a piece of gauze or tissue to remove excess fluid.

7. Hold the pipet in a vertical position with the delivery tip against the inside of the original vessel. Carefully allow the liquid in the pipet to drain by gravity until the *bottom of the meniscus* is exactly at the calibration mark. (The meniscus is the concave or convex surface of a column of liquid as seen in a laboratory pipet, buret, or other measuring device.) To do this, do not entirely remove the index finger from the suction-hole end of the pipet, but, by rolling the finger slightly over the opening, allow a slow drainage to take place.

8. While still holding the pipet in a vertical position, touch the tip of the pipet to the inside wall of the receiving vessel. Remove the index finger from the top of the pipet to permit free drainage. Remember to keep the pipet in a vertical position for correct drainage. In pipets calibrated to deliver, a small amount of fluid will remain in the delivery tip.

9. To be certain that the drainage is as complete as possible, touch the delivery tip of the pipet to another area on the inside wall of the receiving vessel.

10. Remove the pipet from the receiving vessel and place it in the appropriate place for washing (see under Cleaning Laboratory Glassware).

General considerations in pipetting

Laboratory accidents frequently result from improper pipetting techniques. The greatest potential hazard is when mouth pipetting is done instead of mechanical suction. Caustic reagents, contaminated specimens, or poisonous solutions are all pipetted at one time or another in the laboratory, and every precaution must be taken to ensure the safety of the person doing the work (see under Safety in the Laboratory).

After the pipet has been filled above the top graduation mark, removed from the vessel, and held in a vertical position, the meniscus must be adjusted. The pipet should be held in such a way that the calibration mark is at eye level. The delivery tip is touched to the *inside wall* of the original vessel, not the liquid, and the meniscus of the liquid in the pipet is eased, or adjusted, down to the calibration mark.

When clear solutions are used, the bottom of the meniscus is read. For colored or viscous solutions, the top of the meniscus is read. All readings must be made with the eye at the level of the meniscus (Fig. 1-14).

Before the measured liquid in the pipet is allowed to drain into the receiving vessel, any liquid adhering to the outside of the pipet must be wiped off with a clean piece of gauze or tissue. If this is not done, any drops present on

Fig. 1-14. Reading the meniscus.

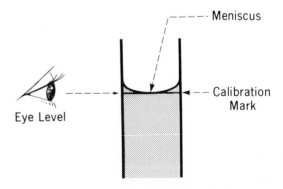

the outside of the pipet might drain into the receiving vessel along with the measured volume. This would make the volume greater than that specified, and an error would result.

TITRATION

Another method of quantitative analysis is the volumetric technique known as *titration*. Titration is a method of measuring the concentration of one solution by comparing it with a measured volume of a solution whose concentration is known. If the concentration of a solution is unknown, it can be found by measuring the volume of the unknown solution that will react with a measured amount of the solution of known concentration (called a standard solution). This process is known as titration. In the clinical laboratory, titration is used to determine the concentrations of acids and bases, as the analytical tool for certain laboratory procedures with body fluids, and in the preparation of some reagents.

This technique is often used to determine the concentration of an unknown acid or an unknown base by means of comparison with a known base or a known acid. In this case the quantity of hydronium ions that react with hydroxyl ions to form water is measured. However, numerous reactions, other than the neutralization reaction between an acid and a base, are used in titrations to determine the concentration of a solution. For example, in chloride determinations, which will be described in Chap. 2 (see under Chloride), mercury ions of a known amount and concentration are titrated with chloride ions of an unknown concentration and known amount; mercury chloride is the end product in this case.

When titration is used to determine concentration, the concentration is traditionally expressed in terms of normality or equivalents. Normality is employed because it is a unit that provides a basis for direct comparison of strength for all solutions. Normality is the number of gram equivalents per liter of solution. A gram equivalent is the amount of a compound that will liberate, combine with, or replace one gram atom of hydrogen. Therefore, 1 equiv of any compound will react with exactly 1 equiv of any other compound. For example, 1 equiv of any acid will exactly neutralize 1 equiv of any base. It is very convenient to have laboratory solutions of such concentrations that any chosen volume of one reagent reacts with an equal volume of another reagent. The system of equivalents or equivalent weights provides this useful tool. The equivalent weight of a substance is calculated by dividing the gram molecular weight of the substance by the sum of the positive valences. A solution that contains 1 gram equivalent weight of substance in 1 L of solution is called a normal ($1\,N$) solution (see under Laboratory Calculations).

In any titration procedure there are certain things that must always be present: (1) a standard solution of known concentration, (2) an accurately measured volume of the standard solution or unknown, (3) an indicator to show when the reaction has reached completion, and (4) a buret (or similar device) to measure the volume of solution required to reach the end point.

Standard solutions of a desired normality may be prepared by weighing on the analytical balance the exact amount of substance calculated to give that normality, dissolving this in a small amount of deionized water, and then diluting the solution to the number of liters required in the original calculation. Standard solutions prepared in this way (by direct weighing on the analytical balance) are known as primary standards. The chemical substances used in the preparation of standard solutions must be pure, must have a high molecular weight, and must not take up or give off moisture. Oxalic acid meets these requirements and is often used as a primary standard. A solution of hydrochloric acid prepared from constant-boiling HCl is also often used as a primary standard. Bases are not often used as primary standards because they take up moisture when exposed to the air, which makes the measurement inaccurate.

The point at which equal concentrations of the standard and the unknown are present is called the end point of the titration. In the case of acid-base titrations, the end point is where neutralization occurs. Various means of detecting the end point are used, depending on the procedure. Sometimes the formation of a precipitate indicates that the end point has been reached. A change in color of one of the reacting solutions can also indicate the end point. The most common method of detecting the end point is through the use of an indicator solution. An indicator solution is a third solution added in the titration procedure (in addition to the standard solution and the unknown solution). The indicator solution is added in measured amounts to the titration flask. Most indicators are solids dissolved in water or alcohol. Phenolphthalein (0.1%) is commonly used as the indicator in acid-base titrations. Phenolphthalein is made up in a solution of alcohol. It is generally best to arrange the titration procedure so that one titrates from a colorless solution to the first sign of a permanent color rather than from a colored to a colorless solution. Phenolphthalein is colorless in an acid solution and red in an alkaline solution. When one is near the end point, the addition of a single drop from the buret may overrun the true end point considerably. This can cause significant error in the titration of small amounts of solutions. To avoid this *drop error*, the titrating solution should be added in split drops as the end point approaches. It is possible to control the flow from the buret with careful manipulation of the stopcock so that only part of a drop goes into the titration flask.

The device that is most often employed to measure the volume required to reach completion of the reaction in a particular titration procedure is the buret. The buret is basically a graduated pipet with a stopcock near the delivery tip to facilitate better control and delivery of the solution (Fig. 1-15). Burets may be obtained in many different capacities and tolerances. The particular buret capacity and tolerance used in a particular procedure will be determined by the degree of accuracy that is desired. To ensure that the buret used is employed with maximum accuracy, a very specific technique or procedure must be followed. Mastery of this technique will come only with practice. It is essential that chemically clean, well-calibrated volumetric equipment be used throughout the procedure to ensure reliable results.

Fig. 1-15. Method of titration.

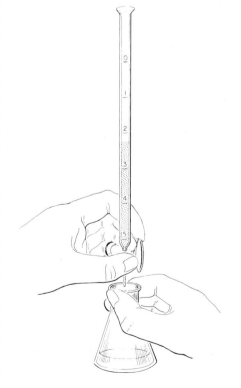

General procedure for titration

1. Use the buret clamp to fasten the buret, which must be clean and free from chips or cracks, to the buret stand, which will support it during the titration procedure. Fasten the clamp to the stand about halfway up the rod.

2. Lightly grease the buret stopcock. The stopcock should turn easily and smoothly, but an excess of lubricant will plug the stopcock capillary bore and prevent emptying of the buret. To grease a clean stopcock properly, apply a bit of grease with the fingertip down the two sides of the stopcock away from the capillary bore. Then insert the stopcock in the buret and rotate it until a smooth covering of the whole stopcock is obtained. If the buret is equipped with a Teflon plug, the stopcock need not be lubricated.

3. Rinse the buret with the titrant. In the case of an acid-base titration with phenolphthalein as the indicator, the titrant (or solution to be added and measured by means of the buret) will always be the base. In rinsing the buret, fill it completely with the titrant, and then let it drain. Discard the rinse solution. Fill the buret slowly and carefully to prevent air bubbles from forming in the narrow buret tube. It is essential that the buret be absolutely clean if the results are to be accurate. A clean buret will drain without any solution clinging to its sides; if the buret is dirty, there will be droplets of liquid clinging to the sides. After rinsing the buret several times with the titrant solution, fill it past the zero mark, and then bring the meniscus exactly to the zero mark by draining, using the stopcock to control the flow (Fig. 1-15).

4. Into an Erlenmeyer flask, pipet the stated amount of the second solution to be employed in the titration. Pipet this solution with a volumetric pipet, using great care to ensure maximum accuracy.

5. Add the required amount of the indicator solution employed to show when the titration reaction has reached completion. (At this point, approximately 5-10 ml of water is often added to the Erlenmeyer flask to dilute the indicator and make the end point more visible. The volume of this diluent is not critical, since it does not enter into the reaction or affect the volumes of the solutions that are being titrated.)

6. Titrate each flask in the following manner:

a. Inspect the buret to be sure that there are no air bubbles trapped in the capillary tube or tip. Air bubbles will add to the apparent volume required to reach the end point, leading to erroneous results. If bubbles are present, drain the buret and refill it with the titrant until there are no bubbles.

b. Inspect to see that the meniscus is exactly at zero, or record the actual buret reading immediately before beginning the titration.

c. Add the solution in the buret to the flask by rotating the stopcock carefully. A right-handed person encircles the buret stopcock with the left hand, using the right hand to swirl the flask during the titration (Fig. 1-15). This will be awkward at first, but when mastered it will become natural.

d. With the buret tip well within the titration flask, the titrant may be added fairly rapidly at first, but as the reaction nears completion, the titrant is added drop by drop and finally by only portions of drops (split drops). Clues that the reaction is nearing completion depend on the particular reaction and indicator being employed. In the case of an acid-base titration with phenolphthalein as the indicator, there is a change from a colorless to a red solution. The phenolphthalein is colorless in acid solutions and red in alkaline solutions. In the neutralization reaction itself hydronium ions react with hydroxyl ions to form water. The reaction begins with an excess of hydronium ions in the Erlenmeyer flask, and the titration is performed until all the hydronium ions have been neutralized by the hydroxyl ions added from the buret. The titration should be stopped at the actual point of neutralization, or as close to it as possible.

In practice, a pink color will appear when the alkali is added to the acid. This color will disappear on shaking. As the titration nears completion, the pink color will remain for a longer time. The base is then added slowly, by split drops, until a faint pink color remains. When the pink color no longer disappears but remains for more than 30 seconds, the end point (or neutralization) has been achieved. It is essential that any titration, using any indicator, be stopped at the actual end point, which is the first faint but permanent color change, or the results will be inaccurate.

e. Immediately on reaching the end point, record the buret reading. Be sure to record a figure that is significant considering the tolerance of the particular buret being used.

7. Clean the buret by rinsing thoroughly with tap water and then with deionized water. Remove any grease from the stopcock with ether. The titrant should not be left standing in the buret. Alkali will "freeze" the stopcock to the buret, and the concentration of the titrant will increase because of evaporation. When the buret is clean, it can be stored either in an inverted position on the buret clamp or in an upright position filled with deionized water.

8. Use the buret readings obtained in the titration procedure to determine the concentration of the unknown solution.

General considerations and calculations

Chemically clean, well-calibrated volumetric equipment, including flasks, pipets, and burets, must be used in every titration procedure. Accurately prepared standard solutions are essential for accurate results. These are weighed analytically and diluted volumetrically. Indicators must be employed to show when the particular reac-

tion has reached completion. These are often color indicators, which change from colorless to a faint permanent color when the reaction has reached completion. However, such instruments as pH meters may also be employed, where the end point is a particular hydronium ion concentration as recorded on the pH meter (see under pH in Chap. 5).

In acid-base titrations in the clinical laboratory, the most commonly used alkali is $0.1\ N$ sodium hydroxide (NaOH). This is relatively stable and can be used to determine the concentration of an acid. However, sodium hydroxide is not absolutely stable and it should be checked daily against a standard acid to be considered reliable.

The acids most commonly used in titration are oxalic acid, hydrochloric acid (HCl), sulfuric acid (H_2SO_4), and nitric acid (HNO_3). A $0.1\ N$ solution of hydrochloric acid made from constant-boiling hydrochloric acid may be used as the reference, or primary standard, in the clinical laboratory. Constant-boiling hydrochloric acid is obtained by distillation and collection of the constant-boiling mixture. The constant-boiling acid is then weighed on an analytical balance and diluted volumetrically. When prepared in this manner, using constant-boiling acid weighed analytically, the primary standard $0.1000\ N$ HCl is accurate within ±0.0004.[12] Further standardization is not necessary. The acid standard prepared in this manner is used for the standardization of alkalis and other reagents.

To find the concentration of a solution, the following information must be available: a standard solution of known concentration, the volume of the standard solution, and the volume of the undetermined solution required to reach completion in the particular reaction. As mentioned previously, the concentration is usually expressed in terms of normality, which permits direct comparison of solutions. Normality is the number of gram equivalents per liter of solution, or milliequivalents per milliliter of solution. However, in practice, 1 L of a solution is rarely used; instead, parts of 1 L are used. Therefore, the number of equivalents is actually the normality of the solution times the volume that is used in the titration. All the ingredients required for the equation to determine the concentration of a solution in any titration are now present. If the equivalents of solution 1 are equal to the equivalents of solution 2, and if the number of equivalents of a particular solution is actually the normality of the solution times the volume, it follows that the normality of solution 1 times the volume of solution 1 is equal to the normality of solution 2 times the volume of solution 2. Or in equation form:

Equivalents of solution 1

$$= \text{equivalents of solution 2}$$

or

$$N_1 \times V_1 = N_2 \times V_2$$

In the case of a typical acid-base titration, assume that 2 ml of a standard $0.1000 \, N$ HCl solution required 1.50 ml of NaOH, added from a buret, to reach the first permanent pink color. What is the normality of NaOH?

$$N_{acid} \times V_{acid} = N_{base} \times V_{base}$$

$$0.1000 \, N \times 2 \text{ ml} = N_{base} \times 1.50 \text{ ml}$$

$$N_{base} = \frac{0.1000 \, N \times 2 \text{ ml}}{1.50 \text{ ml}} = 0.1333$$

That is, the normality of the sodium hydroxide is 0.1333.

The titration technique has numerous uses in the clinical laboratory. It is the means of checking the concentrations of new reagents before they are used in the clinical laboratory. When weaker acids or bases are prepared from more concentrated solutions, the actual normality of the new solution must be determined by titration. In addition, titration is the basis for several chemical determinations that are performed in the clinical laboratory.

PHOTOMETRY

In the clinical laboratory there is a continual need for the use of quantitative techniques. By using a quantitative method, the exact amount of an unknown substance can be determined accurately, and this is the basis for many laboratory determinations, especially in the chemistry department. There are various methods for measuring substances quantitatively, and one of the techniques used most frequently in the laboratory is photometry. Photometry, or colorimetry, employs color and color variation to determine the concentrations of substances.

Photometry is perhaps the most frequently used quantitative method in the laboratory (although not as accurate as titration), and it is imperative that any student learning clinical laboratory techniques know and understand thoroughly the principles of photometry. Probably no measurement technique is used as much but understood as little as photometry. Although photometry is often less precise than other procedures, it has the advantage of being very simple to use. In most laboratories today there is a need for greater efficiency, and through the use of photometry the results of certain tests can be obtained simply and quickly.

Nature of light

To understand the use of photometry, one must first understand the fundamentals of color. To understand color, one must also understand the nature of light and its effect on color as we see it. Light is a type of radiant energy and it travels in the form of waves. The distance between waves is the wavelength of the light. The term *light* is used to describe radiant energy with wavelengths visible to the human eye and with wavelengths bordering on those visible to the human eye.[13] The human eye responds to radiant energy, or light, with wavelengths between about 400 and 750 nm (or mμm). A nanometer or a millimicrometer is 1×10^{-9} m. With modern photometric apparatus shorter (ultraviolet) or longer (infrared) wavelengths can be measured.

The wavelength of light determines the color of the light seen by the human eye. Every color that is seen is light of a particular wavelength. A combination, or mixture, of light energy of different wavelengths is known as daylight, or *white light*. When light is passed through a filter, prism, or diffraction grating, it can be broken into a spectrum of visible colors ranging from violet to red. The visible spectrum consists of the following range of colors: violet, blue, green, yellow, orange, and red. If white light is diffracted or partially absorbed by a filter or prism, it becomes visible as certain colors. The different portions of the spectrum may be identified by wavelengths ranging from 400 to 750 nm for the visible colors. Wavelengths below 400 nm are ultraviolet and those above 750 nm are infrared; these light waves are not visible to the human eye.

The color of light seen in the visible spectrum depends on the wavelength that is not absorbed. When light is not absorbed, it is transmitted. A colored solution has color because of its physical properties, which result in its absorbing certain wavelengths and transmitting others. When white light is passed through a solution, part of the light is absorbed and that remaining is transmitted. A rainbow is seen when there are droplets of moisture in the air that refract or filter certain rays of the sun and allow others to pass through. The colors of the rainbow range from red to violet—the visible spectrum.

Absorption and transmittance: Beer's law

As mentioned above, many solutions contain particles that absorb certain wavelengths and transmit others. Solutions appear to the human eye to have characteristic colors. The wavelength of light transmitted by the solution is recognized as color by the eye. The following are the visible colors of the spectrum and their respective wavelength ranges: violet (400–440 nm), blue (440–500 nm), green (500–580 nm), yellow (580–600 nm), orange (600–620 nm), and red (620–750 nm). A blue solution appears blue because particles in the solution absorb all the wavelengths except blue; the blue is the color transmitted and seen. A red solution appears red because all other wavelengths except red have been absorbed by the solution, while the red wavelength passes through.

The use of photometry, or colorimetry, as a means of quantitative measurement depends primarily on two factors, the color itself and the intensity of the color. Any substance to be measured by photometry must be colored to begin with or must be capable of being colored. An example of a substance that is colored to begin with is hemoglobin (determined by use of photometry in the hematology laboratory). Sugar, specifically glucose, is an example of a substance that is not colored to begin with but is capable of being colored by use of certain reagents and reactions. Sugar content can therefore be measured by photometry.

Measurement by photometry is based on the reaction between the substance to be measured and a reagent, or chemical, used to produce color. The amount of color produced in a reaction between the substance to be measured and the reagent depends on the concentration of the substance. Therefore, the intensity of the color is proportional to the concentration of the substance. Beer's law (or the Beer-Lambert law) states this relationship: color intensity at a constant depth is directly proportional to concentration. Beer's law is the basis for the use of photometry in quantitative measurement. Using this law, if one saw a solution with a very intense red color, one would be correct in assuming that the solution had a high concentration of the substance that made it red. Another way of putting Beer's law is that any increase in the concentration of a color-producing substance would increase the amount of color seen.

As the law states, the depth at which the color is determined must be constant. The depth of the solution is regulated by the cuvette used to hold it. Increasing the depth of the solution through which the light must pass (by using a cuvette with a larger diameter) is the same as placing more particles between the light and the eye, thereby creating an apparent increase in the concentration, or intensity, of color. To avoid this alteration of the actual concentration, only cuvettes with a constant diameter can be used. The use of special tubes calibrated for photometry is discussed under Calibration of Cuvettes for the Photometer.

When using photometry as a method for quantitative measurement, the undetermined colored substance is compared with a similar substance of known strength (a standard solution), based on the principle that the intensity of the color is directly proportional to the concentration of the substance present. The device used to show the quantitative relationship between the colors of the undetermined solution and the standard solution is called a photometer, or colorimeter. Standard solutions will be discussed further under Ensuring Reliable Laboratory Results.

Most of the instruments used in photometry have some means of isolating a narrow wavelength, or range, of the color spectrum for measurements. Instruments using filters for this purpose are referred to as filter photometers, while those using prisms or gratings are called spectrophotometers. Both types are used frequently in the clinical laboratory. In older colori-

metric procedures, visual comparison of the color of an unknown with that of a standard was used. Visual colorimetry has been replaced by the more specific and accurate photoelectric methods.

There are many types of photometers in common use in the clinical laboratory. The principle of most of these machines is the same, in that the amount of light transmitted by the standard solution is compared with the amount of light transmitted by the solution of unknown concentration. There are two common methods of expressing the amount of light transmitted (or absorbed) by a solution. The units used to express the readings obtained by the electronic measuring device (see under General Parts Essential to All Photometers) are either absorbance units or percent transmittance units. Another term for absorptance is optical density (OD). The term optical density is generally an outdated one. Most photometers give the readings in both units. Absorbance units are difficult to read directly from the reading scale because it is divided logarithmically rather than in equal divisions. Absorbance values are directly proportional to the concentration and therefore they may be plotted on linear graph paper to give a straight line (see under Standardization of a Procedure and Use of a Standard Curve in Chap. 2). Most photometers also give the percent transmittance readings on the viewing scale. Percent transmittance is the amount of light that passes through a colored solution compared with the amount of light that passes through a blank solution (see under Ensuring Reliable Laboratory Results). Percent transmittance varies from 0 to 100 (it is usually abbreviated $\%T$), with equal divisions on the viewing scale. As the concentration of the colored solution increases, the amount of light absorbed increases and the percentage of the light transmitted decreases. The transmitted light does not decrease in direct proportion to the concentration or color intensity of the solution being measured. There is a logarithmic relationship between percent transmittance and concentration (see under Standardization of a Procedure and Use of a Standard Curve). Absorbance (or optical density) and percent transmittance are related in the following way: absorbance = 2 minus the logarithm of the percent transmittance, or $A = 2 - \log \%T$. Therefore, 2 is the logarithm of $100\%T$. It is possible to obtain a convenient conversion table for transmittance and absorbance from a standard reference textbook.

Precise, accurate methods are needed to accomplish the numerous determinations required of the modern laboratory. The photometer is one piece of equipment that is essential and can be considered to be of prime importance. Photometers are also known as *photoelectric colorimeters* or *spectrophotometers*. The many available photometers have their own technical variations, but all operate according to the same general principles.

General parts essential to all photometers

There are certain parts necessary to all photometers (Fig. 1-16). These are:

1. *Light source.* Each photometer must have a light source. This can be a light bulb constructed to give the optimum amount of light. The light source must be steady and constant; therefore, use of a voltage regulator or electronic power supply is recommended. The light source may be movable or stationary.

2. *Wavelength isolator.* Before the light from the light source reaches the sample of solution to be measured, the interfering wavelengths must be removed. A system of isolating a desired wavelength and excluding others is called a *monochromator*. In doing this the light is actually being reduced to a particular wavelength. Filters can be used to accomplish this. Some are very simple, composed of one or two pieces of colored glass. Some are more complicated. The more complicated filters are found in the better photometers. The filter must transmit a color that the solution *can* absorb. A red filter transmits red, and a green filter transmits green. Filters are available to cover almost any point in the visible spectrum, and each filter has inscribed on it a number that indicates the wavelength of light that it transmits. For example, a filter inscribed with 540 nm absorbs all light except that of wavelengths around 540 nm. Since the filter must transmit a color that the solution can absorb, for a red solution the filter chosen should not be red (all colors *except* red are absorbed). The wavelength of light transmitted is, then, the important thing to consider in choosing the correct filter for a procedure.

Light of a desired wavelength can also be provided by other means. One of the more commonly used machines employs a diffraction grating with a special plate and slit to reduce the

Fig. 1-16. Parts essential to all photometers.

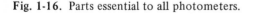
or filter

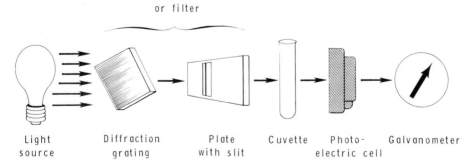

Light source   Diffraction grating   Plate with slit   Cuvette   Photo-electric cell   Galvanometer

spectrum to the desired wavelength. The grating consists of a highly polished surface with numerous lines on it that break up white light into the spectrum. By moving the spectrum behind a slit (the light source must be movable), only one particular portion of the spectrum is allowed to pass through the narrow slit. The particular band of light, or wavelength, that is transmitted through the slit is indicated on a viewing scale on the machine. Certain wavelengths are more desirable than others for a particular color and procedure. The wavelength chosen is determined by running an absorption curve and selecting the correct wavelength after inspecting the curve obtained. Only when new methods are being developed is it necessary to run an absorption curve.

3. *Cuvettes, absorption cells, or photometer tubes.* Any light (of the wavelength selected) coming from the filter or diffraction grating will next pass on to the solution in the cuvette. Glass cuvettes are relatively inexpensive and are satisfactory, provided they are matched or calibrated. Calibrated cuvettes are tubes that have been optically matched so that the same solution in each will give the same reading on the photometer. In using calibrated cuvettes, the depth factor of Beer's law is kept constant. The means by which these tubes can be obtained will be discussed under Calibration of Cuvettes for the Photometer. Depending on the concentration and thus the color of the solution, a certain amount of light will be absorbed by the solution, and the remainder will be transmitted. The light not absorbed by the solution is transmitted. This light next passes on to an electronic measuring device of some type.

4. *Electronic measuring device.* In the more common photometers the electronic measuring device consists of a photoelectric cell and a galvanometer. The amount of light transmitted by the solution in the cuvette is measured by a photoelectric cell. This cell is a most sensitive instrument, producing electrons in proportion to the amount of light hitting it. The electrons are passed on to a galvanometer, where they are measured. The galvanometer records the amount of current (in the form of electrons) that it receives from the photoelectric cell on a special viewing scale on the photometer. The results are reported in terms of percent transmittance. In some cases, the readings are made in terms of absorbance (or optical density). The percent transmittance is dependent on the concentration of the solution and its depth. If the solution is very concentrated (the color appearing intense), less light will be transmitted than if it is dilute (pale). Therefore, the reading on the galvanometer viewing scale will be lower for a more concentrated solution than for a dilute solution. This is the basis for the comparison of color intensity with the photometer.

Several types of photometers are available for use in the clinical laboratory. Some of these are Bausch and Lomb, Beckman, Coleman Junior, Evelyn, Klett-Summerson, and Leitz. For teaching purposes the Coleman Junior Spectrophotometer has proved to be very satisfactory (Fig. 1-17). As the name implies, a spectrophotometer is really two instruments in a single case, a spectrometer (device for producing light of a specific wavelength, the monochromator) and a photometer (device for measuring light intensity). Because of its common use, the operation of this specific machine is outlined below.

Operation of the Coleman Junior Spectrophotometer*

1. Mount the selected scale panel in the galvanometer viewing window. A general-purpose scale panel is usually used. These are several types of scale panels available, depending on the use to which the spectrophotometer is to be put.

---

*From the "Operating Directions for the Coleman Model 6A and 6C Junior Spectrophotometer," Coleman Instruments Corporation, Maywood, Ill., September 1966.

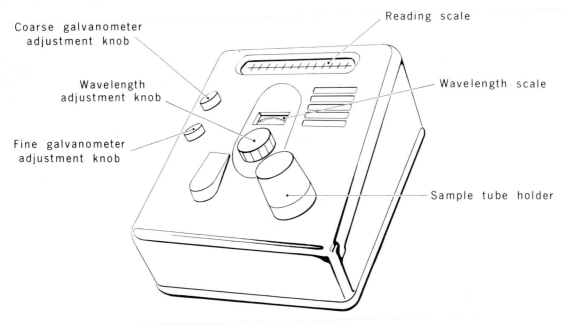

Fig. 1-17. Coleman Junior Spectrophotometer.

The scale panel is calibrated both in percent transmittance and optical density (absorbance).

2. Insert in the cuvette well the cuvette adapter of the proper size to accommodate the type of cuvette specified in the analytical procedure.

3. Turn on the switch located on the back of the instrument. Allow the instrument to warm up for 5 minutes.

4. Verify the galvanometer zero setting, and readjust if necessary. The indicator line on the galvanometer spot should register at zero on the percent transmittance scale. The zero adjustment level for this instrument is located under the raised housing just to the left of the cuvette well. If the spectrophotometer is not disturbed and its position is not altered, this galvanometer adjustment remains very stable.

a. To check the zero position, darken the photo-electric cell by inserting a cuvette adapter in the cuvette well turned 90° from the calibration marker. In this position, the body of the adapter completely blocks the pathway of

light. A piece of opaque paper may also be slipped in the adapter well; in this way the light pathway is also completely stopped.

b. Cover the well with the light shield or other suitable cover.

c. With a pencil point move the galvanometer adjusting lever so that the indicator line on the galvanometer spot reads zero on the left zero index of the selected scale panel.

d. Complete the adjustment by sliding the scale panel until the index is *exactly* at zero on the scale.

5. Adjust the wavelength knob so that the specific wavelength is set. Different procedures will call for different wavelengths. The wavelength to be used will be specified in the procedure.

6. Cuvettes used for reading in the spectrophotometer must be free from scratches. Before placing the cuvette in the adapter for reading, it must be free of finger marks and bubbles; the spectrophotometer does not recognize the cause of light impediment and will respond similarly to

a scratched tube, lint, bubbles, finger marks, and the absorbance of the solution being examined. Therefore, wipe the cuvettes with a clean, dry, soft cloth or gauze before reading.

All cuvettes must contain a certain volume of solution, called the *minimum volume*. Various-sized cuvettes need various minimum volumes to ensure that the light passes through the solution rather than through the empty space in the tube.

7. Place the cuvette containing the reagent blank in the adapter first. For more information on the use of blank solutions, see under Means of Control of Laboratory Error. The calibration mark (or trademark, if precalibrated Coleman cuvettes are used) must face the light source to ensure constancy of the light path. Adjust the galvanometer control knobs (labeled *GALV Coarse* and *GALV Fine*) until the galvanometer index on the viewing scale reads 100%T for the "blank" tube.

8. Remove the blank tube.

9. Place the next polished cuvette containing the solution to be read in the adapter well, again taking note of the calibration mark. Place this mark in a position facing the light source.

10. Record the galvanometer reading to the nearest $\frac{1}{4}$%T reading.

11. Remove the cuvette, and reinsert the blank tube.

12. Observe the reading for the blank tube on the galvanometer scale. It should still read 100%T. If it does, remove the blank tube and proceed with the next tube to be read. If the blank tube does not read exactly 100%T, adjust it to read 100%T with the GALV Coarse and GALV Fine knobs. Then read the next tube. The blank tube should be reinserted between all readings, and it should always read 100%T.

13. Read all tubes, and record results to the nearest $\frac{1}{4}$%T reading. Fractional parts (in fourths) of percent transmittance readings are recorded with the numerator figure only. For example, if a reading is $75\frac{1}{2}$ $(= 75\frac{2}{4})$, the result is recorded as 75^2%T. For a reading of $75\frac{3}{4}$ the result is

recorded as 75^3, and for a reading of $75\frac{1}{4}$ the result is recorded as 75^1.

14. When finished, return the galvanometer index to the original position by turning both the GALV Coarse and GALV Fine knobs completely counterclockwise, and turn off the machine switch.

15. Clean up the area around the instrument, wipe up anything spilled on the machine, and cover the spectrophotometer with the protective cover provided. For cleaning cuvettes see under Cleaning of Laboratory Glassware.

A special adaptation available for Coleman Junior Spectrophotometers is called a Coleman Vacuvette Cell Assembly. This is designed to increase the speed with which samples can be introduced into and discharged from the photometer. Another name for an assembly of this kind is a *flow-through apparatus*. Instead of using separate cuvettes for each sample read in the photometer, the sample is poured directly into a specially designed cuvette incorporating a funnel for easy pouring. The sample is read in the same way as in the regular cuvette method and is then evacuated from the photometer by means of a capillary tubing attached to a discard bottle. When a suitable vacuum system is attached to the cuvette-capillary tubing assembly, rapid and automatic discarding of the sample is possible. This assembly apparatus must be periodically cleaned to maintain its proper operation. A flow-through apparatus can be used for reading samples when the sample can be discarded. It cannot be used to read multiple values on the same sample as the sample is lost once it is poured into the special cuvette. The Coleman Instrument Company manufactures this specially designed cuvette in various sizes so that varying amounts of sample may be read in the photometer. This device is another example of how many laboratory functions have been made more efficient so that time can be saved and results can be sent out more quickly.

For the operation of machines other than the Coleman Junior Spectrophotometer, the student is referred to the manuals supplied with photometers by the manufacturer.

General care and use of photometers

When using a photometer, error caused by color in the reagents used must be eliminated. Since color is so important and since the color produced by the undetermined substance is the desired one, any color resulting from the reagents themselves or from interactions between the reagents could cause confusion and error. By using a blank solution, a correction can be made for any color because of the reagents used. The blank solution contains the same reagents as the unknown and standard tubes with the exception of the substance being measured. The use of blank solutions will be discussed further under Ensuring Reliable Laboratory Results.

A photometer, as is the case with any expensive, delicate instrument, must be handled with care. The manufacturer supplies a manual of complete instructions on the care and use of a particular machine. Care should be taken not to spill reagents on the photometer. Spillage could damage the delicate instrument, especially the photoelectric cell. Any reagents spilled must be wiped up immediately. Photometers with filters should not be operated without the filter in place, as the unfiltered light from the light source may damage the photoelectric cell and the galvanometer. A photometer should be placed on a table with good support, where it will not be bumped and jarred.

In general, photometers employing filters are called *filter photometers*, and those with diffraction gratings are called *spectrophotometers*. Photometers utilize an electronic device to compare the actual color intensities of the solutions measured.

Visual colorimetry

Before photometers became readily available for quantitative measurements, another type of color-comparing device was in common use. This device utilized the human eye to compare color intensity differences and was called a *visual colorimeter*. Visual colorimetry is now used only rarely and has been replaced by photometry. In visual colorimetry, the human eye acts as the instrument for color comparison (in the photometer, the photoelectric cell and galvanometer accomplish this).

The human eye is a poor instrument for measuring light intensity. It is difficult for the human eye to measure accurately shades of color or intensity. There is an error of 5 percent or more even with experience and proper technique, which is one of the reasons why visual colorimetry is inadequate for today's laboratory procedures. Interfering spectra will often cause an even greater error. Such interference often can be reduced or eliminated by the use of a filter.

The visual colorimeter has several other disadvantages. One of these is that more time is required to carry out the desired procedure. In the modern laboratory, many tests are run and speed is important. The temperature of the surrounding area and the order of adding the reagents can also affect the visual colorimeter. In using visual colorimetry, there is a need for deep colors, which requires a larger quantity of the specimen and more reagents. It is not always possible to obtain enough specimen (blood, for example) to run the test satisfactorily with a visual colorimeter.

The names of some of the visual colorimeters used in years past are the Klett, Duboscq, and Dennison colorimeters.

Calibration of cuvettes for the photometer

Essential in photometry is the use of calibrated tubes, or cuvettes (also called absorption tubes). It is necessary that the depth of the tubes used in the photometer be constant (for Beer's law to apply). Only by checking each tube used can its depth be made certain. Cuvettes for the photometer can be purchased precalibrated, but these are expensive. Precalibrated cuvettes must also be checked before being put into actual use in the laboratory. Most laboratories, especially those involved with teaching, calibrate cuvettes for the photometer. As noted previously, these cuvettes have been optically matched so that the same solution in each will give the same percent transmittance reading on the galvanometer viewing scale.

In calibrating cuvettes for use in photometry, the cuvette is carefully checked to see that the solution gives the same reading in that cuvette as it did in a previously calibrated cuvette. To check cuvettes for uniformity, the same solution, such as a stable solution of copper sulfate or cyanmethemoglobin, is read in many cuvettes. Readings are taken and cuvettes that match within an established tolerance are reserved for use. Since cuvettes may not be perfectly round, they are rotated in the cuvette well to observe any changes in reading with position in the well. The cuvette is etched at the point where the reading corresponds with the established tolerance for the absorption reading. Those that do not agree or do not correspond are not used for photometry. Different-sized cuvettes can be used, depending on the photometer. One of the more common sizes of cuvettes, especially for the Coleman Junior Spectrophotometer, is 19 by 105 mm. The Coleman Junior Spectrophotometer can be adapted to use several different-sized cuvettes in the same machine. For each size, a special cuvette adapter is used, enabling the cuvette to fit securely in the cuvette holder. Only when the cuvette fits securely will the readings obtained be precise and accurate.

Procedure for calibrating cuvettes

1. Use only clean, dry cuvettes for calibration.
2. Filter a portion of the chosen colored solution to be placed in the cuvettes. One solution used frequently for calibration is 5% copper sulfate. Filter enough solution to fill the cuvettes to be calibrated. The cuvettes should be filled to approximately the same level.
3. Fill the uncalibrated cuvettes to approximately the same level with the filtered solution.
4. Polish the cuvettes with a gauze or tissue.
5. Calibrate the new cuvettes against previously calibrated tubes.

a. Fill four or five calibrated cuvettes with the same filtered solution to approximately the same level. Polish the cuvettes thoroughly and read in the photometer, noting the readings in percent transmittance for each (see steps 6 to 9).

b. Read the uncalibrated cuvettes in the same manner, following the directions given in the next steps.

6. Set the wavelength at 550 nm (or other suitable wavelength chosen for this procedure).
7. Prepare the photometer for reading cuvettes by following the directions for the particular machine being used.
8. Pick an arbitrary setting on the galvanometer reading scale against which to read the cuvettes. Usually a setting near the center of the viewing scale is chosen (50, 60, or 70%T, for example).
9. Read the previously calibrated cuvettes first, checking the arbitrary setting between each reading. Adjust and reread, if necessary. Record these readings. All the readings for the previously calibrated cuvettes should be within $\frac{1}{2}$%T of each other on the galvanometer scale.
10. To calibrate the new cuvettes:

a. Check the arbitrary center setting; adjust if necessary.

b. Place the polished uncalibrated cuvette in the tube holder; note the reading on the galvanometer viewing scale.

c. If the reading is the same as for the standard cuvettes read previously, mark the cuvette with a wax pencil at the place corresponding to the mark on the calibrated cuvettes (that is, the side of the cuvette facing the light source); this mark will later be permanently etched on the cuvette.

d. If the reading is not the same as for the

precalibrated cuvettes, slowly rotate the cuvette in the holder until the same reading is obtained. Mark the cuvette with a wax pencil as in step 10c. If the reading is not obtained after a complete rotation in the cuvette holder, the new cuvette cannot be used with this particular set of calibrated cuvettes. Set it aside to be calibrated with a different set.

e. Etch the cuvettes with a glass etcher, making a well-defined mark where the wax pencil mark was made. The cuvettes are now ready to be washed and used.

FLAME PHOTOMETRY

Flame emission photometry is used most commonly for the quantitative measurement of sodium and potassium in body fluids. In flame emission analysis by emission photometry, a solution containing metal ions is sprayed into a flame. The metal ions are energized to emit light of a characteristic color. Atoms of many metallic elements, when given sufficient energy (such as that supplied by a hot flame), will emit this energy at wavelengths characteristic of the elements. Lithium produces a red, sodium a yellow, potassium a violet, and magnesium a blue color in a flame. Sodium and potassium are the metal ions most commonly measured in biological specimens, but lithium, which is not normally present in serum, may also be measured in connection with the use of lithium salts in the treatment of some psychiatric disorders. The intensity of the color is proportional to the amount of the element burned in the flame. Flame photometers are laboratory instruments that make use of this principle. Details of the operation of a specific flame photometer should be obtained from the manufacturer, but there are a few general principles and components that are common to most instruments.

An atomizer is needed to spray the sample as fine droplets into the flame. Another name for the atomizer is a nebulizer (Fig. 1-18). The atomizer creates a fine spray of the sample and

Fig. 1-18. Essential parts of a flame photometer.

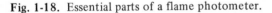
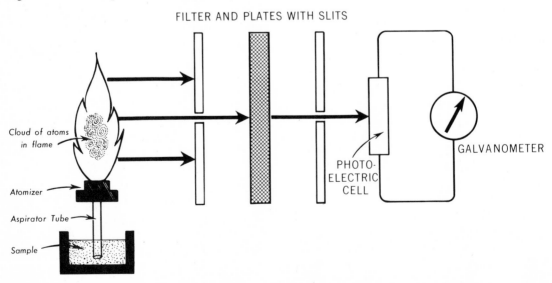

feeds this spray into a burner. The fine spray is produced by combining a stream of sample with a stream of air. A total-consumption burner feeds the entire sample directly into the flame. A premix atomizer mixes the fuel gases and the sample in a mixing chamber before sending this mixture to the flame. Both types of atomizers are available in modern machines.

In most flame photometers the fuel usually consists of various combinations of acetylene, propane, oxygen, natural gas, and compressed air. The combinations and types of fuel used determine the temperature of the flame. For sodium and potassium determinations, a propane-compressed air flame appears entirely adequate. The atomizer and the flame are critical components of a flame photometer. The most important variable in the flame itself is the temperature, since the energy emitted by the metal ions is measured and the number of energized metal ions is dependent on the temperature of the flame. Frequent standardization of flame photometers is essential because thermal changes occur and affect the operation of the instrument and subsequent measurements with it.

Flame photometers must also have a filter, prism, grating, or other device for selecting light of the appropriate wavelength for the element to be measured. These devices spread or disperse the light into its spectral components. The desired wavelength is selected by means of a narrow slit. In this respect the flame photometer is similar to the spectrophotometer. In fact, the light source described for the spectrophotometer has been replaced with an atomizer-flame combination in the flame photometer. The flame photometer must also have an electronic measuring device to detect the intensity of the emitted light. Photocells or phototubes are used to detect the light intensity by converting the light into an electrical current. The amount of current generated is proportional to the quantity of light that reaches the detector. The amount of current is measured by a galvanometer or other recording device (see under Photometry).

The intensity of color is proportional to the amount of the element burned in the flame. When measuring an unknown sample, its intensity of color is compared with that of a standard solution of the element being measured. For example, a standard solution of potassium is used for measuring potassium. This is an example of a flame photometer that operates on an absolute or direct principle.

In another commonly used method of flame photometry, the principle of the *internal standard* is applied. Most modern flame photometers employ an internal standard. In this method, another element, usually lithium, is added to all solutions analyzed—blanks, standards, and unknowns. Lithium is usually absent from biological fluids and it has a high emission intensity. It also emits at a wavelength sufficiently distant from that of potassium or sodium to permit spectral isolation. In flame photometry using the internal standard principle, the emission of the unknown element (sodium or potassium) is compared with that of the reference element lithium. By measuring the ratios of the emissions, any change in gas or air pressure, line voltage, flame temperature, rate of atomization, or other small variable will be minimized because both the unknown element and the reference element are affected simultaneously. A specially designed adaptation of the machine is used for this purpose, and the ratio of the reference lithium and unknown metal emissions is measured by two detectors. Two filter systems are set up, one for the unknown and one for the lithium reference. Lithium does not function as a "true" standard in its use as a reference solution. Therefore, various known concentrations of potassium or sodium are prepared and used to establish calibration curves. The use of lithium as the reference solution can cause problems, however, because lithium salts are now being given to certain patients treated for manic-depressive psychosis. In these patients, the lithium level must be measured.

AUTOMATION IN THE LABORATORY

One of the most revolutionary changes in the clinical laboratory has been the introduction of automated analysis. The demand for laboratory data has grown to such an extent, through the use of the data by physicians in the diagnosis and treatment of disease, that automation has become essential to process the increasing number of requests for laboratory determinations. Physicians have become more and more dependent on the clinical laboratory for accurate, fast results. The first practical automated system was introduced into the clinical laboratory in 1957.[14] Automation provides a means by which an increased work load can be processed rapidly and reproducibly. It does not necessarily improve the accuracy of the results.

Numerous instruments for automation have been devised since 1957, when the first system, employing the *continuous-flow* principle, was conceived by Skeggs. This system was introduced commercially as the AutoAnalyzer (Technicon Instruments Corp., Tarrytown, N.Y.) and has since been used extensively by many laboratories. It has undergone several refinements and modifications, so that the latest units have much more versatility than the original instrument. In the continuous-flow system, samples follow each other in sequence through a channel. Another group of instruments employs the principle of *discrete-sample processing.* Each specimen is processed separately, generally in steps, somewhat as in the conventional manual method. A third principle recently developed makes use of *centrifugal force* to transfer and mix samples and reagents.

All of these automated systems must include some kind of sampling device, a mechanism to add the necessary reagents and sample, modules that can incubate when necessary, measuring modules (usually a photometer), and a recording device. These steps are all necessary in a manual procedure, and generally these same steps must be carried out in the automated system. Auto-

matic analyzers usually employ the same reagents and principles as do the manual methods. The precision is greater in automatic systems, however, because the operation of the machine is under better control and manual intervention has been replaced by mechanical intervention. These systems essentially perform the same chemistry as the manual methods do. Almost any manual method can be adapted to an automatic analyzer. As with any piece of laboratory equipment, the manufacturer's instructions must be followed exactly to ensure proper use of the apparatus.

Whether a laboratory determination is done manually or automatically, certain individual steps are necessary. It is generally advisable to perform as many steps as possible without manual intervention to increase efficiency. The usual steps followed include: collecting and labeling the specimen, transporting the specimen to the laboratory, properly processing the specimen before analysis, measuring the desired constituents, and reporting the results to the physician. Several of these steps can be automated for faster and more accurate results. Some methods and procedures have been partially automated, or semiautomated, by use of mechanical pipetting and diluting devices. Full automation reduces the possibility of human errors that arise from repetitive and boring manipulations done by laboratory technicians, such as pipetting errors in routine procedures.

Originally, automation was used for the tests done most frequently in the clinical laboratory. Automation is used in many areas of the laboratory, and in many larger laboratories today, very few procedures are done manually. Perhaps the chemistry department is the area in which the advent of automation has made the greatest difference. In hematology, automation has also made a great change in the work done. Electronic cell counters have replaced manual counting of white blood cells, red blood cells, and platelets in many laboratories. There is a completely automated system for Wright staining of blood smears. For coagulation studies several automated and semiautomated units are available. Prothrombin time and activated partial thromboplastin time determinations can be done automatically on various instruments. Semiautomatic instruments are also used, especially for dilution. Several instruments are available for precise and convenient diluting, which both aspirate the sample and wash it out with the diluent. Some automatic diluters dispense and dilute in separate processes. There is also an automated instrument for performing routine urinalysis determinations.

To ensure the accuracy of results obtained with automated systems, there must be frequent standardization of methods. Once the standardization has been done, a well-designed automated system maintains or reproduces the prescribed conditions with great precision. Frequent standardization and running of control specimens is essential to ensure this accuracy and precision. If an automated system is basically sound and in good working order, there are many advantages to its use: large numbers of samples may be processed with minimal technician time, two or more methods may be performed simultaneously, precision is superior to that of a manual method, and calculations may not be required. Sometimes the automatic systems are so impressive in their appearance that laboratory technicians put too much faith in them and are misled about their shortcomings. These machines must be understood and their potential problems noted and remembered. Some problems that may arise with many automated units are: (1) there may be limitations in the methodology that can be used

(sometimes a compromise must be made that results in less accurate, although often more precise, values than are obtained with manual methods); (2) with automation, technicians are often discouraged from making observations and using discretion about potential problems; (3) many systems are impractical to use for small numbers of samples, and therefore manual methods are still necessary as backup procedures for emergency individual analyses; (4) backup procedures must be available in case of instrument failures; (5) automated systems are expensive to purchase and maintain—regular maintenance requires technician time as well as the time of trained service personnel; and (6) there is often an accumulation of irrelevant data because it is so easy to produce the results—that is, tests are run that are not always necessary.

The fact that automation has found its way into the clinical laboratory does not mean that the technician is not important. There still are many laboratories where manual procedures are used, especially in smaller hospitals, where the number of laboratory determinations does not always justify the purchase of an automated system. Many smaller hospital laboratories do lease these units, however, and so the size of the hospital does not always limit the use of automated equipment. Backup manual procedures are always necessary in case of equipment failure, and these procedures must be set up and ready to use when needed. The emphasis of the laboratory has turned to speedy results, with accuracy and precision maintained. Automation has enabled the laboratory to accommodate the increased demand for determinations.

ENSURING RELIABLE LABORATORY RESULTS

Results obtained through laboratory determinations are used by the physician both to discover the existence of disease in an individual and to follow his or her progress under treatment. In turn, it is the responsibility of the clinical laboratory to the patient and the physician to ensure that the results reported are reliable and to give the physician an estimate of what constitutes a normal individual.

When describing the *reliability* of a particular

procedure, two terms are commonly used: *accuracy* and *precision*. The reliability of a procedure depends on a combination of these two factors, although they are different and are not dependent on each other. The *accuracy* of a procedure refers to the closeness of the result obtained to the true or actual value, while the *precision* refers to repeatability or reproducibility—that is, the ability to get the same value in subsequent tests. It is possible to have great precision, where all laboratory personnel performing the same procedure arrive at the same answer, without accuracy, if the answer does not represent the actual value being tested for. On the other hand, a procedure may be extremely accurate, yet so difficult to perform that individual laboratory personnel are unable to arrive at values that are close enough to be clinically meaningful.

Sources of variance (error)

In general, it is impossible to obtain exactly the same result each time a determination is performed on a particular specimen. This may be described as the variance (or error) of a procedure. Variance is a general term that describes all of the factors or fluctuations that affect the measurement of the substance in question. These many factors include limitations of the procedure itself and limitations related to the sampling mechanism used.

One of the major difficulties in guaranteeing reliable results involves the sampling procedure. Only a very small amount of sample is taken—for example, 5-10 ml of a total blood volume of 5-6 L, approximately $\frac{1}{1000}$ of the total blood volume. Other sources of variance that involve the sample include the time of day at which the sample is obtained, the patient's position (lying down or seated), the patient's state of physical activity (in bed, ambulatory, or physically active), the interval since last eating (fasting or not), and the time interval and storage conditions

between obtaining the specimen and processing by the laboratory.

Still other sources of variance involve aging of the sample, chemicals, or reagents; personal bias or limited experience of the person performing the determination; and laboratory bias because of variations in standards, reagents, environment, methods, or apparatus. There may also be experimental error resulting from changes in the method used for a particular determination, changes in instruments, or changes in personnel.

The clinical laboratory must make use of a variety of tools to ensure reliable results. These will be described more fully later in this section. In very general terms, accuracy can be aided by the use of the following: (1) properly standardized procedures, (2) statistically valid comparisons of new methods with established reference methods, (3) the use of samples of known values (controls), and (4) participation in proficiency testing programs. Precision can be measured by the proper inclusion of standards, reference samples, or control solutions, statistically valid replicate determinations of a single sample, or duplicate determinations of sufficient numbers of unknown samples. Day-to-day and between-run precision is measured by inclusion of blind samples and control specimens.

What is normal?

Before physicians can determine whether an individual is diseased, they must have an idea of what is normal. This is not an easy task, yet it is the responsibility of the clinical laboratory to supply the physician with this information. Much attention is being paid to the description of what constitutes normal, yet our knowledge remains quite limited. Many factors enter into this determination. There are variations because of such factors as age, sex, race, geographic location, and ethnic, cultural, and economic characteristics, plus internal factors related to the actual analytical methods and practices used by a particular laboratory. To complicate matters, an individual may show daily physiological variations within his or her normal range, to say nothing of normal changes with age. Biometrics (the science of statistics applied to biological observations) is a rapidly expanding field that attempts to describe these variations. The selection of a group on which to base "normals" is another problem confronting the individual laboratory. Traditionally, normals have been defined by testing such groups as blood donors, persons who are working and "feeling healthy," medical students, student nurses, and medical technologists. Many of the old established normals reported in the medical literature have questionable validity because of such factors as poor sampling techniques, questionable selection of the normal group, and questionable use of clinical methods. In developing normal values the proper statistical tools of sampling, selection of the normal comparison group, and analysis of data must be used. Such statistical tools are relatively well defined; however, such a statistical description is beyond the scope of this text.

Statistically, the range of normal for a particular measurement is in most cases related to a normal bell-shaped curve (see Fig. 1-19). Such a distribution has been shown to be correct for virtually all types of biological, chemical, and physical measurements.[15] A statistically valid series of individuals who are thought to represent a normal group are measured and the average

value is calculated. This mathematical average is defined as the mean ($\bar{X}$). The distribution of all values around the average for the particular group measured is statistically described by the standard deviation (SD). In any normal population, 68 percent of the values will be clustered above and below the average and defined statistically as falling within the first standard deviation (±1 SD). The second standard deviation represents 95 percent of the values falling equally above and below the average; while 99.7 percent will be included within the third standard deviation (±3 SD). [Again, variations occur equally above and below the average value (or mean) for any measurement.] Thus, in determining normal values for a particular measurement, a statistically valid series of individuals is chosen and is assumed to represent a normal group. These persons are then tested and all results are averaged. The limits (or range) of normal are then defined in terms of the standard deviation from the average value.

In evaluating an individual's state of health, values outside the third standard deviation value are considered clearly abnormal. Values within the first (68 percent) and second (95 percent) standard deviation limits are considered normal, while those between the second (95 percent) and third (99.7 percent) standard deviation limits are questionable. Thus, normal values will be stated as a range of values. In the past this stated range has been in terms of standard deviation units. Recently, normals have become increasingly described in terms of 95 percent confidence limits. Normal values or confidence limits should also be described in terms of age range and sex.

It is important to realize that so-called normals will vary with innumerable factors, but especially between laboratories and between geographic locations. Thus, it is necessary for each laboratory to give the physician information concerning the range of normals for that particular laboratory. The values will be related to an overall normal, yet they may be more refined or narrow and they may be skewed in the particular situa-

Fig. 1-19. Normal bell-shaped curve.

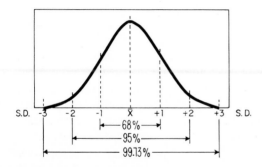

tion in question. Although several textbooks are available that describe normal values for virtually all laboratory measurements, and generally accepted normal values are given in such books, the most important indicator of disease is the situation in the clinician's particular institution and locale.

Finally, it is hoped that increasing standards and improving the quality of all clinical laboratories will bring all of these normals closer to an overall value, while parameters describing what constitutes a physiologically normal situation will become established as biometry is further advanced.

Means of control of laboratory error (variance)

Every clinical laboratory must have a means of ensuring that a particular procedure is performed in such a way that the day-to-day results are within the established precision for the procedure, and that the values reported to the physician represent the true clinical condition of the patient. Control of laboratory error is influenced and maintained by the following factors. The physician must depend on the laboratory values and will complain if these values are not those expected from the clinical diagnosis. Thus, the laboratory must be sure that the results it gives for any determination are clinically correct. This is done primarily through the use of a *quality control program*, which makes use of standards and control samples. Other factors influencing the control of laboratory variance are expanding state and federal regulations and participation in various proficiency testing programs, either voluntarily or because of legal mandate.

In controlling the reliability of laboratory determinations, the objective is to reject results when there is evidence that more than the permitted amount of error has occurred. The clinical laboratory has several ways of controlling the reliability of the results it turns out. When chemical determinations are performed, the term *batch* or *run* is often used. A batch or run is a collection of any number of specimens to be analyzed plus any or all of the following aids for ensuring reliable results—that is, controlling the variance of the procedure:

1. Standard solutions
2. Blanks (these are used only for photometric procedures)
3. Control specimens
4. Duplicates
5. Recoveries (these are used only occasionally)

Standard solutions

To determine the concentration of a substance in a specimen, there must be a basis of comparison. For analyses that result in a colored solution, a photometer is used to make this comparison (see under Photometry). The buret is also used in the clinical laboratory for comparison, in titration for volumetric analysis (see under Titration).

A standard solution is one that contains a known, exact amount of the substance being measured in the sample. The standard solution is measured accurately and then treated as if it were a specimen with contents to be determined. Standard solutions are prepared from high-quality chemicals that have been dried and placed in a desiccator. The standard chemical is weighed on the analytical balance and diluted volumetrically. This standard solution is usually most stable in a concentrated form, in which case it is usually referred to as a *stock* standard. Working standards (a more dilute form of the stock standard) are prepared from the stock, and sometimes an intermediate form is prepared. The working standard is the one employed in the actual determination. Stock and working standards are usually stored in the refrigerator. The accuracy of the procedure is absolutely dependent on the standard solution used; therefore extreme care must be taken whenever these solutions are prepared or used in a clinical laboratory.

To use the standard solution as a basis of comparison in quantitative analysis with the photometer, a series of calibrated colorimeter cuvettes (or tubes) are prepared. Each cuvette has a different amount of the standard solution. In this way, a series of cuvettes is available containing various known amounts of the standard. Standard cuvettes are carried through the same developmental steps (usually from the filtrate stage) as cuvettes containing specimens to be measured. This set of standard cuvettes is read in the photometer and the galvanometer readings are recorded. These readings can be recorded in percent transmittance or in absorbance units (see under Photometry).

Blanks

For every procedure using the photometer, a blank must be included in the batch. The blank contains reagents used in the procedure, but it does not contain the substance to be measured. It is treated with the same reagents and processed along with the undetermined specimens and the standards. The blank solution is set to read $100\%T$ on the galvanometer viewing scale. In other words, the blank tube is set to transmit 100 percent of the light. The other cuvettes in the same batch (undetermined specimens and standards, for example) transmit only a fraction of this light, because they contain particles that absorb light (particles of the unknown substance), and thus only part of the 100 percent is transmitted. Using a blank solution corrects for any color that may be present because of the reagents used or an interaction between those reagents.

Control specimens

Some type of control system to ensure reliable results in the clinical laboratory is essential, a fact that has been proved by numerous laboratory accuracy surveys. Control specimens have long been routinely included in the clinical chemistry laboratory as well as in routine hemoglobin determinations. More recently, all clinical laboratory departments, such as the urinalysis laboratory, have recognized the need for quality control programs and specimens.

The use of control specimens is based on the fact that repeated determinations on the same or different portions (or aliquots) of the same sample will not, as a rule, give identical values for any particular constituent. There are many factors that can produce variations in laboratory analyses. However, with a properly designed control system, it is possible to be aware of the variables and to keep them under control. The control system that is used in most laboratories is the *quality control program.* The quality control program for the laboratory makes use of a *control specimen*, which is similar in composition to the unknown specimen and is included in every batch or run. It must be carried through the entire test procedure, treated in exactly the same way as any unknown specimen, and will be affected by any or all of the variables that affect the unknown specimen. If the value of the control specimen for a particular method is not within the predetermined acceptable range, it must be assumed that the values obtained for the unknown specimens are also incorrect. After the procedure has been reviewed for any indication of error, and the error has been found and corrected, the batch must be repeated until the control value falls in the acceptable range.

If the control value in a determination is out of the acceptable range (out of control), one or more of the following factors may be responsible: (1) deterioration of reagents or standards, (2) faulty instrument or equipment, (3) dirty glassware, (4) lack of attention to timing or incubation temperature, (5) use of a method not suited to the needs and facilities of the laboratory, (6) use of poor technique by the technician because of carelessness or lack of proper training, and (7) statistics: a certain percentage of all determinations will be statistically out of control.

Control specimens can be divided into two main categories: those prepared commercially and those prepared by the individual laboratory.

Commercially prepared controls can be purchased from a manufacturer. These control solutions are obtained in small samples, called *aliquots*, prepared originally from a large pooled supply of serum or plasma. Commercial controls are usually obtained in a lyophilized (or dried) form. Care must be taken in reconstituting the material to add exactly the correct amount of diluent (usually deionized or distilled water) and to make certain that the material is completely dissolved and well mixed. Commercial control solutions generally have an expiration date, the date by which they must be used in order to give reliable results. Controls should not be used after the expiration date. Reconstituted control solutions must be used within a relatively short period of time, which is generally specified by the manufacturer. Commercial control material may be purchased either assayed or unassayed. Assayed control preparations have been tested by the manufacturer and stated values are given for each of the constituents. The manufacturer should provide information concerning the analytical method and statistical procedures used in arriving at the stated values, so that the laboratory can determine the appropriateness of the material for its particular methods and practices. If unassayed control preparations are used, the laboratory will have to establish its own range of acceptable results for each constituent being measured. The method of arriving at this acceptable range is the same as that used in establishing limits for "homemade" control solutions, to be described later. Tentative standards for manufacturers of control preparations were established in 1972 by the National Committee for Clinical Laboratory Standards (NCCLS).

Control solutions can also be prepared by the individual laboratory. In the case of control specimens for most chemistry determinations,

excess serum or plasma is saved at the end of each day and frozen. Such control solutions are particularly practical for larger laboratories; it may be impossible for the smaller laboratory to collect enough serum or plasma to make a control pool. In this case, the commercially prepared product is preferable. After a pool of the serum or plasma has accumulated that amounts to about 2 or 3 L, the control specimens for daily use can be made. Only normal serum or plasma is saved (not lipemic or hemolyzed, for example). When enough serum has been saved, it is thawed and mixed thoroughly. After thorough mixing, the pool is divided into aliquots of a convenient size. Aliquots of 2–3 ml in a small tube or vial are satisfactory. These samples are then stored in a freezer. When such a pool is prepared it is always possible that it may be contaminated with serum hepatitis virus, as shown by a positive test for hepatitis B antigen. Therefore every effort should be made to exclude serum from the pool from patients with hepatitis. In addition, the final pool should be tested for hepatitis B antigen by a radioimmunoassay technique. Such tests of commercially prepared sera have been shown to be positive for hepatitis B antigen; thus both homemade and commercial sera should be handled with proper precautions.

The preceding paragraphs have described control preparations for use in the clinical chemistry laboratory. However, control solutions or preparations are available commercially or may be prepared for all departments in the clinical laboratory. The use of such control material will be further described in subsequent sections of this book.

Once a control solution has been prepared or chosen, it is necessary for the laboratory to determine the acceptable control range for a particular analysis. There are various ways of establishing such a range, and one commonly employed method will be described; however, any method must adhere to statistically acceptable methods. In establishing the control range, an aliquot of the pooled serum or a commercial control specimen is processed along with the regular batch of tests for 15–25 days. It is imperative to thoroughly mix the thawed aliquot since the sample layers as it freezes. In testing the control sample it is important that it be treated exactly like an unknown specimen; it must not be treated any more or less carefully than the unknown specimen.

As mentioned previously, repeated determinations on different aliquots of the same sample will not give identical values for any particular constituent. However, it has been shown that if a sufficient number of repeated determinations are made, the values obtained will fall into a normal bell-shaped curve, as described under What Is Normal? (see Fig. 1-19). When a statistically sufficient number of determinations have been run (the number is different for averaged duplicate determinations and single tests) the mathematical mean ($\bar{X}$) or average value can be calculated. The acceptable limits or variation from the mean for the control solution are then calculated on the basis of the standard deviation from the mean, using certain statistical formulas. Most laboratories use two standard deviation units (2 SD) above and below the mean as the allowable range of the control specimen, while others use this range as a warning limit. Referring back to the normal bell-shaped curve (Fig. 1-19), setting 2 SD as the allowable range for the control sample means that 95 percent of all determinations on that sample will fall within the allowable range, while 5 percent will be out of control. It may not be desirable to disallow this many batches, so the third standard deviation may be chosen as the limit of control, or the action limit. Once the range of acceptable results has been established, one of the control specimens is included in each batch of determinations. If the control value is not within the limits established, the procedure must be repeated, and no results may be given to the physician until the control value is within the allowable range.

It is conventional in most laboratories to plot the daily control specimen values on a quality control chart, as shown in Fig. 1-20. The control chart is made on a rectangular sheet of linear graph paper. Monthly control charts are prepared, with the days of the month marked on the horizontal axis and units of concentration for the determination in question marked on the vertical axis. The mean value for the determination in question is then indicated on the chart in addition to the limits of acceptable error. The 2 and 3 SD values might be indicated with the 2 SD value as a warning limit and the 3 SD value an action limit. Each day the control value is plotted on the chart, and any value falling out of control can easily be seen.

The control chart serves as a visual representation of the information derived from using control specimens. A different control chart is plotted for each substance tested for by the laboratory. It is possible to observe trends leading toward trouble by plotting the control values daily. When procedural changes such as the addition of new reagents, standards, or instruments are made, they are also noted on the control chart. Such a chart can assist in preventing difficulties and can aid in troubleshooting. If all is going well, the plotted control values should be distributed equally above and below the established mean value. A regular weekly visual inspection of the control chart is particularly useful for observing trends before control specimen values are actually out of the established acceptable limits. Generally, an excess of more than five control value results on one side of the mean indicates a trend, although not all such trends need action.[16]

It should be remembered that for the control specimen to have meaning in terms of the reliability of all results reported by the laboratory, it must be treated exactly like any unknown specimen. It does the patient and physician no good to have the control specimen within the allowable range if the value reported for the unknown is not accurate and precise. Once again, the use of quality control specimens is an indication of the overall reliability (both accuracy and precision) of the results reported by the laboratory.

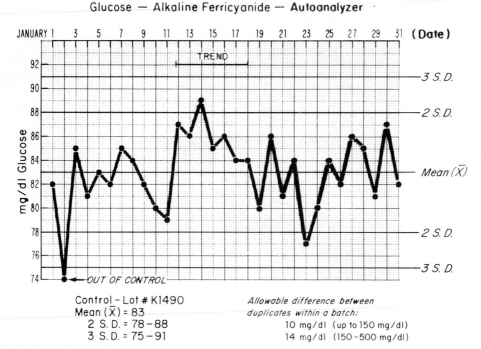

Fig. 1-20. Monthly control chart.

Duplicate determinations

In each batch of determinations, one of the specimens is measured in duplicate. This specimen is chosen at random from those to be tested. Often control specimens are measured in duplicate. If this is done, the allowable range for duplicates is less than that for single determinations. The use of duplicates checks the manual technique used—that is, the precision, or repeatability, of the method. Duplicates do not measure accuracy. It is possible to have grossly inaccurate duplicate results that agree perfectly. The allowable difference between duplicate determinations varies and must be established for each determination performed by the laboratory. This is done using certain statistical formulas; the standard deviation is calculated from the differences between a certain number of duplicate determinations. Duplicate determinations are also part of the quality control program.

Recovery solutions

Recovery solutions are used as an indicator of the accuracy of a particular determination. To any specimen in the batch (or to a control solution), in addition to the regular specimens, a measured amount of the pure substance being analyzed is added. Theoretically, the amount of substance added should be recovered at the end of the determination if the method is an accurate one. Recoveries are not used routinely with most procedures, but are often used to evaluate a new procedure. One method to be discussed in this text, the blood urea nitrogen determination, uses a recovery solution as part of the regular batch.

Recovery solutions are another part of the quality control program.

Proficiency surveys

Proficiency surveys are a means of establishing quality control between laboratories. Both state and national agencies have established programs to help laboratories maintain their quality control programs. Proficiency testing programs are available through the College of American Pathologists (CAP), the Center for Disease Control (CDC), the American Association of Bioanalysts (AAB), and various state health departments. These proficiency programs periodically send specimens to laboratories that choose to participate in the program. The laboratory analyzes the sample, using its routine procedures, and sends the results to the program administrator. Each participating laboratory is furnished with an evaluation of its results compared to those of all other laboratories participating in the survey. Participation in at least one proficiency survey is an important part of a laboratory's quality control program.

Quality control programs

Mentioning a quality control system immediately brings to mind the inclusion of a control sample in each batch or run of determinations. As discussed previously, the control sample may be obtained commercially or prepared by the individual laboratory. The most important consideration is that it be routinely included with each group of laboratory determinations, or in certain instances at least each day, by each person performing the determinations. However, the quality control program established by a laboratory involves much more than the use of control samples. We have already discussed the use of standards, blanks, duplicates, and recoveries as part of the quality control program. The use of automated procedures in place of manual methods often requires the inclusion of additional standards and controls both between specimens and at the end of the run. Other components of a quality control program will now be considered and reviewed.[17,18]

First, consider the specimen itself—how it is collected, transported to the laboratory, received, identified, processed, and stored. The specimen should be visually inspected for hemolysis or lipemia, as these might affect or invalidate certain determinations. Certainly their presence should be recorded with the final result. Later, in photometric procedures, the technician should look at the final solution in the cuvette for turbidity or inappropriate color development.

Another part of the quality control program concerns the way new procedures are validated before they are included among the methods routinely used by the laboratory. Each laboratory must determine the reproducibility (or confidence limits) for each procedure used and establish acceptable limits of variation for control specimens. The quality control program includes calculation of the mean (or average value) and standard deviation and preparation of control charts for each procedure.

The program should include a means of independent monitoring to minimize bias on the part of the technician. This may be done by using blind controls, such as commercial control solutions labeled as patient unknowns, or dividing patient specimens into different aliquots to be processed blindly and independently on the same day, or carried over to another day if the constituent is stable. Another valuable quality control technique is to look at the data generated for each patient and inspect them for relationships between the results obtained by the laboratory. There are many relationships, such as the mathematical relationship between anions and cations in the electrolyte report, the correlation between protein and casts in urine, and the relationship between hemoglobin and the hematocrit and the appearance of the blood smear in hematologic studies.

Each laboratory must have an assessment routine for all procedures to be done on a daily, weekly, and monthly basis to detect problems such as trends and shifts of the established mean value. When such problems are indicated, it is most important that they be corrected and not ignored. Many of these ingredients of the quality control program are the responsibility of the laboratory supervisor and/or director. However, every technician has an important role in ensuring reliable laboratory results, either by running the control specimen or by calling potential problems to the attention of the supervisor. Finally, in addition to the internal quality control program, each laboratory should take part in at least one external proficiency testing program.

COLLECTION, PRESERVATION, AND PREPARATION OF LABORATORY SPECIMENS

The accuracy of the many laboratory tests done on biological specimens from patients depends on proper collection, preservation, and preparation of the samples actually analyzed. The laboratory test can be no better than the specimen on which it is performed. If the specimen is improperly collected, is not stored correctly, or is generally mishandled in some way, the most quantitatively perfect determination is of no use because the results are invalid and cannot be used by the physician in diagnosis or treatment.

All samples sent to the laboratory must be handled initially according to certain general rules. Each division of the laboratory will have unique requirements for specimens used in that division, but there are several general statements that apply to all specimens. Special requirements for the collection, preservation, and preparation of laboratory specimens will be discussed where appropriate in subsequent chapters.

Initial identification of the patient is extremely important. It is essential that a specimen from a particular patient is placed in the container labeled for that patient. The patient's name, hospital identification number, and room number are commonly found on the label. All specimens sent to the laboratory must be properly labeled. An unlabeled container or one labeled improperly should never be accepted by the laboratory. Some labels must also include the time of collection of the specimen and the type of specimen.

A properly completed request slip should accompany all specimens sent to the laboratory.

Several different kinds of specimens are handled routinely in the clinical laboratory. The specimen most often thought of in connection with the clinical laboratory is blood. It is true that blood represents a large percentage of the specimens sent to the laboratory, but urine specimens are also sent in great numbers. Blood and urine specimens will be discussed throughout this book under the various laboratory departments covered.

Laboratory specimens

Many pathological conditions may be associated with the fluid that accumulates in the various cavities of the body. Laboratory examination of the fluid may yield useful information regarding its formation and constituents. The physician can also be alerted to the type of disease process present by the information obtained from the laboratory analysis of a patient's various body fluids. In addition to blood and urine, some of the body fluids examined in the laboratory are pleural, pericardial, peritoneal, synovial, and cerebrospinal.

Urine

The urine specimen has been referred to as a liquid tissue biopsy of the urinary tract that is painlessly and easily obtained. Urine yields a great amount of valuable information quickly and economically but, as for all other human specimens used in the laboratory, the specimen must be carefully collected, preserved, and handled for the information to be regarded as reliable. A routine urine analysis (urinalysis) is included with virtually all hospital admissions.

The composition of urine in random samples collected at different times during the day is likely to vary considerably, because the work of the kidney is so variable. It is not practical to collect an entire day's specimen (24-hour specimen), as it would take too long for any results to be ready for the physician; also, as urine stands, many of the more important constituents found in it disappear or are altered. A 24-hour specimen is required only when it is necessary to know the entire day's volume of urine output, or for quantitative tests in which the exact amount of urine must be known so that the exact amount of substance present may be reported.

Since a 24-hour collection is not necessary for a routine urinalysis, any random specimen that is passed during the day may be used. The first urine voided in the morning is usually recommended as most suitable. This is true primarily because the first morning specimen is the most concentrated one passed during the day. It is more concentrated because less fluid (or water) is excreted during the night, while the same amount of solid or dissolved substance must be excreted for the kidney to perform its function of maintaining the composition of the extracellular fluid. When testing for the presence of urine sugar, the best specimen to use is one voided 2–3 hours after a meal. This is the one exception to the recommended use of the first morning specimen.

It is of prime importance that the containers used to collect the urine specimen be clean and dry. Several types of containers are suitable for this purpose. Glass jars, disposable paraffined containers, and plastic bags or jars are most often used. Disposable wax-coated paper specimen con-tainers and disposable plastic containers are available in several sizes and are preferred by many for routine screening urinalysis. Conical containers are less likely to tip over. Sterile kits for collecting urine for microbiological studies (cultures) are available. There are also special pediatric urine-collecting bags made of clear polyethylene. If a 24-hour pediatric specimen is required, a special tube can be attached to the bag, which is in turn connected to a collection bottle.[19] Large glass or plastic containers with wide mouths and screw caps are used to collect 24-hour samples from adults, usually with added preservatives. The collection bottles may be refrigerated between voidings. Any bedpans that are used to collect voided urine must be scrupulously clean.

Preservation of urine specimens

If a fresh specimen of urine is left at room temperature for a period of time, the urine rapidly undergoes changes. It is for this reason that a good routine urinalysis should include the use of a *fresh specimen*. Decomposition of urine begins within $\frac{1}{2}$ hour after collection. The various laboratory tests to be done on a specimen of urine should be done within $\frac{1}{2}$ hour after collection, if possible; no longer than 1 or 2 hours should elapse before the tests are done unless the urine is preserved in some way.

If it is impossible to examine the urine specimen when fresh or if a 24-hour collection is required, the *urine must be preserved*. Various methods of preserving urine are available, most of which inhibit the growth of bacteria, thus preventing many of the alterations from occurring. One such method is refrigeration. If a chemical preservative is not added, the specimen may be kept 6–8 hours under refrigeration with no gross alterations. Several chemical preservatives are available, one of which is toluene. This is a liquid that works by preventing the growth of bacteria. A thin layer of toluene is added, just enough to cover the surface of the urine. The toluene should be skimmed off or the urine pipetted from beneath it when the urine is examined. Toluene, or the commercially available product toluol, is the best all-around preservative, because it does not interfere with the various tests done in the routine urinalysis. Other common preservatives for urine specimens are formaldehyde (or Formalin), chloroform, thymol, and boric acid. Thymol, a crystalline substance, works to prevent the growth of bacteria. However, thymol may interfere with tests for urine protein and bilirubin. Formalin, a liquid preservative that acts by fixing the formed elements in the urinary sediment, may also be used. It may, however, interfere with the reduction tests for urine sugar and may form a precipitate with urea that interferes with the microscopic examination of the sediment. Preservative tablets that produce formaldehyde are commercially available. These include Urokeep, Cargille Urinary Preservative Tablets, and Kingbury Clark Urine Preservative Tablets. The tablets are more convenient to use than the liquid Formalin and do not interfere with the usual chemical and microscopic examination.

Various disposable collecting systems are available commercially for collecting, storing, transporting, and testing urine specimens. New systems are continually introduced to the market.

In general, it should be remembered that a fresh urine specimen is best for urinalysis tests. It is the easiest to collect and will give the most satisfactory results.

Obtaining the urine specimen

As stated previously, the specimen for urinalysis should be collected in a clean, dry container, and the specimen should be fresh. For routine screening and for most bacteriologic examinations, a fresh, freely flowing voided urine specimen is usually suitable (see under Microbiology). The first morning specimen is the one of choice as it is the most concentrated, since the patient has not been drinking water while asleep. For most routine urinalysis, including protein content and urinary sediment constituents, the concentrated specimen is the most satisfactory one to use.

Occasionally it may be necessary to obtain a catheterized urine specimen, but this procedure is not encouraged because of the risk of patient infection. These urine specimens are obtained by introducing a small tubular instrument called a catheter into the bladder, through the urethra, for the withdrawal of urine. This procedure should be avoided whenever possible, as there is always a risk of introducing bacteria into an otherwise sterile bladder. This could initiate a urinary tract infection. Catheterized specimens are necessary when contamination by vaginal contents in female patients may alter the examination (especially during menstruation). It may also be necessary for obtaining urine specimens for bacteriologic examination when a sterile sample is needed. Under many conditions, however, a freely flowing voided specimen is satisfactory for bacteriologic cultures. Urine obtained by means of catheterization should be *handled very carefully* in the laboratory. Remember that it is an unpleasant procedure for the patient and it does involve some degree of risk.

When both a bacteriologic culture and a routine urinalysis are needed on the same specimen, the culture should always be done first and then the routine tests.

Since many urine specimens are usually sent to the laboratory on a single day, it is especially important that each container be properly labeled when it is collected from the patient. Each specimen must be accompanied by a request slip.

When a 24-hour urine specimen is sent to the laboratory, it must be ascertained first that it has been properly collected. A preservative must have been added at the beginning of the collection time, and the correct collection time must have been used (24 hours total time). In the laboratory, the total volume of specimen is measured and recorded, the urine is thoroughly mixed, and an aliquot is withdrawn for analysis.

Miscellaneous extravascular (body) fluids

When fluids normally found in small amounts in various spaces in the body increase in amount and mechanically inhibit the action of certain key organs such as the heart or lungs, or when such a fluid is needed for diagnostic purposes, the fluid is aspirated. The procedure is done under sterile conditions by a physician. Fluids aspirated from the chest, abdomen, joints, cysts, or abscesses are often brought to the laboratory for various types of tests. The origin of the fluid and the tests to be done should be noted on the container and request slip along with the usual label information required (patient name, hospital number, etc.). Many different tests can be ordered on body fluids, including chemistry determinations, cultures, cell counts and differentials, and examination for tumor cells.

The various types of extravascular fluids, or body fluids, are examined in various departments of the clinical laboratory, depending on what test is to be done and what type of fluid is to be examined. Cell counts are done on most body fluid specimens. For this reason, in many hospitals, body fluid specimens are brought first to the hematology laboratory, and are either examined there or sent on from there to a specific department.

Most normal body fluids are pale and straw-colored. As the cell count and any abnormal debris and constituents increase, the fluid becomes more turbid. All body fluids are to be received in the laboratory in a tube containing Sequestrene (EDTA) or balanced oxalate as an anticoagulant. Synovial fluid requires EDTA as an anticoagulant. The test for mucin on synovial fluid requires that no anticoagulant be added.

Since cell counts are done on many body fluid specimens, the specimen must be a fresh one. If it is not fresh, cell disintegration will occur. No cell counts may be done on a clotted specimen; anticoagulants must be used to prevent coagulation of the specimen when a cell count is needed. Specific gravity tests must also be done on a clot-free specimen. Tests for mucin and protein, however, can be done on clotted specimens. When a glucose determination is ordered, the specimen must be immediately preserved with sodium fluoride to prevent glycolysis. Body fluid specimens to be cultured should be sent to the microbiology laboratory. Specimens to be tested for a chemical constituent should be sent to the chemistry laboratory as soon as possible. Sometimes only one specimen is sent to the hematology laboratory, and several tests are required; except for culture, cell counts should always be done before other tests. For cell counts, the anticoagulant of choice is EDTA. For examination for tumor cells, the fluid may be collected in EDTA or heparin. If the fluid is collected without any anticoagulant, clotting may be observed. The presence of clotting indicates a substantial inflammatory reaction. Sometimes so much fluid is aspirated that it must be collected in a gallon jug instead of the usual tube. It is important to remember that the suitable anticoagulant must be placed in this large container just as in the tube. Most laboratory tests cannot be done on a clotted specimen of body fluid. All body fluids should be considered contaminated, and all equipment must be decontaminated with phenol after being used.

All body fluids are either *transudates* or *exudates*. Transudates are ultrafiltrates resulting from a difference in osmotic pressure across a membrane. Exudates are fluids that occur as a result of an inflammatory condition that leads to an increase in the permeability of a membrane. Generally, a transudate has a specific gravity below 1.018, a protein value of less than 2.5 g/dl, and very few cells. An exudate has a specific gravity above 1.018, a protein value greater than 2.5 g/dl, and many cells. These values often overlap in certain inflammatory states and can cause confusion about whether the fluid is a transudate or an exudate.

Synovial fluid

One special body fluid is called synovial fluid. It is the fluid that lines the joints. Normal synovial fluid resembles uncooked egg white. It is straw-colored, viscous, and does not clot. Examination of this fluid from the joints provides information about joint diseases such as infections, gout, and rheumatoid arthritis. Tests on synovial fluid include cell counts, cell differentials, crystal studies (done on fluid preserved with EDTA), and cultures (done on fluid collected in a sterile heparin tube). To test for clot formation (the mucin clot test), the fluid must be collected in a tube without anticoagulant. Glucose determination requires collection in sodium fluoride.

Cerebrospinal fluid

Cerebrospinal fluid is the most frequently tested body fluid other than blood or urine. It fills the ventricles of the brain, the central canal of the spinal cord, and the subarachnoid spaces of the brain and spinal cord. It is formed in the ventricles and has many of the same characteristics as plasma, since most of its components are derived from the blood plasma. The only known function of the cerebrospinal fluid is a mechanical one—providing protection for the brain and spinal cord. Examination of the spinal fluid is important in the diagnosis of neurological disorders, inflammatory diseases, and hemorrhage in the meninges.

The cerebrospinal fluid, or spinal fluid, is obtained by puncturing one of the spaces between the lumbar vertebrae with a needle. It is collected by lumbar puncture into the L3 or L4 lumbar interspace to avoid damaging the spinal cord. This procedure is done by a physician. The spinal fluid is usually collected into three or four sterile containers (numbered according to the order of collection), each containing between 1 and 3 ml of fluid. It is essential that the containers be properly labeled and handled with extreme care as the procedure of collection cannot be easily repeated. There is a certain risk to the patient in this procedure and for this reason the specimen is extremely precious and must be treated with the utmost care. Cerebrospinal fluid is also considered contaminated, and precautions must be taken to decontaminate all equipment used in connection with the specimen. A 5% phenol or 70% alcohol solution can be used for decontamination. There is always the danger of contracting meningitis if cerebrospinal fluids are not handled properly. Cell counts on a spinal fluid specimen must be done as soon as possible after the spinal tap has been completed, since the cells present will disintegrate within a short time. Tests for glucose in spinal fluid must also be performed immediately to prevent glycolysis. The use of sodium fluoride will slow down the glycolytic process. For the chemical tests ordered, the specimen should be sent to the chemistry laboratory.

Normal cerebrospinal fluid appears clear and colorless. If the fluid is grossly bloody or blood-tinged, the patient may have a serious brain or spinal injury. Sometimes, however, a drop of blood gets into the sample from the puncture needle. It is important for this reason to observe the collected tubes and to note the order in which they were collected. If blood has gotten into the tube from a traumatic tap (blood from the needle, skin, or muscle) the tubes will progressively clear. That is, the first tube collected will have blood in it and the successive tubes will have less. This is one reason why it is important to observe *all* the tubes collected, not just one. If all the tubes are bloody to the same degree, a hemorrhage in the brain or spinal cord is more likely. If the spinal fluid in the tubes appears cloudy, there is good reason to suspect an infection in the central nervous system. Most conditions for which spinal fluid is requested are very serious and require immediate diagnosis and treatment. This is why the laboratory tests are so important and speed is essential.

Swabs for culture

Cotton swabs with samples of specimens from wounds, abscesses, throats, and so forth are brought to the laboratory in a sterile tube for culture. These swabs are potentially from infectious areas and should be treated very carefully in the laboratory. Again, the tube with the swab in it must be properly labeled and the culture done immediately (see under Microbiology). Most bacteria will die if stored on a dry cotton swab, so if the culture cannot be done immediately some means to keep the swab moist and cool must be used. Most organisms can live for many hours if stored properly. Immediate culture is still the best plan, however. Proper technique for disposal of contaminated material must be used.

Feces

Feces, or stool specimens, should be collected in a clean container made of cardboard, preferably plastic-covered. The specimen should be collected and covered without being contaminated with urine. The amount collected depends on the test to be done. The container should be labeled properly, including the time of collection (24-hour specimen, for example) and the laboratory tests desired.

Blood

As discussed previously, blood represents a large percentage of the total specimens used in laboratory determinations. In many cases, laboratory personnel collect the blood specimens. It is important, therefore, to include a thorough discussion of the proper means for collecting, preserving, and handling blood samples. Because it is relatively easy to obtain a blood sample, numerous studies are done on blood in diseased and normal states. Much valuable information is readily available at relatively low cost and with little discomfort to the patient. Certain routine blood studies are now part of every new hospital admission. Many of these studies are carried out in the hematology and chemistry departments (see under Hematology and Chemistry). Blood is also cultured in the microbiology department.

Approaching the patient

Anyone who plans to assume a duty or occupation where contact with patients is required must consider several factors. These persons are providing a service to the patient. Adequate performance of this service involves not only technical knowledge but sincere and concerned interest in humans. This is a quality that, unfortunately, cannot be taught readily. It is a quality that each one must learn as a part of reaching maturity. Those in the medical laboratory field must be not only academically capable but also psychologically adjusted.

A patient in the hospital experiences several emotions, including anxiety and fear. The patient is also probably not feeling well, is concerned about his or her physical condition, may be afraid of what is going to happen next, and is separated from familiar surroundings. For these and other reasons, the patient's mental state is probably at its worst during hospitalization. It is extremely important that the patient be shown kindness and understanding. The collection of blood specimens is one area where laboratory personnel have an opportunity to meet patients. It is essential, therefore, that those doing the blood collecting strive for a real understanding of what the patient is feeling. Try to imagine what it would be like if you were the patient, and act accordingly. Try to talk to patients the way you would like someone to talk to you—be friendly, pleasant, and outgoing.

When approaching a patient for the first time, there are certain procedures to remember. First, make certain that the patient on whom the test is being done is actually the right patient. Checking the hospital number of the patient is essential. Check the wrist tag of the patient to make certain it is the right patient. Ask the patient's name—this is also a good way to start conversation. A mix-up in labeling tubes or drawing blood from the wrong patient can be disastrous. Always label the tubes of blood at the bedside of the patient, as well as any slides, hemoglobin pipets, white blood cell pipets, or other materials used for taking specimens. Proper and immediate labeling is essential.

When working with a pediatric patient, you must first gain the patient's confidence. This may be the first time a child has blood drawn. If this first experience is a bad one, it will be remembered and feared for years to come. It is therefore important to take some extra time to gain the child's confidence before going ahead with the collection procedure. Get acquainted with the child by using a book or a toy, for example. Keep your equipment tray as inconspicuous as possible. Be frank with the child. Sometimes you may be able to tell a story about what you are doing. It is important in working with pediatric patients to bolster their morale as much as possible. Ask for help in restraining a very small or uncooperative child.

Older children may be more responsive when permitted to "help," by holding the gauze, for example. If your technique is efficient and you talk to the patients convincingly, you will be able to "take a picture from their finger" before they realize what has happened. Handling a child often involves handling the parents also. This is best accomplished by allowing the parents to know, by your attitude, that you are kind but very definitely in charge of the situation. This attitude, which is so basic for laboratory personnel, can be developed only with practice.

In the nursery, each hospital will have its own rules, but a few general precautions apply. After working with an infant in a crib, be sure to put up the crib sides. If an infant is in an Isolette, keep the portholes closed. When an oxygen tent is in use, do not forget to close the openings when you have finished with the baby. Never leave laboratory equipment, especially blades or needles, in the bed or room.

Adult patients must be told briefly what is expected of them and what the test involves. With adults and especially when dealing with children, complete honesty is most important. It is unwise to say that a finger puncture will not hurt, when it really will. However, if possible, avoid saying that the puncture will hurt.

Greet the patient in a friendly and tactful manner. Do not become overly familiar; carry on any conversation in a pleasant and calm manner. Tell the patient why you are there and what you are going to do. Speak quietly at all times. Discuss personal information the patient relates to you softly; this is being told to you in confidence. Respect the religious beliefs of the patient. Keep all laboratory reports confidential, and also keep any personal information about the patient confidential. Firmly refuse information about other patients or physicians. If you see the same patient frequently, become familiar with his or her interests, hobbies, or family and use these as topics of conversation. Many patients in the hospital are lonely and need a friend. Occasionally you will find, especially with the extremely ill, that patients do not wish to talk at all; in this case, respect their wishes. Do not irritate the patient. It is important to be honest, but boost the patient's morale as much as possible. Smile, be cordial, and leave the room in a friendly fashion.

Even if the patient is disagreeable (and many are), remain pleasant. It is important to repeat at this point that it is most helpful if you enter the patient's room wearing a pleasant expression; a smile will often work miracles. Be firm when the patient is unpleasant, remain cheerful, and express confidence in the work to be done. Young children who do not understand words seem pacified by the sound of a confident voice. Talking pleasantly to every patient is essential.

In a hospital setting, check before leaving the patient's room to see that you have returned everything to your laboratory tray. Keep the tray holding your supplies and equipment out of reach of the patient. This is especially important when working with children, but it applies to all patients.

Always follow the orders of the hospital or patient station regarding the procedure for isolation patients. Generally there are two types of isolation. One, called *protective* isolation, is used to protect the patient from outsiders. For example, a burn patient is very susceptible to infection, so that anyone entering the room of this type of patient must use isolation procedure. When collecting specimens from patients with leukemia, severe burns, organ transplants, body radiation therapy, and plastic surgery, who must be protected from exposure to pathogens and other bacteria, a sterile gown, cap, gloves, and mask should be worn. Shoe coverings may also be required. With a patient having a kidney transplant or dialysis, protective isolation technique should be used for the sake of the patient and extremely careful collecting technique for the sake of the laboratory. These are examples of protective isolation.

The other type of isolation is *strict* isolation. This is used to prevent the spread of a communicable disease from a patient. Strict isolation is used in cases of hepatitis B, active tuberculosis, meningococcal meningitis, polio, and certain other infectious diseases such as measles or mumps. In these instances, a gown and often a mask and gloves should be worn. When coming in contact with patients who have diseases that are spread by direct contact with a wound or discharge, such as gangrene, abscesses, impetigo, and dysenteries, a gown should be worn; gloves are often an added precaution. When in contact with patients with hepatitis B, venereal disease, or dermatosis, gloves should be worn. After collecting blood samples from any patient, but especially from patients in the high-risk categories, the hands should always be washed. Any spilled blood should be immediately wiped up with a disinfectant to prevent the spread of the disease. Whether protective or strict isolation is observed, a nurse on the station will provide instructions about procedure. Always follow these instructions explicitly.

Collection of blood specimens

Any discussion concerning blood specimens must begin with collection procedures for blood. There are two general sources of blood for clinical laboratory tests: peripheral, or capillary, blood and venous blood. This applies to all areas of the clinical laboratory. For small quantities of blood for some hematologic or microchemical determinations, capillary blood is suitable. This is obtained from the capillary bed by puncture of the skin. The tip of the finger is the site most commonly punctured. For larger quantities of blood, a puncture is made directly into a vein, using a sterile syringe and needle or vacuum tube and needle system. A vein in the upper forearm (or antecubital fossa) area is most often chosen for venipuncture as these veins are easily palpable and fairly well fixed (Fig. 1-21).

Peripheral or capillary blood

For the small quantities of blood required for most hematologic procedures and for micro-

Fig. 1-21. Major veins of the arms.

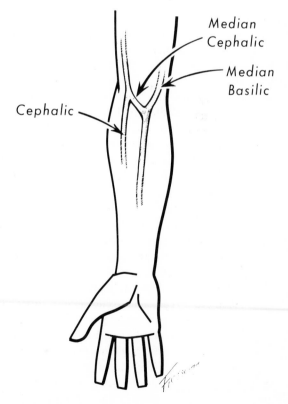

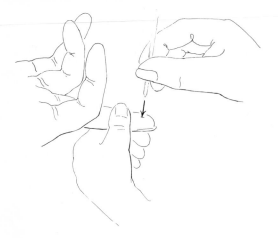

Fig. 1-22. Finger puncture technique.

techniques requiring serum or plasma, an adequate blood sample may be obtained from the capillary bed by puncture of the skin. From certain patients, such as babies, burned patients, or amputees, it may be necessary or desirable to draw only a very small amount of blood. This can be accomplished quite easily by means of capillary puncture. This blood is collected into suitable capillary tubes or pipets or used directly to prepare blood films. In adults and older children, the tip of the finger is punctured (Fig. 1-22); in infants, the plantar surface of the heel or the large toe is punctured. In general, the earlobe should be avoided for puncture because there is a slower flow of blood there and the concentration of cells and hemoglobin will be greater. Blood obtained by puncturing the earlobe has been found to contain a higher concentration of hemoglobin than fingertip or venous blood and also is not reliable for white blood cell counts.[20] The earlobe is sometimes the desirable source of blood for the preparation of blood films used to study leukocyte abnormalities, since larger cells are frequently trapped in the capillary bed because of the slow circulation. Blood obtained by skin puncture of these types is generally called capillary blood, but it is closer to arteriolar blood in its composition. The results

of tests from venous and capillary (fingertip) blood compare well if the capillary blood is free-flowing. To ensure free flow of capillary blood, the finger must be warm.

Various types of lancets or blades are used for skin puncture. The best type of blade to use is one that is disposable. Use of nondisposable blades is obsolete because of the risk of hepatitis B infection. Some blades require the operator to gauge the depth of the puncture, while others have a safety gauge on them. It is important that all used blades be discarded and that none remain in the laboratory. Infectious hepatitis B can be transmitted if blades are reused or improperly discarded (see under Safety in the Laboratory).

Procedure for finger puncture

1. Assemble the necessary equipment: lancet, alcohol pad, dry gauze, slides, and capillary tubes or other supplies necessary to receive the blood.

2. Be sure that the patient is seated comfortably.

3. Choose an area for the puncture that is free from calluses, edema, or cyanosis. Warm the puncture site if it is cold by immersing it in warm water or by rubbing it.

4. Cleanse the skin of the puncture site on the third or fourth finger vigorously with a pad soaked in 70% alcohol. This will remove dirt and epithelial debris, increase the circulation, and leave the area relatively sterile. Allow the area to air dry.

5. Grasp the finger firmly and make a quick, firm puncture about 2–3 mm deep with the sterile disposable lancet (Fig. 1-22). This puncture should be made at right angles to the fingerprint striations on the patient's finger midway between the edge and midpoint of the fingertip. The puncture should not be made too far down on the finger and should not be too close to the fingernail. A deep puncture hurts no more than a superficial one and it gives a much more satisfactory flow of blood.

6. Discard the lancet in the appropriate disposal container. Dirty lancets should never be

left lying on the work area. They should be discarded immediately after use and should not be touched again. Used lancets must be autoclaved before final disposal.)

7. Wipe away the first drop of blood, using a clean piece of dry gauze or tissue. This drop is contaminated with tissue fluid and will interfere with laboratory results if used. The succeeding drops are used for tests.

8. If a good puncture has been made, the blood will flow freely. If it does not, use gentle pressure to make the blood form a round drop. Excessive squeezing will cause dilution of the blood with tissue fluid.

9. Collect the specimens by holding a capillary tube to the blood drop or by touching the drop to a glass slide. Rapid collection is necessary to prevent coagulation, especially when several tests are to be done using blood from the same puncture site.

10. When the blood samples have been collected, have the patient hold a sterile, dry piece of gauze or cotton over the puncture site until the bleeding has stopped.

Precautions to be noted when obtaining capillary blood

If the patient's fingers are cold, slight rubbing may help to warm them. The finger or heel must not be squeezed excessively, because tissue fluid may dilute the blood sample or cause the blood to clot faster than it normally would. The first drop of blood is always removed because it contains tissue fluid, alcohol, or perspiration, which will dilute the blood. Immediately after an operation, patients with low blood pressure and those in surgical shock may require more than one puncture. Only one sterile blade is used at a time. The tip of the blade should not touch anything until it punctures the skin of the patient. Contaminated blades are thrown away and new ones used. After the puncture is made, the blade is discarded. Clean hands are essential when working with patients.

When blood is to be collected from patients on high-risk stations, such as kidney dialysis or renal transplant, extra precautions must be taken to avoid exposure to possible hepatitis B virus. Rubber gloves must be worn and any drops of blood adhering to the outside of collecting pipets or capillary tubes wiped off with alcohol. The laboratory should be alerted to the fact that these specimens may be contaminated. The request slips themselves are sometimes contaminated with blood, and this should be avoided at all cost. All persons collecting blood samples must wash their hands between patients.

Using capillary blood for hematologic studies

For the hematology laboratory, when blood is taken for blood cell counts and the hemoglobin determination (these tests involve the use of special diluting pipets), the tip of the pipet is placed in the drop of blood. The pipet is not touched to the skin. Usually the hemoglobin test is taken first. The blood measured in the hemoglobin pipet must be put into the diluent immediately and mixed well. It can be read in the photometer later. Hemoglobin pipets require more blood than the red or white cell diluting pipets; that is, a larger drop of blood is required.

White and red cell counts are done next. Blood measured in the red and white cell diluting pipets must be diluted immediately with the proper diluting fluid. After dilution, the pipets must be immediately shaken for 15 seconds. If blood and diluent are not shaken immediately, proper mixing will not occur and clots may form. The pipets can then be placed in the equipment tray until there is time to shake them for 5 minutes in the laboratory before doing the cell counts.

Special disposable micropipets are available, especially for some of the routine hematologic determinations. This system uses a self-filling pipet and a polyethylene reagent reservoir for dilution of the blood (see under Hematology). This unit is called a Unopette (Becton, Dickinson & Co.). This pipet can be used with either capillary or venous blood, and the general unit has been adapted for several chemical and hematologic determinations.

After the red and white cell counts, any other tests, such as reticulocyte counts, are done. Platelet counts are always done first. The blood films are prepared last, following the directions given under Cell Morphology in Chap. 3.

Venous blood

Blood may be obtained directly from a vein by using a sterile syringe and needle or a vacuum tube and needle system. Veins in the forearm are most commonly used. The three main veins in the forearm are the cephalic, median cephalic, and median basilic (Fig. 1-21). The median cephalic vein is usually chosen for venipuncture. The median basilic might roll or move, and the skin over the cephalic might be tougher to penetrate. Other sites may be used when necessary.

The veins that are generally used for venipuncture are those in the forearm, wrist, or ankle. The first choice for a venipuncture site is a vein in the forearm. They are larger than those in the wrist, hand, or ankle regions. The wrist, hand, and ankle veins are used only if the forearm site is not available. Venipuncture must be performed with great care and concern. The veins of the patient are the main source of blood for testing, and the entry point for medications, intravenous solutions, and blood transfusions. A patient has only a limited number of accessible veins, and it is important that everything possible be done to preserve their good condition and availability. Part of this responsibility lies with the person doing the blood drawing.

The venipuncture may be made by either the syringe method or the vacuum tube method. In the syringe method, a needle is attached to a syringe and inserted into the vein. The plunger of the syringe is drawn back, which creates suction, drawing the blood into the syringe. In the vacuum tube method, one end of a two-way needle is partially attached to the rubber stopper of a specially purchased vacuum tube. The other end of the two-way needle is inserted into the vein. Once in the vein, the needle in the rubber stopper is pushed through the stopper to make a direct connection to the vacuum tube. The vacuum tube creates suction, which draws the blood into the tube. One commercially available vacuum tube system is called a Vacutainer tube (Becton, Dickinson & Co.).

The majority of clinical laboratory determinations are done on whole blood, plasma, or serum. Many of these are done in the hematology or chemistry laboratories, but many other areas of the laboratory require venous blood at some time or other. Most venous blood specimens are drawn from fasting patients. Most fasting blood is drawn in the morning before breakfast. This means that the food from the previous meals has been completely digested and absorbed and any excess has been stored. Food intake, medication, activity, and time of day can all influence the laboratory results for blood specimens. Some of these facts are rarely taken into account by the persons interpreting the laboratory results. The fasting state is one fact that is carefully noted, however, especially for glucose and phosphorus determinations. Through numerous studies it has been found that the average meal has no significant effect on the concentration of most blood constituents, with certain exceptions, such as tests for glucose, phosphorus, and triglycerides. Eating significantly affects blood glucose and triglycerides, giving a falsely high result, and phosphorus, giving a falsely low result. Because it is the most efficient time of day to draw specimens for the laboratory, most of the blood collecting is done early in the morning, and for this reason most of the patients are in the fasting state. Fasting specimens, however, are not necessary for many laboratory determinations. Blood should not be collected while intravenous solutions are being administered, if possible.

When doing a venipuncture, the technician should remain in a standing position, which gives the greatest freedom of movement. The patient should assume a comfortable position. Bed patients should remain lying down, and ambulatory patients should be seated comfortably. The seated patient should put an arm on a table or other firm support and extend it for the technician.

Application of the tourniquet

The use of a tourniquet is desirable to enlarge the veins, so that they become more prominent. A strip of flat tubing (about 1 in wide) serves as a tourniquet. It is applied around the arm just above the bend in the elbow and should be just tight enough to stop the blood flow (Fig. 1-23). The patient should also be instructed to clench the fist, to aid in building up the blood pressure in the area of the puncture. The proper way to apply a tourniquet is as follows:

1. Place the tourniquet under the patient's arm just above the bend in the elbow.

2. Grasping the ends of the tourniquet, pull up so that tension is applied to the tourniquet. This tension must be maintained throughout the procedure.

3. With the proper tension, tie a loop in the tourniquet. Do not tie a bow or a knot. The loop must be made in such a way that it can

Fig. 1-23. Application of a tourniquet.

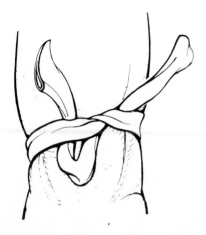

easily be released when the tourniquet is to be removed (Fig. 1-23).

4. Do not leave the tourniquet on for long periods of time because this will cause stoppage of the circulation (stasis). Prolonged stasis results in gross alterations in the blood constituents. Stasis should be allowed for a minimum time only.

The most prominent vein is usually chosen for venipuncture. If the veins are difficult to find, have the patient open and close the fist a few times; this will build up more pressure. Veins may be made more prominent by allowing the arm to hang down for 2-3 minutes, by massaging the vein toward the trunk of the body, or by lightly slapping the site of the puncture. Veins may be hardened or rubbery in elderly persons or in those who have had repeated venipuncture. Rolling veins may be held in place by putting the thumb and index finger on the vein so that 2-5 cm of vein lies between them. As soon as the vein is entered, the thumb and finger are removed. The veins can be felt by touching or palpating with the index finger. They reveal themselves as elastic tubes under the surface of the skin. By pressing up and down on the vein gently several times, the path of the vein can be felt.

Once the site for venipuncture has been chosen and the vein observed or palpated, the area is cleansed with an antiseptic solution. One suitable antiseptic is 70% medicated alcohol. The area of puncture is rubbed thoroughly with the antiseptic. After application of the antiseptic, the area must not be touched until after the actual puncture is made.

To insert the needle properly into the vein, the index finger is placed alongside the hub of the needle with the bevel of the needle facing up. The vein is fixed by grasping the patient's arm with the other hand and pulling the skin taut. This can be accomplished by placing the thumb about 1 or 2 in below the puncture site (Fig. 1-24). The needle should be pointing in the same direction as the vein. The syringe or vacuum tube

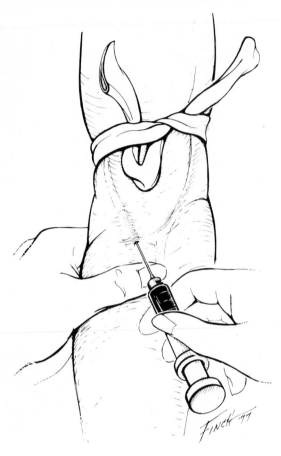

Fig. 1-24. Venipuncture technique.

apparatus should be held so that it makes a 30-40° angle with the patient's arm. The tip of the needle is then placed on the vein and pushed deliberately forward. When the vein has been punctured and a suitable amount of blood removed into the tube or syringe, the patient releases the clenched fist, the tourniquet is released, dry gauze is placed over the puncture site, and the needle is withdrawn slowly. After removing the needle, pressure may be applied on the puncture site, using gauze.

If difficulty is experienced in entering the vein (no blood appears in the tube or syringe) and especially if a hematoma (collection of blood under the skin) starts to form, release the tourni-

quet and promptly withdraw the needle, applying pressure to the wound. It is best to select an alternate site for repeated venipunctures on the same patient.

It is most important that the tourniquet be released *before* the needle is removed from the skin. If this is not done, excessive bleeding will occur. If the venipuncture is poorly done (if there is trauma to the tissues), a hematoma may result. This should be avoided, if at all possible.

Procedure for venipuncture

1. Assemble the necessary equipment:

a. For a vacuum tube system (the Vacutainer method). Thread the short end of the double-pointed needle into the holder and tighten securely. Place the vacuum tube in the holder and push the tube forward until the top of the stopper meets the guide mark on the holder. The point of the needle will thus be embedded in the stopper without puncturing it and losing the vacuum in the tube.

b. For a needle and syringe system. Remove the syringe from its protective wrapper and the needle from the vial and assemble them, allowing the vial to remain covering the needle when not in use. Attach the needle so that the bevel faces in the same direction as the graduation marks on the syringe. Check to make sure the needle is sharp, the syringe moves smoothly, and there is no air left in the syringe.

2. Identify the vein to be entered, preferably one in the antecubital fossa area of the arm. These veins are usually easily palpable and fairly well fixed in place.

3. Apply the tourniquet so that it can be easily released. The tourniquet should not be left in place unless the technician is ready to proceed immediately with the venipuncture.

4. Cleanse the skin at the venipuncture site thoroughly by rubbing well with 70% medicated alcohol.

5. With the patient's cooperation, grasp the elbow with your left hand and hold the arm fully extended. Anchor the vein with your thumb, drawing the skin tight over the vein to prevent the vein from moving. Ask the patient to open and close the fist.

6. Using the assembled vacuum tube system or syringe and needle, try to enter the skin first and then the vein, at a 30–40° angle. Enter the vein with the bevel of the needle up (Fig. 1-24).

7. With the Vacutainer system, when in the vein, push the vacuum tube into the needle holder all the way so that the blood flows into the tube. Blood will fill the tube under this vacuum.

8. With the syringe and needle system, if the vein has been entered, blood will spontaneously enter the syringe. In persons with low venous pressure, the plunger of the syringe is withdrawn slightly to make certain the needle has entered the vein. Blood should enter the syringe if the needle is in the vein properly. Withdraw the blood by using the left hand to pull back the plunger while steadying the syringe with the right hand.

9. When sufficient blood has been withdrawn, release the tourniquet. Place a dry gauze pad over the needle and puncture site and gently withdraw the needle.

10. Instruct the patient to hold the gauze pad over the venipuncture site for 2 or 3 minutes.

11. With the Vacutainer system, remove the tube from the Vacutainer holder and, if anti-coagulation is used, invert several times gently to mix the blood with the anticoagulant. Label the tubes with the patient's name, hospital number, and other information required by the hospital.

12. With the syringe and needle system, re-move the needle from the syringe and gently expel the blood into the tube. Avoid foaming or rupture of the cells by using gentle pressure on the plunger of the syringe. Stopper the tube and invert gently to mix anticoagulant with the blood, if anticoagulant is used. If a Vacutainer tube is used to hold the blood, push the needle through the stopper and allow the blood to collect in the tube under the vacuum in the tube. Label the tube properly.

13. Reinspect the venipuncture site to ascertain that the bleeding has stopped. If bleeding has stopped, apply a Band-Aid over the wound; otherwise continue to apply pressure until the bleeding stops. Do not leave the patient until the bleeding stops.

General considerations for venipunctures

The Vacutainer system is an ideal means of collecting multiple samples with ease. A multiple-sample needle is used. After blood has filled the first tube, remove the tube from the needle holder, leaving the needle in the vein, and insert a second tube. Blood will fill the second tube just as it did the first. Remember to thoroughly mix any anticoagulated blood right away to ensure proper mixing of the anticoagulant and blood. The multiple-sample needle has a special adaptation that prevents blood from leaking out during the exchange of tubes. Be certain to label all the tubes collected in this manner.

If blood must be drawn from a patient who has intravenous equipment attached to one arm, the blood sample should be drawn from a vein in the other arm. If neither arm is free, an ankle vein is the site of choice for the venipuncture.

In weak or elderly patients, the venous pressure may be so low that the pressure of the needle or the negative pressure of the vacuum tube may collapse the vein. In these cases it is advisable to use a syringe, for then the negative pressure can be controlled.

If the patient's clothing is too tight above the venipuncture site, it will slow down the flow of blood and it may cause a hematoma. If the tourniquet is too tight it will cause the arterial flow to stop. The radial pulse should be felt with the tourniquet in place correctly. A tight tourniquet can cause cyanosis, and it pinches the skin, causing unnecessary discomfort to the patient. It may also cause the vein to disappear before the puncture is made. When this happens the vein has collapsed, and the tourniquet should be released for a few minutes and the procedure repeated.

The placement of the needle—the angle of entry and the entry itself—is important. The angle of entry with the skin should be 45° or less. If the skin and vein are penetrated at one time, the needle may go straight through the vein. It is best to make the penetration in two steps: the skin first and then the vein. The bevel of the needle must always be covered by skin before the vacuum tube is fully engaged, otherwise the vacuum in the tube is lost. If there is a poor flow of blood, the needle may be half into the vein or the bevel may be partly occluded. To correct this problem, turn the needle gently, push in gently, or press down gently to keep the vein wall off the bevel. The needle must be in line with the vein to have a good flow of blood.

Blood drawn for culture in the microbiology laboratory must be collected in a special way. Extreme care must be taken to prevent contamination from the skin of the patient, from the person collecting the specimen, and from the equipment used. For this reason, a special skin-cleansing procedure is used that involves more careful and lengthy cleaning of the venipuncture site with a 2% tincture of iodine solution. Blood is collected into a special blood culture bottle using a blood-collecting set. Regular syringe and needle or vacuum tube systems are not used to collect blood for cultures. Culture bottles are labeled and brought to the laboratory.

Circulation of blood

Blood, although a liquid, can correctly be called a tissue. It circulates throughout the body, acting as a transportation system. As it circulates through the system of blood vessels (the vascular system), oxygen is transported from the lungs to the tissues of the body, products of digestion are absorbed in the intestine and carried to the various body tissues, and substances produced in various organs are transferred to other tissues for use. Cellular elements of the blood may also be transported to fight infection or aid in the coagulation of the blood. At the same time, waste products from the body tissues are picked up by the blood, and these end products of metabolism are then excreted through the skin, kidneys, and lungs.

The heart is the pump that forces the blood, under pressure, out through the arteries to all parts of the body. If an artery is cut, blood spurts out in small bursts each time the heart contracts. Near organs and muscles, the arteries branch out into smaller and smaller blood vessels called arterioles. Still smaller branches from the arterioles are called capillaries. In the tiny capillaries, the blood cells give up the oxygen they have been carrying and exchange it for the waste product from the body tissues, carbon dioxide. The capillary blood carrying carbon dioxide flows into larger vessels called venules, and then into still larger vessels called veins. The veins carry the blood back to the heart. As the blood flows through the capillaries, it gradually loses pressure. In the veins it has still less pressure. Therefore, if a vein is cut the blood oozes out; it does not spurt out. After the veins have carried the blood back to the heart, the blood is pumped into the alveoli, or air sacs of the lung. In the alveoli the carbon dioxide is removed from the red blood cells, which take up oxygen in its place. The blood then returns to the heart to be pumped out to the body once again through the arteries. It is important to understand the basics of the blood circulation so that the proper sites for blood collection are used.

The chemical compound in the red blood cells that actually picks up the oxygen and exchanges it for carbon dioxide is hemoglobin. When hemoglobin is saturated with oxygen, it is bright red in color. When oxygen is replaced by carbon dioxide, the hemoglobin becomes darker red. When blood from an artery is compared with blood from a vein, the arterial blood is visibly brighter red because of the nature of the hemoglobin compound just described.

Anticoagulants

Blood is a combination of formed elements (red cells, white cells, and platelets) in a liquid portion called plasma. *In vivo* (in the body) the blood is in a liquid form, but *in vitro* (outside the body) it will clot in a few minutes. Blood that is freshly drawn into a glass tube appears as a translucent, dark red fluid. In a matter of minutes it will start to clot, or coagulate, forming a semisolid jellylike mass.[21] If left undisturbed in the tube, this mass will begin to shrink, or retract, in about 1 hour. Complete retraction normally takes place within 24 hours. When coagulation occurs, a pale yellow fluid called serum separates from the clot and appears in the upper portion of the tube. During the process of coagulation certain factors present in the original blood sample are depleted or used up. Fibrinogen is one important substance found in the circulating blood (in the plasma portion) that is necessary for coagulation to occur. Fibrinogen is converted to fibrin when clotting occurs, and the fibrin lends structure to the clot in the form of fine threads in which the red cells (erythrocytes) and white cells (leukocytes) are embedded. Serum is used extensively for chemical, serological, and other laboratory testing, and can be obtained from the tube by gently rimming the clot and centrifuging without waiting for clot retraction to take place (see under Specimens—General Preparation in Chap. 2).

If coagulation is prevented by the addition of an anticoagulant, the formed elements of the blood—the red cells, white cells, and platelets—can be separated from the plasma. If the anticoagulated blood is centrifuged, it separates into three main layers: the red cells, the buffy coat (consisting of white cells and platelets), and the plasma (see Fig. 3-3). Hematologic studies are done primarily on whole anticoagulated venous blood or on capillary blo▮ everyone involved in coll▮ thoroughly understands t▮ anticoagulant. Use of the▮ lant is essential, and to▮ determination to be done ▮ be written on the request s▮p.

The anticoagulants chosen for specific determinations must be such that they do not alter the blood components and do not affect the laboratory tests to be done. The following are some adverse effects of using an improper anticoagulant or using the wrong amount of anticoagulant.

1. The anticoagulant may contain a substance that is the same as, or reacts in the same way as, the substance being determined. An example would be the use of sodium oxalate as the anticoagulant for a determination of sodium.
2. The anticoagulant may remove the constituent to be measured. An example would be the use of an oxalate anticoagulant for a calcium determination; oxalate removes calcium from the blood by forming an insoluble salt, calcium oxalate.
3. The anticoagulant may affect enzyme reactions. An example would be the use of sodium fluoride as an anticoagulant in an enzyme determination. Fluoride destroys many enzymes.
4. The anticoagulant may alter cellular constituents. An example would be the use of oxalate in cell morphology studies in hematology. Oxalate distorts the cell morphology; red cells crenate, vacuoles appear in the granulocytes, and bizarre forms of lymphocytes and monocytes appear rapidly when oxalate is used as the anticoagulant. Another example is the use of heparin as an anticoagulant for blood to be used in the preparation of blood films that will be stained with Wright's stain in hematology. Unless stained within 2 hours, heparin gives a blue background with Wright's stain.

too little anticoagulant is used, partial clotting will occur. This interferes with cell counts in hematology.

6. If too much liquid anticoagulant is used, it dilutes the blood sample and thus interferes with certain quantitative measurements.

Several anticoagulants are available, in the form of powders or liquids, for various purposes in the clinical laboratory. Some of the more commonly used anticoagulants are:

1. *Sodium fluoride.* This is a powder, used primarily for blood glucose specimens since it is also an enzyme poison (preventing glycolysis, or destruction of glucose). More information on the use of this anticoagulant will be found under Glucose in Chap. 2.

2. *Potassium oxalate.* This is a powder, used commonly in the chemistry laboratory for the determination of blood urea nitrogen, bicarbonate, chloride, creatinine, glucose, and many other substances. The oxalate in the anticoagulant precipitates calcium from the blood, interfering with the clotting mechanism. When calcium ions are combined with oxalate and are therefore not available to participate in clotting, the blood does not clot.

3. *Ammonium and potassium oxalate.* Also called balanced oxalate, or double oxalate, this combination is a powder. It is used for some hematology work. It is not used in chemistry, as a rule, because the presence of ammonium in the anticoagulant interferes with some of the chemistry determinations. This anticoagulant has become obsolete in most laboratories since the advent of EDTA.

4. *EDTA (ethylenediaminetetraacetic acid), Versene, or Sequestrene.* This is a liquid or dry anticoagulant used primarily in the hematology laboratory. It is the anticoagulant of choice for blood to be used in cell counts, hematocrit, hemoglobin, and cell differentials on stained blood films, to name but a few tests, because it preserves the morphological structure of the blood cell elements. EDTA removes calcium ions from the blood.

5. *Sodium citrate.* This anticoagulant is widely used for coagulation procedures, including prothrombin times and partial thromboplastin tests. It prevents coagulation by inactivating calcium ions. The citrate helps to prevent the rapid deterioration of labile coagulation factors such as factor V and factor VII.[22]

6. *Sodium oxalate.* This anticoagulant is also used for coagulation studies. It combines with calcium, forming insoluble calcium oxalate.

7. *Heparin.* This liquid is theoretically the best anticoagulant, because it is a normal constituent of blood and introduces no foreign contaminants in the blood specimen. It is, however, expensive, and has only a temporary effect as an anticoagulant. It prevents coagulation for approximately 24 hours by neutralizing thrombin, thus preventing the formation of fibrin from fibrinogen. Only a small amount of heparin is needed, so that simply coating the insides of tubes or syringes is often enough to give a good anticoagulant effect. Heparin is used for blood gas determinations and pH assays.

Laboratory handling of blood specimens

As discussed previously, if no anticoagulant is used, serum is obtained. After being placed in the tube, the blood is allowed to clot. The serum is then removed from the clot by centrifugation and is placed in a clean, dry tube. Serum can be used in the chemistry laboratory for tests for sodium, potassium, calcium, phosphorus, acid and alkaline phosphatase, cholesterol, uric acid, and liver function, to mention but a few. Serum is also used for serology testing.

It is important to remove the plasma or serum from the remaining blood cells, or clot, as soon as possible. Since biological specimens are being handled, the need for certain safety precautions is stressed. All blood specimens represent a potential contamination problem, especially with the hepatitis B virus (see under Safety in the Laboratory). Blood specimens should ideally be handled while wearing rubber gloves. The outsides of the tubes may be bloody, and initial laboratory handling of all specimens necessitates direct contact with the tubes. The rubber corks on the tubes must be removed carefully and not popped off, as this could cause infection by inhalation or by contact of the infectious aerosol with mucous membranes. Corks should be twisted gently while covering them with gauze to minimize the risk from aerosol. To separate the serum and plasma from the remaining blood cells, the tube must be centrifuged. It is generally best to remove the serum and plasma as quickly as possible to prevent alterations from taking place in the sample to be tested. It is especially important to remove the plasma quickly from the cell layer when potassium oxalate has been used as the anticoagulant, because the salt (potassium oxalate) shrinks the red blood cells and the intracellular water diffuses into the plasma (fluid inside the red cell leaves the cell and thus causes shrinkage). Tubes should be covered while in the centrifuge to protect the worker from the specimens, and the centrifuge should be placed as far from laboratory personnel as possible. The safest procedure for separating the centrifuged serum or plasma from the cell mass left in the tube is by pipetting instead of pouring. Pipet the serum or plasma by using mechanical suction and a disposable pipet. All serum and plasma tubes, as well as the original blood tubes, should be discarded properly when they are no longer needed for the determination.

Appearance of blood specimens

Those working with specimens in the laboratory must be able to recognize the appearance of normal as opposed to abnormal plasma or serum. Normally, serum or plasma is straw-colored, but various shades of yellow are also normally seen.

Abnormal-appearing serum and plasma can be clinical indications of serious disorders. Also, the use of such abnormal specimens can interfere with determinations, especially chemistries.

Hemolysis in specimens is perhaps the most common cause of the abnormal appearances to be considered in this section. A specimen that is hemolyzed appears red, usually clear red, because the red blood cells have been lysed and the hemoglobin has been released into the remaining portion of the blood. Often the cause of hemolysis in specimens is the technique used for venipuncture. A poor venipuncture, with excessive trauma to the blood vessel, can result in a hemolyzed specimen. Collecting the blood in dirty tubes or tubes that are not entirely dry can also result in hemolysis. In these cases, carefully repeating the venipuncture and using clean, dry equipment will produce a normal-appearing specimen that can be used for chemical determinations. Hemolysis of blood can also be caused by freezing, prolonged exposure to warmth, unnecessarily forceful spraying of blood from the needle of a syringe when transferring it to a specimen tube, or allowing the serum or plasma to remain too long on the cells before removing it to another tube. Hemolyzed serum or plasma is unsuitable for several chemistry determinations. The procedure to be done should always be checked first to see if abnormal-appearing specimens can be used.

Jaundiced serum or plasma is another specimen with an abnormal-looking hue. When serum or plasma takes on a brownish yellow color, there has most likely been an increase in bile pigments, namely bilirubin. Excessive intravascular destruction of red blood cells, obstruction of the bile duct, or impairment of the liver leads to an accumulation of bile pigments in the blood, and the skin becomes yellow. When this occurs, the skin of the patient is said to be *jaundiced*. The serum or plasma can also be jaundiced, or yellow. Those performing clinical laboratory determinations should note any abnormal appearance of serum or plasma and record it on the report slip. Another term for jaundiced is *icteric*. Jaundiced serum or plasma is seen in patients with hepatitis. Once again, we stress the importance of being observant in all areas of laboratory work—noticing things like jaundiced specimens can assist the physician in making a diagnosis.

When the blood, serum, or plasma takes on a milky white appearance, the specimen is said to be *lipemic*. The presence of lipids, or fats, in the serum causes this abnormal appearance. A blood specimen drawn from a patient soon after a meal may often appear lipemic. Lipemic specimens, for the most part, do not interfere with chemical determinations.

The handling of individual serum or plasma tubes will depend on the analysis to be done and the time that will elapse before it. Serum or plasma may be kept at room temperature, refrigerated, frozen, or protected from light, depending on the circumstances and the determination to be done. Some specimens must be analyzed immediately after they reach the laboratory, such as specimens for blood gas and pH analyses. Blood specimens for hematology studies can be stored in the refrigerator for 2 hours before being used in testing. After storage, anticoagulated blood, serum, or plasma must be thoroughly mixed after it has reached room temperature.

Plasma and serum can be frozen and preserved satisfactorily until the determination can be done. Whole blood cannot be frozen as the red blood cells rupture on freezing. Freezing preserves most chemical constituents in serum and plasma and provides a method of sample preservation for the laboratory. In general, refrigerating specimens retards alterations of many constituents. With all biological specimens, however, preservation should be the exception rather than the rule. A laboratory determination is best done on a fresh sample.

Other specimens

Other types of specimens such as gallstones, kidney stones, sputum, seminal fluid, or tissue samples may be sent to the laboratory for certain analyses. Each of these requires special treatment and handling.

VOCABULARY OF THE LABORATORY

Every specialty has a vocabulary of its own. The clinical laboratory is no different. Progress in learning the vocabulary of the laboratory and of medicine in general will come with experience, but some introductory information is important for anyone coming into the laboratory for the first time.

Most modern medical words are made up of parts derived from Greek or Latin, some with changes that have gradually been made over the years as the ancient words were adopted into English. All but the simplest medical terms are made up of two or three parts. For example, *pathology* is the study of disease or suffering. The root word is *pathos-*, from the Greek, meaning suffering or disease. The suffix *-logy* is also from the Greek word, *-logia*, from *logos*, mean-

ing the study of. By examining the root word along with the prefix and/or suffix, the meaning of most medical words can be understood.

Medical stem words, prefixes, and suffixes

Many of the common stem words, prefixes, and suffixes are listed below.[23]

Prefix	Meaning
a-, an-	lack, not
ab-, a-	away from, outside of
ad-	to, toward
ambi-, ambo-	both
amyl-, amylo-	starch
angi-, angio-	vessel, vascular

Prefix	Meaning	Prefix	Meaning
ante-	before, preceding, in front of	heter-, hetero-	other, another, different
arteri-, arterio-	artery, arterial	hex-, hexa-	six
arthr-, arthro-	joint	hom-, homo-	common, like, same
aur-, auri-, auro-	ear	hydr-, hydro-	water, hydrogen
bi-	two, twice, double	hyp-, hypo-	deficiency, lack, below
bi-, bio	life	hyper-	excessive, above normal
brachi-, brachio-	arm, brachial	hyster-, hystero-	uterus, uterine, hysteria
brady-	slow	icter-, ictero-	icterus, jaundice
bronch-, broncho-	bronchus, bronchial	immuno-	immune, immunity
cardi-, cardia-, cardio-	heart, cardiac	in-, im-	not, in, into
cephal-, cephalo-	head	inter-	between, among
cerebr-, cerebri, cerebro-	cerebrum, cerebral, brain	intra-	within, inside
cervic-, cervico-	neck, cervix, cervical	is-, iso-	equality, similarity, uniformity
chol-, chole-, cholo-	bile, gall	juxta-	near, next to
circum-	around, about	kerat-, kerato-	horn, horny, cornea
co-, com-, con-, cor-	with, together	ket-, keto-	presence of the ketone group
col-, coli-, colo-	colon	kilo-	thousand
contra-, counter-	against, opposite	lact-, lacti-, lacto-	milk, lactic
crani-, cranio-	cranium, cranial	lapar-, laparo-	flank, abdomen
cyan-, cyano-	dark blue, presence of the cyanogen group	laryng-, laryngo-	larynx, laryngeal
		latero-	lateral, to the side
cyst-, cysti-, cysto-	gallbladder, urinary bladder, pouch, cyst	leuk-, leuc-, leuko, leuco-	white, colorless, leukocyte
de-	undoing, reversal	levo-	left, on the left
dec-, deca-	ten, multiplied by ten	lith-, litho-	stone
deci-	tenth, one-tenth of	lymph-, lympho-	lymph, lymphatic
derm-, derma-, dermo-	dermis, dermal, skin	macr-, macro-	large, great, long
dextr-, dextro-	toward, of, or pertaining to the right	mal-	wrong, abnormal, bad
		mamm-, mammo-	breast
di-, dis-	two, twice, double	medi-, medio-	middle, medial, median
dipl-, diplo-	twofold, double, twin	meg-, mega-	large, extended, enlarged, one million times as large as
dis-, di-	separation, reversal, apart from		
dys-	abnormal, diseased, difficult, painful, unlike	micr-, micro-	small, minute, one-millionth
		mon-, mono-	single, one, alone
en-, em-	in, inside, into	morph-, morpho-	form, structure
end-, endo-	within, inner, internal	multi-	many, much, affecting many parts
enter-, entero-	intestine, intestinal		
ep-, epi-	upon, beside, among, above	my-, myo-	muscle
erythr-, erythro-	red	myel-, myelo-	marrow
eu-	good, well, normal, true	nas-, naso-	nose, nasal
ex-, e-, ef-	out, away, without	ne-, neo-	new, recent
extra-	outside of, beyond the scope of	necr-, necro-	death
		nephr-, nephro-	kidney
ferri-	ferric, containing iron(III)	neur-, neuro-	neural, nervous, nerve
ferro-	ferrous, containing iron(II)	nitr-, nitro-	nitrogen
fibr-, fibro-	fiber, fibrous	non-	not, ninth, nine
gastr-, gastro-	stomach, gastric	normo-	normal
gluc-, gluco-	glucose	nucle-, nucleo-	nucleus, nuclear
glyc-, glyco-	sweet, sugar, glucose, glycine	oo-	egg, ovum
gyne-	female, woman	orth-, ortho-	straight, direct, normal
hem-, hema-, hemo-	blood	ost-, oste-, osteo-	bone
hemi-	half, partial	ot-, oto-	ear
hepat-, hepato-	liver, hepatic	oxy-	oxygen

Prefix	Meaning
par-, para-	near, beside, adjacent to
path-, patho-	pathological
peri-	about, beyond, around
phag-, phago-	eating, feeding
pharyng-, pharyngo-	pharynx, pharyngeal
phleb-, phlebo-	vein, venous
phon-, phono-	sound, speech, voice
phot-, photo-	light
physi-, physio-	natural, physical, physiological
phyt-, phyto-	plant, vegetable
plasm-, plasmo-	plasma, protoplasm, cytoplasm
pneum-, pneumo-	air, gas, lung, respiratory
poly-	multiple, compound, complex
post-	after, behind
pre-	before
pro-	front, forward, before
proct-, procto-	rectum, anus
prot-, proto-	first, primitive, early
pseud-, pseudo-	false, deceptively resembling
psych-, psycho	psyche, psychic, psychology
pulmo-	lung, pulmonary
py-, pyo-	pus
pyel-, pyelo-	renal pelvic
pykn-, pykno-, pycn-, pycno-	compact, dense
pyr-, pyro-	fire, heat
radio-	radiation, radioactivity
re-	again, back
ren-, reni-, reno-	kidney, renal
retro-	back, backward, behind
rhin-, rhino-	nose, nasal
rubr-, rubri-, rubro-	red
sarc-, sarco-	flesh, fleshlike, muscle
semi-	half
ser-, seri-, sero-	serum, serous
sub-	under, less than
super-	above, upon, extreme
supra-	upon, above, beyond, exceeding
syn-, sym-	together, with
tachy-	rapid, quick, accelerated
thorac-, thoraci-, thoracico-, thoraco-	thorax, thoracic
thromb-, thrombo-	clotting, coagulation, blood platelets
thyr-, thyreo-, thyro-	thyroid
tox-, toxi-, toxo-	toxic, poisonous

Prefix	Meaning
trache-, tracheo-	trachea, tracheal
trans-	through, across
trich-, tricho-	hair, filament
un-	not, without
uni-	one
ur-, uro-	urine, urinary
uter-, utero-	uterus, uterine
vas-, vasi-, vaso-	vessel, vascular
ven-, vene-, veni-, veno-	vein, venous

Suffix	Meaning
-algia	a painful condition
-ase	enzyme
-ation	action, process
-blast	sprout, shoot, germ, formative cell
-cele	tumor, hernia, pathological swelling
-cyte	cell
-desis	binding, fusing
-ectomy	surgical removal
-emia	blood
-esthesia	feeling, sensation
-gram	drawing, record
-graph	something written, recorded
-itis	inflammation
-logy	field of study
-lysis	dissolving, loosening, dissolution
-megaly	abnormal enlargement
-oma	tumor, neoplasm
-opia, -opy	defect of the eye
-osis	process, state, diseased condition
-pathy	disease, therapy
-penia	deficiency
-phil, -phile	having an affinity for
-plasty	plastic surgery
-rrhage, -rrhagia	abnormal or excessive discharge
-scope	viewing instrument
-scopy	inspection, examination
-stoma	mouth, opening
-stomy	operation establishing an opening into a part
-tomy	cutting, incision, section
-uria	of or in the urine

REFERENCES

1. U.S. Department of Labor, Occupational Safety and Health Administration, Occupational Safety and Health Standards, *Fed. Regist.*, vol. 39, no. 125, pt. II, 1974.

2. G. M. Ederer and J. M. Matsen, We're Going All Out Against Hepatitis, *Medical Laboratory Observer*, p. 42, November–December 1973.

3. U.S. Department of Labor, Occupational Safety and Health Administration, Occupational Safety and Health Standards—Carcinogens, *Fed. Regist.*, vol. 39, no. 20, pt. III, pp. 3756–3757, 1974.

4. William Gasser, Converting to the Metric System, *Cadence*, vol. 7, no. 12, pp. 53–54, March–April 1976.

5. "Metric Guide for Educational Materials: A Handbook for Teachers, Writers and Publishers," American National Metric Council, Washington, D.C., 1976.

6. Israel Davidsohn and John Bernard Henry (eds.), "Clinical Diagnosis by Laboratory Methods," 15th ed., p. 553, W. B. Saunders Company, Philadelphia, 1974.

7. Testing of Glass Volumetric Apparatus, *Natl. Bur. Stand. (U.S.) Circ.* 602, 1959.

8. Norbert W. Tietz (ed.), "Fundamentals of Clinical Chemistry," 2d ed., p. 7, W. B. Saunders Company, Philadelphia, 1976.

9. Testing of Glass Volumetric Apparatus, *op. cit.*

10. Barbara A. Brown, "Hematology: Principles and Procedures," 2d ed., p. 13, Lea & Febiger, Philadelphia, 1976.

11. Tietz, *op. cit.*, pp. 27–29.

12. *Ibid.*, p. 40.

13. *Ibid.*, p. 103.

14. L. T. Skeggs, Jr., An Automated Method for Colorimetric Analysis, *Am. J. Clin. Pathol.*, vol. 28, p. 311, 1957.

15. Davidsohn and Henry, *op. cit.*, p. 2.

16. *Ibid.*, p. 6.

17. Richard J. Henry, Donald C. Cannon, and James W. Winkelman, "Clinical Chemistry, Principles and Techniques," 2d ed., p. 307, Harper & Row, Hagerstown, Md., 1974.

18. Tietz, *op. cit.*, p. 99.

19. Davidsohn and Henry, *op. cit.*, pp. 78–80.

20. G. Brickman, Blood from the Ear Lobe, *J. Lab. Clin. Med.*, vol. 27, p. 487, 1942.

21. Bong Hak Hyun, John K. Ashton, and Kathleen Dolan, "Practical Hematology," p. 2, W. B. Saunders Company, Philadelphia, 1975.

22. *Ibid.*, p. 185.

23. Leslie Lee, "The Lab Aide," pp. 103–108, C. V. Mosby Company, St. Louis, 1976.

BIBLIOGRAPHY

American Red Cross: "Advanced First Aid and Emergency Care," Doubleday & Company, New York, 1973.

Annino, Joseph S. and Roger W. Giese: "Clinical Chemistry, Principles and Procedure," 4th ed., Little, Brown and Company, Boston, 1976.

Benenson, A. S., H. L. Thompson, and M. R. Klugerman: Application of Laboratory Controls in Clinical Chemistry, *Am. J. Clin. Pathol.* vol. 25, p. 87, 1955.

Copeland, B. E.: "Quality Control in Clinical Chemistry," rev. ed., Chicago Commission on Continuing Education, American Society of Clinical Pathologists, Washington, D.C., 1973.

Davidsohn, Israel and John Bernard Henry (eds.): "Clinical Diagnosis by Laboratory Methods," 15th ed., W. B. Saunders Company, Philadelphia, 1974.

"Dorland's Pocket Medical Dictionary," 22d ed., W. B. Saunders Company, Philadelphia, 1977.

Freier, E. and V. Rausch: Quality Control in Clinical Chemistry, *Am. J. Med. Technol.*, vol. 24, p. 195, 1958.

Henry, Richard J., Donald C. Cannon, and James W. Winkelman: "Clinical Chemistry, Principles and Techniques," 2d ed., Harper & Row, Hagerstown, Md., 1974.

International System of Units, *Natl. Bur. Stand. (U.S.) Spec. Publ.* 330, 1972.

Kanter, Muriel W.: "Clinical Chemistry—Allied Health Series," Bobbs-Merrill Company, Inc., Indianapolis, 1975.

"Laboratory Safety Guide," California Association of Public Health Laboratory Directors, April 1976.

"Manual of Laboratory Safety," Fisher Scientific

Company, Pittsburgh (available without charge).

McFate, Robert P.: "Introduction to the Clinical Laboratory," 3d ed., Year Book Medical Publishers, Inc., Chicago, 1972.

Pattison, C. P., K. M. Boyer, J. E. Maynard, and P. C. Kelly: Epidemic Hepatitis in a Clinical Laboratory, *J. Am. Med. Assoc.*, vol. 230, p. 6, 1974.

Radin, N.: What Is a Standard? *Clin. Chem.*, vol. 13, p. 55, 1967.

Raphael, Stanley S. et al.: "Lynch's Medical Laboratory Technology," 3d ed., vol. I, W. B. Saunders Company, Philadelphia, 1976.

Roach, Gregory C.: "Laboratory Safety," American Society for Medical Technology in association with Interpersonal Associates, Inc., Bellaire, Tex., 1975.

Steere, N. V. (ed.): "Handbook of Laboratory Safety," 2d ed., Chemical Rubber Company, Cleveland, 1971.

"Safety in Handling Hazardous Chemicals," Matheson, Coleman, and Bell, Norwood, Ohio (available without charge).

Tietz, Norbert W. (ed.): "Fundamentals of Clinical Chemistry," 2d ed., W. B. Saunders Company, Philadelphia, 1976.

U.S. Department of Labor, Occupational Safety and Health Administration: Occupational Safety and Health Standards—Toxic Substances, Ketones, *Fed. Regist.*, vol. 40, no. 90, pt. II, 1975.

Winstead, Martha: "Reagent Grade Water: How, When and Why?" no. 1. The American Society of Medical Technologists, 1967.

TWO
CHEMISTRY

The field of laboratory medicine is expanding rapidly, and with it the specialty of clinical chemistry. Perhaps chemistry is the area in which changes are occurring most rapidly, because of the many automated devices available. The uses and general principles of some of the automated methods and apparatus found in the clinical chemistry laboratory are discussed in this chapter and in Chap. 1 (see under Automation in the Laboratory). For this reason there is an increased demand for well-trained, qualified laboratory personnel to perform the routine chemistry determinations.

The techniques of most chemical procedures performed in the laboratory are not in themselves difficult, but their proper execution requires genuine interest, reliability, and a good basic knowledge of the principles involved. It is essential, therefore, that the basic principles as well as the techniques used in clinical chemistry be mastered by the student.

From this chapter, the student should gain enough knowledge and instruction in basic skills to be able to perform accurately and conscientiously the routine chemical determinations done in a clinical laboratory. This instruction covers the basic theory of chemical determinations, use and care of laboratory equipment and apparatus, application of quantitative measurement, proper preparation of reagents, recognition of problems when they arise, proper collection and handling of laboratory specimens, reporting of results obtained, and, perhaps most important, the need for care and accuracy when performing any procedure in the laboratory.

If one's basic knowledge is adequate, other, more complicated chemistry determinations can be learned more easily. In this chapter specific methods are discussed for the determination of urea nitrogen, glucose, chloride, amylase, and bilirubin. The general principles of the use of flame photometry in analyses

for sodium and potassium are discussed. These determinations were chosen to illustrate techniques and types of methods used routinely in the clinical chemistry laboratory. There are many other procedures that are not covered, but other methods and procedures for the analysis of different constituents use these same basic techniques. In each method illustrated, principles involved in most other laboratory determinations are applied. It is inevitable that the medical laboratory technician will be called on to perform chemistry tests other than those described in this textbook. The technician should be able to apply the basic knowledge learned here to new laboratory tests.

Each new procedure should be approached with a definite pattern in mind. The technician should be aware of the type of specimen required for the test and should make certain that it is collected, prepared, and preserved properly. Any reagents needed for the procedure must be prepared by following the directions carefully. The technician should review the procedure beforehand, and it is worthwhile to look up clinical implications and background material for the determination in textbooks. The principle of the test, why the reagents are used and what they do in the reactions that occur, the stepwise method to be followed, technical factors and sources of error for the particular method, calculations, reporting of results to the physician, and normal values for the substance to be measured are all essential information for the person performing the test. The procedures discussed in this chapter (chloride, glucose, amylase, bilirubin, urea nitrogen, and sodium and potassium) were approached with this pattern in mind. By reviewing these procedures and noting how they are discussed, the student will be better able to approach a new procedure and to perform an accurate laboratory analysis.

A procedure should never become a "cookbook" method. Specific directions are necessary in performing any laboratory determination, but there is so much to know about even the simplest procedure that the directions alone are not enough. It is the job of the well-trained laboratory technician to do some additional research if necessary to gain as much knowledge as possible about every laboratory test that is performed.

To attain any degree of proficiency, practice and experience are necessary. Repeated practice with the laboratory tools discussed in this chapter and in Chap. 1 will result in a much better understanding of clinical chemistry and, eventually, a keen appreciation of honest and accurate performance in the chemistry laboratory.

Clinical applications are discussed throughout the chapter. In this way it is hoped that the student will not lose sight of the most important aspect of the chemistry determinations performed—the reason for making them in the first place—the patient.

SPECIMENS—GENERAL PREPARATION

Accurate chemical analysis of biological fluids depends on proper collection, preservation, and preparation of the sample, in addition to the technique and method of analysis used. The most quantitatively perfect determination is of no use if the specimen is not properly handled in the initial steps of the procedure. Each chemical method has unique problems of its own, but in general the collection, means of preservation, and initial preparation or processing of samples follow a similar pattern, regardless of what the final analysis is to be (see under Collection, Preservation, and Preparation of Laboratory Specimens in Chap. 1).

Once the blood has been collected and brought to the laboratory, a series of steps is carried out before the analysis is done. Ideally, all laboratory measurements should be performed within 1 hour after collection. When this is not practical, and it often is not, the specimens should be processed to the point where they can be properly stored so that the constituents to be measured will not be altered. There are two additional reasons for storing specimens: each sample should be retained long enough after analysis to permit a repeat analysis if necessary, and specimens collected in a timed sequence should be stored until they can be analyzed at the same time.

Processing includes separation of cells from serum or plasma, preparation of protein-free filtrates, observation of specimen color, refrigeration, and freezing.

Most chemical determinations are done on venous whole blood, plasma, or serum. Arterial blood is primarily used for blood gas determinations. Plasma is the liquid portion of the circulating blood and it contains fibrinogen. Serum is plasma with the fibrinogen removed, which is usually accomplished by the clotting mechanism.

Some chemical constituents change rapidly after the blood is removed from the vein. The best policy is to perform tests on fresh specimens. When the specimen must be preserved until the test can be done, there are ways to retard alteration. For example, sodium fluoride is used to preserve blood glucose specimens, since it prevents glycolysis.

With few exceptions, the lower the temperature, the greater the stability of the chemical constituents. Furthermore, the growth of bacteria is considerably inhibited by refrigeration and is completely inhibited by freezing. Room temperature is generally considered to be 18-30°C, the refrigerator temperature about 4°C, and freezing about −5°C or less. Refrigeration is a simple and reliable means of retarding alterations, including bacteriologic action and glycolysis, although some changes still take place. Refrigerated specimens must be brought to room temperature before chemical analysis. Removing cells from plasma and serum is another means of preventing some changes. Some specimens needed for certain assays, such as bilirubin, must be shielded from the light or used immediately. Bilirubin is a light-sensitive substance.

Serum or plasma may be preserved by freezing. Whole blood cannot be frozen satisfactorily because freezing ruptures the red cells. Freezing preserves enzyme activities in serum and plasma. Serum and plasma freeze in layers with different concentrations, and for this reason these specimens must be well mixed before they are used in a chemical determination.

Every precaution must be taken to preserve the chemical constituents in the specimen from the time of collection to the time of testing in the laboratory if the results are to be meaningful to the physician. In general, tubes for collecting blood for chemical determinations do not have to be sterile, but they should be chemically clean. Serum is usually preferred to whole blood or plasma when the constituents to be measured are relatively evenly distributed between the intracellular and extracellular portions of the blood.

To obtain serum, the blood is collected in a plain tube, using no anticoagulant, and allowed to clot for at least 15-20 minutes at room temperature. The clot may adhere to the wall of the tube, so that rimming the tube gently with a wooden applicator stick is necessary before centrifugation. A gentle sweep should be made around the inside walls of the tube with the stick. Excessive rimming is not necessary and can actually hemolyze the red blood cells. This problem is usually eliminated if serum Vacutainer tubes are used to collect the blood, because these tubes are usually siliconized to minimize hemolysis and to prevent the clot from adhering to the wall of the tube. By allowing the clot to retract for longer than 20 minutes, hemolysis is minimized and the yield of serum is greater. However, if the serum remains on the clot for too long, glycolysis can occur and other constituents are altered—there can be a shift of substances from the cells to the serum, for instance. Therefore, the time to allow for clot retraction depends on the determination to be done. After clotting has taken place, the tube is centrifuged and the supernatant serum is removed. It is important to remind those handling blood specimens in all steps of the laboratory analysis to treat the specimens as if they might be contaminated. Many laboratories require all persons handling specimens in any way to wear rubber gloves. Rubber corks must be carefully removed from blood specimens, centrifuges must be covered and placed in a shielded area, all serum and plasma samples must be pipetted by mechanical suction, and all specimen tubes and supplies must be discarded properly.

It is pertinent at this point to describe a new process for the separation of serum and plasma from cells. With so many automated methods, processing the blood often takes longer than the actual analysis. A faster, more efficient way of separating serum from cells was also needed. Several systems have been devised for this purpose. In one, regular vacuum serum tubes are used for collecting the blood, and then a special unit is placed on the tube of blood before centrifugation. This unit dispenses a silicone mixture during centrifugation that forms an inert barrier between the serum and the cells. The serum can easily be poured off into another container for analysis without having to worry about contamination with cells. With other units it is necessary to purchase a special blood-collecting tube, which resembles an ordinary vacuum tube but contains inert silicone gel. The gel is displaced up inside the tube during centrifugation and forms a barrier between the serum and the cells. The serum can easily be poured or pipetted off into the appropriate container for testing. These products are all designed to save valuable time for the technician.

Hemolyzed serum or plasma is unfit as a specimen for several chemistry determinations. Hemolyzed serum appears red, usually clear red. Several constituents, such as the enzymes acid phosphatase, lactate dehydrogenase (LDH), and serum glutamic-oxaloacetic transaminase (SGOT), are present in large amounts in the red blood cells, so that hemolysis of these cells will significantly elevate the value obtained for these substances in serum. Hemoglobin is released during hemolysis and may directly interfere with a reaction or its color may interfere with photometric analysis of the specimen. The procedure to be done should always be checked to see whether abnormal-looking specimens can be used.

Jaundiced serum or plasma takes on a brownish yellow color. The technician should be especially careful in handling such a specimen. Gloves can be worn and the hands should be washed frequently. Jaundiced serum is a good indication of the presence of hepatitis, which is very infectious. The abnormal color of the serum can interfere with photometric measurements.

Lipemic serum takes on a milky white color. The presence of lipids in serum or plasma can cause this abnormal appearance. Often, however, the lipemia results from collecting the blood from the patient too soon after a meal. Lipemic serum interferes with photometric readings for some tests.

Blood drawn from patients on certain types of medication can give invalid chemistry results for some constituents. Drugs can alter several chemical reactions. Drugs can affect laboratory results in two general ways: some action of the drug or its metabolite can cause an alteration (*in vivo*) in the concentration of the substance being measured, and/or some physical or chemical property of the drug can alter the analysis directly (*in vitro*). The number of drugs that affect laboratory measurements is increasing.

Collecting microspecimens for chemistry

There are instances where only small amounts of blood can be collected, and many laboratory determinations have been devised for very small amounts of sample. In general, the same procedure is followed as for any other drawing of capillary blood (see under Capillary Blood in Chap. 3). For chemistry procedures, blood can be collected in a capillary tube by touching the tip of the tube to a large drop of blood while the tube is being held in a slightly downward position. The blood enters the tube by capillary action. Several tubes (approximately 4 by 75 mm) can be filled from a single skin puncture. Tubes are capped and placed in a test tube to be transported and centrifuged. Careful centrifugation technique must be used because capillary tubes tend to break easily. When the analysis is delayed, the tube is scratched with a file and broken just above the junction of serum and cells. The serum portion of the tube is then recapped and refrigerated.

Preparation of a protein-free filtrate

Biological fluids are very complex in their composition. There are hundreds of detectable substances in urine and blood, for instance. Chemical analysis would be impossible if it were necessary to completely isolate each substance before it could be measured. An optimal method is one that can test for a specific substance while the other substances remain. A test is said to be specific when none of the other substances interfere. In chemical analysis, however, almost all determinations are subject to some interference. Sometimes the interference is small enough or constant enough that it does not significantly alter the accuracy or precision of the test results. Sometimes the interference does affect the results, and in such cases the specimen must be specially treated before the analysis can take place. That is, the substances causing the interference must be isolated, or removed, from the specimen.

Whole blood is made up of cells and plasma. The red cells are largely composed of protein and the plasma also contains a significant amount of protein. Protein molecules tend to have many electrically charged areas, and since chemical reactions involve the transfer of charges, the presence of so many charged protein molecules may interfere with reactions. It therefore may be necessary to remove the proteins before continuing with the determination. Removing proteins also has the effect of preserving the specimen since it removes enzymes, which are protein in nature.

If proteins are left in the specimen, they can interfere with the determination by causing turbidity, foaming, or precipitation, or by directly interfering with color reactions. Any of these effects can lead to errors in many clinical determinations. Therefore many determinations require preliminary treatment to remove proteins. Proteins may be removed by precipitation with chemicals (acids or salts of heavy metals) or by passing the serum through a dialyzing membrane that allows only the smaller particles through. Acids often used to precipitate proteins are trichloroacetic, tungstic, and picric. Salts of heavy metals that can be used to precipitate proteins are sodium sulfate, ammonium sulfate, and zinc sulfate. Ethyl alcohol and methyl alcohol are two organic chemicals used in protein precipitation.

The dialyzing membrane is used in many automated methods, but the chemical filtrate methods are used for most determinations done manually in the laboratory. Chemistry procedures requiring initial removal of protein will specify how it should be done.

The term *protein-free filtrate* is used to describe the solution left after treatment of a specimen to remove the protein. Some techniques leave behind residual proteins ranging in concentration from 1 to 5 mg/dl.[1] Many separations of protein are accomplished by means of precipitation. Either the substance being determined is removed by precipitation, or the interfering materials are precipitated. The precipitate is isolated by filtration or centrifugation. Chemical precipitation of serum, plasma, whole blood, urine, or cerebrospinal fluid is thus followed by either filtration or centrifugation and subsequent decantation of the crystal-clear protein-free filtrate. Proteins are easily precipitated, and the techniques used include the use of heat, acids, bases, organic solvents, alcohols, salts, metal ions, or a combination of these. Some common methods for the precipitation of proteins, yielding protein-free filtrates, are the Folin-Wu, Haden modification of the Folin-Wu, trichloroacetic acid (TCA), and Nelson-Somogyi methods.

The classical method for the preparation of a protein-free filtrate is the Folin-Wu method.[2] Water is added to whole blood, followed by sulfuric acid (H_2SO_4), which converts hemoglobin to acid hematin, and finally sodium tungstate (Na_2WO_4), which precipitates the proteins. This method gives a slightly acid filtrate. The original method devised by Folin and Wu calls for 1 ml of blood, 7 ml of water, 1 ml of 0.66 N H_2SO_4, and 1 ml of 10 g/dl Na_2WO_4. The color change that occurs in this reaction, from blood red to chocolate brown, signifies conversion of hemoglobin to methemoglobin (acid hematin). Complete precipitation is indicated by the absence of foaming and by a clicking sound when the mixture is shaken against the rubber stopper. If the brown color does not appear the change is not complete; this can be remedied by dropwise addition of 10 ml/dl H_2SO_4 with vigorous shaking after each drop until the change is complete.

Haden's modification of the Folin-Wu method is much more commonly used today. The advantage of this method is that the reaction is practically immediate and the filtration step can be carried out right away. In the Haden modification the acid and water are combined to give a single $0.083\ N\ H_2SO_4$ reagent. It has been further suggested that the water, sodium tungstate, and acid be combined to form a single reagent, tungstic acid, but this reagent is stable for only 2 weeks and requires a waiting period for the precipitate to turn chocolate brown. The Haden modification is described below.

Procedure for Haden modification of the Folin-Wu filtrate method[3]

1. Into a test tube pipet 8 ml of $0.083\ N$ H_2SO_4.
2. Using an Ostwald pipet, pipet 1 ml of well-mixed blood into the test tube. Blow out the last drop from the pipet. If serum or plasma is used, choose a volumetric pipet for measuring the sample into the test tube. If centrifugation is to be used for the separation, use a centrifuge tube, which is specifically constructed to withstand centrifugal force.
3. Place a rubber stopper in the tube and mix by gentle inversion four or five times. In this initial step, the hemoglobin is converted to acid hematin (a dark brown color is seen). Thorough mixing is important after each new reagent is added.
4. Into the test tube, pipet 1 ml of 10 g/dl Na_2WO_4 (a graduated pipet may be used) to complete the precipitation of the protein.
5. Stopper the tube again and mix well. Shake the tube until a metallic click is heard. During this step the actual precipitation of protein is accomplished; thorough shaking is of primary importance.
6. Remove the insoluble protein by filtration or centrifugation. For whole blood filtration is the means usually employed, while for serum or plasma centrifugation is generally used.

a. Filtration method. Place filter paper in a funnel and place a clean, dry test tube under the funnel. Pour the mixture into the filter paper, being careful that none of it spills down the sides of the funnel. Allow *all* of the fluid to collect in the test tube under the funnel before any is used for analysis. The fluid collected in the test tube is the *filtrate*. Before pipetting any of the filtrate, mix it well. It should be water-clear and colorless. This filtrate is protein-free.

b. Centrifugation method. Place the tube in the centrifuge, being certain to balance the tube with another, similar tube. Centrifuge for at least 5 minutes at 3000 r/min. After centrifugation, the protein will be packed at the bottom of the tube; the clear supernatant solution at the top is free of protein and can be pipetted for eventual analysis. This solution too should be clear and colorless.

The Haden modification of the Folin-Wu method yields a nearly neutral filtrate. The acid is used up in the protein precipitation. If the solution is too acid or too alkaline, the protein will not be completely precipitated. The reaction occurring in this procedure has two steps:

$$Na_2WO_4 + H_2SO_4 \longrightarrow$$
$$Na_2SO_4 + H_2WO_4 \text{ (tungstic acid)}$$

$$H_2WO_4 + \text{protein (in blood,}$$
$$\text{serum, plasma, etc.)} \longrightarrow$$
$$\text{protein tungstate (insoluble)}$$

Other protein-precipitating methods

TCA is another common protein-precipitating agent. It produces a strongly acid filtrate, which may not be desirable in some quantitative methods. It may also result in filtrates that are not as clear as the Folin-Wu filtrates. In some analyses an organic filtrate may be needed. Alcohol-ether or alcohol-acetone mixtures may be used.

The Nelson-Somogyi method involves successive addition of aqueous solutions of barium hydroxide and zinc sulfate to the sample. The proteins are precipitated as zinc salts. This method provides a very clear, protein-free filtrate. It also removes other substances (uric acid and some creatinine) that might interfere in the copper reduction methods for glucose determination. The Nelson-Somogyi method is therefore often used with glucose determinations involving copper reduction (see under Glucose).

The centrifugation method of removing precipitated protein usually gives greater recovery of protein-free solution. When filtration is used, some solutes can be lost by adsorption onto the filter paper, or the paper itself can introduce new solutes into the mixture.

It is important in all methods for protein precipitation that the filtrate be examined carefully for the presence of any foaming or cloudiness, which would indicate incomplete removal of protein. Two variables are important for maximal precipitation: the pH of the reaction mixture, and the concentration of the precipitant. There must be sufficient reagent to combine with the protein in the blood. Ordinarily a safe excess is used. If desired, proteins may be put back into solution, by acidification in the case of metal proteinates and by making the mixture strongly alkaline in the case of protein salts.

The protein-free filtrate can be analyzed quantitatively by photometric or volumetric methods. The directions for specific procedures will list the agents to be employed for the removal of protein and will state how to analyze the resulting protein-free filtrate.

STANDARDIZATION OF A PROCEDURE AND USE OF A STANDARD CURVE

Once a series of standard tubes have been read in the photometer, the galvanometer readings and standard concentrations are plotted on graph paper. This is the first step in the use of a standard curve, a most essential tool in the majority of chemistry determinations.

"Precalibrated" test procedures are commercially available; however, they should *not* be used. Each laboratory must include standards for each batch of determinations whenever possible. Failure to do so can result in errors resulting from the use of new reagents, deterioration or contamination of old reagents, the use of incorrect filters, and changes in instruments.

Semilogarithmic graph paper is the type most commonly used to plot the readings from the photometer. The horizontal axis of this graph paper is a linear scale, and the vertical axis is a logarithmic scale. The concentration in the standard cuvettes is plotted on the horizontal axis. The readings from the photometer are plotted along the vertical axis. In most cases the percent transmittance readings are used (as opposed to optical density readings). These readings can be plotted directly on the logarithmic scale, as the concentration is proportional to the logarithm of the galvanometer reading. In this way percent transmittance readings are converted to the appropriate numbers on the logarithmic scale. Using semilogarithmic graph paper is simple and convenient for most laboratory purposes. When percentages are plotted against concentrations on semilogarithmic graph paper, the proportional relationship is direct, and a straight-line graph is obtained when the individual standard points are connected. The criteria for a good standard curve are that the line is straight, that the line connects all points, and that the line goes through the origin, or intersect of the two axes. The origin of the graph paper is the point on the vertical and horizontal axes where there is $100\%T$ and zero concentration.

Another type of graph paper, called *linear* graph paper, is available for plotting standard curves. This graph paper has both horizontal and vertical linear scales. If linear graph paper is used to construct a standard curve, the percent transmittance readings must first be converted to logarithmic values and the logarithmic values plotted on the vertical axis. If percent transmittance readings are converted to optical densities (or absorbance units), or if the galvanometer scale is calibrated in optical density units, the optical density readings can be plotted directly against the concentration. Again, a straight-line graph must be obtained. To eliminate the conversion of percent transmittance to optical density in order to obtain the necessary straight-line graph, the use of semilogarithmic graph paper is suggested.

When plotting points on graph paper, whether they represent concentrations or galvanometer readings, care must be taken to note the intervals on the graph paper. Many errors result from carelessness in the initial plotting of points on the graph paper.

When a graph is prepared, the axes must also be properly labeled. Additional information usually recorded on the paper includes the name of the person constructing the graph, the procedure for which the graph was prepared, the date, the photometer used, and the wavelength setting used.

Once the standard curve has been plotted, it is used to calculate the concentrations of any unknowns that were included in the same batch as the standards used to make the graph. To find the concentration of a solution, there must be some way of comparing it with a solution of known concentration. An example of the construction and use of a standard curve is given in Fig. 2-1.

Three standard solutions are prepared with the following concentrations of standard: standard 1 (S_1), 0.02 mg; standard 2 (S_2), 0.04 mg; and standard 3 (S_3), 0.06 mg. These concentrations are plotted on the linear, horizontal scale of the graph paper. The three standard tubes are read in a photometer, giving the following readings in

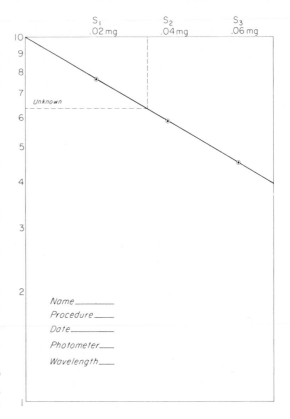

Fig. 2-1. Construction of a standard curve.

percent transmittance: S_1, 76^2; S_2, 58^3; and S_3, 45^1. The percent transmittance readings are plotted under their respective concentrations on the logarithmic, vertical scale of the paper. The points are connected, using a ruler. An undetermined substance gives a reading of $63^2 \%T$. Using the graph in Fig. 2-1, the 63^2 point on the vertical scale is found, followed horizontally to the graph line just drawn, and then followed vertically to the concentration scale. The degree of accuracy with which an unknown concentration can be read depends on the concentrations of the standards used. In this example, the unknown concentration is 0.0343 mg (the figure in the fourth decimal place is approximate).

Using standard solutions to standardize the

analyses of each batch, rather than relying on a permanently established calibration curve, allows the clinical laboratory to produce more reliable results. It compensates for variables such as time, temperature, the age of the reagents, and the condition of the instruments. It is always best to use several different concentrations of the standard solution, not just one. To obtain reliable photometric information about the concentration of a substance, standards must be used as the basis for comparison.

Standard solutions are also used in quantitative analytical procedures in which the photometer is not employed. For example, whenever titration is used to measure concentration, a standard solution must be employed. There must be some basis for comparison in this technique also (see under Titration in Chap. 1).

GLUCOSE

The most commonly performed procedure in the clinical chemistry laboratory is the determination of blood glucose. Blood glucose tests are performed in all sorts of clinical laboratories, in hospitals, independent laboratories, clinics, and private physicians' offices. They are used primarily for the diagnosis and then treatment (or control) of diabetes mellitus. Although several different methods are used to quantitatively measure the amount of glucose in a blood specimen, most methods depend on the formation or disappearance of color in a solution and employ the photometer for this measurement. Several of the methods have been automated, but the same principles apply as for the manual methods. Because tests for blood glucose are so common, and because the techniques involved in most of the methods are basic to so many other types of chemistry determinations, blood glucose determinations are discussed here in some detail.

Glucose determinations may be performed on specimens taken from patients in a fasting state, on specimens taken 2 hours after the patient has eaten 100 g of carbohydrate (postprandial), or as part of various glucose tolerance tests, depending on the physician's instructions. The methods used for glucose determinations can be divided into three categories: oxidation methods, which depend on the reducing ability of glucose; aromatic amine methods, which involve a reaction between the aldehyde group of glucose and the amino group of an aromatic amine; and enzymatic methods, which are based on the enzymes glucose oxidase and hexokinase. Since many additional substances that normally occur in the blood either are measured as glucose or interfere with various tests, the term *true blood glucose* is often encountered when tests of blood glucose are described.

Before considering the various types of tests for blood glucose and describing two specific methods, we discuss carbohydrates, carbohydrate metabolism, and the clinical significance of glucose in the following sections.

Carbohydrates

Carbohydrates are organic compounds composed of carbon, hydrogen, and oxygen. They are the principal source of energy for the life processes carried on by the body, glucose being the ultimate source of food energy. The carbohydrates include simple sugars and substances that, when decomposed, break down into simple sugars. Carbohydrates are grouped as monosaccharides, disaccharides, and polysaccharides. The monosaccharide group contains simple sugars only. A simple sugar is one that cannot be broken down further and still retain the characteristics of a sugar. Glucose, also known as dextrose, is the primary monosaccharide of the body and of the blood. Fructose and galactose, two other monosaccharides, are absorbed through the intestine and into the blood, where they are converted to glucose before they are utilized by the body for energy. Glucose is the sugar given when an intravenous solution of sugar is administered. Disaccharides are made up of two monosaccharides. Examples of disaccharides are maltose, lactose, and sucrose, or common table sugar. Sucrose is the primary source of sugar in the American diet. Polysaccharides are made up of many monosaccharide units linked together. Examples of polysaccharides are starch and glycogen, both dietary sources of carbohydrates. Glycogen is the storage form of sugar in the body.

Under ordinary conditions, the concentration of glucose in the blood is kept within a narrow range by an elaborate system of mechanisms collectively called carbohydrate metabolism. Some of the mechanisms used by the body to keep the glucose within this range are absorption of glucose by the intestine, storage and breakdown of glycogen (the form in which glucose is stored in the body) by the liver, storage of glucose as glycogen by the mass of skeletal muscles, and production and release of the hormone insulin by the pancreas. Other hormones that affect the blood glucose level are produced by the adrenal cortex, and by the pituitary and thyroid glands.

Metabolism of carbohydrates

In the mouth, the powerful enzyme salivary amylase begins the digestion of starch to maltose. The activity of amylase is inhibited at the acid pH of the stomach. However, when food leaves the stomach, pancreatic amylase in the duodenum continues the hydrolysis or breakdown of starch and glycogen to maltose. The maltose, along with ingested lactose and sucrose, is further split by the disaccharidases formed in the intestinal mucosa, forming the monosaccharides glucose, galactose, and fructose. These monosaccharides are then absorbed through the wall of the small intestine into the blood, the major portion going into the portal circulation and to the liver. Thus, conditions that decrease the absorptive surface of the intestine or interfere with its enzyme production result in decreased absorption of monosaccharides. Thyroxine increases absorption of monosaccharides, and therefore changes in thyroid function may affect the rate and amount of absorption. Once absorbed from the intestine and passed on to the liver, galactose and fructose are converted to glucose. Virtually all blood sugar is in the form of glucose, and it is glucose metabolism that chiefly concerns us.

Glucose is the ultimate source of energy for all body cells. Energy is provided by the oxidation of glucose, ultimately to carbon dioxide and water, through the process called glycolysis. Glycolysis, or glucose oxidation, depends on the presence of *insulin*. Therefore the absence of insulin will result in an increased concentration of glucose in the blood (clinically, the condition diabetes mellitus). Insulin is responsible for maintaining a healthy level of glucose in the blood. This is done in a variety of ways, including the processes of glycogenesis and glycolysis. *Glycolysis* is the breakdown or oxidation of glucose. Other forms of glucose utilization, or breakdown, that are also dependent on insulin are the synthesis of fatty acids and amino acids (the building blocks of protein). *Glycogenesis* is the formation of glycogen from glucose. Glycogen is the form in which glucose is stored in the body, primarily in the liver. Thus, insulin regulates the concentration of blood glucose by either oxidation (glycolysis) or storage (glycogenesis). The secretion of insulin is stimulated by increased blood glucose concentrations.

Glucose can also be provided to the blood by the process of *gluconeogenesis*, the production of glucose from fat and protein. This takes place in the liver, where glucose is derived from certain amino acids (protein) and glycerol (from fat) by glucocorticoid hormones produced by the adrenal cortex. Decreased blood glucose and decreased glycogen storage in cells stimulate this process.

Only a certain amount of glucose can be stored

as glycogen. The excess glucose is converted to fatty acids and stored as triglycerides in body fat. Insulin is also necessary for the formation of fat (*lipogenesis*) in the liver and the *adipose tissue* or body fat.

Although glucose is also stored in the muscles as glycogen, this cannot contribute to the blood glucose concentration, as muscle glycogen can be oxidized only within the muscle cell.

After a period of fasting, the usual amount of glucose in the blood is between 60 and 100 mg per deciliter of blood, depending on the method of analysis.[4] The blood glucose level usually increases rapidly after carbohydrates are ingested, but returns to normal in $1\frac{1}{2}$-2 hours. Aside from this increase after eating, the level of glucose in the blood is kept within a remarkably narrow range. This regulation of the blood glucose level is largely dependent on the activity of the liver. After a heavy meal, the glucose produced from digested carbohydrates is absorbed and the blood sugar rises. Some of this glucose may be oxidized at once for energy. However, the liver removes a large portion and stores it as glycogen, while some is carried to muscles, where it is also stored as glycogen for later use for immediate energy by the muscles. Some of the glucose diffuses into the tissue fluids and provides a direct source of energy for cell activity. After these immediate needs of the body have been supplied, the remainder is converted to fat and stored in the adipose tissue of the body. If the blood glucose level is so great that these control mechanisms cannot remove the excess glucose, the kidneys exert a regulating effect by excreting sugar in the urine. The blood glucose concentration above which glucose is excreted in the urine is called the *renal threshold*. For most individuals the renal threshold for glucose is 160-170 mg/dl.

As a result of these metabolic processes, the blood glucose gradually returns to its fasting level. Since the body continues to utilize glucose for energy during normal activity, the blood glucose has a tendency to drop. This stimulates the liver to convert stored glycogen to glucose

(*glycogenolysis*), maintaining the normal level of blood glucose.

In summary, the various reactions that make up glucose metabolism are catalyzed by very specific enzymes. In addition, the combined efforts of a number of hormones influence the ability to maintain normal levels of blood glucose. Only one hormone, insulin, which is produced by the beta cells of the islets of Langerhans in the pancreas, decreases the blood glucose concentration. This is done in a number of ways, including glycogenesis, the formation of glycogen in the liver and muscles; lipogenesis, the formation of fat from carbohydrates; and glycolysis, the utilization of glucose, probably by increasing the permeability of the body cells to glucose. When there is a deficiency in the amount or effectiveness of insulin (as in diabetes mellitus), the blood glucose level increases. This increase in blood glucose level is referred to as *hyperglycemia*. Although there is plenty of glucose in the blood in diabetes mellitus, the body is unable to utilize it for energy, as its utilization is dependent on the presence of insulin. For this reason, in diabetes mellitus there is starvation of the body cells when there is plenty of glucose in the blood, or starvation in the face of plenty.

Several hormones have the effect of raising the blood glucose concentration. The actions of *growth hormone* and *adrenocorticotropic hormone* (ACTH), which are secreted by the anterior pituitary, are opposite (antagonistic) to that of insulin and tend to raise the blood glucose level. *Hydrocortisone* and other steroids produced by the adrenal cortex stimulate gluconeogenesis, the production of glucose from fat and protein. *Epinephrine*, which is secreted by the adrenal medulla, stimulates glycogenolysis, the conversion of glycogen to glucose. *Glucagon* is secreted by the alpha cells of the pancreas, and acts to increase blood glucose by stimulating glycogenolysis in the liver. Finally, *thyroxine*, which is secreted by the thyroid, also stimulates glycogenolysis and contributes to an increased blood glucose level, besides increasing the rate of absorption of glucose from the intestine.

Clinical significance

Glucose is one of the few chemical constituents of the blood that can change rapidly and dramatically in concentration. Many diseases cause a change in glucose metabolism, but the most frequent cause of an increase in blood glucose is diabetes mellitus. This disease is associated with a relative or absolute deficiency of insulin. This deficiency results in an inability of the body to oxidize glucose, as glucose is unable to enter muscle and liver cells. Diabetes mellitus is a chronic metabolic disorder with deficiencies in carbohydrate, lipid, and protein metabolism. Changes in fat metabolism resulting from diabetes mellitus can be life-threatening when they result in *ketoacidosis*, a condition in which there is an increased concentration of ketone bodies (which are derived from fat catabolism) in the blood and an accompanying decrease in blood pH, or acidosis. Other complications include increased cholesterol in the blood; atherosclerosis, a vascular disease with deposits of fat in the blood vessels; and kidney disease. There are approximately 2 million recognized diabetics in the United States, which is probably only half of the overall incidence, or 2 percent of the entire population.[5] There is a strong family tendency to the disease, although the exact mechanism of acquisition is unknown. Early diagnosis is important, as proper treatment may delay or minimize the complications of the disease.

Diabetes mellitus is controlled clinically through a number of factors. These include various dosages of insulin, oral drugs, and the composition of the diet. The result of uncontrolled diabetes mellitus is a high blood glucose level, with glucose subsequently appearing in the urine.

In a diabetic patient the glucose concentration can be very high or very low. At either extreme the patient may be in a state of unconsciousness. It is therefore necessary for the physician to know whether the unconsciousness results from a high glucose concentration (*diabetic coma*) or a low glucose concentration (*insulin shock*). It is often not obvious from the physical appearance of the patient which condition exists; however, prompt and appropriate treatment is mandatory. It is the responsibility of the laboratory to get the result of the glucose determination to the physician as soon as possible, so that the correct treatment can be started. In this type of emergency glucose determination, the test must be done rapidly but with the utmost accuracy, as an error or delay may have a serious effect.

In many cases high blood glucose values are caused by conditions other than diabetes mellitus. Some of these are traumatic injury to the brain; febrile disease; certain liver diseases; overactivity of the adrenal, pituitary, and thyroid glands, which produce hormones that increase blood glucose levels; or the ingestion of a heavy meal.

There are also conditions that cause low blood sugar, or *hypoglycemia*. These include liver disease in which the metabolism of glycogen is impaired, and conditions that result in an increased concentration of insulin in the blood (*hyperinsulinemia*). A decrease in blood glucose is life-threatening because the brain and cardiac cells are dependent on glucose in the blood and interstitial fluids. Hypoglycemia may result in muscle spasms, unconsciousness, and death. High concentrations of insulin can result from an overdose of insulin in the diabetic or from certain pancreatic tumors.

Specimens

Because the amount of glucose in the blood increases after a meal, it is important that the test be done only on fasting blood specimens. A random sample of blood is of little value for a glucose determination. The blood should be drawn long enough after the last meal that the food has been completely digested and absorbed and any excess has been stored. The specimen for a blood glucose test is usually drawn in the morning before breakfast and is called a *fasting blood sugar* (FBS). The term fasting in this case means that the patient has had no breakfast, no cream or sugar, no tea or cola drink, no drugs that might affect the blood glucose level, and no emotional disturbances that might cause liberation of glucose into the blood.

Glucose determinations may be performed on specimens of whole blood, plasma, or serum. They may be requested on other body fluids, especially urine and cerebrospinal fluid. In the past, glucose determinations were usually performed on whole blood; however, for several reasons plasma or serum is now preferred. The glucose concentration in whole blood is not identical to that in plasma or serum. There is a uniform concentration of glucose throughout the water portion of plasma and red blood cells, but there is more water in the plasma than in the red cells, which also contain hemoglobin. Since plasma (or serum) contains approximately 10–15 percent more water than whole blood, the total glucose in plasma (or serum) is about 10–15 percent greater than in whole blood.[6] The exact value can be calculated for any specimen; however, it is dependent on the method of analysis used and the hematocrit, or percentage of packed red blood cells per unit volume of blood.

There are other reasons for using plasma (or serum) rather than whole blood.[7] It is easier to interpret values obtained from a single-component system such as plasma than from a two-component system such as whole blood. It is necessary to mix whole blood thoroughly before sampling. This is a particular problem with automated methods, where samples stand in the sample tray for a period of time before being tested. There are several substances in blood that interfere with tests for blood glucose, either because they are measured as glucose or because they interfere in enzyme procedures. These substances are more concentrated within red blood cells, so tests on plasma tend to be more specific for glucose. As indicated above, values on whole blood tend to vary with the hematocrit. Glucose is more stable in plasma than in whole blood, as many glycolytic enzymes are present in the red blood cell. Finally, plasma or serum is easier to handle, to pipet precisely, and to store than whole blood.

An advantage of using whole blood is the convenience of measuring glucose directly on capillary blood, such as that taken from infants, or in mass screening programs for the detection of diabetes mellitus. Capillary blood must be thought of as essentially arterial rather than venous. In the fasting state the arterial (capillary) blood glucose concentration is 5 mg/dl greater than the venous concentration.

Another factor that must be taken into account in considering specimens for glucose determinations is the *stability of glucose in body fluids*. Many enzymes present in the blood, particularly in the red cells, affect glucose. As whole blood is allowed to stand at room temperature in a test tube, these enzymes destroy glucose. This action is called glycolysis, and it occurs at an average rate of approximately 7 mg/dl per hour.[8] Plasma that is removed from the red cells after moderate centrifugation contains leukocytes, which also metabolize glucose. However, cell-free plasma, prepared by adequate centrifugation, shows no glycolytic activity. When unhemolyzed serum or plasma is separated from the cells, the glucose concentration is generally stable for up to 8 hours at room temperature, and up to 72 hours at 4°C. Cerebrospinal fluids are frequently contaminated with bacteria or other cellular constituents such as leukocytes that may cause the breakdown of glucose. Thus, cerebrospinal fluids should be analyzed for glucose without delay. Refrigeration or the addition of a small amount of sodium fluoride to the fluid may retard glycolysis for a few hours.

Keeping these considerations in mind, there are several ways to prevent or retard glycolysis in a specimen to be analyzed. Samples for glucose analysis should be delivered to the laboratory as soon as possible after being drawn from the patient. Whole blood glucose determinations should be performed within $\frac{1}{2}$ hour after collection of the specimen, or a protein-free filtrate should be prepared within this time, if a preservative has not been added to the blood. In the filtrate stage, the concentration of glucose is relatively stable. If plasma or serum is to be used for the glucose determination, it must be separated from the cells or clot within $\frac{1}{2}$ hour after the blood is drawn.

Using a special anticoagulant, usually sodium fluoride, seems to be the best way to preserve blood glucose specimens. Sodium fluoride acts in two ways to preserve glucose: as an anticoagulant by tying up calcium and thus preventing clotting, and as an enzyme inhibitor that prevents glycolytic enzymes from destroying the glucose. However, clotting may occur after several hours, so it is advisable to use a combined fluoride-oxalate mixture. When the blood sample is placed in sodium fluoride tubes, it must be thoroughly mixed to ensure the proper effect, and the tubes should be kept at room temperature until tested. It must be remembered that a specimen containing sodium fluoride cannot be used in any determination involving an enzyme that might be inhibited by fluoride. For example, in the urea nitrogen method the enzyme urease would be inhibited by fluoride.

Glucose determinations may also be required on 24-hour collections of urine. Here again glycolysis must be prevented. This may be done by adding 5 ml of glacial acetic acid to the container before collection to inhibit bacterial activity by lowering the pH to 5 or 6. Another effective urine preservative is 5 g of sodium benzoate. Preservatives that have reducing ability must be avoided if a method that depends on the reducing ability of glucose is to be used.

Glucose tolerance tests

We have described tests for blood glucose on fasting blood specimens. However, in the detection and treatment of diabetes it is often necessary to have more information than can be obtained from this one determination. Patients with mild or diet-controlled diabetes may have fasting blood glucose levels within the normal range, but they may be unable to produce sufficient insulin for prompt metabolism of ingested carbohydrates. As a result, the blood glucose rises to abnormally high levels and the return to normal levels is delayed. Since early detection and management of diabetes is important to avoid the many complications of the disease, it is desirable to detect these early cases of diabetes or prediabetes. For these reasons, the physician may request a glucose tolerance test.

There are many glucose tolerance tests, but they are based on the same basic principles. The test begins with the patient in a fasting state, and blood is sampled and tested as a baseline control. Glucose is then administered, by either ingestion or injection, and samples are obtained at timed intervals. The amount of glucose administered and the collection intervals depend on the tolerance test used. Urine specimens may also be tested at fasting and timed intervals coinciding with the blood sampling. In many tolerance tests samples are taken at intervals of $\frac{1}{2}$, 1, 2, and 3 hours. In a less complicated procedure fasting specimens are collected, the desired load of glucose is administered, and a sample is taken in exactly 2 hours. This 2-hour sample is referred to as a 2-hour *postprandial* sample. Interpretation of glucose and insulin tolerance tests is rather complicated, but curves obtained from such tests have been described as normal, diabetes mellitus, hyperinsulinism, and hypoglycemic curves. When the 2-hour postprandial test is used, normal individuals show blood glucose levels at or slightly below normal at 2 hours.

Methods for quantitative determination of glucose

The various methods for the quantitative determination of glucose can be divided into three general categories: oxidation methods, aromatic amine methods, and enzymatic methods.

Oxidation methods

Oxidation methods for blood glucose depend on the fact that glucose contains an aldehyde group as part of its chemical structure. The presence of this aldehyde gives glucose its reducing properties (Fig. 2-2).

Other substances in blood also have reducing properties. Some of these *nonglucose reducing substances (NGRS)* are glutathione and ergothioneine, which are found within red blood cells, and other materials such as uric acid, creatinine, ascorbic acid, certain amino acids, homogentisic acid, creatine, phenols, glucuronic acid, and sugar phosphates. These nonglucose reducing substances are also referred to as *saccharoids.* The methods for determining blood glucose differ primarily in the way they handle the nonglucose reducing substances. When the nonglucose reducing substances are removed as part of a glucose determination, the resulting value is called the *true glucose* value.

Nonglucose reducing substances are removed in glucose determinations both by improvements in methodology and by precipitation of protein, which removes other interfering substances by coprecipitation. In the Folin-Wu method, which is a copper reduction method, the protein is removed with tungstic acid. This is not recommended because it gives a filtrate that contains significant amounts of nonglucose reducing substances, especially glutathione. The barium hydroxide and zinc sulfate method of removing protein is preferred, as it removes most of the nonglucose reducing substances and gives values only slightly higher than those obtained with the glucose oxidase and hexokinase techniques, which are specific for glucose. When glucose is analyzed with automated devices such as the AutoAnalyzer, the protein is separated from the specimen by means of a dialyzer. Of the many methods available for the determination of blood glucose, one reduction method employs potassium ferricyanide and another uses alkaline copper solutions. In either case, the glucose acts to reduce the reagent to a lower oxidation product. This product is then analyzed photometrically.

Alkaline copper reduction methods for glucose depend on the reduction of copper(II) [Cu(II)] to copper(I) [Cu(I)] while the aldehyde group of glucose is oxidized to gluconic acid.

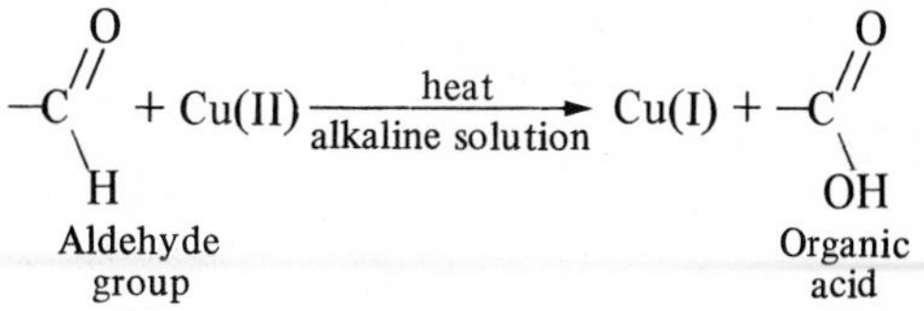

Fig. 2-2. Glucose molecule.

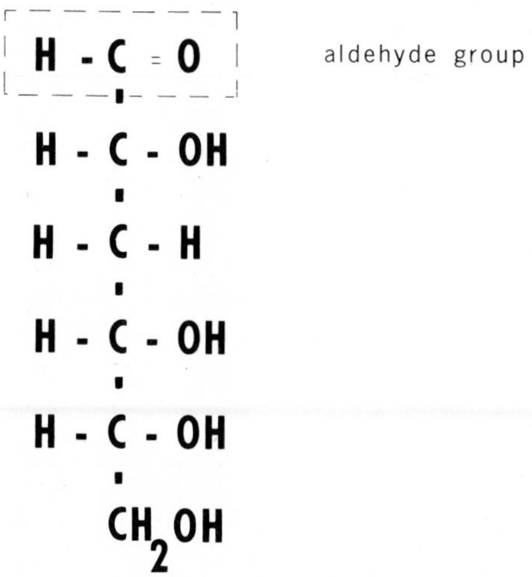

$$
\begin{array}{l}
\boxed{H - C = O} \quad \text{aldehyde group} \\
H - C - OH \\
H - C - H \\
H - C - OH \\
H - C - OH \\
CH_2OH
\end{array}
$$

$$
-\overset{\overset{O}{\|}}{C}\diagdown_H + Cu(II) \xrightarrow[\text{alkaline solution}]{\text{heat}} Cu(I) + -\overset{\overset{O}{\|}}{C}\diagdown_{OH}
$$

Aldehyde group   Organic acid

These were among the original methods of testing for glucose. Two classic examples of alkaline copper reduction methods are the Folin-Wu method and the Nelson-Somogyi method. With the older Folin-Wu method, an alkaline copper solution is added to a tungstic acid protein-free filtrate and heated. The copper(II) ion is reduced to copper(I). The copper(I) ion so formed then reduces a solution of phosphomolybdic acid to form a blue solution, which is measured photometrically. The Folin-Wu method is rather nonspecific for glucose, however, as it measures both glucose and nonglucose reducing substances. In the Nelson-Somogyi method barium hydroxide and zinc sulfate are used for the precipitation of proteins. This is a significant improvement, as the filtrate is virtually free of all nonglucose reducing substances. A disadvantage of all copper reduction methods is the reoxidation of copper(I) ions to copper(II) ions by air. Therefore, steps must be taken to minimize reoxidation in the procedure.

Other procedures that make use of the reducing ability of glucose are the *alkaline ferricyanide methods.* In these methods, a hot alkaline ferricyanide solution, which is yellow, is reduced by glucose to a ferrocyanide solution, which is colorless. The decrease in the yellow color is proportional to the glucose concentration. The reaction may be followed by measuring the loss of yellow color, or by adding ferric ions, which react with ferrocyanide to form Prussian blue. In this case the formation of a blue color is measured. An advantage of ferricyanide methods is that they are not as subject to reoxidation by air as the copper reduction methods. The ferricyanide method has been automated for use on the AutoAnalyzer.

Aromatic amine methods

These methods depend on the fact that various aromatic amines react with glucose in hot acetic acid to form colored derivatives. The aromatic amine commonly used is *ortho*-toluidine (*o*-toluidine). The methods involve a reaction between the aldehyde group of glucose and the amino group ($-NH_2$) of the aromatic amine. The *o*-toluidine method is replacing oxidation meth-

ods for the determination of glucose because it is highly specific, is easily performed, and can be adapted to serum or plasma without deproteinization. It has an advantage over the specific enzymatic methods in that it is not susceptible to enzyme inhibitors.[9] Several such procedures are available, and one will be included in this section. The manual procedures have been adapted for automated techniques.

Enzymatic methods

The use of enzymes is a means of achieving absolute specificity in the determination of glucose concentration. The two most widely used enzyme methods are based on the enzymes glucose oxidase and hexokinase. Glucose oxidase catalyzes the oxidation of glucose to gluconic acid and hydrogen peroxide. In some methods the amount of hydrogen peroxide produced or oxygen used is measured by an electrode process. In others a second enzyme, peroxidase, catalyzes the oxidation of a chromogen such as *o*-toluidine to a colored product; in this case the color that is formed is proportional to the amount of glucose present. When peroxidase is used in these procedures, the test is subject to interference from a number of substances such as ascorbic acid, uric acid, bilirubin, glutathione, and hemoglobin, which react with hydrogen peroxide, resulting in falsely low results. Many of these interfering substances can be removed by the use of a Nelson-Somogyi filtrate. Glucose oxidase methods have been adapted for automated procedures; Dextrostix (Ames Co., Elkhart, Ind.) is a commercial strip semiquantitative test that makes use of a glucose oxidase-peroxidase-chromogen system.

Another enzyme used in glucose tests is hexokinase. These methods are less subject to interference than the glucose oxidase-peroxidase methods. They have also been automated.

Sodium fluoride cannot be used as a preservative in any of the enzymatic methods, as it is an enzyme inhibitor.

Nelson-Somogyi method[10,11,12]

The Nelson-Somogyi method is widely used in clinical laboratories. It employs the reduction of an alkaline copper solution.

Principle

In this method use is made of the fact that glucose contains an aldehyde group and thus has reducing properties. Other nonglucose reducing substances may be present in the specimen, as described previously. These saccharoids may be removed by the preparation of a protein-free filtrate. There are many ways of precipitating protein; the Nelson-Somogyi method calls for the use of barium hydroxide and zinc sulfate, which form zinc hydroxide and barium sulfate. This method produces filtrates that are almost free from reducing substances other than glucose. Uric acid and protein are completely removed in this procedure. Thus, this filtrate gives a nearly true glucose value only slightly higher (2–3 mg/dl) than that obtained with enzymatic techniques.[13] The filter paper used in the precipitation step must be checked and must be free from outside contamination.

The Nelson-Somogyi method is accurate, simple, and convenient. It can be used with specimens of whole blood, serum, plasma, or cerebrospinal fluid.

After the protein-free filtrate has been prepared, the reduction step takes place. In a hot alkaline solution, the glucose present in the filtrate reduces cupric [Cu(II)] salts to cuprous [Cu(I)] salts. The amount of cuprous salts formed is directly proportional to the amount of glucose present in the specimen. Heat is provided by a boiling-water bath. Alkalinity is provided by the working copper reagent, which is prepared fresh daily.

Arsenomolybdic acid is employed as a color-producing reagent. It is partly reduced by the cuprous salts that are formed in the reduction step to lower oxidation products of a blue color.

The amount of blue present is measured in a photometer. The intensity of the blue color is a measure of the amount of copper reduced to the cuprous state and therefore of the amount of glucose originally present in the blood specimen. The intensities of the colors of the specimens to be measured are compared in a photometer with the color formed in a series of standard tubes.

The reactions taking place in the Nelson-Somogyi method are given below in equation form:

$$\text{Glucose (in filtrate)} + Cu(II) \xrightarrow[\text{solution}]{\text{hot, alkaline}}$$

$$Cu(I) + \text{oxidized glucose}$$

$$Cu(I) + \text{arsenomolybdic acid} \longrightarrow$$

$$Cu(II) + \text{reduced arsenomolybdate}$$
$$\text{(blue, stable color)}$$

Reagents

For the preparation of the protein-free filtrate:

1. Zinc sulfate (5 g/dl). Dissolve 100 g of $ZnSO_4 \cdot 7H_2O$, and dilute to 2000 ml in a graduated cylinder, using deionized water.
2. 0.3 N barium hydroxide. Dissolve 90 g of $Ba(OH)_2 \cdot 8H_2O$ in water and dilute to 2000 ml in a graduated cylinder. Filter if cloudy. Store in tight polyethylene containers filled to capacity.

Concentrations of the solutions of zinc sulfate and barium hydroxide are not as important as the fact that they exactly neutralize each other. To titrate, measure 10 ml of zinc sulfate solution into a 250-ml flask and add 50 ml of water and 4 drops of 1% phenolphthalein. Add barium hydroxide dropwise from the buret, using continual agitation, until the end point is reached. If the barium hydroxide is added too rapidly, a false end point will be reached. Dilute the stronger solution so that 10 ml of zinc solution requires 10 ml of barium solution ±0.05 ml.

For the reduction process:

1. Copper reagent, solution A. Dissolve 50 g of anhydrous sodium carbonate (Na_2CO_3), 50 g of Rochelle salts (potassium sodium tartrate), 40 g of sodium bicarbonate ($NaHCO_3$), and 400 g of anhydrous sodium sulfate (Na_2SO_4) in about 1600 ml of deionized water, and dilute to 2 L. Filter if necessary. Store this solution where the temperature will not fall below 20°C. A sediment may form after a few days. This may be filtered off without detriment to the reagent.

2. Copper reagent, solution B. Dissolve 150 g of copper sulfate ($CuSO_4 \cdot 5H_2O$) in 1 L of deionized water. Add 0.5 ml of concentrated H_2SO_4.

3. Alkaline copper reagent. This must be prepared fresh each day. Measure 4 ml of solution B into a 100-ml volumetric flask and dilute to 100 ml with solution A. Mix well.

    This reagent provides the copper ions necessary for the glucose to be oxidized. It contains sodium carbonate to provide the proper alkalinity and Rochelle salts to keep the copper in solution.

4. Glucose stock standard (10 mg/ml glucose). Dissolve 1 g of standard, pure, anhydrous glucose in a small amount of deionized water, and dilute to 100 ml with saturated benzoic acid. A saturated solution of benzoic acid can be prepared by dissolving 10 g of benzoic acid in 1 L of heated deionized water. Some crystals of benzoic acid should remain to ensure that the solution is saturated.

5. Glucose intermediate standard (0.5 mg/ml glucose). Dilute 5 ml of glucose stock standard to 100 ml with saturated benzoic acid. Prepare this solution once a week.

6. Glucose working standards. These must be prepared daily. Prepare four working standards by pipetting 1, 2, 3, and 4 ml of intermediate glucose standard into four 10-ml volumetric flasks. Dilute to volume with deionized water. The glucose concentrations in these working standards are 0.05 mg/ml (S_1), 0.10 mg/ml (S_2), 0.15 mg/ml (S_3), and 0.20 mg/ml (S_4). The working standards are used to construct the standard curve from which the unknown values are calculated. The working standards deteriorate and cannot be used for more than 1 day.

7. Control solution. This is commercially obtained or made by the laboratory by pooling glucose filtrates over a period of time, freezing, thawing, and mixing, dividing into 5-ml aliquots, and using as a control after establishing the control limit of values.

For the color development stage:

Arsenomolybdate color reagent. Dissolve 100 g of ammonium molybdate in 1800 ml of deionized water, add 84 ml of concentrated H_2SO_4, and mix. Add 12 g of sodium arsenate ($Na_2HAsO_4 \cdot 7H_2O$) dissolved in 100 ml of water. Mix, and place in an incubator at 37°C for 24–48 hours. Store in a glass-stoppered brown bottle. This reagent is stable indefinitely.

Procedure

Results with the Nelson-Somogyi method are precise within 5%. This method can be used for spinal fluid glucose determinations as well as for serum, plasma, or whole blood.

Preparation of protein-free filtrate of serum, plasma, or blood

1. Prepare a barium hydroxide-zinc sulfate filtrate by pipetting the following into a clean, dry test tube, corking and mixing well after each addition: 7.5 ml of deionized water; 0.5 ml of serum, plasma, or blood; 1.0 ml of $Ba(OH)_2$; and 1.0 ml of $ZnSO_4$.

2. Filter through filter paper into a labeled test tube. Other dilutions may be made when necessary. The filtrate should be clear and colorless.

Preparation of protein-free filtrate from capillary blood specimens

1. Pipet 1.5 ml of 1 mg/ml sodium fluoride (NaF) into a centrifuge tube.

2. Pipet 0.1 ml of blood from the patient and add to NaF in the centrifuge tube.

3. Prepare a filtrate by adding the following to the centrifuge tube: 0.2 ml of $Ba(OH)_2$ (mix with a glass stirring rod) and 0.2 ml of $ZnSO_4$ (mix as before).

4. Let stand for 5 minutes, then centrifuge. Place a small wisp of cotton on the tip of a 1-ml volumetric pipet before removing the supernatant fluid (filtrate) into the pipet.

Preparation of protein-free filtrate from cerebrospinal fluid specimens

1. Prepare a filtrate from cerebrospinal fluid as soon as possible after collection to prevent glycolysis. Cerebrospinal fluid glucose tests must be done in conjunction with glucose tests on blood or plasma collected at the same time as the spinal fluid, as normal values for spinal fluid glucose are 20 mg/dl less than those for blood. Prepare the filtrate by pipetting the following into a clean, dry centrifuge tube, mixing by rotating the tube after each addition: 5 ml of deionized or distilled water, 1 ml of spinal fluid, 2 ml of $Ba(OH)_2$, and 2 ml of $ZnSO_4$.

2. Centrifuge. Decant and save the supernatant fluid (filtrate).

Preparation of reagents

These are to be made fresh daily.

1. Alkaline copper reagent
2. Working glucose standards (S_1, S_2, S_3, and S_4)

Reduction of copper(II) to copper(I) by glucose

1. Pipet 1-ml portions of filtrates, controls, and working standards into Folin-Wu tubes. Pipet 1 ml of deionized water into one tube to serve as a blank. Folin-Wu tubes are specially constructed tubes with a constriction near the bulb end to prevent air from getting into the contents of the tube. Any oxygen present would tend to reoxidize the copper as it is being reduced by the glucose. The reduction process takes place in the Folin-Wu tube. The fluid level in the tube must be below the constriction and below the boiling-water level.

2. Add 1 ml of alkaline copper reagent, and mix well by hitting the tube against the hand.

3. Place the tubes in a boiling-water bath for 20 minutes. During boiling the copper is reduced by glucose, with the aid of heat and alkalinity, from its cupric form to cuprous oxide. This settles as a fine yellow or orange precipitate.

4. Remove the tubes from the boiling-water bath after 20 minutes, and immediately place them in a cold-water bath for 1 minute. The timing of boiling and cooling is critical and must be watched carefully. If overcooled, copper(I) will be reoxidized to copper(II) by the oxygen in the air.

Color development

1. Add 1 ml of arsenomolybdate color reagent to all tubes, and mix by hitting against the hand. The color develops very rapidly and will be completely developed by the time mixing and evolution of carbon dioxide are complete (carbon dioxide evolves as the color develops). The mixture will appear to foam during this process. Vigorous agitation is necessary to ensure complete reaction. The arsenomolybdate should be added to the Folin-Wu tubes as soon as possible.

2. A deep blue color is the result of reduction of arsenomolybdate. This color is stable indefinitely. The intensity of the blue color is directly proportional to the amount of glucose originally present in the specimen.

3. Dilute the solution in the Folin-Wu tubes to 25 ml (these tubes have a calibration mark to assist in the dilution step) with deionized water.

Cork and mix thoroughly. Transfer to labeled calibrated cuvettes for reading in the photometer.

Reading tubes in the photometer

1. Polish the cuvettes.
2. Read in the photometer at a wavelength setting of 505 nm.
3. The color is very stable, and the tubes may therefore be read in the photometer at any time.
4. Enter galvanometer readings for standards, controls, and unknowns on a work sheet. Prepare a standard graph, and calculate the milligrams of glucose per 100 ml of blood.

Calculations

Blood glucose results are reported in units of milligrams of glucose per 100 ml of blood, or mg/dl. These units are used to report many of the common chemistry values determined in the laboratory. The calculating of glucose results, like other results, is a stepwise procedure:

1. *To determine how much of the specimen was actually used in the procedure:*

In this procedure, 0.5 ml of blood is used to prepare the protein-free filtrate. This 0.5 ml is diluted to a total of 10 ml by the addition of 7.5 ml of water, 1.0 ml of $Ba(OH)_2$, and 1.0 ml of $ZnSO_4$. Of the resulting protein-free filtrate, 1 ml is pipetted into the Folin-Wu tube for the reduction process. These factors must be taken into consideration in the final calculation. The 1 ml of filtrate used in the Folin-Wu tube is the actual amount of specimen treated in the determination steps: copper reduction, color development, and analysis in the photometer. Using the following formula, the amount of blood actually being measured in the photometer cuvette and the amount represented by the percent transmittance reading is found:

$$\frac{0.5 \text{ ml of blood}}{10 \text{ ml of filtrate}} = \frac{x \text{ ml of blood}}{1 \text{ ml of filtrate}}$$

$$x = 0.05 \text{ ml of blood}$$

The final result is reported in units of glucose present in 100 ml of blood (mg/dl), however, so another step is necessary in the calculation.

2. *To determine how many milligrams of glucose is present in 100 ml of blood (mg/dl):*

The value read from the standard graph is the milligrams of glucose in 1 ml of filtrate or in 0.05 ml of blood. Using the following formula, the glucose value in milligrams per deciliter may be found:

$$\frac{\text{mg of glucose}}{0.05 \text{ ml of blood}} \text{ (read from standard graph)}$$

$$\times \frac{100 \text{ ml of blood}}{0.05 \text{ ml of blood}} = \text{mg}/100 \text{ ml (mg/dl)}$$

If any other dilutions have been made during the procedure, this must be taken into consideration in the calculations. In cases of high blood glucose values, dilutions are often made.

For any specimen with a glucose concentration that is higher than that of the most concentrated standard, special steps must be followed. The value of such a specimen cannot be read from the standard graph for this batch. If this be the case, a dilution of the filtrate is made. For a 1:2 dilution, use 1 ml of filtrate and 1 ml of deionized water. For a 1:5 dilution, use 1 ml of filtrate and 4 ml of deionized water. The dilution made will depend on the concentration of glucose present in the specimen. One milliliter of this dilution is pipetted into a Folin-Wu tube, and this is analyzed, along with a blank, standards, and controls, in the regular manner. The standard graph is prepared and the unknown value read from it. The additional dilution factor must be applied in the final calculation of the glucose value. Making a dilution of the colored solution in the cuvette is not enough. A filtrate dilution must be made. In cases of high blood glucose levels, there is not enough copper in the copper reagent to be completely reduced by the glucose present in the specimen. To allow for this possibility, a diluted filtrate is recommended.

o-Toluidine glucose determination

As mentioned previously, determinations of glucose with o-toluidine[14,15] are replacing procedures such as the Nelson-Somogyi method that depend on the reducing ability of glucose. o-Toluidine methods depend on the reaction between the aldehyde group of glucose and the amino group of the aromatic amine o-toluidine. These methods have the advantages that they are highly specific, easily performed, adaptable to serum or plasma without deproteinization, and not susceptible to enzyme inhibitors. They have also been automated. The following procedure is a micromethod, adapted for situations where there is a limited amount of specimen.

Principle

This method makes use of the fact that aldohexoses react specifically with o-toluidine in glacial acetic acid in the presence of heat to produce a blue-green color. Because aldohexoses other than glucose are usually present in very small concentrations in body fluids, results obtained by this method approach the true value for glucose. The method has the additional advantage that it can be performed directly on serum, plasma, cerebrospinal fluid, or urine without deproteinization. When whole blood is used, or when the specimen is moderately hemolyzed, it must be deproteinized. The procedure can be used on capillary blood.

Reagents

These reagents are for both direct methods and those utilizing a protein-free filtrate.

1. Glucose stock standard (10 mg/ml glucose). Dissolve 1.000 g of standard, pure, anhydrous glucose in a small amount of deionized water, and dilute to 100 ml with saturated benzoic acid. (See under Nelson-Somogyi Method for preparation). Benzoic acid serves as an effective glucose preservative.

2. Glucose working standards. Prepare four working standards daily: S_1, 0.5 mg/ml; S_2, 1.0 mg/ml; S_3, 2.0 mg/ml; and S_4, 3.0 mg/ml. Prepare S_2, S_3, and S_4 by pipetting 1, 2, and 3 ml of the glucose stock standard into three 10-ml volumetric flasks and diluting to volume with deionized water. To prepare S_1 (0.5 mg/ml), dilute 5 ml of the 1.0 mg/ml (S_2) standard to 10 ml in a 10-ml volumetric flask.

3. Trichloroacetic acid (3 g/dl). Quickly weigh 30 g of reagent-grade TCA, transfer to a 1-L flask, and dilute to volume with deionized water. Store at 4°C.

4. o-Toluidine reagent (6 ml/dl). Add 1.5 g of reagent-grade thiourea to 940 ml of reagent-grade glacial acetic acid. Dissolve completely before adding 60 ml of o-toluidine. Mix well and store in an amber glass reagent bottle at room temperature. Thiourea is added as a stabilizer; with it the reagent can be used only after aging overnight. After this aging the reagent retains stability for several months.

Procedure

Direct determination on specimen without deproteinization

1. Measure 0.05 ml of each sample (serum, plasma, standards, control, and water for a blank) into screw cap tubes.

2. Add 3.0 ml of o-toluidine reagent to each tube and mix well.

3. Stopper with Teflon-lined screw caps and heat in a boiling-water bath or a heating block preset at 100°C for 12 minutes. Remove from heat and cool in an ice bath for 5 minutes. Remove from ice and bring to room temperature. This requires about 10 minutes in a 25°C water bath. The tubes are stoppered with Teflon-lined screw caps to prevent contamination from the steam of a boiling-water bath. Maximum color development is reached after 10–12 minutes at

100°C; 16 minutes or longer results in lower absorbance readings.

4. Transfer the color reaction mixture to cuvettes, polish, and read the absorbances of the standard and the unknown against the blank at 630 nm. The color is stable for at least 1 hour.

5. For samples reading lower than the last standard, dilute the color reaction mixture 1:2 with glacial acetic acid. Dilute the blank similarly, and read the diluted sample against the diluted blank. To calculate the results, multiply the value on the graph by 2.

Determination on specimen with deproteinization

1. Prepare protein-free filtrates by adding 0.5-ml portions of sample (blood, serum, plasma, urine, or spinal fluid), control, working standards, and water (for the blank) to 4.5-ml portions of TCA. Mix and set aside for at least 5 minutes. Filter. Filtration is preferred to centrifugation since it is difficult to remove particulate matter from the supernatant fluid by centrifugation and the apparent clarity of the supernatant fluid may be deceptive. Tungstic acid, barium hydroxide, zinc sulfate, and TCA filtrates yield approximately the same results; perchloric acid filtrates hinder color development.

2. Transfer 0.5 ml of each clear filtrate (specimens, blank, and standards) into appropriately marked tubes. To each tube add 3 ml of o-toluidine reagent. Mix well. Cap with Teflon-lined screw caps.

3. Boil the mixtures in a water bath or heating block (100°C) for 12 minutes. Remove from heat and cool in an ice-water bath for 5 minutes. Remove from the ice bath and bring to room temperature by placing in a 25°C water bath for about 10 minutes.

4. Transfer the reaction mixture to cuvettes and read against the blank at 630 nm. The color is stable for at least 1 hour.

5. For samples reading lower than the last standard, dilute the color reaction mixture 1:2 with glacial acetic acid. Dilute the blank similarly, and read the diluted sample against the diluted blank. To calculate the results, multiply the value on the graph by 2.

Calculations

Blood glucose results are reported as milligrams of glucose per 100 ml of blood, or mg/dl. To calculate the results, plot the percent transmittance against the glucose concentration of the standards on semilogarithmic graph paper. The line joining the plotted points should be straight and should pass through the origin. The glucose concentrations of the unknown samples can be read directly from the graph as the same amount of sample and standard is measured in both the direct and the filtrate procedure, namely 0.05 ml. In the direct color development, 0.05 ml of blood and working standard solution is used. In the procedure involving preparation of a protein-free filtrate, 0.05 ml of blood is also tested, as shown by the following:

$$\frac{0.5 \text{ ml of blood}}{5 \text{ ml of filtrate}} = \frac{x \text{ ml of blood}}{0.5 \text{ ml of filtrate}}$$

$$x = 0.05 \text{ ml of blood}$$

The milligrams of glucose present in 100 ml of blood is calculated as follows:

$$\frac{\text{mg of glucose}}{0.05 \text{ ml of blood}} \text{(read from standard graph)}$$

$$\times \frac{100 \text{ ml of blood}}{0.05 \text{ ml of blood}} = \text{mg/dl}$$

Therefore, multiply the reading from the graph (mg/0.05 ml blood) by 2000 (100 ÷ 0.05) to convert to mg/dl. If any other dilutions have been made during the procedure, this must be taken into consideration in the calculations.

Technical factors and sources of error

There are many causes of poor agreement between duplicates or of inaccurate results. Pipetting errors in preparing the filtrates; in transferring the standards, controls, and filtrates; or in preparing the reagents are one major cause of inaccurate results. Pipetting errors are greater with whole blood than with serum or plasma. Adequate mixing is important, and insufficient mixing can lead to difficulties. Whenever a reagent is added to another mixture (copper reagent or arsenomolybdate reagent, for example), adequate mixing of the contents of the tube is essential. If the photometer is not used correctly or if the blank tube is not adjusted properly at the beginning of the readings, the end results will be inaccurate.

Sodium fluoride is the anticoagulant of choice for blood glucose determinations. If another type of anticoagulant is used, the plasma must be separated from cells or the protein-free filtrate must be set up within 30 minutes after the blood has been drawn.

It is important that the timing during reduction of copper in the water bath be watched carefully. It is also important that the water be actually boiling to ensure complete reduction. The cold-water bath is also essential, as it stops the reaction.

The standards used for the procedure must be in good condition. They must be analyzed at the same time as the rest of the batch, and if another batch is analyzed later in the day, new standards must be also.

Reporting results and recording laboratory data

Glucose results, in mg/dl, are usually reported to the nearest whole number. The laboratory retains the standard graphs and the galvanometer readings obtained for a particular procedure for a period of time. The actual results are kept by the laboratory indefinitely as a permanent record. The results are reported to the physician only when the control values check out.

Normal values

For whole blood glucose, fasting:
65-90 mg/dl (Nelson-Somogyi)
60-100 mg/dl (*o*-toluidine)
For plasma or serum glucose, fasting:
70-110 mg/dl (*o*-toluidine)
For cerebrospinal fluid glucose:
40-75 mg/dl (Nelson-Somogyi)
40-80 mg/dl (*o*-toluidine)

CHLORIDE

One of the procedures in the chemistry laboratory in which titration is used as a means of quantitative measurement is the determination of chloride. Because titration is an important volumetric technique in the clinical laboratory, the chloride procedure will be described in some detail.

Chloride is one of the electrolytes found in the body. As used in the clinical chemistry laboratory, the term *electrolytes* refers primarily to sodium, potassium, chloride, and bicarbonate, because these substances are the major ions in the body. These four electrolytes are often discussed together because changes in the concentration of one of them are almost always accompanied by changes in the concentration of one or more of the others. Electrolytes are substances that form or exist as ions or charged particles when dissolved in water. One example of an electrolyte is sodium chloride, which forms Na^+ and Cl^- in water. The ions Na^+ and Cl^- are also called electrolytes. The sodium ion is called a *cation* because it is attracted by a negatively charged electrode or cathode, and the chloride ion is called an *anion* because it is attracted by a positively charged electrode or anode. All charged particles are either anions (negatively charged) or cations (positively charged).

Chloride is found in serum, plasma, cerebrospinal fluid, tissue fluid, and urine. There is very little chloride inside the cells of the body, with the exception of the red cells, which contain some chloride. The chief extracellular anions are chloride and bicarbonate, and there is a reciprocal relationship between them; that is, when there is a decrease in the amount of one, there is an increase in the amount of the other. In the blood, two-thirds of the chloride is found in the plasma and only one-third in the red cells. Because of the difference in chloride concentration between the red cells and the plasma, the test for chloride is routinely performed on plasma (or serum) and not on whole blood. Physiologically, only the concentration of chloride in the extracellular fluid is important. This is another reason why plasma or serum is chosen as the specimen for this determination.

Clinical significance

The chloride ion is the most important anion of the extracellular fluids in the body. It is the major anion that counterbalances the major cation, sodium, to maintain the electrical neutrality of the body fluids. Electrical neutrality is maintained at all times in the body fluids. This means that the sum of all the cations (positively charged particles) equals the sum of all the anions (negatively charged particles).

Chloride has two main functions in the body: it is important in determining the osmotic pressure, which controls the distribution of water between cells, plasma, and interstitial fluid, and it is important in maintaining the acid-base balance. Chloride also plays an important role in the buffering action when oxygen and carbon dioxide exchange in the red blood cells. This activity is known as the *chloride shift*. When blood is oxygenated, chloride travels from the red blood cells to the plasma, and at the same time bicarbonate leaves the plasma and enters the red cells. Water travels in the same direction as chloride, and the red blood cells become dehydrated when the blood is oxygenated. Whenever bicarbonate goes from the red blood cells to the plasma, as it must do during carbon dioxide transport, the bicarbonate anions are replaced by an equivalent amount of chloride anions.

An example of the chloride shift in the laboratory is the replacement action that occurs when a specimen for a chloride determination is allowed to stand for a while before the cells and plasma are separated. When whole blood comes into contact with air, carbon dioxide (and thus bicarbonate) escapes from the blood. As carbon dioxide leaves the plasma, chloride diffuses (or shifts) out of the red cells to replace it. The contact between whole blood and air, therefore, has the effect of lowering the plasma carbon dioxide and raising the plasma chloride. Specimens of whole blood left in contact with air may therefore give falsely high plasma or serum chloride values.

Under Collection, Preservation, and Preparation of Laboratory Specimens, the proper general handling of blood specimens was discussed. The cells must be removed from the plasma by centrifugation as quickly as possible. Once separated from the cells, the serum or plasma has a very stable chloride concentration.

The other important function of chloride is to regulate the fluid content of the body and its influence on the kidney. The kidney maintains the electrolyte concentration of the plasma within very narrow limits. This regulation is necessary for life. Renal function is set to regulate the composition of the extracellular fluid first and then the volume. Consequently, if the body loses salt (sodium chloride), it loses water.

Low serum or plasma chloride values may be seen in nephritis where salt is lost, as in chronic pyelonephritis. A low chloride value may also be seen in the types of metabolic acidotic conditions that are caused by excessive production or diminished excretion of acids, as in diabetic acidosis and renal failure. Prolonged vomiting, from any cause, may ultimately result in a decrease in serum and body chloride.

High serum or plasma chloride values are seen in dehydration and in conditions that cause decreased renal blood flow, such as congestive heart failure. Excessive treatment with or dietary intake of chloride ions also results in high serum levels.

As discussed above, the electrolytes are the major charged particles present in the extracellular fluid. The chief negatively charged constituents are chloride and bicarbonate. The chief positively charged constituents are sodium and potassium. There are other electrolytes, but those mentioned are the ones most likely to show variation in electrolyte problems. Collectively, the four charged particles chloride, bicarbonate, sodium, and potassium make up the electrolytes. It is essential that the positively charged particles balance, or electrically neutralize, the negatively charged particles. When this balance is not achieved, electrolyte imbalance occurs; this is extremely dangerous for the patient and can be fatal. Therefore, to assess electrolyte balance, the laboratory must often perform electrolyte determinations. A set of electrolyte determinations consists of tests for chloride, bicarbonate, sodium, and potassium. These determinations are often done as emergency procedures, for electrolyte imbalance cannot be tolerated by the patient for long. Treatment to remedy the imbalance must be started as quickly as possible.

Specimens

Because two-thirds of the chloride in blood is found in the plasma, plasma or serum is ordinarily used for analysis of chloride. After venipuncture, the blood is placed in a properly labeled tube. Blood should be collected for a chloride determination in tubes that are free of even trace contamination. There are many sources of chloride in the laboratory, and even tap water may contain a significant amount of chloride. Glassware and pipets used for the chloride determination must also be free from any contamination with chloride. The anticoagulant used most frequently is potassium oxalate, but ethylenediaminetetraacetic acid (EDTA) can also be used. Heparin is a very good anticoagulant for this purpose, but it is very expensive and is therefore not used as a rule. Sodium fluoride cannot be used for the chloride determination, because the fluoride is a halogen (as is chloride), and both react in the same way in the analysis. If sodium fluoride were used a falsely high chloride value would be obtained because the fluoride would also be measured. If serum is used, the blood is placed in a labeled tube containing no anticoagulant and is allowed to clot. The serum or plasma should be removed from the red cells as soon as possible after the blood is drawn to prevent the chloride shift from occurring. Moderate hemolysis does not significantly affect the concentration of chloride in the serum.

Methods for quantitative determination

Most analyses for chloride employ some type of titration procedure. The titrations can be carried out manually or potentiometrically. Manual titration methods for the detection of chloride include the Cavett and Bolderidge method, the Volhard method, the Whitehorn method, and the Schales and Schales method. One commonly used potentiometric titration method employs the

Buchler-Cotlove Chloridometer. Chloride is also measured colorimetrically by the AutoAnalyzer method, which is used in many laboratories.

Schales and Schales chloride method[16]

Principle

The interfering proteins are first removed by precipitation with tungstic acid (the modified Folin-Wu filtrate method). Proteins, if present, will interfere with color detection and with the reaction. Titration is the next step. The chloride in the protein-free filtrate is titrated with mercuric nitrate [$Hg(NO_3)_2$], using diphenylcarbazone to indicate when the end point has been reached. When all the chloride in the filtrate has reacted with the mercuric nitrate, the diphenylcarbazone indicator changes color from orange-red to faint blue-violet.

In the titration with mercuric nitrate, the reaction taking place is

$$2NaCl + Hg(NO_3)_2 \longrightarrow 2NaNO_3 + HgCl_2$$

When all the chloride ions have reacted with the mercuric nitrate, the first excess of mercuric ions react with the indicator to form a faint blue-violet complex salt. The reaction is complete when the end point is reached—that is, when the first blue-violet color is produced by the addition of a drop or a split drop of mercuric nitrate. The first, faintest, permanent blue-violet is the end point. It is most important to use caution in titrating, as even a fraction of a milliliter of overtitration will result in grossly inaccurate results. The amount of standard mercuric nitrate used in the titration is an index of the chloride content.

Reagents

For the preparation of the protein-free filtrate:

1. 0.083 N H_2SO_4.
2. Sodium tungstate [10 g/100 ml (or 10 g/dl)].

Ten grams of $Na_2WO_4 \cdot H_2O$ is dissolved and diluted to 100 ml with deionized water.

For titration of chloride in the filtrate:

1. Mercuric nitrate. Weigh 3.0 g of $Hg(NO_3)_2$, and dissolve it in 200 ml of deionized water and 20 ml of 2 N nitric acid (HNO_3). Quantitatively transfer the solution to a 1-L volumetric flask, and dilute it to the calibration mark. Mix well.

   The mercuric nitrate solution is used in the buret for titrating the chloride ions. It is necessary to know the concentration of the mercuric nitrate if the concentration of the chloride is to be determined. It is difficult to weigh mercuric nitrate accurately, since it takes up water readily. Therefore, it is weighed approximately and its concentration is checked against a known, stable, standard solution of sodium chloride each time a batch of chlorides is analyzed. The addition of a specific amount of nitric acid in the initial preparation of the reagent serves to sharpen the end point of the reaction. If more or less nitric acid is added, the end-point color will not be as sharp.

2. Standard sodium chloride. Weigh 584.5 mg of NaCl analytically; dissolve and dilute it to 1 L with deionized water in a volumetric flask.

   This reagent is used to find the concentration (normality) of the mercuric nitrate solution. This standard can be weighed accurately on the analytical balance. Chemically pure (CP) sodium chloride is dried at 120°C and stored in a desiccator. This is the chemical that should be used to prepare the standard solution. The concentration of the sodium chloride expressed in normality is 0.01 N. The concentration can also be expressed as 0.01 equiv/L, or 0.01 meq/ml.

3. Diphenylcarbazone indicator. Dissolve 100 mg of diphenylcarbazone (Eastman Kodak number 4459) in 100 ml of 95% alcohol.

   This reagent must be stored in the dark, preferably in the refrigerator. In the daylight, the orange-red solution turns yellow in a few days and cannot be used. Even in the dark, its color changes slowly to cherry red. Because it is unstable to this degree, this reagent is prepared fresh each month. If the indicator is cherry red, it is no longer suitable for use in this procedure.

Procedure

Results with this procedure are precise within 1 percent. This method is applicable to the determination of chloride in a variety of biological fluids (serum, plasma, urine, and cerebrospinal fluid).

Preparation of protein-free filtrates

1. Prepare duplicate Folin-Wu filtrates from serum, plasma, or control specimens by pipetting the following into centrifuge tubes, corking and mixing well after each addition: 8 ml of 0.083 N H_2SO_4; 1 ml of plasma, serum, or control; and 1 ml of 10 g/dl Na_2WO_4. Cork and mix well.

2. Centrifuge for 5 minutes at 2000–3000 r/min.

3. From the centrifuge tube, pipet 2 ml of the clear, supernatant filtrate into a labeled 25-ml Erlenmeyer flask. Pipet a duplicate aliquot into another labeled 25-ml Erlenmeyer flask. Each filtrate is always pipetted in duplicate.

Titration of standard sodium chloride to determine normality of mercuric nitrate solution

1. Into duplicate 25-ml Erlenmeyer flasks pipet 2-ml samples of the NaCl standard solution. To each of the flasks add 0.06 ml of diphenylcarbazone indicator *just before* titration (indicator is made up in alcohol and will evaporate if exposed to the air for too long).

2. From a buret containing $Hg(NO_3)_2$, add reagent until the blue-violet end point is reached.

As the end point is approached, add the $Hg(NO_3)_2$ in split drops.

3. Titrate each of the 2-ml samples of standard solution, and record the amount of reagent needed to reach the end point. The duplicate titrations must agree within the allowable range established. This range will depend on the size of the buret used. For a 5-ml buret with 0.02-ml calibrated divisions, the titrations of duplicate solutions must agree within 0.02 ml. If this agreement is not achieved, additional samples must be pipetted and titrated until the duplicates do agree.

Titration of chloride in the filtrate

1. To each of the flasks containing 2 ml of filtrate of unknown concentration, add 0.06 ml of diphenylcarbazone just before titrating.

2. Titrate with the mercuric nitrate in the buret until the blue-violet end point is reached. Again, the final end point is approached by addition of split drops from the buret. Record the buret readings. Duplicate titrations must agree within the established range to be considered accurate.

Calculations

When the titration has been completed, the results are calculated. Chloride results are usually reported in units of milliequivalents per liter (meq/L). These units are used because the major functions of chloride in the body are associated with osmotic pressure regulation and acid-base balance.

1. *To calculate the normality of standard sodium chloride solution:*

The standard sodium chloride was weighed analytically and diluted volumetrically: 584.5 mg of NaCl was diluted to 1 L with deionized water; this is the same as 0.5845 g/L. A 1 N NaCl solution would contain 58.45 g/L, or 58.45 mg/ml. For the standard solution used in this procedure

$$\frac{58.45 \text{ g}}{1 \text{ } N} = \frac{0.5845 \text{ g}}{x \text{ } N}$$

$$x = 0.01 \text{ } N \text{ for standard NaCl}$$

0.01 N NaCl is the same as 0.01 equiv/L, or 0.01 meq/ml, so 1 ml of the standard sodium chloride solution contains 0.01 meq of NaCl.

2. *To calculate the normality of the mercuric nitrate solution:*

Two milliliters of the standard sodium chloride is titrated with the mercuric nitrate reagent, and the volume of mercuric nitrate (in milliliters) required to reach the end point is recorded. Using the following equation, the normality of the mercuric nitrate can be calculated:

$$N_{std\,\text{NaCl}} \times V_{std\,\text{NaCl}} = N_{\text{Hg(NO}_3)_2} \times V_{\text{Hg(NO}_3)_2}$$

$$0.01 \times 2 \text{ ml} = x \times \text{ml used for titration}$$

$$x = \text{normality of mercuric}$$
$$\text{nitrate solution}$$

where N = normality
V = volume

3. *To calculate the normality of unknown serum or plasma:*

The filtrate was prepared with 1 ml of serum or plasma, 8 ml of 0.083 N H_2SO_4, and 1 ml of 10 g/dl Na_2WO_4. In the final filtrate, there is 1 ml of serum in a total volume of 10 ml, or 0.1 ml of serum in 1 ml of filtrate. The measured 2-ml aliquot titrated therefore contains 0.2 ml of serum or plasma. The following equation is used to calculate the normality of the unknown:

$$N_{\text{Hg(NO}_3)_2} \times V_{\text{Hg(NO}_3)_2} = N_{\text{serum}} \times V_{\text{serum}}$$

Normality from step 2 $\times$ buret reading

$$= x \times 0.2 \text{ ml}$$

$$x = \text{normality of serum or plasma}$$
$$(\text{meq/ml or equiv/L})$$

4. *To calculate the chloride value in milliequiva-*

lents *per liter (desired units for report to physician):*

One equivalent equals 1000 meq. Therefore multiplying the result obtained in step 3 by 1000 converts the value to the desired units (meq/L). Results are rounded off and reported to the nearest whole number.

Technical factors and sources of error

Pipetting errors can cause inaccurate results. This is probably the major source of error. Pipetting is involved in preparing the protein-free filtrates, transferring the filtrate to the Erlenmeyer flask for titration, and measuring the standard solutions and diphenylcarbazone indicator. A pipetting error in any of these steps can cause the entire determination to be in error.

Poor titration techniques are also a cause of error. Improper handling of the buret or carelessness in detecting the end point are common causes of errors.

All reagents used in the chloride determination must be free from any outside chloride contamination. No anticoagulant containing a halogen (chloride, bromide, fluoride, or iodide) can be used in the determination because it would give falsely high results. Glassware and pipets must be chemically clean. Sources of chloride contamination in the laboratory are many (including tap water, which contains significant amounts). For this reason, all glassware must be rinsed well with deionized water, and all reagents must be prepared with deionized water.

Buchler-Cotlove Chloridometer method[17]

Principle

The accuracy of the manual titration methods, such as the Schales and Schales method, depends on the technician's skill and judgment in determining the visual end point of the titration reaction. To eliminate the factor of human judgment, methods for measuring the end point electrically have been developed. One such method involves the use of the Buchler-Cotlove Chloridometer.

In the Buchler-Cotlove Chloridometer, silver ions are released from a silver wire when a current is generated in an electrode. The silver ions combine with chloride in the specimen to form insoluble silver chloride. The potential of the solution being titrated changes at the equivalence point, since the solution goes from having an excess of chloride ions to having an excess of silver ions. There must be a sufficient volume of sample that the electrodes are fully immersed in the solution. A small stirrer attached to the electrode assembly thoroughly mixes the specimen as it is being analyzed.

When all the chloride is used, the change in potential is used to shut off the machine. In this way the end point is detected automatically. The lapsed time for each titration is automatically recorded on a timer. Since the rate of release of silver ions is constant, the amount of time during which they are released is directly proportional to the amount of chloride in the sample. That is, the more chloride present in the sample, the longer it takes to generate enough silver ions to combine with all of it. In the calculations the titration time for the unknown is compared with the titration time for a standard sodium chloride solution. Modern instruments read directly in milliequivalents per liter.

The Chloridometer method is one of the most accurate methods available for determining chloride in the clinical laboratory. Other halogens do interfere with this method, just as they do with other methods for chloride. The Chloridometer can be used with plasma, serum, cerebrospinal fluid, sweat, and urine specimens. Specimens are diluted in a mixture of acetic and nitric acids containing a small amount of gelatin. The nitric acid provides good electrolytic conductivity and the acetic acid provides a sharper end point. All reagents must be prepared with chloride-free water (distilled or deionized). An automatic diluter is convenient for delivering the acid reagent and the standard or unknown samples into the titration vials. The electrodes of the machine must be rinsed well after each analysis.

Reagents

1. Chloride standard (100 meq/L). Dilute 5.845 g of NaCl to 1 L with deionized water.
2. Chloride standard (25 meq/L). Dilute 1.461 g of NaCl to 1 L with deionized water.
3. Diluent, 0.1 N HNO_3-10 ml/dl acetic acid. To 900 ml of deionized water, add 6.4 ml of concentrated HNO_3 and 100 ml of glacial acetic acid.
4. Gelatin indicator. Thoroughly mix the following dry pulverized chemicals in the weight ratio of 60:1:1:
   a. Gelatin, Knox Unflavored Gelatin number 1 (Chas. B. Knox Gelatin Company, Inc., Johnstown, N.Y.), or any USP grade.
   b. Thymol blue, water-soluble.
   c. Thymol crystals, reagent grade.
   To 6.2 g of dry mixture, add approximately 1 L of hot deionized water and heat gently with continuous swirling until the solution is clear. Dispense into vials and refrigerate; remove a fresh vial for each day's analyses, immersing it in hot water to liquefy the gelatin.

Procedure

For electrode maintenance:

1. New silver wire should be adjusted daily or when the wire becomes pointed. Loosen the binding post holding the silver wire in place and advance the silver wire. Cut it with a wire cutter and position the anode so that it is almost flush with the upper edge of the stirrer. For proper generation of silver ions an adequate surface area

of the generator anode must be immersed in the solution.

2. Tighten the binding post against the silver wire. The generator anode must make a secure electrical connection with the binding post above and to the right of the electrode assembly.

3. Polish the new surface of the advanced wire, since machine oil deposited in fabricating the wire temporarily insulates the anode and prevents the generation of silver. Polishing may also be required if the blank time is excessive. To polish the electrodes, rub a small amount of silver polish on a strip of dampened cloth. Do not use sandpaper, emery paper, or any other strongly abrasive material. Using a shoeshine motion, scrub the electrode until it is thoroughly clean and bright. When polishing the indicator electrodes, also scrub the bottom end of the nylon parts in contact with the sample during titration. Although the performance of the instrument will not be impaired unless a film thick enough to conduct current is collected on the bottom end, it is advisable always to polish the end of the rod whenever the electrodes are scrubbed. When the polishing procedure is finished, rinse well with deionized water and blot dry.

4. Pipet 0.05 or 0.1 ml of standard into a titration vial, using a micropipet. Add four drops of gelatin and titrate the standard to condition the electrodes. Discard the result.

5. Between titrations, rinse the electrodes with deionized water and blot dry with a gauze square.

6. When the titrations are finished, rinse the electrodes, blot dry, and place them in a clean dry vial.

For sample analysis:

1. To 0.05 or 0.1 ml of biological fluid (depending on the instrument used), add 4 ml of nitric-acetic diluent and 4 drops of gelatin indicator in a titration vial.

2. Prepare blanks containing 4 ml of acid diluent and 4 drops of gelatin indicator.

3. Prepare standards containing 0.05 or 0.1 ml of standard solution, 4 ml of acid diluent, and 4 drops of gelatin indicator.

4. Polish all four electrodes before using the instrument. See steps 1 to 4 in the maintenance procedure above.

5. Turn the *titration rate* switch to the proper rate for the chloride level to be analyzed.

6. Place the sample titration vial in position and turn the titration switch to position 1.

7. Set the adjustable pointer of the meter-relay 10 divisions above the indicating pointer after the indicating pointer has reached a stable position below 5 microamperes.

8. Set the *seconds* and/or *meq/L* indicator dials to 000.0.

9. Turn the titration switch to position 2 to start titration.

10. Record seconds and/or meq/L at the end of the titration.

11. Remove the vial and rinse the electrodes with deionized water.

12. Reset the seconds and/or meq/L indicator dials to 000.0.

Calculations

The use of an auxiliary readout accessory, found on many of the Chloridometers used today, eliminates the calculation of chloride concentration from titration time. In each titration, when set properly, it automatically subtracts the reagent blank time and shows the net titration time in milliequivalents per liter on a digital register. To manually calculate the values for the unknown samples, the following method is used when readings are in seconds rather than milliequivalents per liter.

1. Titrate the reagent blank, standard, control, and unknown samples as described above and record the reading in seconds.

2. Calculate the average value in seconds for the reagent blank and subtract this from the values in seconds for the standard, control pool, and unknown samples.

3. Calculate the factor:

$$\frac{\text{Concentration of standards (meq/L)}}{\text{Average corrected seconds value of the standards}}$$

4. Multiply the corrected values in seconds for the control pool and unknown samples by this factor, and record the results in milliequivalents per liter.

AutoAnalyzer method

Principle

In this method, the specimen being analyzed for chloride is diluted with a solution of mercuric thiocyanate after being dialyzed to remove the proteins. Ferric nitrate reagent is also added. Mercuric thiocyanate, like mercuric chloride, is undissociated. The chloride ions compete successfully with thiocyanate ions for mercuric ions. The resulting free thiocyanate ions combine with ferric ions to produce a red complex, $Fe(SCN)_3$. This color is measured colorimetrically in the automated analyzer. The amount of color is proportional to the amount of chloride present in the specimen.

Chloride in other body fluids

Chloride may be measured in other body fluids, such as urine or cerebrospinal fluid. The chloride content in urine can be quite variable, and an amount of specimen should be used in the procedure that will give a suitable titration reading. Urine and cerebrospinal fluid can be used in the Buchler-Cotlove Chloridometer with good results. If the Schales and Schales method is used, 0.2 ml of the cerebrospinal fluid is diluted with 1.8 ml of distilled water, and this is substituted for the usual sample (2 ml of protein-free filtrate) in the 25-ml Erlenmeyer flask. The calculations are the same as for serum or plasma.

For urine specimens, 0.2 ml of specimen is diluted with 1.8 ml of distilled water and this is titrated as before with mercuric nitrate. Often a very alkaline urine specimen will produce a purple-pink color as soon as the titration has begun. If this happens, 10 ml/dl acetic acid or 1 N nitric acid is added dropwise until the color disappears. This mixture is then titrated as before. The amount of specimen used must be taken into consideration in the calculations.

The chloride content of sweat is now used in the diagnosis of cystic fibrosis of the pancreas and other organs. Sweating can be induced and an adequate sample of sweat can be obtained by several methods. Sweat is collected on filter paper or another suitable test paper and weighed. An extract of the sweat is made and is titrated by the Schales and Schales method or the Chloridometer method. In 98 percent of patients with cystic fibrosis, the secretion of chloride in sweat is two to five times above normal. The determination of chloride in sweat, as well as the other electrolytes, is considered the most reliable single test in the diagnosis of cystic fibrosis. The chloride content of normal sweat varies with age.

Reporting results and recording laboratory data

Chloride results are usually reported to the physician in milliequivalents per liter, to the nearest whole number. Laboratory records, however, are recorded in milliequivalents per liter to the first decimal place. Results are reported to the physician only when the control specimen value is within the established limits.

Normal values[18]

For serum and plasma:
  98-109 meq/L
For cerebrospinal fluid:
  122-132 meq/L

For urine:
  170–250 meq/L (varies greatly)

For sweat:
  5–30 meq/L

SODIUM AND POTASSIUM

As described in the preceding section, the measurement of the major electrolytes, sodium (Na^+), potassium (K^+), bicarbonate (HCO_3^-), and chloride (Cl^-), is an important function of any clinical chemistry laboratory. These substances are the major ions of the body and are often considered together. Changes in the concentration of one of them are almost always accompanied by changes in the concentration of one or more of the others (see under Chloride).

Clinical significance

Sodium is the cation, or positively charged particle, found in the highest concentration in extracellular fluid. It is important in maintaining the osmotic pressure and in electrolyte balance. Sodium is associated with the levels of chloride and bicarbonate ion, and for this reason it has a major role in maintaining the acid-base balance of the body cells. A low serum sodium level is called hyponatremia and a high one is called hypernatremia. Low sodium levels are found in a variety of conditions, including severe polyuria (as in diabetes insipidus), metabolic acidosis (as in diabetic acidosis), Addison's disease (where the supply of adrenocortical hormones is inadequate—these hormones have a strong influence on the level of sodium), diarrhea, and some renal tubular diseases. An increased sodium level is found in Cushing's syndrome (where there is hyperactivity of the adrenal cortex and more hormones than normal are produced), severe dehydration caused by primary water loss, certain types of brain injury, diabetic coma after therapy with insulin, and after excess treatment with sodium salts.

Potassium is the chief intracellular cation, but it is also found extracellularly. It has an important influence on the muscle activity of the heart. Since potassium is largely excreted by the kidney, it becomes elevated in kidney failure and shock. Like sodium, potassium is influenced by the presence of the adrenocortical hormones and is associated with acid-base balance. An elevated potassium level in serum is called hyperkalemia and a decreased one is called hypokalemia. High serum potassium levels are generally seen in cases of oliguria, anuria, or urinary obstruction. In renal tubular acidosis, there is increased retention of potassium in the serum. One important purpose of renal dialysis is the removal of accumulated potassium from the plasma. Low serum potassium levels can result from prolonged diarrhea or vomiting, or from inadequate intake of dietary potassium. Even in potassium deficiency, the kidney continues to excrete potassium. The body has no effective mechanism to protect itself from excessive loss of potassium, so a regular daily intake of potassium is essential.

Specimens

Serum specimens are used most commonly for the determination of sodium, although plasma can be used. Sodium is stable in serum for at least 2 weeks at room temperature or in the refrigerator. Since flame photometry is usually used to analyze sodium levels, scrupulous care is necessary. The slightest contamination of specimens or equipment will drastically alter the results. Glassware used for sodium determinations must be clean and free from sodium contamination; when possible, plastic containers should be used to avoid contamination. If plasma is to be analyzed, siliconized tubes may be used to collect the blood, or lithium heparin or lithium oxalate anticoagulants may be used. Sodium can be measured in 24-hour urine specimens and in cerebrospinal fluid.

The collection of blood for potassium studies requires special attention and technique. If plasma is used, an anticoagulant containing potassium cannot be used. Since the concentration of potassium in the red blood cell is about 20 times that in serum or plasma, it is imperative that hemolysis be avoided. To avoid a shift of potassium from the red cells to the plasma or serum, it is important to separate the cells from the plasma or serum as quickly as possible. When blood is collected for a potassium test, opening and closing of the fist before venipuncture should be avoided, since this muscle action may result in an increase in plasma potassium levels of 10–20%. Potassium levels in plasma are about 0.1–0.7 mmol/L lower than those in serum because of the release of potassium from ruptured platelets during the coagulation process. Potassium in serum is stable for at least 2 weeks at room or refrigerator temperature. Potassium levels in urine vary with dietary intake and are measured in a 24-hour collection.

Methods for quantitative determination

There are several methods for determination of sodium and potassium levels in serum or plasma. The older chemical methods have been replaced almost entirely by the use of flame emission photometry, which is rapid, easy to use, accurate, and precise. An automated flame photometry method is also used in some laboratories, where the sample is automatically diluted and presented to a flame photometer equipped with a recorder or readout device. Since the details of the analyses for potassium and sodium vary with the flame photometer used, they are not included in this discussion. The technician should consult the instruction manual provided with the instrument. Basic information on flame photome-

try as a quantitative technique in the laboratory may be found under Flame Photometry in Chap. 1. The accuracy of the results depends on following the manufacturer's instructions explicitly.

Flame emission photometry is based on the principle that when atoms of many metallic elements, especially sodium and potassium, are given sufficient energy in one form or another, they will emit this energy at particular wavelengths that are characteristic for the element. Dilute solutions of serum or another biological fluid (such as urine) are atomized into a flame and burned. The elements in these solutions are excited by the flame and emit characteristic spectra. By the use of appropriate filters, the emission from potassium or sodium may be isolated and focused on a photocell, which responds linearly to the light energy directed on it. Since light is emitted in direct proportion to the concentration of sodium or potassium in the unknown fluid, the response of the photocell is directly related to the concentration, and unknowns may be determined by comparing the response with that of known standard solutions.

Sodium always produces a yellow color in a flame and potassium produces a violet color. The amount of color is measured with a detector and read with a meter (Fig. 1-18). In most cases, the internal standard method of flame photometry is used: an exact amount of lithium is added to each sample, and the intensity of the sodium or potassium color in the flame is compared by the instrument with the intensity of the red color from the lithium internal standard. The use of an internal standard (lithium) helps to compensate for changes in the condition of the flame and in the levels of interfering substances in the sample being measured.

It is necessary to dilute samples to be measured in a flame photometer. The extent of dilution depends on the type of instrument used, the type of specimen, and the concentrations of the ions to be measured. Dilution also decreases or eliminates interference by other constituents in the sample.

Standard solutions should be analyzed with the unknown samples. These standards are usually prepared from the chloride salt of sodium or potassium, depending on the element to be measured. Standard solutions should be stored in polyethylene containers to avoid contamination from the sodium that is found in many glass containers.

Water used in preparing reagents should be pure and free from sodium contamination. To check for contamination, water may be aspirated into the flame photometer and any appearance of a yellow color noted. A yellow color would suggest sodium contamination.

The flow of fuel into the flame must be strictly controlled. A change in the rate of flow of fuel or oxidant changes the flame temperature and flame size and thus affects the sensitivity of the test procedure. The use of combustible gases for fuel requires special handling and precautions in the laboratory. Work areas should be well-ventilated.

Normal values[19]

For sodium:
    Serum: 135-155 mmol/L (or meq/L) for adults
    Urine: 27-287 mmol/L in 24 hours (urine sodium is variable and it depends on intake; these values are for persons on a "normal" diet)
    Cerebrospinal fluid: 135-155 mmol/L
For potassium:
    Serum: 3.6-5.5 mmol/L
    Urine: 26-123 mmol/L in 24 hours (urine potassium is dependent on intake; there is also a large diurnal variation, the output during peak daytime activity being as much as five times that at night during sleep)
    Cerebrospinal fluid: 2.3-3.1 mmol/L

CLINICAL ENZYMOLOGY

Clinical enzymology is a complex and rapidly developing field in clinical chemistry. A thorough understanding of the chemistry of enzymes is not expected of the technician, but it is necessary to be introduced to the field of clinical enzymology in general. Procedures involving enzyme determinations or involving the use of enzymes as reagents are performed under highly controlled conditions (see under Amylase and Urea Nitrogen).

Enzymes are the catalysts that accompany all biological processes in living organisms. Organisms must carry out most of these processes at a moderate temperature and usually at a nearly neutral pH. Enzymes make this possible by modifying the speed of the reactions without being used up themselves. The organic enzyme catalysts are produced by living cells, but they act independently of the cells that produce them. There are hundreds of enzymes in the human body, and in larger hospital laboratories today enzyme assays may account for as much as 20-25 percent of the work load. As many as 12-18 enzymes are measured routinely in many clinical laboratories.

Enzymes increase the speed of biochemical reactions without themselves undergoing any permanent change: they are neither used up in the reaction nor do they appear as a reaction product. They greatly accelerate a chemical reaction by lowering the activation energy needed of the reaction. Enzymes are proteins and are therefore susceptible to denaturation by heat or chemical agents. Like other catalysts, enzymes are needed in very small amounts, and their activity is usually quite specific.

In the clinical laboratory enzymes are utilized in two different ways. They may be employed as analytical tools. That is, an enzyme may be used as a reagent to bring about some desired chemical reaction. The enzyme urease is used in this way in the urea nitrogen procedure (see under

Urea Nitrogen). When an enzyme is used as a reagent, the unknown factor is not the action of the enzyme on its substrate. Enzymes may also be analyzed for diagnostic purposes (see under Amylase). The measurement of enzymes present in body fluids is expressed in terms of *activity units*, not concentration units. The activity of an enzyme can be described as the amount of substrate it converts to reaction product per unit of time.

The particular substances on which enzymes act are called *substrates*. In the urea nitrogen procedure utilizing urease, the substrate is the urea. The new substance formed as a result of the enzyme activity is called the *end product*. The end product formed by the action of urease on urea is ammonium carbonate. Each enzyme catalyzes a special reaction for only a certain type of substrate.

Nomenclature

At one time enzymes were usually named by adding the ending *-ase* to the substrate. As more enzymes became known and more information about them became available, this naming system became inadequate and a more detailed nomenclature was devised. Often the old names for the enzymes are still used, such as urease, amylase, and lipase. The new nomenclature system provides a practical basis for identifying all enzymes now known as well as enzymes that have yet to be discovered. The International Union of Biochemistry studied systems for identifying enzymes beginning in 1955, and the results of their studies, including a new system of nomenclature, were published in 1964 and revised in 1972.[20] Their proposals have been accepted by all workers in the field and provide a systematic classification for all enzymes.

Two names are provided for each enzyme, a systematic name, which clearly describes the nature of the catalyzed reaction, and a working or practical name, which may be the same as the systematic name or may be a modification of that name for everyday use. Each enzyme is designated by a numerical code consisting of four numbers separated by periods, such as 1.3.2.4. The first of the four numbers defines the class to which the enzyme belongs. All enzymes belong to one of six classes, characterized by the type of reaction they catalyze:

1. *Oxidoreductases* catalyze oxidation-reduction reactions.
2. *Transferases* catalyze transfer of a group other than hydrogen.
3. *Hydrolases* catalyze the hydrolysis of esters, ethers, peptides, and so on.
4. *Lyases* catalyze removal of a group from a substrate by mechanisms other than hydrolysis, leaving double bonds.
5. *Isomerases* catalyze interconversion of optical, geometric, or positional isomers.
6. *Ligases* catalyze the linkage of two compounds while breaking a pyrophosphate bond.

These six major classes are divided into subclasses. The second and third numbers in the enzyme code indicate the subclass and sub-subclass to which the enzyme is assigned. The last number is the specific serial number given to each enzyme in its sub-subclass.

The systematic name for each enzyme consists of two parts: the first gives the name of the substrate or substrates acted on, and the second, a word ending in -ase, indicates the type of reaction catalyzed by all enzymes in the group. Because of the rules governing the terminology of enzymes, an enzyme can be identified by both its code number and its systematic name. This nomenclature for enzymes will appear complicated to the novice, but it becomes understandable with use. The important thing to remember about the naming of enzymes is that enzyme names end in -ase (except for an occasional old name still in use), the part of the name before the -ase gives the type of reaction catalyzed by the enzyme, and the part before that gives the name of the substrate acted on (examples are lactate dehydrogenase and glutamic pyruvic transaminase).

In some laboratories it has become a common and convenient practice to use capital letter abbreviations for the names of certain enzymes. This practice has not been universally standardized, however.

Factors affecting enzymes

Many chemical and physical factors affect the action of enzymes. The *concentration of the substrate* is one factor that can affect the action of the enzyme. If the concentration of the substrate is gradually increased in an enzyme reaction system, keeping all other factors constant, the rate of reaction will increase until a maximum value is reached. After this point, an increase in substrate concentration has no further effect on the reaction rate.

The *concentration of the enzyme* is very important. The speed of the reaction is proportional to the concentration of the enzyme. Therefore, in a clinical laboratory procedure employing enzyme reactions, the concentration of the enzyme must be constant.

The *pH* is also important. Every enzyme has an optimal pH, at which it is most efficient. The optimal pH for urease activity is approximately 7. A buffer is present in the urease solution used in most urea nitrogen procedures to ensure that the pH is kept constant. Extremely high or low pH values generally result in complete loss of activity for most enzymes.

The *temperature* used for the enzyme reaction is another important factor. There is a definite relation between temperature and enzyme activity—that is, the speed of enzyme reactions is increased two to three times for each 10°C rise in temperature. This rate of increase is known as the Q^{10}. Each enzyme has its own particular Q^{10}, but the value is around 2 for most enzymes. A Q^{10} of 2 means that for each 10°C rise in temperature the activity of the enzyme is doubled. A Q^{10} of 3 means that for each 10°C rise in temperature the activity of the enzyme is tripled. Each enzyme also has its optimal temperature—the temperature at which the greatest amount of substrate is changed per unit time. In other words, the highest temperature at which the enzyme will react without danger of being inactivated is its optimal temperature. Of the many factors affecting the activity of enzymes, temperature is one of the most critical. Increasing the temperature beyond the optimal temperature for a particular enzyme may result in denaturation of the enzyme. Over a period of time, enzymes will be deactivated or denatured at even moderate temperatures. Enzymes should be stored at or below 5°C to maintain their activity. For example, the optimal temperature for urease is 48-50°C. Above 55°C, urease begins to be destroyed because of its protein nature.

There is a definite relation between *time* and enzyme activity. A particular amount of enzyme will decompose a particular amount of substrate (urea, in the case of urea nitrogen) per minute. Therefore, the enzyme reaction must be stopped at a definite time.

The presence of *enzyme poisons or inhibitors* must be avoided in any procedure employing enzyme reactions. If such an inhibitor is present, the reaction will not take place satisfactorily. One enzyme inhibitor already discussed is fluoride, which is present in the anticoagulant sodium fluoride used in some glucose procedures. For this reason, sodium fluoride must not be used as an anticoagulant for specimens in any enzyme procedure (such as amylase) or procedures employing enzymes (such as urea nitrogen). Other enzyme inhibitors are heavy metals such as mercury, gold, and silver. Even a trace of these heavy metals will make the enzyme assay invalid, because the activity of the enzyme is inhibited. Denaturation of enzymes can also be caused by vigorous shaking or by ultraviolet radiation, as in sunlight. Any substance that precipitates protein would also stop an enzyme reaction.

Measurement of enzyme activity

Enzymes are essential to life and health, and abnormal enzyme activity may be a sign of disease. Measurements of the activity of digestive enzymes in body fluids as an aid to diagnosis date back to the early 1900s, and some of the earliest observations are still useful. One of these early observations was made on amylase in urine, first studied by Wohlgemuth in 1908. Measurements of enzyme activity in serum began in the 1920s and 1930s with studies on alkaline phosphatase in bone and liver disease.

All the factors that influence enzymes *in vivo*—such as the concentrations of the substrate and the enzyme, the pH, the temperature, and the presence of inhibitors—must be considered when enzyme determinations are performed *in vitro*. Since enzyme activity is easily influenced by changes in the environment, laboratory determinations must be carried out under carefully controlled conditions.

Concentrations of enzymes are measured in the laboratory in terms of activity units in a convenient volume or mass of the specimen analyzed. For example, one activity unit for amylase in the Somogyi method is the amount of the enzyme that, in 30 minutes at 40°C, converts an excess of starch to substances that have the reducing ability of 1 mg of glucose. These units are referred to as Somogyi units of amylase.

Since enzymes are active in all parts of the body, determination of enzyme activity is important in the diagnosis and treatment of certain diseases. Some of the more common enzyme determinations that have become valuable diagnostic tools are described below.

1. *Lipase.* Lipase, which is found in the pancreas, hydrolyzes fats into fatty acids and glycerol. Increased amounts of this enzyme indicate disease and inflammation of the pancreas.

2. *Alkaline phosphatase.* Phosphatase enzymes carry out hydrolysis of the phosphate esters into inorganic phosphorus. Alkaline phosphatase is present in high concentration in the bone and in somewhat lower concentration in the liver. Serum alkaline phosphatase activity is increased in bone and liver disease.

3. *Acid phosphatase.* Acid phosphatase also hydrolyzes phosphate esters, but is active at a pH of about 5.0. The largest source of acid phosphatase is the prostatic tissue of the male. Metastatic carcinoma of the prostate gland produces very high serum acid phosphatase levels.

4. *Transaminase.* Transamination is a function of tissue in general. The enzyme activity of transaminase in the serum of normal persons remains relatively constant from day to day. If tissues become infarcted because of stoppage of blood flow to them, transaminase is released into the bloodstream and there is an increase in serum transaminase. In heart muscle and liver infarction, serum glutamic-oxaloacetic transaminase (SGOT) is increased. The amount of increase measured is an indication of the extent of the infarction.

5. *Amylase.* Amylase is formed in the pancreas and is found in increased amounts in the serum in varying degrees of pancreatic disturbance. Normally only small amounts of amylase are found in the blood. Increased amounts of pancreatic amylase are found in the blood during the early stage of acute pancreatitis. Amylase catalyzes the hydrolysis of starch into simpler molecules, with maltose as the end product. The measurement of serum amylase is one of the most common laboratory tests for enzyme activity and is described in the next section.

AMYLASE

The measurement of serum amylase is one of the most common enzyme tests done in the laboratory. It is used in this section to illustrate a clinical enzymatic determination. Normally, only a small amount of amylase is found in the serum. Increased amounts are seen during the early stage of acute pancreatitis, and they are clinically very significant.

In the body, amylase is present in a number of organs and tissues. The greatest concentration of amylase is in the pancreas, where the enzyme is synthesized and secreted into the intestinal tract for digestion of starches. Amylase is also secreted by the salivary glands and is present in saliva, where it initiates hydrolysis of starches while the food is still in the mouth and the esophagus. The enzyme found in normal serum is predominantly of pancreatic and salivary origin.

Clinical significance

Assays of amylase activity in the serum are of interest clinically in relation to diseases of the pancreas and in the evaluation of pancreatic function. In acute pancreatitis (with symptoms of severe abdominal pain), amylase activity increases from the normal range of 40-140 units/dl to about 550 units/dl and sometimes as much as 2000-3000 units/dl. It is difficult to establish normal values for this determination because of the variations in the molecular weight of the starch molecules used in different procedures, so only values over 200 units/dl are considered clinically significant.

The onset of pancreatitis may be swift and severe, and the measurement of amylase activity is often an important diagnostic test. It is essential that this test be performed accurately and rapidly. The blood amylase activity may fluctuate rapidly and dramatically during an attack and may subside to near-normal levels shortly after one. Because of this rapid change in the blood amylase activity, physicians often order emergency amylase determinations for a patient having an attack of acute abdominal pain. In these cases, the laboratory report on amylase activity is often an essential factor in determining the treatment to be used for the patient.

Blood amylase activity may also be elevated in patients with mumps, in which there may be secondary involvement of the pancreas.

Specimens

Amylase is quite stable. The activity loss is negligible at room temperature for 1 week and at refrigerator temperatures for 2 months. All the common anticoagulants, except heparin, inhibit the activity of this enzyme. Citrate, EDTA, and oxalate inhibit it by as much as 15 percent. Because of this inhibition problem, the test for amylase activity should be performed only on serum or on heparinized plasma. If urine is used, it should be a timed specimen and should be diluted 1:2 with saline before it is used in the procedure.

Methods for quantitative determination

Methods for measurement of amylase can be divided into two main groups: saccharogenic methods and amyloclastic methods. Since amylase hydrolyzes starch to sugars, one approach to measuring amylase activity is to let the sample act on a starch substrate and measure the sugar produced, using an ordinary method such as that of Nelson and Somogyi. This is basically what happens in a saccharogenic amylase method. The most serious problem in these methods is the instability of starch solutions. Starches vary considerably in their proportions of amylose and amylopectin, and the length of the starch molecule (and therefore its molecular weight) depends on how it was manufactured and how the substrate was prepared by the manufacturer. Starch does not disperse in water to form a true solution, but instead forms a colloidal solution. The degree of dispersion of starch in solution varies with temperature. It is therefore essential that the starch substrates be prepared and treated in exactly the same manner if the data from different batches used in the laboratory are to be comparable. Starch solutions deteriorate rapidly because of the formation of mold and should be refrigerated.

When the reducing materials (sugars) have been formed by the action of amylase on the starch substrate, the quantity of the reducing substances formed is measured. This may be accomplished by any of the common methods for measuring reducing substances (Folin-Wu or Nelson-Somogyi). The quantities of reducing sugars produced are determined on protein-free filtrates of the reaction mixtures. With some starch solutions, it is difficult to obtain clear filtrates. If the turbidity of the filtrate is caused by starch and not incompletely precipitated proteins, it will not affect the assay, as it will clear up during a later stage of the procedure.

Success of the saccharogenic methods depends greatly on control of the starch substrate solutions. One saccharogenic amylase method is that devised by Somogyi and modified by Henry and Chiamori. In this method, the unknown sample is incubated with a buffered starch solution for a timed period (30 minutes). A protein-free filtrate is prepared, and the reducing substances are determined by reaction with alkaline copper solution and arsenomolybdate color reagent (see under Glucose). Somogyi defined the unit of amylase activity in the saccharogenic assay as that quantity of enzyme that liberates reducing substances with a reducing value equivalent to that of 1 mg of glucose in the course of a 30-minute reaction at 40°C and at a pH of 6.9-7.0.[21] The concentration is expressed as the number of units per 100 ml of blood, or units per deciliter. Most methods use the Somogyi units for reporting results, although not all methods involve measurements at 40°C. The Somogyi method is used as a reference method for most other amylase procedures. Most saccharogenic methods can measure amylase activity only up to 450–500 Somogyi units. If higher values are indicated or suspected, the specimen must be diluted with saline, or preferably with dilute albumin (5 mg/dl) in saline, before the incubation with starch solution. Several automated saccharogenic procedures have been described.

Somogyi also described amyloclastic methods for the determination of amylase activity. Starch forms a blue-black color with iodine, and the amyloclastic methods use this to measure the time required for all the starch to be hydrolyzed. As the starch is hydrolyzed, its capacity to give the blue-black color with iodine is lost. Amyloclastic methods are based on the disappearance of the blue-black color given by iodine and starch-enzyme solutions. In the method devised by Caraway, the concentration of amylase is determined by the action of the enzyme on a stable starch substrate; the amount of starch remaining is determined by measuring the absorbance of the colored complex formed with iodine in the photometer.[22] This type of method measures the decrease in starch substrate concentration rather than the product formed, as in the saccharogenic methods.

Several dye-labeled amylase substrates have been introduced commercially in recent years. Three such commercial products are Maylochrome (Roche Diagnostics, Nutley, N.J.), Amylose-Azure (Calbiochem, Los Angeles, Calif.), and Phadebas (Pharmacia Laboratories, Inc., Piscataway, N.J.). All three dye substrates are water-insoluble. Their suspensions, in buffer solutions, are attacked by the enzyme to produce small, water-soluble fragments that contain blue dye. These can be measured in the photometer after being separated by centrifugation or filtration from the water-insoluble unreacted substrate. There is no direct relation between Somogyi units and the enzyme activity units measured by these amyloclastic methods or with the commercially available products. Somogyi units are so generally accepted in this country that values obtained by other procedures are usually multiplied by an appropriate factor to convert them into equivalent Somogyi units.

One common source of error in amylase determinations is contamination by saliva. Coughing, sneezing, or even talking near the specimen can cause an apparent increase in serum amylase activity. With modern pipetting techniques, using mechanical suction, there should be no introduction of saliva. This is a real problem, however, and should be kept in mind when doing this assay.

Controls should be analyzed with each batch of specimens. Commercial control serum or laboratory-prepared control serum can be used. A control serum can be prepared in the laboratory by adding clear saliva (containing amylase) to a pooled serum specimen to raise the amylase activity to about 250–300 Somogyi units. Aliquots of 1 ml can be pipetted into tubes and frozen until used. The control tube for each day's use can be thawed by immersion in water at $40°C$ and should be mixed well before the sample for the procedure is pipetted.

As in any enzyme procedure, careful attention must be paid to the control of temperature and pH. A change in pH can result from improper cleaning of laboratory glassware.

Somogyi amylase method, modified by Henry and Chiamori[23,24]

Principle

The assay of amylase activity involves incubation of the specimen (serum, plasma, urine, or other biological fluid) with the starch substrate under controlled conditions of pH, time, and temperature. In this saccharogenic method, the concentration of the starch cleavage products is determined by their ability to reduce copper in the Nelson-Somogyi method. Products of the non-enzymatic breakdown of starch and preexisting reducing substances in the specimen are simultaneously corrected for with the specimen blank. Chloride ion, which is necessary for amylase activity, is found in the buffer solution. The presence of the chloride ion maintains the optimal pH of 6.9–7.0 for the amylase enzyme.

Amylase activity is reported in Somogyi units per 100 ml of blood, or units per deciliter. One Somogyi unit is the amount of enzyme that, in 30 minutes at $37.5°C$ (the temperature for this method), converts an excess of starch to substances that have the reducing ability of 1 mg of glucose.

Reagents

1. Purified cornstarch. Heat approximately 1800 ml of 0.25 g/dl sodium hydroxide (NaOH) in a 2000-ml beaker to 50-$55°C$. Discontinue heating and add approximately 200 g of cornstarch, using a mechanical stirrer for agitation. Continue agitation for about 1–2 hours. Allow the starch to settle overnight. Decant the yellow liquid. Suspend the starch in water. Agitate for a while and again let the starch settle overnight. Decant the water. Repeat the washing with water twice more. Allow the starch to dry at room temperature.

2. Buffer-NaCl solution. Dissolve 2.25 g of potassium phosphate monobasic (KH_2PO_4), 2.40 g of sodium phosphate dibasic anhydrous (Na_2HPO_4), 2.5 g of NaCl, and 2.0 g of NaF in about 800 ml of water, and dilute to 1 L with water. This solution should have a pH of about 6.8.

3. Working starch suspension (1.5 g/dl). In a 1-L beaker, make a smooth paste of 15 g of purified cornstarch and 100 ml of buffer-NaCl solution. Heat 900 ml of buffer-NaCl solution to boiling in an Erlenmeyer flask. Add the hot solution to the starch suspension gradually with vigorous agitation. The final pH is about 7.0.

4. 0.2 N barium hydroxide. Dissolve 90 g of $Ba(OH)_2 \cdot 8H_2O$ in water and dilute to 2000 ml with water.

5. Zinc sulfate (5 g/dl). Dissolve 100 g of $ZnSO_4 \cdot 7H_2O$ in water and dilute to 2000 ml with water.

The concentrations of the barium hydroxide and zinc sulfate solutions are not as important as the fact that they exactly neutralize each other. To titrate, measure 10 ml of $ZnSO_4$ solution into a 250-ml flask; add 50 ml of water and 4 drops of phenolphthalein solution. Titrate by adding barium hydroxide solution dropwise with continual agitation. *Too rapid addition of barium hydroxide will give a false end point.* Dilute the stronger solution so that 10 ml of $ZnSO_4$ requires 10 ± 0.05 ml of $Ba(OH)_2$ solution for neutralization.

6. Solution A. Dissolve 50 g of anhydrous Na_2CO_3, 50 g of potassium sodium tartrate (Rochelle salt), 40 g of $NaHCO_3$, and 400 g of anhydrous Na_2SO_4 in about 1600 ml of water and dilute to 2 L with water. Filter if necessary. A sediment may form after a few days; this may be filtered off without detriment to the reagent. Store this solution where the temperature will not fall below $20°C$.

7. Solution B. Dissolve 15 g of $CuSO_4 \cdot 5H_2O$ in water and dilute to 100 ml with water. Add 0.5 ml of concentrated H_2SO_4.

8. Alkaline copper reagent. Prepare on the day of use by diluting 4 ml of solution B to 100 ml with solution A in a volumetric flask. Turbidity appears when solution A is first added; swirl the flask to dissolve this precipitate before diluting the contents to volume.

9. Arsenomolybdate color reagent. Dissolve 100 g of ammonium molybdate in 1800 ml of water. Add 84 ml of concentrated H_2SO_4 and mix. Add 12 g of $Na_2HAsO_4 \cdot 7H_2O$ dissolved in 100 ml of water and mix. Place in an incubator at $37°C$ for 24–48 hours. The reagent should be stored in a glass-stoppered brown bottle. It is stable indefinitely.

10. Glucose stock standard (10.0 mg/ml). Dissolve 1.000 g of pure anhydrous glucose in saturated benzoic acid solution (0.25 g/dl) and dilute to 100 ml with the same solution. Store at refrigerator temperature. Pure glucose is available from the National Bureau of Standards.

11. Glucose intermediate standard (0.500 mg/ml). Dilute 5 ml of glucose stock standard to 100 ml with saturated benzoic acid solution. Prepare fresh weekly.

12. Glucose working standards (0.025, 0.05, 0.100, 0.150, and 0.200 mg/ml). Dilute 1, 2, 3, and 4 ml of glucose intermediate standard to 10 ml with water, using four volumetric flasks. To make the 0.025 mg/ml standard, dilute 5 ml of the 0.05 mg/ml standard to 10 ml with water in a volumetric flask. Prepare fresh daily.

Procedure

For each specimen to be analyzed, carry out the following steps:

1. Pipet 5.0-ml portions of starch suspension into the specimen activity tube and the specimen blank tube. Swirl before pipetting.

2. Warm in a $37.5°C$ water bath for a minimum of 5 minutes.

3. Note the exact time and add 0.5 ml of specimen to the *specimen activity tube*, stopper the tube, and mix rapidly inverting twice.

4. Incubate both tubes for exactly 30 minutes in the $37.5°C$ water bath.

5. Add 2.0 ml of $Ba(OH)_2$ to both tubes.

6. Mix and remove from bath.

7. Add 0.5 ml of specimen to the *specimen blank tube* and mix.

8. Add to each tube 0.5 ml of water. Mix.

9. Add 2.0 ml of $ZnSO_4$ to each tube and shake vigorously. Let stand 5 minutes.

10. Filter or centrifuge.

11. Pipet into Folin-Wu tubes 1 ml of water for a blank, 1 ml of each of the working glucose standards, and 1 ml of each of the filtered or centrifuged solutions prepared above.

12. Add 1 ml of alkaline copper reagent to each Folin-Wu tube. *Mix the contents well by hitting the tube against the hand.*

13. Place all the tubes in a rack. Place the rack

in a boiling-water bath for 20 minutes, immersing the contents of all of the tubes for *exactly* the same length of time; do not place the tubes into the bath one at a time. When removing the tubes from the bath, remove all of them at the same time—that is, remove the whole rack. *Immediately* place the rack of tubes in cold water for exactly 1 minute.

14. Quickly terminate the cooling period by adding 1 ml of arsenomolybdate reagent to each tube.

15. Mix the contents well by hitting each tube against the palm of the hand. Mix until the evolution of CO_2 is complete.

16. If the solutions are cloudy, let stand for 5 minutes to hydrolyze the residual starch.

17. Dilute each tube to the 25-ml mark with water. Mix well by tipping, and transfer to colorimeter tubes.

18. Read the color intensity in the photometer at 555 nm. The color is very stable, and may therefore be read at the technician's convenience.

19. Record the readings for the blank, standards, controls, and unknown.

20. Construct a standard line on graph paper, using the standard readings.

Calculations

Plot the concentrations of the glucose standards, expressed as milligrams per Folin-Wu tube, against the galvanometer readings. Read the concentrations of the unknowns, in milligrams per Folin-Wu tube, from the straight line. For each specimen, subtract the value for the specimen blank tube from the value for the specimen activity tube. Convert to Somogyi units by the formula:

$$\frac{mg}{Folin\text{-}Wu\ tube}\ (\text{corrected for blank}) \times \frac{10}{1} \times \frac{100}{0.5}$$

= Somogyi units per 100 ml of specimen (units/dl)

When analyzing urine specimens, calculate both Somogyi units per 100 ml of specimen and Somogyi units excreted during the period of time over which the specimen was collected.

Technical factors and sources of error

If an anticoagulant is used to obtain plasma for this determination, it must be heparin. The enzyme is destroyed by the other commonly used anticoagulants. Many anticoagulants chelate calcium, and compounds that chelate calcium are powerful enzyme inhibitors. Serum is the specimen most often used for this determination. Care must be taken to not contaminate the specimen with saliva, either through careless pipetting or by accidentally coughing or talking near the specimen. Saliva contains amylase and would cause a falsely high measurement.

Since this is an enzyme measurement, care should be taken to keep the reaction time, temperature, and pH constant. The starch substrate must be fresh and prepared correctly.

Reporting results and recording laboratory data

Tests for amylase are accurate, but the results, although reliable, are arbitrary measurements of amylase activity. The amylase activity actually depends on the enzyme concentration and the concentrations of activators and inhibitors that may be present. There is a significant difference between normal values for males and females, those for females being somewhat higher. The results of amylase determinations are reported in terms of the activity of the enzyme, usually in Somogyi units. Different methods give somewhat different values, but the Somogyi unit is the reference unit for other methods. Values obtained by methods other than the Somogyi saccharogenic method are usually converted to equivalent Somogyi units by multiplying by a suitable factor. Laboratory results are not reported to the physician unless the control values for the determination check out within the established range. If the amylase activities determined turn out to be greater than 200 units/dl in serum or duodenal fluid or greater than 400 units/dl in urine, the supernatant fluid should be diluted and the procedure repeated from that step. The dilution depends on the enzyme activity, but the usual dilution is 1:2, using water or saline as the diluent.

Normal values[25]

For serum amylase (males):
  38-118 Somogyi units/dl
For serum amylase (females):
  46-141 Somogyi units/dl
For serum amylase (overall):
  40-140 Somogyi units/dl
For urine amylase:
  66-870 Somogyi units/dl, or 43-245 Somogyi units/hour
For duodenal fluid amylase:
  100-800 Somogyi units/dl

UREA NITROGEN

The determination of urea nitrogen in the serum, plasma, or whole blood is a widely used screening test for the evaluation of kidney function. Tests for urea nitrogen and creatinine are often requested together as the simultaneous determination of these two substances can aid in the differential diagnosis of several renal diseases.

Clinical significance

Increases in urea nitrogen may result from prerenal, renal, or postrenal causes. Prerenal causes include cardiac involvement, water depletion because of decreased intake or excessive loss, or protein breakdown problems. Renal causes include acute glomerulonephritis, chronic glomerulonephritis, polycystic kidney, and nephrosclerosis. Postrenal causes include all types of obstruction of the urinary tract (stones, enlarged prostate gland, or tumors). Urea is, in general, a waste product of protein metabolism, being removed from the blood in the kidneys. Accumulation of urea in the blood above a certain amount may indicate a flaw in the filtering system of the kidneys. Urea is a principal waste product of protein catabolism. Its chemical formula is NH_2CONH_2. It is sometimes difficult

to determine urea in the laboratory, but it is relatively simple to analyze for the nitrogen in the urea. It is common practice, therefore, to determine urea nitrogen in the chemistry laboratory.

Aside from protein itself, the major nitrogen-containing compounds in the blood are urea, amino acids, uric acid, creatinine, creatine, and ammonia, listed in order of their quantitative importance. These substances are collectively referred to as nonprotein nitrogen (NPN). They may be measured as NPN, or determined separately; they are commonly measured separately. Whole blood, serum, or plasma is used. For these determinations it is often necessary to remove protein from the sample before the analysis. A protein-free filtrate may be prepared by either the tungstic acid or the barium hydroxide-zinc sulfate method.

Nitrogen (N) exists in the body in many forms, mostly in components of complex substances. Nitrogen-containing substances are classified into two main groups: protein nitrogen (protein substances containing nitrogen) and nonprotein nitrogen (nonprotein substances containing nitrogen). The NPN substances are not precipitated by the usual protein-precipitating reagents; they remain in the filtrate after the protein has been removed.

The major NPN component is urea nitrogen. Normally, urea comprises about 45 percent of the total NPN. The concentration of NPN is therefore determined predominantly by the concentration of urea. In a healthy individual, amino acids comprise about 20 percent, uric acid about 20 percent, creatinine about 5 percent, and creatine about 5 percent of the total NPN.

Since urea is the chief component of the NPN material in the blood, it is also quantitatively the most important. It is distributed throughout the body water and is equal in concentration in the intracellular and extracellular fluid. Whole blood, plasma, or serum may therefore be used for urea nitrogen determinations. Gross alterations in the NPN usually reflect a change in the concentration of urea. Because the concentration of urea is directly related to protein metabolism, the protein content of the diet will affect the amount of urea in the blood. The ability of the kidneys to remove urea from the blood will also affect the urea content. However, the urea concentration is primarily influenced by the protein intake. In the normal kidney, urea is removed from the blood and excreted in the urine. If kidney function is impaired, urea will not be removed from the blood and the result will be a high urea concentration in the blood. Considerable deterioration must usually be present before the blood urea nitrogen (BUN) level rises above the normal range of 8-26 mg/dl (or 8-26 mg/100 ml). The condition of abnormally high BUN is called uremia. Decreased BUN levels are usually not clinically significant, unless a case of liver damage is suspected. During pregnancy, lower than normal urea nitrogen is often seen.

The liver is the sole site of urea formation; it is the only organ that contains all the enzymes needed. As protein breakdown occurs (as amino acids undergo deamination, for example), ammonia is formed in increased amounts. This potentially toxic substance is removed in the liver, where the ammonia combines with other amino acids and is finally converted to urea. The amount of urea in the blood is determined by the amount of dietary protein and by the kidney's ability to excrete urea. If the kidney is impaired, the urea is not removed from the blood, and as it accumulates the BUN level increases. Since the urea concentration is also influenced by the diet, people who are undernourished or who are on low-protein diets may have BUN levels that are not accurate indications of kidney function. Because of this problem, the test for creatinine is sometimes considered a better test for kidney function.

One of the most important chemical tests done to detect kidney damage and kidney disease is the test for urea nitrogen. Urea nitrogen may be determined in plasma, serum, whole blood, urine, and most other biological fluids. This test is performed routinely in all laboratories and is one that every student of clinical laboratory procedures should learn to do accurately. The techniques used in the urea nitrogen test are basic to many other procedures done in the chemistry laboratory. The methods discussed in this section employ the photometer for accurate quantitative measurements, a direct reaction with a colorimetric reagent, and an enzyme reaction procedure.

Specimens

Urea nitrogen may be determined directly in serum, plasma, urine, or other biological specimens. If whole blood or plasma is used, the sample of blood must be properly anticoagulated. The choice of anticoagulant is very important. An anticoagulant containing nitrogen (such as ammonium and potassium oxalate, double oxalate) must not be used as it would give falsely high results (the nitrogen in the ammonium salt would be measured along with the urea nitrogen). Direct measurement of ammonia is involved in some methods. If the method involves an enzymatic reaction—for example, using the enzyme urease to convert urea to ammonium carbonate—sodium fluoride cannot be used as the anticoagulant. Fluoride is an enzyme inhibitor and actually destroys some enzymes. One anticoagulant that can be used with good results is potassium oxalate. EDTA can also be used.

Since urea can be lost through bacterial action, the specimen should be analyzed within a few hours after collection or should be preserved by refrigeration. Refrigeration preserves the urea nitrogen without measurable change for up to 72 hours. Urine urea is particularly susceptible to bacterial action, so in addition to refrigeration of the urine specimen, crystals of thymol may be added to help reduce the loss of urea. Protein-free filtrates are stable for long periods of time, so if the protein must be removed before analysis, the filtrate can be prepared and stored indefinitely until the analysis is done.

The urea nitrogen concentration in serum or plasma is approximately 2 mg/dl higher than that in whole blood. The decision to use whole blood, serum, or plasma can be left to the laboratory.

BUN is a measure of nitrogen and not of urea. To convert milligrams of urea nitrogen to milligrams of urea, the BUN value is multiplied by 2.14, or 60/28. The molecular weight of urea is 60, and it contains two nitrogen atoms with a combined weight of 28.

Methods for quantitative determination

A wide variety of methods have been devised for the determination of urea nitrogen. Some of them may be performed directly on whole blood, serum, or plasma, while others require a protein-free filtrate. The variety of methods available indicate that the ideal method has not yet been found.

A group of manual methods used frequently to determine the urea nitrogen concentration, which are very reliable, require the addition of the enzyme urease to whole blood, serum, or plasma. During incubation, urea is converted to ammo-

nium carbonate $[(NH_4)_2CO_3]$ by urease. The ammonia in the ammonium carbonate is analyzed in one of several ways.

The enzyme urease is obtained from jack beans, sword beans, or soybeans. It can be purchased in tablet or powder form. At a certain pH and temperature, urease hydrolyzes urea to ammonium carbonate according to the reaction

$$CO(NH_2)_2 + 2H_2O \xrightarrow{\text{urease}} (NH_4)_2CO_3$$
$$\text{Urea} \qquad\qquad\qquad \text{Ammonium carbonate}$$

This reaction is complete and highly specific. The amount of urease recommended in the procedure used, along with the incubation times and temperature, is adequate to deal with any concentration of urea that may occur in human blood. Urease obeys the general laws of most enzymes (see under Clinical Enzymology). Enzymes are protein in nature; therefore, urease is a protein. Any of the urease that is not used in the hydrolysis is removed in the protein-precipitation step. In the urea nitrogen procedure that utilizes an enzyme reaction, the substrate is urea, and the end product is ammonium carbonate.

The method of Bertholet, modified by Chaney and Marbach, measures the ammonium carbonate by reacting it with a phenol-hypochlorite solution to yield a deep blue color which can be measured colorimetrically. The intensity of the blue color is proportional to the quantity of urea in the specimen. Sodium nitroprusside acts as a catalyst in the reaction. The urease solution used is buffered with EDTA, which complexes any metal ions that might interfere with the enzymatic reaction. In this method, because a high dilution of sample is used, it is not necessary to precipitate and remove the proteins before measurement. Protein-free filtrates may be used, however.

Another method, devised by Gentzkow, measures the amount of ammonium carbonate formed by reacting it with Nessler's solution. Before nesslerization, a protein-free filtrate is prepared by the modified Folin-Wu method. Nessler's reagent converts the ammonium carbonate to ammonia and carbon dioxide. The reagent then reacts with the ammonia to produce a yellow color, which can be measured colorimetrically. The intensity of the yellow color is directly proportional to the amount of urea present in the specimen.

One commonly used method for urea nitrogen involves a nonenzymatic reaction. Urea will react directly with diacetylmonoxime to produce a yellow compound that can be measured colorimetrically. This method has been adapted for both manual and automated analyses; both yield comparable results and use essentially the same reagents. Because so many laboratories are automated for chemistry analyses and the diacetylmonoxime method is used in automatic analyzers, we describe the manual method here. Samples for this assay need not be treated to remove protein before the analysis because of the specificity of the reagents. Many reagent kits available commercially use this method.

Three manual methods for urea nitrogen are described in this chapter: the modified Bertholet urease method, the Gentzkow nesslerization method, and the diacetylmonoxime method. Because urease is used in the Bertholet and Gentzkow methods, enzymes and their general characteristics should be reviewed (see under Clinical Enzymology). We describe three different methods for urea nitrogen for a number of reasons. The Gentzkow nesslerization method includes the use of a recovery solution, which is a general check on the accuracy of the method. The use of recoveries and recovery theory are part of quality control in the laboratory, especially in the initial evaluation of a new procedure. The Bertholet urease method was devised for microsamples of specimen. In some cases only a microsample is available for analysis, and in other cases the laboratory chooses micromethods for general use. The nonenzymatic diacetylmonoxime method involves yet another way of quantitatively measuring urea nitrogen. It eliminates the need to use an enzyme solution, which can be unstable, and it is similar to

automated methods that use the same reagents and principle of reaction.

Blood urea nitrogen—Gentzkow urease nesslerization method[26]

Principle

Whole blood (preserved with potassium oxalate) is incubated with urease, which breaks down urea to form ammonium carbonate. From this incubated blood, a modified Folin-Wu filtrate is prepared. Nessler's reagent is added to the protein-free filtrate. In the alkaline pH of Nessler's reagent, the ammonium carbonate forms ammonium ions and carbon dioxide. The ammonium ions combine with the mercury-potassium iodide complex in Nessler's reagent to form a yellow compound. The intensity of the yellow color developed is compared with the intensity of the color in a series of standard tubes containing ammonium sulfate that has been nesslerized.

The reactions taking place in this procedure are given below.

$$CO(NH_2)_2 + 2H_2O \xrightarrow{\text{urease}} (NH_4)_2CO_3$$

Urea (in whole blood) → Ammonium carbonate

$$(NH_4)_2CO_3 + \text{Nessler's reagent} \xrightarrow[\text{pH}]{\text{alkaline}}$$

$$NH_4^+ + CO_2$$

NH_4^+ + mercury-potassium iodide complex $\longrightarrow$
(In Nessler's reagent)

yellow compound

A protein-free filtrate is prepared by the modified Folin-Wu method.

Reagents

Note: all reagents must be made with ammonia-free water.

1. 0.095 N H_2SO_4.
2. Sodium tungstate (10 g/dl). Dissolve 100 g of $Na_2WO_4 \cdot 2H_2O$ in ammonia-free water and dilute to 1 L.
3. $M/15$ primary phosphate solution. Dissolve 9.08 g of KH_2PO_4 in ammonia-free water and dilute to 1 L.
4. $M/15$ secondary phosphate solution. Dissolve 17.88 g of $Na_2HPO_4 \cdot 7H_2O$ in ammonia-free water and dilute to 1 L.
5. $M/15$ phosphate buffer, pH 7.0. Mix 389 ml of $M/15$ KH_2PO_4 with 611 ml of $M/15$ Na_2HPO_4. Check the pH of the buffer on a pH meter. The acceptable pH range is 6.95–7.05.
6. Stock urease (2 g/dl suspension). Dissolve 2 g of urease in ammonia-free water and dilute to 100 ml. Mix gently. Use practical-grade, type II, jack bean urease powder (available from Sigma Chemical Co., St. Louis, Mo.).
7. Working urease suspension. Prepare fresh daily. Mix gently: 1 part stock urease suspension, 2 parts $M/15$ phosphate buffer, pH 7.0, and 2 parts ammonia-free water.
8. Stock urea solution (10 mg/ml nitrogen). Dissolve 2.143 g of urea in ammonia-free water and dilute to 100 ml.
9. Working urea solution (1 mg/ml nitrogen). Dilute 10 ml of stock solution to 100 ml with ammonia-free water. Prepare weekly.
10. Ammonium sulfate stock standard solution (1 mg/ml nitrogen). Dissolve 4.7165 g of desiccated $(NH_4)_2SO_4$ in ammonia-free water and dilute to 1 L.
11. Working ammonium sulfate standard solution (0.01 mg/ml nitrogen). Dilute 1 ml of the stock solution to 100 ml with ammonia-free water.
12. Stock Nessler's solution. Prepare commercially available Nessler's compound (reagent-grade, Koch-McMeekin formula) according to the instructions on the label. This compound is available from Scientific Products, a division of American Hospital Supply Corp. (McGaw Park, Ill.).
13. Potassium gluconate (1 g/dl). Dissolve 2 g of potassium gluconate in ammonia-free water and dilute to 200 ml. Store at 4°C. Prepare fresh weekly.
14. Potassium persulfate (2.5 g/dl). Use a salt containing 0.001% or less nitrogen, such as Mallinkrodt low nitrogen or British Drug House ANALAR. Dissolve 5 g of $K_2S_2O_8$ in ammonia-free water and dilute to 200 ml. The salt is not readily dissolved and a magnetic stirrer may be used to aid in dissolving it. Store at 4°C. Prepare fresh weekly. During warm weather, remove this solution from the refrigerator only long enough to measure the amount required, because decomposition is rapid at high temperatures.
15. Working Nessler's solution. Mix well: 1 part 1 g/dl potassium gluconate solution and 1 part 2.5 g/dl potassium persulfate solution. Add this mixture to 2 parts stock Nessler's solution and mix well. Use this mixture within 15 minutes after preparation.

Reagent notes

Stock urease may be made from soybean meal instead of jack bean meal. It may also be made from urease tablets. The tablets are ground finely and mixed with a specific amount of water. Ammonia-free (double-distilled) water is very important in this procedure and must be used whenever water is needed.

The addition of the persulfate and gluconate solution to Nessler's reagent helps to stabilize the final color reaction. The sulfuric acid used in the protein-precipitating step (0.095 N) is more concentrated than the acid usually used in the modified Folin-Wu filtrate (0.083 N). It must be more concentrated to correct for the water present in the urease solution.

Comments on procedure for direct nesslerization method–Use of recovery check

Since there are many variables in an enzyme method, it is advisable to periodically check the accuracy of the method through the use of a recovery solution. An accurately measured amount of recovery solution is added to one of the control blood samples in a batch. It is best to choose a blood sample that is known to be in the normal range for urea nitrogen. The recovery solution is a quantitatively prepared solution of the substance that is being measured in the unknown patient samples. The recovery solution for the urea nitrogen determination is a solution of urea.

This procedure requires the use of a recovery solution, along with a control sample, to ensure that the results will be reliable. The measured sample of recovery solution is added to a control sample or to a known normal blood sample. Theoretically, the amount of nitrogen in the recovery solution added to the control should be recovered at the end of the procedure. That is, none should be lost or gained along the way. The use of a recovery solution checks the accuracy of the method. For this procedure, the recovery solution is a solution of urea that has been accurately prepared and measured.

Procedure

Incubation with urease

1. Pipet 1 ml of well-mixed whole blood into labeled test tubes, using an Ostwald pipet. Treat undetermined specimens and control sample alike. Pipet a duplicate sample of one undetermined specimen and the control.

2. To one of the control tubes (labeled R) pipet 0.2 ml of working urea solution (the recovery solution). This must be done very carefully, as the accuracy of the whole batch depends on it. Mix well.

3. To each of the tubes add 1 ml of working urease solution (this solution must be prepared fresh each day). Mix by shaking. Do not invert.

4. Immediately place tubes in a water incubator at 48-50°C.

5. Incubate the tubes for 15 minutes. Shake the tubes every 5 minutes. Do not invert. At the end of the 15 minutes, remove the tubes, and immediately go on with the next step.

Preparation of protein-free filtrates

1. Immediately after removing the tubes from the incubator, add 7 ml of 0.095 N H_2SO_4. Cork and mix well by inversion.

2. Add 1 ml of 10 g/dl Na_2WO_4. Cork the tubes and shake vigorously.

3. Pour mixture into filter paper previously placed in funnels, and filter into labeled test tubes. The filtrate should be clear and colorless.

Preparation of reagents

These are to be made fresh daily.

1. Working urease.

2. Working Nessler's reagent. This is stable for only 15 minutes.

Color development

1. Into labeled photometer cuvettes, pipet:

Cuvette	Ammonia-free water (ml)	Standard $(NH_4)_2SO_4$ (ml)	Filtrate (ml)
Blank	5		
Standard 1	4	1	
Standard 3	2	3	
Standard 5		5	
Control	4		1
Recovery	4		1
Unknown	4		1

2. Cover the cuvettes with Parafilm (American Can Co., Greenwich, Conn.), hold them firmly, and invert the mixture several times.

3. Prepare working Nessler's reagent.

4. To each photometer cuvette, add 1 ml of working Nessler's reagent. Mix immediately after

each addition. Set a timer for 15 minutes after the addition of Nessler's reagent.

5. The color formed is stable for at least 1 hour and may be stable for up to 3 hours. Read the photometer cuvettes at the end of the 15-minute waiting period, using a wavelength setting of 505 nm.

Reading cuvettes in the photometer

1. Polish the cuvettes.
2. Read them in the photometer at a wavelength setting of 505 nm.
3. Enter galvanometer readings (%T or absorbance) for standards, control, recovery solution, and unknown specimens on a work sheet. Prepare a standard graph and calculate the milligrams of urea nitrogen per 100 ml of blood (mg/dl).

Calculations

Urea nitrogen results are reported in milligrams per deciliter, or milligrams of urea nitrogen per 100 ml of blood. Several factors must be considered before the final results can be calculated. The calculation of final results is accomplished by reviewing the steps in the procedure:

1. *To determine how much of the specimen was actually present in the protein-free filtrate:*

In this procedure, 1 ml of whole blood is incubated with 1 ml of working urease solution. After incubation, 7 ml of $0.095 N$ H_2SO_4 and 1 ml of 10 g/dl Na_2WO_4 are added. This is a total of 10 ml in the tube. Of this 10 ml, 1 ml of filtrate is pipetted into the photometer cuvette. Using the following formula, the amount of blood actually being treated in the photometer cuvette and the amount represented by the percent transmittance reading is found:

$$\frac{10 \text{ ml of filtrate}}{1 \text{ ml of blood}} = \frac{1 \text{ ml of filtrate}}{x \text{ ml of blood}}$$

$$x = 0.1 \text{ ml of blood}$$

The result read from the graph therefore represents the milligrams of urea nitrogen in 0.1 ml of blood.

2. *To determine how many milligrams of urea nitrogen are present in 100 ml of blood (mg/dl):*

As stated above, the result read from the graph is the milligrams of urea nitrogen present in 0.1 ml of blood. The following formulas may be used to find the result in milligrams per deciliter:

$$\frac{\text{Graph reading, mg of urea N}}{0.1 \text{ ml of blood}}$$

$$= \frac{x \text{ mg of urea N}}{100 \text{ ml of blood (mg/dl)}}$$

or

$$\text{Graph reading, mg of urea N} \times \frac{100}{0.1}$$

$$= x \text{ mg of urea N per 100 ml of blood (mg/dl)}$$

If any other dilutions have been made during the procedure, they must be accounted for in the calculations.

3. *To calculate the recovery concentration:*

In the beginning of the procedure, 0.2 ml of working urea recovery solution was added to one of the control tubes, labeled R. The concentration of the working urea solution is 1 mg/ml nitrogen. Therefore, in the 0.2 ml of recovery solution that was added, there is 0.2 mg of nitrogen. The 0.2 mg of urea nitrogen was added to tube R and should be measured (or recovered) at the end of the procedure. This tube was diluted through the incubation and preparation of protein-free filtrate, as the other tubes were. The resulting total amount in tube R is, however, 10.2 ml, not 10 ml as in the rest of the tubes (the other tubes do not have the added 0.2 ml of working urea solution). To calculate the amount of urea in the 1 ml of filtrate pipetted into the photometer cuvette for tube R, use the following formula:

$$\frac{10.2 \text{ ml of filtrate}}{0.2 \text{ mg of urea N}} = \frac{1 \text{ ml of filtrate}}{x \text{ mg of urea N}}$$

$x = 0.0196$ mg of N added to recovery tube

Taking this into consideration, tube R should have 0.0196 mg of nitrogen *more* than the control tube (the same specimen as used for tube R, but no recovery solution added). The control value read from the graph is subtracted from the value for tube R read from the graph. One hundred percent recovery is 0.0196 mg of nitrogen. Calculate the percent recovery, with 0.0196 mg of nitrogen as 100 percent, using the following formula:

$$\frac{0.0196 \text{ mg of N}}{100\%}$$

$$= \frac{\text{mg of N actually recovered in determination}}{x\% \text{ recovery}}$$

The acceptable recovery range is 90–110 percent. If the percent recovery is outside these limits, the procedure must be repeated and the results must not be given out until the recovery is within the limits established. The use of a recovery solution tells just how good the method really is.

Technical factors and sources of error

The blood specimens must contain no fluoride or ammonium salts. Both will interfere with the final results (fluoride will give low results and ammonium salts high results). The glassware used must be free from contamination by substances such as mercury, fluoride, and ammonia compounds. Ammonia-free water must be used to prepare all reagents and for any step in the procedure requiring the use of water. Ammonia-free water can be purchased commercially or prepared from tap water by double distillation.

The protein-free filtrates must be clear and colorless. If the urea content is high, the filtrate will be colored with hemoglobin, because the ammonium carbonate formed by the action of the urease will neutralize part of the acid, leaving an insufficient amount for the precipitation of the protein. To a colored filtrate, $2\,N\,H_2SO_4$ is added in small drops until all the color disappears.

Dilutions of the filtrates must be prepared whenever an unknown filtrate gives a galvanometer reading lower than the most concentrated standard solution used (S_5, in most cases). Using ammonia-free water, a 1:5 or 1:10 dilution of the filtrate is prepared. The color is developed using 1 ml of this diluted filtrate, and a reading is taken with a new set of standards and a blank. This additional dilution factor must be taken into consideration in the final calculations.

Incubation time, temperature, and pH are critical factors in any enzyme reaction. These factors must be watched carefully to ensure good results.

Reporting results and recording laboratory data

Urea nitrogen results are usually reported in milligrams per deciliter, to the nearest whole number. The laboratory retains the standard graph and the work sheet with the galvanometer readings obtained with a particular procedure for a time. The results for the various specimens are recorded permanently in some manner by the laboratory. Results are reported to the physician only when the control values check out and when the recovery is within the acceptable range, 90–110 percent for the urea nitrogen procedure.

Blood urea nitrogen—Bertholet urease method[27]

Principle

During an incubation period, the urea present in the sample is hydrolyzed to ammonium carbonate by the enzyme urease. When the alkali solution reacts with the ammonium carbonate, ammonia is formed. The reaction is buffered by EDTA, which also serves to chelate any heavy metal ions that might otherwise inactivate the urease. Ammonia is estimated by the Bertholet reaction, in which it reacts with phenol and alkaline hypochlorite to form blue indophenol. Sodium nitroprusside $[Na_2 Fe(CN)_5 NO]$ acts as a catalyst. The intensity of the blue color is proportional to the quantity of urea in the specimen. The blue color is measured in a photometer and is stable for several hours.

The reactions that take place in the procedure are given below:

$$H_2N-\overset{\overset{\displaystyle O}{\|}}{C}-NH_2 + 2H_2O + H^+ \xrightarrow{\text{urease}}$$

Urea
in specimen

$$(NH_4)_2CO_3 + H^+ \longrightarrow 2NH_4^+ + HCO_3^-$$

Ammonium
carbonate

$$NH_4^+ + OH^- \longrightarrow NH_3 + H_2O$$

Ammonia

$$NH_3 + NaOCl = 2$$

Ammonia

Indophenol
(blue in dissociated form)

Reagents

All reagents must be prepared with ammonia-free water.

1. Phenol-nitroprusside solution. Place 10 g of pink-white phenol and 0.050 g of $Na_2 Fe(CN)_5 NO \cdot 2H_2O$ in a 1-L volumetric flask containing about 500 ml of ammonia-free water. Dissolve the reagents, dilute to the mark, and mix thoroughly. Store this solution in a dark brown bottle in a refrigerator and discard after 2 months.

2. Alkaline hypochlorite solution. Place 5 g of NaOH in about 500 ml of ammonia-free water in a 1-L volumetric flask. Cool, add 0.42 g of sodium hypochlorite (NaOCl) (commercial bleaches such as Clorox are satisfactory), dilute to the mark, and mix thoroughly. Store in an amber bottle in a refrigerator and discard after 2 months.

3. Sodium ethylenediaminetetraacetic acid (EDTA), pH 6.5 (1 g/dl). Dissolve 10 g of EDTA in about 800 ml of ammonia-free water. Adjust the pH to 6.5 with 1 N NaOH and dilute to 1 L. EDTA binds cations that might interfere with urease activity.

4. Urease stock solution (40 modified Sumner units/ml). Suspend 0.2 g of urease (jack bean, containing 3500–4100 units/g) in 10 ml of water and add 10 ml of glycerol. Store in a refrigerator and discard after 4 months.

5. Urease working solution (0.4 units/ml). Dilute 1 ml of the urease stock with 100 ml of EDTA solution. Store in a refrigerator and discard after 3 weeks.

6. Urea nitrogen stock standard (500 mg urea N/dl). Dissolve 1.0717 g of dry urea in about 50 ml of ammonia-free water in a 100-ml volumetric flask. Add 0.1 g of sodium azide, dilute to the mark, and mix. Sodium azide serves as a preservative. Ammonium sulfate is sometimes used as a standard; it has the advantage of being stable, but the disadvantage of not controlling the enzymatic steps in the procedure.

7. Urea nitrogen working standard (50 mg urea N/dl). Dilute 10 ml of the stock standard to about 90 ml with ammonia-free water in a 100-ml volumetric flask. Add 0.1 g of sodium

azide, dilute to the mark, and mix thoroughly. Store in a refrigerator and discard after 6 months.

Procedure

1. Plasma or serum may be used directly with this method. If plasma is used, it must be obtained with oxalate, citrate, heparin, or EDTA as the anticoagulant to eliminate colorimetric interference of the hemoglobin. If a sample of whole blood is used, the protein must be removed first. If the serum is very lipemic, a special blank tube must be prepared by adding the phenol color reagent to the urease before adding the serum, and then setting the zero absorbance for the lipemic sample with the special blank tube prepared. If a high result is anticipated on clinical grounds, it saves time to prepare a sample of serum diluted 1:5 with saline and run this diluted sample along with the regular sample. Urine may be used with this method. The urine must be treated to remove the ammonia ordinarily present in urine (ammonia would be measured too and give a falsely high urea nitrogen result). To remove ammonia from urine, the specimen is treated with either Lloyd's reagent (sodium aluminum silicate) or Permutit. The ammonia is absorbed by either method. The treated urine sample is filtered and 1 ml is diluted to a total volume of 50 ml in a 50-ml volumetric flask. Ammonia-free water must be used to dilute the sample. The regular aliquot of diluted sample is used in the procedure as described below. The dilution of the urine must be remembered when the final calculations are made. The dilution must be made because urine has about 50 times as much urea nitrogen as serum. Cerebrospinal fluid may be used with this method directly, if necessary.

2. Label a series of tubes for blank, standard, control, control duplicate, and unknowns.

3. Pipet 1.0 ml of urease working solution into each tube.

4. With a micropipet, add 10 μl of unknown serum and working standards to the appropriate tubes. Mix and incubate all tubes for 15 minutes at 37°C.

5. Add rapidly and successively, mixing after each addition, 5.0 ml of the phenol-nitroprusside solution and 5 ml of the alkaline hypochlorite. It is essential that these reagents be added in the stated order.

6. Place tubes in a 37°C water bath for 20 minutes.

7. Transfer the solutions into photometer cuvettes.

8. Measure the absorbances (read %T and use a conversion chart for absorbances) at 560 nm in the spectrophotometer, using the blank as a reference.

9. Record galvanometer readings and calculations on the report sheet.

Calculations

$$\frac{A_u}{A_s} \times 50 \text{ mg/dl of urea N} = x \text{ mg/dl of urea N}$$
$$\text{(in standard)}$$

where A_u and A_s are the absorbances of the unknown and standard, respectively.

Blood urea nitrogen—Diacetylmonoxime method[28]

Principle

This is a direct assay method, which does not require the removal of protein from the sample before testing. The test may be done with protein-free filtrates, however. Serum is the specimen of choice for this method, but plasma may be used if properly anticoagulated. Cells or clot must be removed from the serum or plasma within 1 hour after collection. The method is based on the direct reaction of urea (not ammonia) with diacetyl to form a yellow compound (a diazine derivative). Because diacetyl is unstable, it is replaced by the reagent diacetylmonoxime, which is more stable. The color is intensified by the presence of thiosemicarbazide, which is added to the diacetylmonoxime reagent when it is prepared. Ferric ions increase the rate of the reaction. Since diacetyl reacts directly with urea and not with ammonia, the ammonia does not have to be removed from urine specimens for this method to be used with urine. The same reagents and reactions are used in many automatic analyzer methods, hence this manual method is widely used as a backup procedure in many laboratories. The intensity of the yellow color in the unknowns is compared colorimetrically to that in the standards. The reactions that take place in this method are outlined below:

CH$_3$
|
C=NOH $\xrightarrow{\text{H}_3\text{O}^+}$ C=O $\xrightarrow[\text{urea}]{(\text{H}_2\text{N})_2\text{CO}}$
|
C=O C=O
|
CH$_3$ CH$_3$

Diacetyl-   Diacetyl
monoxime

CH$_3$
|
C=N
| $\rangle$C=O
C=N
|
CH$_3$

Yellow diazine
derivative

Reagents

1. Diacetylmonoxime solution. Dissolve 1 g of diacetylmonoxime (2,3-butanedionemonoxime), 0.2 g of thiosemicarbazide, and 9 g of NaCl in water and dilute to 1 L.
2. Working acid ferric chloride solution. Cautiously add 60 ml of concentrated H$_2$SO$_4$ and 10 ml of 85 ml/dl phosphoric acid to about 800 ml of water. Add 0.1 g of ferric chloride (FeCl$_3$) and dilute to 1 L.
3. Benzoic acid standard diluent: 0.016 M benzoic acid solution. Dissolve 2 g of benzoic

acid in 1 L of water. Add 0.8 ml of concentrated H$_2$SO$_4$ and mix. Use this solution for preparing and diluting stock standards.
4. Stock urea nitrogen standard (10 mg/ml). Place 21.433 g of urea in a 1-L volumetric flask. Add enough standard diluent to dissolve. Dilute to volume with standard diluent.
5. Working urea nitrogen standard. Dilute 1-, 2-, and 3-ml portions of stock standard to 100 ml with the standard diluent. This gives standards with urea N concentrations of 10, 20, and 30 mg/dl, respectively.

Procedure

1. Label photometer cuvettes for a reagent blank, three standards (10, 20, and 30 mg/dl urea N), control, control duplicate, and each unknown.

2. Add 1.0 ml of working diacetylmonoxime solution from the automatic pipettor to all cuvettes.

3. Pipet 10 μl of distilled water to the blank and 10 μl of standards (10, 20, 30 mg/dl), control, and unknowns to the labeled cuvettes. If using 10-μl TC pipets, rinse them out with the reagent in the cuvette. Mix well by shaking.

4. Add 1.0 ml of working acid FeCl$_3$ reagent from the automatic pipettor to all cuvettes and mix well by inversion, using Parafilm.

5. Place in a boiling-water bath (100–105°C) for exactly 12 minutes (this should be timed). Use special boiling racks.

6. At the end of the boiling time, place in a cold-water bath for 2 minutes.

7. Read against the reagent blank at 535 nm *immediately*. Loss of color occurs within 20 minutes. Record %T and/or absorbance (A) readings on the report sheet for the diacetylmonoxime procedure.

8. Plot the standard readings on graph paper (use semilogarithmic paper to plot %T readings). Standards must be read because the color is affected by timing. Calculate the urea nitrogen in milligrams per deciliter from the standard graph.

Calculations

Calculate the results from the standard graph line.

$$\frac{A_u}{A_s} \times \text{concentration of standard}$$

$$= x \text{ mg/dl of urea N}$$

For serum and plasma:
  8–26 mg/dl of urea N
For urine:
  6–17 g of urea N in 24 hours

LIVER FUNCTION—BILIRUBIN

Normal liver function

The liver is a large and complex organ, absolutely necessary for numerous body functions. The liver is responsible for many metabolic, storage, excretory, and detoxifying functions. More specifically, the liver is a major factor in the metabolism of carbohydrates, lipids, and proteins, in terms of both intermediary metabolism and the synthesis of many essential compounds. Many necessary enzymes and coenzymes for carbohydrate, lipid, and protein metabolism are present only in cells of the liver. Glycogen is formed, stored, and converted back to glucose in the liver. Energy derived from food is made available to the cells of the body through the process of glycolysis of the high-energy bonds in adenosine triphosphate (ATP), which were formed by oxidative phosphorylation in the cells of the liver.

The liver is the site of detoxification of various substances. These toxic substances may be formed in normal body metabolism and converted or detoxified by the liver; an example is the formation of urea from the ammonia produced in protein metabolism. Toxic substances introduced into the blood from the intestine (such as dyes, heavy metals, and drugs) are excreted by the liver. The liver is essential in the formation and secretion of bile, bile pigments, and bile salts, which are necessary for digestion. These substances are derived from bilirubin, a major by-product of the destruction of red blood cells. In addition, the liver is the site of forma-

tion and synthesis of many of the factors involved in the clotting of blood.

These important functions of the liver may be altered when the liver is diseased or damaged. Numerous laboratory tests are available to determine both the existence of liver disease and the extent, location, and type of damage so that appropriate treatment can be initiated. There is no one test that will give a complete clinical view of liver function; instead, a carefully selected group of tests may be requested by the physician depending on the process in question. One test of liver function is for the presence and concentration of bilirubin in the blood and the urine. A discussion of bilirubin metabolism follows.

Bilirubin metabolism

Bilirubin is a normal product resulting from the breakdown of red blood cells. Individual red blood cells do not exist indefinitely in the body; they are degraded after approximately 120 days. As part of red blood cell degradation, the heme portion of the hemoglobin molecule is converted to the bile pigment bilirubin by the *reticuloendothelial (RE) system*, primarily by RE cells in the liver, spleen, and bone marrow. A total of approximately 6 g of hemoglobin is released each day as overage red blood cells are eliminated from the body. The cells of the RE system first phagocytize the red cells, then convert the released hemoglobin through a complex series of reactions in which the heme portion of the molecule is finally converted to bilirubin. Bilirubin is a vivid yellow pigment. An increase in the concentration of bilirubin in the blood indicates the presence of jaundice. Although it is useful in the bile, bilirubin is a waste product that must eventually be eliminated from the body. When it is formed by the RE cells, bilirubin is not soluble in water. Therefore it is transported from the RE cells through the blood to the liver cells as a bilirubin-albumin complex. This water-insoluble form of bilirubin is often referred to as *free* bilirubin or *unconjugated* bilirubin.

Bilirubin is normally excreted from the body by the liver by way of the intestine. It is excreted by the liver rather than the kidney because free bilirubin linked to albumin cannot pass through the glomerular capsule of the kidney. When free bilirubin reaches the liver, it is converted to a water-soluble product by the Kupffer cells of the liver. It is made soluble by conjugation with glucuronic acid and some other hydrophilic substances to form bilirubin glucuronide.

Water-soluble bilirubin, often referred to as *conjugated* bilirubin, can be eliminated from the body by way of the kidney or the intestine. Normally, conjugated bilirubin is excreted by the liver into the bile, transported to the common bile duct and then to the gallbladder, where it is concentrated and emptied into the small intestine.

In the intestine, most of the bilirubin is converted to urobilinogen. Bilirubin is reduced to urobilinogen by the action of certain bacteria that make up the intestinal flora. Urobilinogen is actually a group of colorless chromogens, all of which are referred to as urobilinogen. Approximately half of the urobilinogen formed in the intestine is absorbed into the portal blood circulation and returned to the liver. In the liver, most of the urobilinogen is excreted into the bile once again and returned to the intestine.

A very small amount of urobilinogen escapes this liver clearance and is therefore excreted from the body by way of the urine. This represents only about 1 percent of the urobilinogen produced in 1 day. Urobilinogen in the intestine is either eliminated from the body unchanged or oxidized to the colored compound urobilin. Incidentally, urobilin is the substance that gives the feces their normal color. The net effect is that, in normal circumstances, 99 percent of the urobilinogen formed from bilirubin is eliminated by way of the feces.

It is therefore apparent that the urine normally contains only a very small amount of urobilinogen and no bilirubin. As mentioned, unconjugated bilirubin cannot be excreted by the kidney and is absent in urine. However, conjugated bilirubin can pass through the renal glomerulus, and if it is present in abnormal concentration in the blood, it will be excreted by the kidney.

Abnormal bilirubin metabolism: Jaundice

Jaundice is a condition that occurs when the serum bilirubin concentration becomes greater than normal and there is an abnormal accumulation of bilirubin in the body tissues. Since bilirubin is a vivid yellow pigment, an accumulation in the tissues results in a yellow pigmentation of the skin, the sclera or white of the eyes, and the mucous membranes. The causes of jaundice are numerous and must be discovered as soon as possible in order to initiate prompt and proper treatment. There are several schemes for the classification of the various types of jaundice; one such scheme describes three types, namely *prehepatic*, *hepatic*, and *posthepatic or obstructive*.[30]

Prehepatic jaundice is also described as *hemolytic* jaundice. It occurs in conditions in which there is increased destruction of red cells. This type of jaundice is found in infants with blood group incompatibilities, in neonatal physiological jaundice, and with an increased production of free bilirubin. There is an increased formation of conjugated bilirubin and a subsequent increased formation of urobilinogen. While there is an increased concentration of urobilinogen in the stool, the liver cannot pick up or reexcrete the greatly increased amount of urobilinogen returned to the liver by the portal circulation. Therefore, more urobilinogen goes into the general blood circulation and is eliminated in the urine. In summary, prehepatic or hemolytic jaundice is characterized by increased free bilirubin in the blood and increased urobilinogen in the feces and urine.

Hepatic jaundice results from conditions that involve the liver cells directly and prevent normal excretion. Such a condition might be specific damage such as conjugation failure in neonatal physiological jaundice, where there is an enzyme deficiency. Diseases of conjugation failure result in an increased concentration of unconjugated bilirubin in the blood. Disturbances of the transport mechanisms by which conjugated bilirubin is passed into the bile canaliculi also occur in hepatic jaundice. Diffuse or overall hepatic cell involvement occurs in such conditions as viral hepatitis, toxic hepatitis caused by heavy metal or drug poisoning, and cirrhosis. In these cases the ability of the liver cells to remove and conjugate free bilirubin is decreased, resulting in increased amounts of free bilirubin in the blood. Bilirubin that is conjugated by the liver is not excreted into the bile, resulting in increased amounts of conjugated bilirubin in the blood, which can now be eliminated by the kidney. Urobilinogen that is formed and goes into the portal circulation cannot be removed by the liver cells and will also appear in the urine. Thus, urobilinogen in the urine is useful for the detection of early hepatitis; however, as the disease progresses to later stages, the liver is unable to form and pass conjugated bilirubin into the bile, so that the formation, reabsorption, and amount of urobilinogen in the urine are also decreased.

Posthepatic jaundice is also referred to as obstructive jaundice. It occurs when the common bile duct is obstructed by stones, tumors, spasms, or a stricture. As a result, the bilirubin that has been conjugated by the liver is regurgitated back into the liver sinusoids and the blood. If the blockage is sufficiently extensive, liver cell function may be impaired, and both free and conjugated bilirubin are found in the blood. The conjugated bilirubin will be excreted by the kidney, and therefore bilirubin is found in the urine. Since bilirubin conjugated by the liver is unable to reach the intestine, no urobilinogen is formed and none is found in the blood or the urine. Since urobilinogen is not formed, urobilin is absent, and the stools are characteristically chalky white to light brown in color.

Methods for quantitative determination of bilirubin

Tests for serum bilirubin used in the clinical laboratory are based on the reaction of bilirubin with diazotized sulfanilic acid to form azobilirubin, which has a red-purple color. This reaction was first described by Ehrlich in 1883, and the diazo reagent is also referred to as *Ehrlich's* reagent. The basic reaction has been modified by the addition of alcohol, particularly methanol. Azobilirubin has indicator properties in strongly acid or strongly alkaline solutions. Thus, many modifications of the diazo reaction measure the amount of red dye in an acid medium, while others measure the blue color in a strongly alkaline medium. Most procedures involve a modification of the Malloy-Evelyn technique, which utilizes a diazo reaction with methanol added.

As mentioned above, bilirubin is present in serum in two forms: free, and conjugated to glucuronic acid. Since the glucuronide is freely soluble in water, it reacts rapidly with Ehrlich's reagent. A reading made at a specific time (usually 1 minute) after the addition of Ehrlich's reagent is generally taken as a measure of the bilirubin glucuronide (conjugated bilirubin) concentration. Free bilirubin is not soluble in water and reacts with Ehrlich's reagent only after the addition of methanol. A reading made after the addition of methanol and a sufficient waiting period, usually 20 or 30 minutes, is a measure of the concentration of the two forms of bilirubin. The concentration of free bilirubin (also referred to as *indirect* bilirubin) is the difference between the total concentration of bilirubin and the concentration of *direct* or 1-minute bilirubin.

Clinical significance of bilirubin

An increased serum bilirubin concentration may indicate increased destruction (hemolysis) of red blood cells, impaired excretory function of liver cells, or obstruction of the bile flow. In obstructive jaundice there is an increase in total bilirubin; however, this is primarily in the form of conjugated bilirubin, giving a large value for the 1-minute or direct bilirubin. In hemolytic jaundice there is an increase in total bilirubin, primarily free bilirubin; therefore the indirect fraction is increased. With liver damage such as viral hepatitis, both the free and conjugated bilirubin increase, and total, direct, and indirect fractions are elevated.

Elevations in serum bilirubin occur in many infants in the first few days of life. This is especially true of premature infants. Such neonatal physiological jaundice may involve either a deficiency of the enzyme that transfers glucuronate groups onto bilirubin or liver immaturity. Bilirubin cannot be conjugated, and the concentration of free or indirect bilirubin is increased in the blood. This is generally a temporary deficiency, which lasts only a few days, and levels seldom exceed 10 mg/dl. However, blood levels of bilirubin must be monitored carefully to see that toxic concentrations, over 20 mg/dl, do not occur. This is most likely to happen in cases of incompatibility between the blood groups of the mother and the infant, which is largely alleviated through the use of Rh immune globulin (see Chap. 9). Such levels of unconjugated bilirubin are toxic, for if the

binding capacity of plasma albumin for bilirubin is exceeded, the unconjugated bilirubin may cause irreversible brain damage (*kernicterus*). Micromethods have been developed for analyzing the very small amounts of blood available for testing from infants. Treatment of infants with enzyme deficiency involves phototherapy. Blood incompatibility or bilirubin levels approaching 20 mg/dl may require exchange transfusion.

Specimens

Determinations may be done on serum or plasma, although serum is preferred. The blood should be drawn when the patient is in a fasting state to avoid alimentary lipemia. Exposure of serum to light, especially that of wavelengths at the lower end of the visible region, results in the destruction of bilirubin and should be avoided. Specimens stored in short, stoppered tubes and placed in solid wooden blocks under artificial light appear to be protected during the usual delay before analysis. The procedure should be carried out as soon as possible, at least within 2 or 3 hours after the blood has clotted. Specimens can be stored in the dark in a refrigerator for up to 1 week or in the freezer for 3 months without significant loss of bilirubin. The presence of hemoglobin results in the measurement of an erroneously low value for bilirubin by a diazo method. However, it must be kept in mind that it is difficult to see hemoglobin in the presence of increased amounts of bilirubin. Carotenemia, the presence of carotene or vitamin A in the specimen, does not interfere with the determination of bilirubin.

Serum bilirubin method of Malloy and Evelyn (modified)[31, 32]

Principle

Bilirubin reacts with Ehrlich's reagent (diazotized sulfanilic acid plus nitrous acid) to form the red-purple dye azobilirubin. The intensity of the purple color that is formed is proportional to the bilirubin concentration in the serum. Since bilirubin that has been conjugated with glucuronic acid is soluble in water, it reacts with the diazo reagent in aqueous solution to form a color within 1 minute. This conjugated bilirubin is thus referred to as direct bilirubin. Alcohol (methanol) is then added to the test solution. This accelerates the reaction of all forms of bilirubin in the serum—especially the unconjugated bilirubin that did not react in the aqueous solution and is therefore referred to as indirect bilirubin. A value for total bilirubin is obtained after letting the color reaction stand for 30 minutes. The concentration of unconjugated bilirubin is the difference between the concentrations of total bilirubin and conjugated bilirubin.

Results for this bilirubin procedure are calculated from a standard graph prepared by the laboratory. It is advantageous to use a permanent graph from day to day, because the standardization itself is a fairly involved procedure and the standard bilirubin solution is very unstable. When the procedure is standardized sufficiently, pure bilirubin must be used. Commercially available bilirubin varies in purity. Pure crystalline bilirubin is available as a standard reference material from the National Bureau of Standards. Freeze-dried serum standards containing elevated bilirubin levels are also commercially available. When the procedure is standardized, the standard solutions are prepared according to an acceptable method and treated exactly as the unknown in the procedure that follows.* Of course, the appropriate control specimens or reference samples must be included with each set of determinations to ensure the accuracy of the procedure.

---

*For the standardization procedure, refer to a standard chemistry text such as "Fundamentals of Clinical Chemistry," 2d ed., Norbert W. Tietz (ed.), W. B. Saunders Company, Philadelphia, 1976.

Reagents

1. Solution A: sulfanilic acid solution. Dissolve 1.0 g of sulfanilic acid in water. Add 15 ml of concentrated hydrochloric acid (HCl). Dilute to 1 L with deionized water. The solution is stable indefinitely.
2. Solution B: sodium nitrite (0.5 g/dl). Dissolve 1.0 g of $NaNO_2$ in deionized water and dilute to 200 ml in a volumetric flask. Prepare fresh daily.
3. Ehrlich's diazo reagent. Mix 10 ml of sulfanilic acid solution (solution A) with 0.3 ml of $NaNO_2$ solution (solution B). Use the reagent within 30 minutes after preparation.
4. Blank reagent. Dilute 15 ml of concentrated HCl to 1 L with water. The reagent is stable indefinitely at room temperature.
5. Methanol, absolute, analytical reagent grade.

Procedure

For each serum specimen and control specimen to be analyzed, carry out the following:

1. Select two cuvettes for each specimen. Each specimen will have a color development cuvette labeled U (unknown) and a blank cuvette labeled B (blank).
2. Into each blank tube place 9.5 ml of deionized water. To this add 0.5 ml of clear, unhemolyzed serum and mix by gentle inversion.
3. Transfer 5.0 ml of the diluted serum to the color development tube, labeled U.
4. To each blank tube (B), add 1 ml of blank reagent.
5. Using the 540-nm wavelength in the spectrophotometer, adjust the blank reading to 100%T.
6. To the color development tube (U) for each specimen, add 1 ml of Ehrlich's diazo reagent rapidly from a 1-ml serological pipet and mix immediately.
7. *Exactly* 1 minute after the addition of the diazo reagent, read the color development tube against the blank tube for that specimen, which was set at 100%T. This reading will give the conjugated (direct) bilirubin concentration for

each specimen when read from the standard graph.

8. To all cuvettes, both blank and color development, add 6 ml of absolute methanol and mix by gentle inversion.

9. After 30 minutes, read each color development tube at 540 nm against the appropriate blank tube, which was set at 100%T. Be certain that there are no bubbles in the light path when this reading is made. This reading will give the total bilirubin concentration for each specimen.

Calculations

Results for this procedure are read from a previously prepared standard graph, showing %T plotted on semilogarithmic graph paper against bilirubin concentration (milligrams per deciliter of sample reagent in the color development tube).

1. Values for total bilirubin may be obtained directly from the standard graph.

2. Values for conjugated bilirubin (free or direct) may be obtained by dividing the 1-minute value read from the prepared graph by 2. (The solutions at the 30-minute reading have twice the volume of those at the 1-minute reading because of the addition of 6 ml of methanol.)

3. Values for unconjugated (indirect) bilirubin are obtained by subtracting the 1-minute (direct) value from the total bilirubin value.

4. If a specimen gives a reading lower than 10%T, Beer's law no longer applies and the procedure must be repeated using 0.2 ml of serum rather than 0.5 ml. Make up the difference with deionized water and calculate accordingly.

Technical factors and sources of error

The Malloy-Evelyn method is less precise at the low or normal range than when the bilirubin concentration is elevated. The precision is approximately ±10 percent in the low range and approximately ±5 percent when the bilirubin concentration is more than 5 mg/dl. Elevation of the bilirubin concentration may be indicated by the appearance of the specimen; however, a highly colored serum does not necessarily indicate bilirubin. Both hemoglobin and carotene may give a similar appearance. Therefore, no accurate conversion of bilirubin concentration to icterus index is possible. The presence of hemoglobin results in the measurement of an erroneously low value for bilirubin by the diazo method. Errors as great as 25 percent have been reported,[33] and observable hemolysis may cause negative errors of 5-15 percent in most diazo methods.[34] Turbidity should be avoided in the cuvettes; therefore lipemia should be avoided by use of a fasting specimen. It is important that all reagents and samples be added in the exact proportions and sequence described in the procedure. If not, a precipitate may form that will invalidate the results. Proper mixing after each step of the procedure is also essential. Before photometric readings are made, the cuvettes should be checked for the presence of bubbles. These may be dispersed by tapping the cuvette gently or by using a stirring rod.

The diazo reagent is unstable and must be used within 30 minutes after preparation. It is therefore prepared fresh with each set of determinations. The instability is caused by the formation of very unstable nitrous acid when the sulfanilic acid solution (solution A) is added to the sodium nitrite solution (solution B).

The amount of time required for full color development in the total bilirubin reaction varies. Procedures have been described with intervals ranging from 10 to 30 minutes. It is important to consistently use the time specified in a procedure; in this case 30 minutes was chosen.

Since serum bilirubin is relatively unstable, determinations should be made as soon as possible after the specimen is collected and the serum is separated from the clot. The primary source of instability is exposure to light, so specimens should be kept out of the light until the determination is performed. In the frozen state bilirubin in *serum* is stable for several months. However, most prepared bilirubin standards do not appear to have such stability.

A brown color may appear in the diazo reaction with serum from uremic patients. The contribution of this nonspecific color is insignificant with elevated bilirubin concentration, but may be significant in such azotemic serum with normal bilirubin concentrations.

Biliverdin (a green-colored oxidation product of bilirubin) does not interfere with the diazo reaction for bilirubin as it does not react with the diazo reagent. However, bilirubin will convert to biliverdin on standing, giving falsely low results.

Beer's law does not apply when concentrations of bilirubin are present that give percent transmittance readings lower than 10 percent. Therefore the serum must be diluted, or a smaller volume of the serum must be retested, with corresponding corrections for the volume change in the calculations.

Since bilirubin concentrations must be closely followed in infants with jaundice, many microtechniques have been described for the determination of bilirubin. Most of the micromethods proposed are modifications of the Malloy and Evelyn procedure described in this section. The method presented here may be scaled down by using one-tenth of the volumes given in the procedure.

Reporting results and recording laboratory data

Bilirubin results are usually reported in milligrams of bilirubin per 100 ml of serum (mg/dl), to the nearest whole number. Both direct and total bilirubin values are reported. The laboratory retains the work sheet with the galvanometer readings obtained by a particular procedure for a time. The results for the various specimens are recorded permanently in some manner by the laboratory. Results are reported to the physician only when the quality control values are within acceptable limits.

Normal values

Serum bilirubin in healthy adults:
Less than 0.4 mg/dl direct
Less than 1.0 mg/dl total

Infants (based on the Jendrassik-Grof diazo method): [35]

Up to 24 hours: Premature, 1–8 mg/dl total
                 Full-term, 2–6 mg/dl total
Up to 48 hours: Premature, 6–12 mg/dl total
                 Full-term, 6–10 mg/dl total
Days 3–5:   Premature, 10–14 mg/dl total
                 Full-term, 4–8 mg/dl total
After 1 month: As for adults

Other tests of liver function

The bilirubin procedure that has been described is only one of several laboratory determinations that are used by the physician to estimate liver function. The determination of bilirubin concentration may not detect less severe, hidden (or occult) liver disease. Results from several laboratory procedures must be evaluated by the physician before an accurate diagnosis can be made. The physician or institution may have a preferred battery of tests to determine liver function. A brief description of some of the tests most often included in such a liver profile follows. In each case, normal liver function should be kept in mind when considering the rationale behind the use of each test as part of the liver profile.

Bilirubin

Normal bilirubin metabolism and the significance of elevated values have been discussed previously. When liver disease is suspected without the clinical finding of jaundice, a slight elevation of the direct (conjugated) bilirubin can be very significant in detecting occult liver disease.

Serum glutamic-oxaloacetic transaminase

This enzyme, also called *aspartate aminotransferase* (AST), is found primarily in the liver, heart, kidney, and muscle tissue. Acute destruction of tissue in any of these areas results in rapid release of the enzyme into the serum. SGOT is therefore elevated in all forms of hepatitis.

Alkaline phosphatase

This enzyme may be produced in many tissues. It is normally produced in the liver by the bile duct epithelium and in the bone by osteoblasts. The enzyme appears to facilitate the transfer of metabolites across cell membranes and is associated with lipid transport and with the calcification process in bone synthesis. Serum alkaline phosphatase is particularly useful in the diagnosis of hepatobiliary disease and bone disease associated with increased osteoblastic activity.

Protein

In normal healthy individuals, the various plasma proteins are present in delicately balanced concentrations with a normal ratio of albumin to globulin. In liver disease this ratio may be altered. A number of tests for liver function are therefore based on the albumin-globulin relation.

Protein electrophoresis (ELP)

This is the most effective way to demonstrate significant alterations in the protein fractions. Electrophoretic separation of serum proteins is also of value in following the course of liver disease after diagnosis.

Cephalin-cholesterol flocculation

The cephalin-cholesterol flocculation test is used to demonstrate increased gamma globulin and decreased albumin in serum specimens. The amount of turbidity produced in the reaction is usually considered to be directly proportional to the amount of gamma globulin present.

Thymol turbidity

The thymol turbidity test indicates an increase in lipids and beta globulins.

Prothrombin

Another protein formed in the liver is prothrombin. It is necessary for the normal coagulation of blood. If liver function is impaired, less than normal amounts of prothrombin are formed and blood clotting is delayed. A determination of the prothrombin time can be used to test for abnormal liver function.

Bromsulfophthalein test

This test is based on the excretory ability of the liver. Bromsulfophthalein, a derivative of phenolphthalein, is excreted almost entirely by the liver in the normal individual. The normal liver can remove this organic dye from the bloodstream and excrete it into the bile, where it is eliminated by way of the feces. When the liver cells are diseased or damaged, or the flow of blood to the liver is decreased, this function is impaired. In the absence of jaundice, this is a simple, sensitive test of liver function and aids in the early detection of liver disease. It is used when the values for other liver function tests are normal. The dye is injected intravenously and its concentration is determined in serum collected 45 minutes after the injection.

REFERENCES

1. Richard J. Henry, Donald C. Cannon, and James W. Winkelman, "Clinical Chemistry, Principles and Techniques," 2d ed., p. 390, Harper & Row, Hagerstown, Md., 1974.
2. O. Folin and H. Wu, A System of Blood Analysis, *J. Biol. Chem.*, vol. 38, p. 81, 1919.
3. R. L. Haden, *J. Biol. Chem.*, vol. 56, p. 469, 1923.
4. Henry et al., *op. cit.*, p. 1289.
5. Norbert W. Tietz (ed.), "Fundamentals of Clinical Chemistry," 2d ed., p. 234, W. B. Saunders Company, Philadelphia, 1976.
6. *Ibid.*, p. 243.

7. *Ibid.*, p. 243.
8. M. Weissman and B. Klein, *Clin. Chem.*, vol. 4, p. 420, 1958.
9. Henry et al., *op. cit.*, p. 1284.
10. Norton Nelson, A Photometric Adaptation of the Somogyi Method for the Determination of Glucose, *J. Biol. Chem.*, vol. 153, p. 375, 1944.
11. Michael Somogyi, Determination of Blood Sugars, *J. Biol. Chem.*, vol. 160, p. 169, 1945.
12. Michael Somogyi, Determination of Blood Sugars, *J. Biol. Chem.*, vol. 195, p. 19, 1952.
13. Henry et al., *op. cit.*, p. 1283.
14. Roderick P. MacDonald, "Standard Methods of Clinical Chemistry," vol. 6, p. 159, Academic Press, New York, 1970.
15. K. M. Dubowski, An o-Toluidine Method for Body Fluid Glucose Determination, *Clin. Chem.*, vol. 8, pp. 215–235, 1962.
16. O. Schales and S. S. Schales, Simple and Accurate Method for Determination of Chloride in Biological Fluids, *J. Biol. Chem.*, vol. 140, p. 879, 1949.
17. E. Cotlove, H. V. Trantham, and R. L. Bowman, An Instrument and Method for Automatic, Rapid, Accurate and Sensitive Titration of Chloride in Biological Samples, *J. Lab. Clin. Med.*, vol. 50, p. 461, 1958.
18. Henry et al., *op. cit.*, p. 720.
19. *Ibid.*, p. 643.
20. Commission on Biochemical Nomenclature, International Union of Pure and Applied Chemistry and International Union of Biochemistry, "Enzyme Nomenclature (1972)," American Elsevier Publishing Company, Inc., New York, 1973.
21. Tietz, *op. cit.*, p. 630.
22. W. T. Caraway, A Stable Starch Substrate for the Determination of Amylase in Serum and Other Body Fluids, *Am. J. Clin. Pathol.*, vol. 32, p. 97, 1959.
23. M. Somogyi, Modifications of Two Methods for the Assay of Amylase, *Clin. Chem.*, vol. 6, p. 23, 1960.
24. R. J. Henry and N. Chiamori, Study of the Saccharogenic Method for the Determination of Serum and Urine Amylase, *Clin. Chem.*, vol. 6, p. 434, 1960.
25. Henry et al., *op. cit.*, p. 949.
26. C. J. Gentzkow, Accurate Method for Determination of Blood Urea Nitrogen by Direct Nesslerization, *J. Biol. Chem.*, vol. 143, p. 531, 1942.
27. A. L. Chaney and E. P. Marbach, Modified Reagents for Determination of Urea and Ammonia, *Clin. Chem.*, vol. 8, p. 131, 1962.
28. R. T. Evans, Manual and Automated Methods for Measuring Urea Based on a Modification of Its Reaction with Diacetyl Monoxime and Thiosemicarbazide, *J. Clin. Pathol.*, vol. 21, p. 527, 1968.
29. Henry et al. *op. cit.*, p. 517.
30. Tietz, *op. cit.*, pp. 1032–1034.
31. H. T. Malloy and K. A. Evelyn, *J. Biol. Chem.*, vol. 119, p. 481, 1937.
32. Recommendation on a Uniform Bilirubin Standard, in S. Meites (ed.), "Standard Methods of Clinical Chemistry," vol. 5, p. 75, Academic Press, New York, 1965.
33. D. Watson, A Note on the Haemoglobin Error in Some Nonprecipitation Diazomethods for Bilirubin Determinations, *Clin. Chim. Acta*, vol. 5, p. 613, 1960.
34. C. J. McGann and R. E. Carter, The Effect of Hemolysis on the Van den Bergh Reaction for Serum Bilirubin, *J. Pediatr.*, vol. 57, p. 199, 1960.
35. Tietz, *op. cit.*, p. 1040.

BIBLIOGRAPHY

Annino, Joseph S. and Roger W. Giese: "Clinical Chemistry, Principles and Procedures," 4th ed., Little, Brown and Company, Boston, 1976.
Davidsohn, Israel and John Bernard Henry (eds.): "Clinical Diagnosis by Laboratory Methods," 15th ed., W. B. Saunders Company, Philadelphia, 1974.
Dixon, M. and E. C. Webb: "Enzymes," 2d ed., Academic Press, New York, 1964.
Hald, P. M. and W. B. Mason: Sodium and

Potassium by Flame Photometry, in David Seligson (ed.), "Standard Methods of Clinical Chemistry," vol. II, pp. 165–185, Academic Press, New York, 1958.

Henry, Richard J., Donald C. Cannon, and James W. Winkelman: "Clinical Chemistry, Principles and Techniques," 2d ed., Harper & Row, Hagerstown, Md., 1974.

Kanter, Muriel W.: "Clinical Chemistry—Allied Health Series," Bobbs-Merrill Company, Inc., Indianapolis, 1975.

Raphael, Stanley S. et al.: "Lynch's Medical Laboratory Technology," 3d ed., vol. I, W. B. Saunders Company, Philadelphia, 1976.

"Report of the Commission on Enzymes of the International Union of Biochemistry," Pergamon Press, New York, 1961.

Tietz, Norbert W. (ed.): "Fundamentals of Clinical Chemistry," 2d ed., W. B. Saunders Company, Philadelphia, 1976.

THREE
HEMATOLOGY

The word *hematology* comes from the Greek *haima*, meaning blood, and *-logia*, from *logos*, meaning discourse and, hence, the science of or the study of. Hematology is therefore the science, or study, of blood. In a hematology course, one is concerned with the main constituents of the blood. Blood is composed of plasma and cells; the plasma is the fluid portion of the blood.

The total volume of blood in an average adult is about 6 L, or 7–8 percent of the body weight. About 45 percent of this amount is composed of the formed elements of the blood and the remaining 55 percent is the plasma. Approximately 90 percent of the plasma is water; the remaining 10 percent is proteins (albumin, globulin, and fibrinogen), carbohydrates, vitamins, hormones, enzymes, lipids, and salts.

Blood is part of the circulatory system of the body and has several different functions. It carries nutrients to the tissues, the most important nutrient being oxygen, which is carried by the red cells. Waste products (end products of metabolism) are carried by the blood to the organs of excretion. Many natural defense agents circulate continually with the blood supply. Much valuable information can be readily obtained from hematologic tests, and certain routine measurements and examinations are now a part of virtually every hospital admission.

The blood cells, or formed elements, to be discussed in this chapter are the red blood cells (*erythrocytes*), the white blood cells (*leukocytes*), and the platelets (*thrombocytes*). The laboratory tests performed in the area of hematology center around the cells and some of their constituents: their number or concentration, the relative distribution of various types of cells, and the structural or biochemical abnormalities that contribute to disease. The entire range of types of disease is seen: heredi-tary, immunologic, nutritional, metabolic, traumatic, and inflammatory (including infectious, hormonal, and neoplastic). In many instances the hematologic examination is virtually diagnostic, and in many instances it is a major contribution to the eventual solution of a diagnostic problem.

Diseases with a primary hematologic cause are not common, but hematologic manifestations secondary to other diseases are quite common. A wide variety of diseases may show signs or symptoms of a hematologic nature. Many diseases produce anemia, and others produce enlarged lymph nodes. Additional examination will usually indicate the primary involvement of some system besides the blood and lymph nodes.

The major source of the blood cells is the bone marrow, although the lymph nodes and spleen contribute some of the white blood cells. Many other sources make contributions to the blood.

Several hematologic tests are required as part of every patient's initial hospital admission report and are also a part of the physical examination in a physician's office. Many of these tests are considered routine and can be done by a laboratory technician with limited training. The routine admission and office examination tests include hemoglobin, hematocrit, white blood cell count, and cell differential. The differential includes classification of the white blood cells and examination of the red blood cells and platelets. These tests are often referred to as the *complete blood count* (CBC). With the advent of electronic cell counters, other values or tests are also becoming more routine. The red blood cell count and calculated red blood cell indices are now part of the routine CBC in many laboratories. In addition to their use for screening, the CBC results are helpful in the diagnosis of many diseases. They can reflect the body's ability to fight disease and may be used to determine how the patient is progressing in certain disease states such as infection or anemia. That

these tests are done frequently does not mean that they are unimportant. The physician can obtain valuable information about a patient's physical condition from accurately performed routine hematologic determinations.

In this chapter, the student should gain enough basic knowledge about the formed elements of the blood, their enumeration, and their characteristics to perform routine tests accurately and conscientiously in the clinical laboratory. This knowledge should include the basic theory of the determinations, use and care of the equipment used to perform the tests, proper preparation of the reagents, ability to recognize problems when encountered, proper handling of the specimens, calculation of the results, and an appreciation of the need for accuracy and care in performing all hematologic determinations. See under Collection, Preservation, and Preparation of Laboratory Specimens in Chap. 1 for a detailed account of the collection of blood for hematologic studies.

Performing accurate hematologic determinations requires repeated practice. The clinical la-

boratory student should not become discouraged if progress seems slow during the first practice periods in the hematology laboratory. Many of the techniques call for manual dexterity and experience in the manipulation of the equipment. Because the techniques in hematology have greatly expanded in recent years, there has been increased use of automated equipment, which can accurately handle large volumes of work. Some of the automated devices and methods will be discussed in this chapter.

Clinical applications of the hematologic tests will also be discussed here. Again, it is important that the student remember the reason why the laboratory determination was ordered in the first place. The patient is the ultimate concern of the laboratory and of the physician who uses the information provided by the laboratory.

Procedures performed in the hematology laboratory require microscopic observation, macroscopic observation, and, in some instances, a combination of both. In certain of the routine procedures, photometry is used.

SPECIMENS

Capillary blood

Since samples for hematologic study are so often obtained by finger puncture or venipuncture, the student should review the collection of specimens and the approach to the patient in general (see under Collection, Preservation, and Preparation of Laboratory Specimens in Chap. 1).

Capillary blood can be used with good results for morphological studies in hematology. For making differential blood counts and for enumerating cellular elements, capillary or peripheral blood can be obtained from the fingertip, earlobe, heel, or big toe. This kind of sampling is sometimes called microsampling. In newborn infants, blood is generally obtained from the plantar surface of the big toe or heel, since these areas are more accessible than the fingertip. Newborns have a small blood supply, and removing blood by venipuncture would deplete too much of their blood. If blood is needed from very young children, the third or fourth fingertip is generally punctured. In adults who have very poor veins or whose veins cannot be used because intravenous solutions are being administered, the tip of the third or fourth finger is punctured to obtain the blood sample. A free flow of blood is needed for the results obtained with capillary blood to agree with those from venous blood.

Venous blood

Because it is not always practical to obtain capillary blood for hematology, venous blood is often used. More tests can be done with a tube of venous blood, including the measurement of sedimentation rate, which requires more blood than some of the other hematology determinations. There must be some means of preventing coagulation, as clotted blood cannot be used. The types of anticoagulants available and their use are discussed under Anticoagulants in Chap. 1. For most hematologic studies the anticoagulant used is EDTA, or Sequestrene. This preserves the morphology of the cellular elements and prevents coagulation. It is important that the blood be mixed well with the anticoagulant immediately after it is collected to ensure proper anticoagulation. Not even small clots are acceptable for hematology. When refrigerated properly, EDTA specimens can be preserved for several hours until the work can be done. White cell counts, microhematocrit, platelet counts, and sedimentation rates can be measured up to 24 hours after blood is collected in EDTA if it is refrigerated at $4°C$.[1] The EDTA removes the calcium ions from the blood and thus inhibits coagulation.

Only certain anticoagulants are acceptable for hematologic tests. In addition to keeping the blood in a liquid form (preventing clotting), the anticoagulant must maintain the natural appearance of the red blood cells (RBC), white blood cells (WBC), and platelets. Sequestrene is the only anticoagulant in general use that can do all these things. Another anticoagulant that is used in some laboratories is balanced, or double, oxalate. This anticoagulant is a composite of ammonium oxalate and potassium oxalate balanced in such a way that the size and shape of the red blood cells are preserved. Balanced oxalate does not preserve the morphological features of the white blood cells or the platelets, and for this reason it cannot be used for all the hematologic tests.

Immediately after the blood has been properly drawn and placed in the tube containing the anticoagulant, it should be gently mixed by repeated inversion. This is necessary to ensure thorough contact with the anticoagulant. Clotted specimens are absolutely unacceptable for most tests done in the hematology laboratory, especially cell counts. If there is even a tiny clot in a specimen, the cell count will be grossly inaccurate.

Initial laboratory handling of specimens

After the blood specimen has been collected from the patient, it must be transported to the laboratory for analysis. Assuming that the specimen was properly labeled when it was drawn and is in good condition, it is examined in the laboratory as quickly as possible to prevent deterioration. Laboratory tests are done on fresh specimens whenever possible. Special handling of specimens for the various hematologic determinations will be discussed later in this chapter in connection with specific tests.

Immediately before a test is performed on a blood specimen, the blood sample must be mixed by repeated inversion for 5 minutes. This can be accomplished by hand or with a mechanical tube inverter. If the blood sample has stood for a few minutes, it should be mixed again for at least 1 minute.

When a preserved blood specimen is allowed to stand for a period of time, the components will settle into three distinct layers: (1) the plasma, or top layer, (2) the buffy coat, a grayish white cellular layer composed of the nucleated cells and platelets, and (3) the red blood cells, comprising the bottom layer. Some hematologic procedures are based on the ability of the blood specimen to settle into layers when it has been preserved by use of an anticoagulant.

Appearance of specimens

When the blood specimen has been properly drawn and preserved in the prescribed manner, the plasma will have its natural color, a very light yellow or straw hue. There are occasions when the plasma may have an altered color because of a disease process, but color changes can also result from improper handling of the specimen by the laboratory worker. The color change most often seen is the appearance of red in the plasma caused by the release of hemagolobin into the solution when the red blood cells are broken up. This breakup, or rupturing, of the red cells is called *hemolysis*. Hemolysis is one of the changes resulting from alterations in osmotic pressure in the solution surrounding the red cells. It can also occur when the membrane surrounding the red cells has been mechanically ruptured.

The principle of osmotic pressure and osmosis is very important whenever a solution or diluent is used as part of a procedure. In many hematologic procedures, diluents are used. In simple terms, osmosis is the passage of a solvent through a membrane from a dilute solution into a more concentrated one. The difference in concentra-tion between the solutions on each side of the membrane causes the phenomenon called *osmotic pressure*. If the concentrations of these solutions are the same, there will not be any pressure. When the concentration is the same in the diluent solution as it is inside the red blood cell, the diluent is called an *isotonic* solution. If the diluent is less concentrated than the inside of the red blood cell, the solution is called a *hypotonic* one. From the definition of osmosis it can be seen that in the case of a hypotonic solution (dilute), the passage of diluent will be from outside the red cell into the red cell, causing the cell to swell and eventually to rupture, or hemolyze. If the solution outside the red blood cell is more concentrated than that inside it, the outside solution is called *hypertonic*. In the case of a hypertonic solution, the osmosis of the solvent is from the inside of the red cell to the surrounding solution. When this happens, the red cell will shrink from loss of liquid and will become crenated.

When red cells are in plasma, they are in an isotonic solution. For this reason, any diluent used to dilute blood for hematology tests must have the same concentration as plasma. When a solution has the same concentration as, or is isotonic with, plasma, it is called a *physiological solution*. One very common physiological solution used in hospitals is isotonic saline solution, a 0.85 g/dl solution of sodium chloride (NaCl). If red blood cells are placed in an isotonic saline solution, their size is preserved. Hypotonic and hypertonic solutions are unsatisfactory for hematologic studies.

Two types of blood samples are unsuitable for hematology tests: clotted samples and hemolyzed samples. Clotted specimens are not suitable for cell counts because the cells are trapped in the clot and are therefore not counted. A cell count on a clotted sample will be falsely low. In hemolyzed specimens the red cells are no longer intact, and red cell counts on hemolyzed samples will also give falsely low results.

FORMATION AND FUNCTION OF BLOOD CELLS AND COMPONENTS

During early fetal life, blood cells are formed in many of the body tissues. During this period, the liver and spleen are the most active sites of blood cell production, or *hematopoiesis*. At about the fourth month of fetal life, the bone marrow begins functioning as a blood cell producer. Shortly after birth, under normal conditions, the marrow is the only tissue that continues to produce red cells, granular leukocytes (granulocytes), monocytes, and platelets. Until the age of 5, the marrow in all the bones is red and cellular, and actively produces cells. Between 5 and 7 years, the long bones become inactive and fat cells appear to replace the active marrow. Red marrow is gradually displaced by fat cells in the other bones through the maturing years. In other words, red marrow is transformed to yellow marrow. After 18–20 years, red marrow remains only in the vertebrae, the ribs, the sternum, the skull, and partially in the femur and the humerus.

However, the marrow is able to become active again when necessary, as in hemolytic anemias or chronic hemorrhage, when there is an increased loss of red blood cells from the body and a demand for increased red blood cell production. Such increased marrow activity is helpful to normal body function. This is not the case in other instances, as in leukemia or other malignancies, where increased marrow activity of one cell type is detrimental to the body as a whole. Another situation that is incompatible with life occurs when the marrow is suppressed or unable to function normally in cell production. In this case the marrow is said to be *aplastic*. Bone-marrow aspirations may therefore be necessary to detect abnormal changes in the newly formed cells or in their quantity. Early blood disease may be detected by an examination of the bone marrow.

The leukocytes found in normal peripheral blood consist of the granulocytes (neutrophils, eosinophils, and basophils), monocytes, and lymphocytes. The bone marrow produces the erythrocytes, granulocytes, monocytes, and platelets. Lymphocytes are produced primarily by the lymphoid tissue (lymph nodes and nodules, thymus, and spleen); some are also produced in the bone marrow.

These formed elements of the blood go through a normal series of developmental steps or stages in the marrow or lymphoid tissue and are found in the general peripheral blood circulation only when they are sufficiently developed or mature. However, immature cells, or cells in early developmental stages, may appear in the peripheral blood in certain disease states. Each cell type has a normal life span and function. When their normal life span is complete, the formed elements are eliminated from the body by processes in which parts of the cells are reused and parts are eliminated from the body.

When the body is functioning normally, the production and destruction of the formed elements of the blood are balanced so that a constant supply is available. When one of the steps in these processes is not functioning properly or is occurring too rapidly a blood disorder will result, and this will cause alterations in the other steps as well, since they are all closely related. These alterations might reflect diseases of the blood formation system or diseases of non-hematologic origin. For example, chronic bleeding resulting from a nonhematologic cause such as gastric ulcer or carcinoma results in hypochromic anemia. A similar condition of hematologic origin results from simple dietary iron deficiency. When tests are performed in the hematology laboratory, changes in the appearance of the red blood cells or other formed elements or changes in the manner in which whole blood or various components react under certain test conditions are noted to determine whether alterations in function have occurred.

Red blood cell formation and function

In adults, erythrocytes are formed in the bone marrow. The mature red blood cell is often described as a biconcave disk—that is, it is doughnut-shaped, with a depressed area rather than a hole in the center, as shown in Fig. 3-1. It does not contain a nucleus (it is nonnucleated).

The red blood cell begins as a nucleated cell within the bone marrow. As the cell matures in the bone marrow, its diameter decreases and the nucleus becomes denser, smaller, and is finally released from the cell (extruded). While this occurs the concentration of hemoglobin increases and the cytoplasm (cell material other than the nucleus) progressively changes from blue to orange in a stained blood film. The whole sequence of maturation from an early cell precursor to a circulating red cell takes only 3-5 days.

The young red blood cell that has just extruded its nucleus is referred to as a *reticulocyte*. It is about the same size as or slightly larger than a mature red blood cell. Reticulocytes differ from mature red blood cells morphologically because they contain a fine basophilic reticulum or network of RNA (ribonucleic acid), a cytoplasmic remnant that decreases as the cell matures. When stained with Wright's stain, the reticulocyte appears pinkish grey or has a slight bluish tinge. This *polychromasia* (many colors) represents the presence of RNA within the cell. With a special stain such as brilliant cresyl blue or new methylene blue, the basophilic reticulum of RNA appears blue (see under Counting Reticulocytes). Under normal conditions, reticulocytes remain and mature further in the bone marrow for a day or two before they are released into the peripheral blood. Red blood cells are released into the peripheral blood as reticulocytes by squeezing (or insinuating) through an opening in the endothelial cells lining the marrow cavity. These reticulocytes become fully mature—that is, they lose all RNA—within a day or two. Therefore, the number of reticulocytes in the peripheral blood is an indication of the degree of red blood cell production by the marrow. Normally about 1 percent of the circulating red blood cells are reticulocytes.

The main function of the red blood cell is to carry oxygen to all cells of the body. The oxygen is transported in a chemical combination with hemoglobin. Thus, the concentration of hemoglobin in the blood is a measure of its capacity to carry oxygen, on which all cells are absolutely dependent for energy and therefore life. To combine with and therefore transport oxygen, the hemoglobin molecule must have a certain combination of substances, namely heme (which contains iron) and globin. Deficiencies in the presence or metabolism of any of these substances will result in a decrease in hemoglobin and/or oxygen-carrying capacity.

Red blood cells have a total life span of about 120 days, and the body releases new red cells into the circulatory system every day. When red cells are worn out, the body stores the cell components that are reusable, including protein from the globin portion of the hemoglobin molecule and iron, and eliminates the nonreusable components. The heme portion of the hemoglobin molecule is such a waste product. It is converted to bilirubin, concentrated in the bile, and eliminated from the body by way of the feces, and to a much smaller extent the urine, as

Fig. 3-1. Normal red cell.

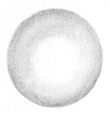

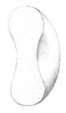

Normal
Red Cell

Side View
of Normal
Red Cell

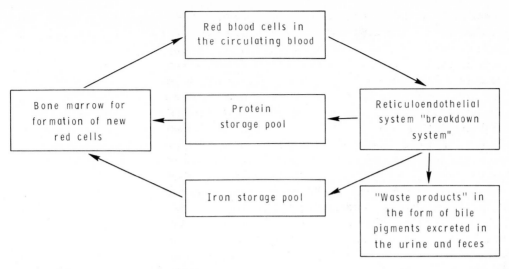

Fig. 3-2. Blood formation and destruction process.

urobilin and urobilinogen. The metabolism and elimination of bilirubin were described in Chap. 2. A schematic representation of the blood formation and destruction process is shown in Fig. 3-2.

Dead red cells are broken down by the reticuloendothelial (RE) system. The RE system is composed of connective tissue cells that carry on *phagocytosis*, a process in which a cell engulfs, or eats, foreign material. The RE cells are located in the blood sinusoids (tiny blood vessels), liver, spleen, bone marrow, and lining of the lymph channels in the lymph nodes. They are important in the body's defense mechanism and in the breakdown of globin to amino acids, which are returned to the protein storage pool of the body. They are also essential for the retention and reuse or storage of iron, which is needed for the formation of hemoglobin and transport of oxygen. A deficiency of iron results in anemia, a condition in which the oxygen-carrying capacity of blood is decreased. Iron deficiency anemia, one of the more common types of anemia, may result from a dietary deficiency of iron or from loss of iron from the body through bleeding.

White blood cell formation and function

The leukocytes are nucleated and are part of the defense mechanism of the body. Unlike the red cells, white cells use the blood primarily for transportation to their place of function in the body tissues. The neutrophils, eosinophils, and monocytes act as phagocytic scavengers—they engulf and destroy invading microorganisms and clear the body of unwanted particulate material such as dead or injured tissue cells. This is the first step in the repair of injured tissue. The lymphocytes and plasma cells act as immunocytes, inactivating foreign antigens by antibody production and by delayed hypersensitivity reactions. Plasma cells are not normally found in the peripheral blood. Lymphocytes and plasma cells are produced primarily in the lymphoid tissue (lymph nodes, nodules, and spleen) and secondarily in the marrow.

Under normal conditions, five types of leukocytes are found in the blood: lymphocytes, neutrophils, monocytes, eosinophils, and basophils. When a blood film is stained with Wright's stain and examined with the microscope, the majority of the cells seen will be red blood cells, which appear as small, rounded, pink or reddish orange bodies. Scattered among the red-staining cells are the less numerous leukocytes. There are normally 600–800 red cells to each leukocyte. The leukocytes are larger and more complex in appearance than the red blood cells. They consist of a nucleus surrounded by cytoplasm. Usually the nucleus is in the center of the cell and is a prominent purple-staining body. It can be round or oval (as in the lymphocyte) or lobulated (as in the neutrophil and eosinophil). The cytoplasm, which gives the cell its shape, stains a variety of colors, depending on its contents. The size of the cell, the shape and size of the nucleus, and the staining reactions of the nucleus and the cytoplasm aid in the identification of leukocytes.

Leukocytes are categorized as granulocytes and nongranulocytes. *Granulocytes* are leukocytes that contain specific granulation, such as neutrophils, eosinophils, and basophils (see also Staining the Blood Film). Nongranulocytes may contain nonspecific granulation, but specific granules are not seen; they include the monocytes and lymphocytes. Granulocytes are cells belonging to the *myeloid* series, but monocytes are also classified as myeloid cells (see also under Origin and Function of Blood Cells Related to Morphological Examination and Alterations).

The five types of leukocytes will be studied more thoroughly under Normal Leukocyte Morphology, but a brief description of each follows.

1. *Neutrophil.* This cell is normally the most numerous and most prominent of the white cells seen in an adult blood film. The nucleus is lobulated (with three to five lobes), and the cytoplasm stains pinkish lavender and contains numerous fine lilac granules.
2. *Lymphocyte.* This cell is the next most numerous in adult blood samples (usually about three neutrophils are seen to each lymphocyte). The nucleus is round or oval, and the cytoplasm stains blue and is usually free from any granules, although nonspecific azurophilic granules may be present. Lymphocytes are further classified as small, medium, and large.
3. *Monocyte.* This is the largest white cell and is often confused with the lymphocyte. It usually has a horseshoe- or kidney-shaped nucleus (although it may be round) that stains lavender. The cytoplasm stains slate gray or muddy blue and can be vacuolated.
4. *Eosinophil.* This cell is easily recognized by the large, red, beadlike granules seen in the cytoplasm. Normally, few eosinophils are present (only about 4 per 100 total white cells counted).
5. *Basophil.* This cell is the one least likely to be seen (only 1 per 100 total white cells counted). It is easily distinguished, however, by the purple-blue beadlike granules seen in the cytoplasm.

Platelet formation and function

The third formed element of the blood is the platelet, or thrombocyte. Platelets are small colorless bodies 1–4 μm in diameter. They are generally round or ovoid, although they may have projections called pseudopods. Platelets have a colorless to pale blue background substance containing centrally located, reddish to violet granules. They are produced in the bone marrow by cells called *megakaryocytes*, which are large and multinucleated. Platelets do not have a nucleus, and are not actually cells—they are portions of cytoplasm pinched off from megakaryocytes and released into the bloodstream. In the bloodstream platelets are an essential part of the blood clotting mechanism. They act to maintain the structure or integrity of the endothelial cells lining the vascular system by plugging any gaps in the lining. They also function in the clotting process by (1) acting as plugs around the opening of a wound, and (2) releasing certain factors that are necessary for the formation of a blood clot.

Blood plasma

The formed elements of blood are suspended in a fluid called blood plasma. Plasma is the protein fraction of the blood, and it contains in solution many substances that are necessary for maintenance of the body. It is a complex mixture including water, proteins, carbohydrates, lipids, electrolytes, and clotting factors, plus enzymes, vitamins, hormones, and trace metals.

Homeostasis and hematology tests

If blood is collected, anticoagulated, and allowed to settle, or centrifuged, three layers will separate and be observed (see Fig. 3-3).

The bottom layer will consist of packed red blood cells and will normally make up 43–47 percent of the total blood volume (the percentage differs in males and females). On top of this layer a thin whitish layer called the *buffy coat* will be seen. This consists of the leukocytes and platelets and normally makes up about 1 percent of the total blood volume. The uppermost layer is a colloidal liquid called plasma. The plasma layer normally represents 52–57 percent of the total blood volume.

All of the fluid and cellular elements that make up the blood are in a constant state of exchange. The overall effect is a state of equilibrium in which the supply is equal to the demand for normal body function. This state of equilibrium within the blood is termed *homeostasis*, and various tests that are done on blood measure the overall state of homeostasis within the body. Many of the constituents of plasma (or serum, if the blood is allowed to clot) are measured in the clinical chemistry laboratory. Some of these tests have been described in Chap. 2.

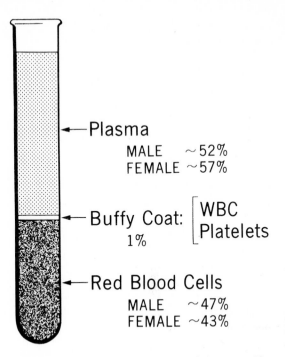

Fig. 3-3. Layers of normal blood (after centrifugation).

Clinical hematology is primarily concerned with testing the formed elements within the blood. The oxygen-carrying capacity of the blood is routinely measured by testing the hemoglobin concentration and the hematocrit (percentage of total blood volume occupied by the red blood cells), counting the red blood cells, and observing the morphology or appearance of the red blood cells on a peripheral blood film. Red blood cell production by the marrow is assessed by means of a reticulocyte count, and examination of the bone marrow may be necessary in certain disease states.

The leukocytes in the blood are routinely assessed by counting the number of cells present in a particular volume, and observing the morphology and determining the percentage of each cell type present in a peripheral blood film. This is referred to as a white blood cell *differential*. Here again, examination of the bone marrow may be necessary in certain cases; however, this is not a routine procedure.

Platelets are also routinely assessed in clinical hematologic studies by observing their number and morphology in the peripheral blood film. If certain disorders are suspected, they may also be counted. The blood clotting mechanism may also be checked, when necessary, by testing for the clotting factors that are present within the plasma.

Since the equilibrium of the blood is affected by a great many factors, hematology tests are useful in the study of all sorts of disease states; of hematologic or other origin. Thus, hereditary, nutritional, metabolic, traumatic, inflammatory and infectious, hormonal, immunologic, neoplastic, drug-induced, and other disease states can be assessed by hematologic studies. The physician will depend on such laboratory results, in combination with the clinical history and physical examination, to determine the state of health or disease of the patient.

HEMOGLOBIN

The determination of hemoglobin is the test ordered most frequently in the hematology laboratory. It is included in the routine complete blood count (CBC) for most new hospital admissions. The measurement of hemoglobin is relatively simple and can be done quickly by the laboratory. Along with the hematocrit measurement, the hemoglobin value is used to follow many disease states, especially the anemias. The measurement of the concentration of hemoglobin in the blood is called *hemoglobinometry*.

Synthesis, structure, and forms of hemoglobin

Hemoglobin synthesis is a complex process, starting in the bone marrow with the production of the erythrocytes. The heme (iron-containing) portion of the molecule combines with globin (the protein portion) and forms an activated form of hemoglobin that is ready to transport oxygen. Each hemoglobin molecule consists of four heme groups and a globin moiety, which is composed of four polypeptide chains (Fig. 3-4).

The heme group is an iron complex containing one iron atom. Iron is essential for the primary function of the hemoglobin molecule—carrying oxygen to the tissues. If iron is lacking, because of either inadequate intake or increased loss from the body, anemia results, since hemoglobin is not formed in sufficient quantity. When reduced hemoglobin is exposed to oxygen at increased pressure, oxygen is taken up at the iron atom until each molecule of hemoglobin has bound four oxygen molecules, one molecule at each iron atom. Since this is not a true oxidation-reduction reaction, the hemoglobin molecule carrying oxygen is said to be oxygenated. The molecule fully saturated with oxygen (four oxygen molecules per hemoglobin) is called *oxyhemoglobin*. It contains 1.34 ml of oxygen per gram of hemoglobin. Oxyhemoglobin carries oxygen from the lungs to the tissues of the body. Hemoglobin returning with carbon dioxide from the tissues is known as *reduced hemoglobin*.

Heme is itself a complex molecule. It is made up of a tetrapyrrole ring, called *protoporphyrin*, with a central iron, as shown in Fig. 3-4. Since the heme molecule is a porphyrin, a group of diseases called the *porphyrias* result from certain disorders of heme synthesis. Normally heme is excreted from the body as bilirubin, which is eventually converted to the various bile salts and pigments. The iron is normally removed and retained by the RE system, stored, and reused in the production of new hemoglobin.

The globin portion of the hemoglobin molecule is a protein substance that consists of four chains of amino acids (polypeptides). Each of the four

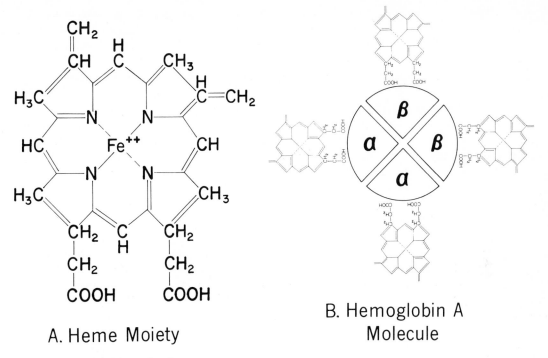

A. Heme Moiety

B. Hemoglobin A Molecule

Fig. 3-4. Hemoglobin molecule.

globin chains is attached to a heme portion to form a single hemoglobin molecule. Different forms of hemoglobin may occur in the red cells. These forms differ in the content and sequence of amino acids in the globin chains. For instance, the principal adult hemoglobin (Hb A) contains two alpha and two beta chains, as shown in Fig. 3-4. In fetal hemoglobin (Hb F) the two alpha chains are paired with two gamma chains. In still another form of hemoglobin (Hb A_2), the alpha chains are paired with two delta polypeptide chains. These are the three normal forms of hemoglobin. Other genetically determined forms of hemoglobin may be demonstrated by means of electrophoresis. Many abnormal forms of hemoglobin lead to clinical illness because they interfere with the oxygen-carrying capacity of the blood.

The combination of Hb A and Hb A_2 should normally make up 95 percent of the hemoglobin in an adult, with Hb F making up 5 percent or less. The Hb F is the major form found during intrauterine life and at birth. Adult hemoglobin (Hb A) is formed in small amounts by the fetus and rapidly increases after birth. Screening for abnormal hemoglobins should be postponed until several months after birth, because only at the age of 6 months does the proportion of adult hemoglobin forms become definitive. Disorders in which the presence of a structurally abnormal hemoglobin is considered to play an important role pathologically are called *hemoglobinopathies.* In some hemoglobinopathies, all the hemoglobin is in one abnormal form. In others, two abnormal forms may be present. In still others, some normal forms and some abnormal forms are present.

One fairly common abnormal hemoglobin is Hb S. It occurs mostly among the black population in and from tropical Africa. Persons with this abnormal hemoglobin form are likely to suffer from sickle-cell anemia. The four clinically important abnormal hemoglobins are Hb S, Hb C, Hb D, and Hb E. These are all hereditary, and the disorders affect the protein portion of the hemoglobin molecule, altering the structure of the polypeptide chain. These abnormal hemoglobins, as well as the normal ones, can be distinguished from each other by electrophoresis.

The circulating blood carries a composite of hemoglobin, oxyhemoglobin, carboxyhemoglobin, (hemoglobin combined with carbon monoxide), and minor amounts of other forms of this pigment. Hemoglobin can combine with other substances besides oxygen, some normally and some abnormally. If hemoglobin is converted to an abnormal hemoglobin pigment, it is no longer capable of oxygen transport, and if this impairment is severe, a condition of *hypoxia*, or *cyanosis*, will occur.

The hemoglobin molecule has a much greater affinity for carbon monoxide than for oxygen and will readily combine with carbon monoxide if it is present even in low concentration. The formation of carboxyhemoglobin is reversible, and if carbon monoxide is removed the hemoglobin will once again combine with oxygen. Carboxyhemoglobin is found normally in small amounts, especially in the blood of smokers; concentrations range from 2 to 10 g/dl.[2]

Methemoglobin is a type of hemoglobin in which the iron has been oxidized from the ferrous to the ferric state and is therefore incapable of carrying oxygen, which is replaced by a hydroxyl radical. The formation of methemoglobin results from the presence of certain chemicals or drugs, and is reversible. Methemoglobin is normally present in the blood in concentrations of 1-2 g/dl.[3]

Another abnormal hemoglobin derivative is *sulfhemoglobin*. Sulfhemoglobin is formed irreversibly and remains for the life of the carrier red blood cell. Its exact nature is not clear, but it is thought to be formed by the action of some drugs and chemicals such as sulfonamides. Sulfhemoglobin is not capable of transporting oxygen.

To measure hemoglobin accurately in the blood, it is necessary to prepare a stable derivative containing all the hemoglobin forms that are present. For this reason, there is one particular method for the determination of hemoglobin, the *cyanmethemoglobin* method. All forms of circulating hemoglobin are readily converted to cyanmethemoglobin, except for sulfhemoglobin, which is rarely present in significant amounts. Another procedure called the *oxyhemoglobin* method has been used, but it does not detect sulfhemoglobin or methemoglobin, and it has been largely replaced by the cyanmethemoglobin method.

Variations in normal values

The normal values for hemoglobin in the peripheral blood vary with the age and sex of the individual. Altitude also affects the hemoglobin measurement, in that the normal hemoglobin concentration is higher at high altitudes than at sea level. At birth, the hemoglobin concentration is normally 17-23 g/dl. It decreases to 9-14 g/dl by about 2 months of age. By 10 years of age, the normal hemoglobin will be 12-14 g/dl. Normal adult values range from 12 to 15 g/dl in women and 14 to 17 g/dl in men. There may be a slight decrease in the hemoglobin level after 50 years of age.[4]

When the hemoglobin value is below normal, the patient is said to be *anemic*. Anemia is a very common condition and is frequently a complication of other diseases (see under Red Cell Alterations in this chapter). In this condition the circulating erythrocytes may be deficient in number, deficient in total hemoglobin content per unit blood volume, or both. A decrease in hemoglobin can result from bleeding conditions, in which the patient loses erythrocytes. An increase in hemoglobin, usually as a result of an increase in the number of erythrocytes (erythrocytosis), is seen in polycythemia and newborn infants.

Specimens

The test for hemoglobin can be done on free-flowing capillary blood obtained from a finger puncture, or on venous blood preserved with an anticoagulant. The anticoagulant of choice for hematologic studies, including hemoglobin determinations, is EDTA or Sequestrene. The hemoglobin content of blood remains unchanged for several days when properly anticoagulated and refrigerated at 4°C.

Measurement of hemoglobin

Hemoglobin is determined as grams of hemoglobin per 100 ml of blood, or grams per deciliter. Reporting hemoglobin as a percentage of a normal value is not satisfactory because there are so many different methods and each method has its own normal value. For example, 80 percent of normal for one method may be the same as 98 percent of normal for another. The values for 100 percent hemoglobin in five different testing methods are listed below.

Sahli   17.3 g/dl
Dare   16.0 g/dl
Haden   15.6 g/dl
Wintrobe   14.5 g/dl
Haldane   13.8 g/dl

Visual hemoglobin methods

Some methods for determining the amount of hemoglobin present in a blood specimen are much more commonly used than others. Many years ago, before the use of the photometer, most hemoglobin methods depended on the human eye to determine the changes in color intensity caused by hemoglobin concentration differences; these methods were not very accurate. Some of the visual methods are the Tallquist, Dare, Haden, Haldane, and Sahli methods. Most of these methods are no longer used.

The Sahli method is now rarely used in the physician's office. In the Sahli method, the hemoglobin in the blood sample is converted to acid hematin by the addition of 0.1 N hydrochloric acid (HCl). The addition of acid to blood converts the red hemoglobin to a brown color. Since brown is more easily matched by the human eye than red, the Sahli method for testing hemoglobin is one of the more acceptable visual methods. The error in a visual method is great, however, and these methods are certainly not recommended.

Gasometric methods

Gasometric analysis with the Van Slyke apparatus is the most accurate method for determining hemoglobin, but it is not used routinely in the clinical laboratory because it is time-consuming and complicated. It is used as a reference method to obtain the hemoglobin concentration in blood samples used for standardization of hemoglobin procedures.

Quantitative photometric methods

As mentioned earlier, a method for measuring hemoglobin must be chosen that will detect all forms of hemoglobin. The one used by most laboratories is the cyanmethemoglobin method. This is now the internationally recognized method of choice. Another method used by some is the oxyhemoglobin method. The oxyhemoglobin method uses 0.04 ml/dl ammonium hydroxide (NH_4OH) solution to hemolyze the red blood cells and convert the hemoglobin to oxyhemoglobin for measurement in the photometer.[5] This conversion is complete and immediate and the resulting color is stable. The cyanmethemoglobin method uses Drabkin's reagent, a combination of three chemicals: sodium bicarbonate ($NaHCO_3$), potassium cyanide (KCN), and potassium ferricyanide [$K_3Fe(CN)_6$]. When Drabkin's reagent is mixed with the blood specimen, the stable pigment cyanmethemoglobin is formed and can be measured in the photometer. Both methods utilize photometry (see under Photometry in Chap. 1), and the one used by the laboratory will depend to some degree on the type of photometer available. Photometric hemolgobin determinations are rapid and can give accurate results. The degree of accuracy will also depend on the basic technique used and the accuracy of the equipment, stability of the reagents, and cleanliness of the glassware.

Various automated and semiautomated techniques have been employed to measure hemoglobin. Automatic pipettors and dilutors are used for portions of the measuring and diluting steps in many procedures. A special flow-through apparatus attached to the Coleman Junior Spectrophotometer enables a faster, more efficient photometric measurement of the unknown hemoglobin solution (see under Operation of the Coleman Junior Spectrophotometer in Chap. 1). This apparatus is designed to increase the speed with which samples can be introduced and discharged from the photometer. One automatic apparatus, the model S Coulter counter (Coulter Electronics, Hialeah, Fla.), measures hemoglobin as well as white cell count, red cell count, hematocrit, and red cell indexes. This automated device has made a significant contribution to the busy hematology laboratory (see under Counting the Formed Elements of the Blood).

Equipment for hemoglobin determination

A special pipet called a *Sahli* pipet can be used for hemoglobin determinations. The Sahli pipet is calibrated to contain 20 μl (or 0.02 ml) of blood. Since it is a to-contain pipet, it must be rinsed with the diluent to ensure proper measurement of the blood sample. The accuracy of hemoglobin pipets must be checked before the pipets can be used for hematologic determinations. This can be done simply by comparing the new pipet with U.S. Bureau of Standards pipets, which have been very carefully calibrated.

When Sahli pipets are used, special rubber

tubing with a mouthpiece (called a sucker) must be attached to the pipet for suction. When this is done, mouth suction is generally used, and this introduces a potential risk to the user. Extreme care must be used if this kind of pipetting is done (see under Safety in the Laboratory in Chap. 1).

Disposable, self-filling, self-measuring dilution micropipets now are commercially available. One such system is called Unopette (Becton, Dickinson & Co., Rutherford, N.J.) (Fig. 3-5). These systems are easy to use and are available with a series of different diluting fluids for different purposes. One system (Unopette), for hemoglobin determination, consists of a self-filling, self-measuring pipet attached to a plastic holder; the pipet fills with blood automatically by capillary action. A plastic reagent container, called the reservoir, is filled with Drabkin's reagent in the hemoglobin Unopette system. The pipet containing the blood is inserted into the reagent reservoir and emptied and rinsed correctly, according to the manufacturer's instructions. The

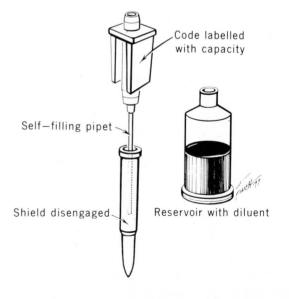

Fig. 3-5. Self-filling disposable pipet and diluent reservoir.

Code labelled with capacity

Self—filling pipet

Shield disengaged

Reservoir with diluent

blood is mixed well with the reagent and is then ready to be read in the photometer.

Another essential piece of equipment for hemoglobin determinations is the cuvette for the photometer. New cuvettes must be carefully tested for optical perfection before they are used for hemoglobin determinations. This is done by comparing them in the photometer with previously calibrated cuvettes (see under Photometry in Chap. 1). Once the cuvettes have been calibrated, they should be carefully washed and stored until used. Using scratched and dirty cuvettes will result in inaccurate hemoglobin values.

Since most hemoglobin determinations employ photometry, a photometer of good quality and in good working order is essential. Most brands of photometers give good results if certain precautions are taken. Before a photometer can be used to determine the hemoglobin concentration, it must be standardized. Since the Coleman Junior Spectrophotometer is in general use and has been discussed in some detail in Chap. 1, the procedure presented in this section for standardization of the photometer will deal specifically with this instrument. However, the same general procedure can be followed for any type of photometer.

Standardization of the Coleman Junior Spectrophotometer

Stable standard cyanmethemoglobin solutions representing 1:250 dilutions of whole blood containing 5, 10, and 15 g of hemoglobin per 100 ml of blood are available commercially and are certified by the College of American Pathologists (CAP). This type of hemoglobin standard is commonly used by all clinical laboratories. When a certified standard (CAP) is used, the following procedure may be followed in setting up the cuvettes for reading in the photometer:

1. Label 11 cuvettes (test tubes may be used if the flow-through type of apparatus is available for the photometer) as follows: blank, 1, 1

duplicate, 2, 2 duplicate, 3, 3 duplicate, 4, 4 duplicate, and 5, 5 duplicate.

2. Using volumetric pipets, pipet the following amounts into the cuvettes:

Tube	Standard (ml)	Drabkin's reagent (ml)
Blank	0	5
1 1 duplicate	1	4
2 2 duplicate	2	3
3 3 duplicate	3	2
4 4 duplicate	4	1
5 5 duplicate	5	0

3. Mix the contents of the cuvettes very well.

4. Read in the photometer, using a wavelength setting of 540 nm.

5. Record absorbance (A) readings directly or record percent transmittance readings and convert to absorbance.

6. Calculate the concentration (C) of hemoglobin (mg/dl) for each of the standard cuvettes (see the original concentration of standard solution used).

7. Calculate the concentration of hemoglobin (g/dl) for each of the standard dilutions.

8. Calculate the K value for each standard ($K = A/C$) and calculate the average K value for the spectrophotometer.

9. Plot the standard line on semilogarithmic graph paper with percent transmittance readings (use linear graph paper for absorbance readings). Draw the straight line through the points that gives the best fit for the graph. Subsequent hemoglobin concentrations can then be read directly from this straight line. Generally, readings between 20 and

80%T are more accurate than readings at either end of the scale. If a patient sample gives a reading greater than 80%T, the test is repeated with twice as much blood. If a patient sample gives a reading less than 20%T, the blood sample is diluted with twice as much diluent and the test is repeated. Volumes must be taken into account in the calculations.

For the oxyhemoglobin or the cyanmethemoglobin method, standards can be prepared in the laboratory by obtaining a sample of blood on which the hemoglobin has already been determined by oxygen capacity or iron content. The oxygen capacity determination is the reference method most frequently used for hemoglobin standardization. It is based on the assumption that 1 g of hemoglobin will combine with 1.34 ml of oxygen. The following formula can be used to find the hemoglobin concentration:

$$\text{Hemoglobin (g/dl)} = \frac{\text{oxygen capacity (ml/dl)}}{1.34 \text{ (ml/g)}}$$

This blood sample is used for the stock standard solution. For the cyanmethemoglobin method, the sample is diluted in a volumetric flask with Drabkin's reagent so that the hemoglobin concentration is approximately 25–30 g/dl. This standard should be stored in a refrigerator until ready for use. From the stock standard, a series of working standards are prepared, including duplicate sets for each of 10 dilutions having a total volume in each cuvette of 10 ml. The first cuvette should contain 10 ml of stock standard only, the second cuvette 9 ml of stock standard and 1 ml of Drabkin's reagent, the third cuvette 8 ml of stock standard and 2 ml of Drabkin's reagent, and so on, ending with the tenth cuvette containing 1 ml of stock standard and 9 ml of Drabkin's reagent. A similar system is used for the oxyhemoglobin method, using the 0.04 ml/dl NH$_4$OH reagent to dilute the standards.

A blank tube containing 5 ml of Drabkin's reagent or 0.04 ml/dl NH$_4$OH is placed in the cuvette well, and the galvanometer beam is adjusted to read 100%T with the wavelength scale set at 540 nm. The percent transmittance for each of the standards is obtained by reading the samples in the photometer, reinserting and reading the blank tube between samples. The readings for the standards are recorded and transcribed on semilogarithmic graph paper as percent transmittance (ordinate) versus concentration of hemoglobin in grams per 100 ml (abscissa). A line is drawn through the plotted points, and a table is prepared from this graph showing the concentration of hemoglobin corresponding to each percent transmittance reading. This table is used to obtain subsequent hemoglobin values for that machine.

An alternative method is to calculate the constant factor $K (= A/C)$ for the instrument (see step 8 above). By using the average K value, hemoglobin concentrations corresponding to all the potential galvanometer readings may be calculated and a standard chart may be prepared.

The standard chart will show the range of hemoglobin concentrations that can be accurately determined with a particular photometer. Only hemoglobin values obtained from the linear portion of the graph may be used to prepare the standard chart. The chart prepared from data obtained with one photometer cannot be used with any other photometer.

Cyanmethemoglobin method[6]

Principle

A 20-μl portion of blood is diluted and hemolyzed in Drabkin's solution, which consists of potassium ferricyanide, potassium cyanide, and sodium bicarbonate. The ferricyanide converts the hemoglobin iron from the ferrous state (Fe^{2+}) to the ferric state (Fe^{3+}) to form methemoglobin. This combines with potassium cyanide to form the stable pigment cyanmethemoglobin. The color reaction takes 5–10 minutes to reach completion. The color intensity of this mixture is measured in a photometer at a wavelength of 540 nm (corresponding to a yellow-green filter). Absorbance is directly proportional to the concentration of hemoglobin. The concentration (C) of hemoglobin (g/dl) can be calculated from $C = A/K$, where K is the constant for the spectrophotometer used in the standardization and A is absorbance. The concentration can also be read directly from a standard line.

Reagents

Drabkin's reagent [1 g of $NaHCO_3$, 0.050 g of KCN, and 0.200 g of $K_3Fe(CN)_6$ —or a previously prepared commercial mixture of these chemicals] is diluted to 1 L with deionized water. This reagent should be prepared fresh at least once a month and should be stored in a brown bottle to prevent deterioration; it is unstable in light. Drabkin's reagent is a clear, pale yellow solution. It should be discarded if it becomes turbid. Although Drabkin's reagent contains only a small amount of cyanide, it is still regarded as a poison and must be treated with caution.

A control solution should be used for every hemoglobin determination. Daily controls should be run using either a commercial control specimen or one prepared by the laboratory. Daily use of control values gives information about the state of the hemoglobin reagent (whether deterioration has occurred), the accuracy of the pipets used, the variation and cleanliness of the calibrated photometer cuvettes, and the variation in the photometer used to measure the amount of hemoglobin in the samples. Technical skills are also checked. When the control value is not within the acceptable limits, hemoglobin values for the unknown patient blood specimens being measured should not be reported until the reason for the control error is found. "Out of control" values are seen with deterioration of reagents, faulty equipment (photometer), dirty glassware, inaccurate standardization of the photometer, deterioration of the control specimen, inaccurate

or broken pipets, or poor technique (see under Ensuring Reliable Laboratory Results in Chap. 1.)

Procedure

1. Allow the spectrophotometer to warm up adequately. Set the wavelength scale at 540 nm.
2. Prepare a blank tube with 5 ml of Drabkin's reagent.
3. Label test tubes for each specimen. Deliver 5 ml of Drabkin's reagent into each test tube. This can be done with an automatic pipetting device if one is available.
4. Draw blood into a Sahli pipet to the 20-μl mark. To use the Sahli pipet properly, attach rubber "sucker" tubing to the end of the pipet. Use careful mouth pipetting for this technique. Have ready a finger cot, to be worn on the end of the finger while adjusting the level of blood in the pipet. This is a precautionary step taken to prevent the spread of hepatitis virus by direct contact with the blood. When initially drawing the blood into the pipet, do not draw it more than 1 mm past the 20-μl mark.
5. If venous blood is used, gently mix the sample by inversion for at least 5 minutes. If capillary blood is used, the pipetting may be done directly from the drop at the puncture site.
6. Wipe the outside of the pipet free of blood and adjust the amount of blood exactly to the calibration mark. This adjusting is done by using capillary action and by tapping the end of the pipet against the finger cot. The pipet should be held in a horizontal position while this is done.
7. Place the pipet at the bottom of the tube with the 5 ml of Drabkin's reagent and discharge the blood by blowing through the sucker and pipet. The pipet must be rinsed with the reagent several times by drawing the solution up into it and blowing it out again. Rinse until all visible evidence of blood inside the pipet is gone.
8. Mix the contents of the tube by inserting the pipet to the bottom of the tube again and blowing vigorously through the pipet. It is most important that the amounts of blood and diluent

be accurately measured and that these solutions be thoroughly mixed.

9. Color development takes 5–10 minutes. After the 10-minute waiting period, read the blank tube in the photometer and adjust to 100%T. Then read the hemoglobin solution. This can be done either by transferring the solution to a photometer cuvette or by pouring it directly into a flow-through system in the photometer.

10. Record all readings.

11. Convert the percent transmittance readings to concentrations by using the calibration curve or table prepared for the photometer (see under Standardization of the Coleman Junior Spectrophotometer).

12. Report hemoglobin results to the first decimal place.

13. Check quality control samples daily and plot the values on the control chart for the machine. Only when the control values check out are the patient values sent out to the physician. Duplicate determinations should agree within 0.4 g/dl or the determinations should be repeated.

Procedure with Unopette system

The only difference in using the Unopette system is in the initial blood sampling and dilution. Instead of the Sahli pipet and tubes of Drabkin's reagent, the Unopette system is employed. This consists of a capillary measuring device and a reagent reservoir. The blood is collected in the self-filling capillary pipet and is emptied into the plastic reservoir containing 5 ml of Drabkin's reagent. The manufacturer's instructions should be followed for this procedure (either capillary or venous blood may be used).

Once the blood is mixed with the diluent in the reservoir, there is the usual 10-minute waiting period for the color to completely develop. The mixture is transferred to a calibrated photometer cuvette or poured into a flow-through apparatus. The readings in percent transmittance are con-

verted to grams per deciliter by use of the prepared standard calibration table.

Precautions, technical factors, and sources of error

Several precautions have already been discussed. Photometric methods for the determination of hemoglobin are rapid and give accurate results only when the equipment is in good working condition. The photometer must be working well, and the pipets and calibrated cuvettes must be clean and free from breaks or scratches. The Sahli pipets must be calibrated before they are used. Drabkin's reagent, if used, must be prepared fresh each month and stored in a brown bottle to prevent deterioration. Photometers must be standardized before being used for the hemoglobin determination. They should be restandardized periodically and the calibrated hemoglobin tables redone when changes occur in the values. Each photometer must have a calibration table.

Before the unknown samples are read in the photometer, they must be crystal-clear. If there is any turbidity, a falsely high result will be read. Turbidity may result from exceptionally high white blood cell counts, the presence of Hb S and Hb C, the presence of abnormal globulins, or lipemic blood specimens.

Blood containing carbon monoxide requires 3 hours for the formation of cyanmethemoglobin from carboxyhemoglobin with Drabkin's reagent.

One of the greatest causes of error is improper pipetting technique. Using precalibrated, self-filling pipets (such as the Unopette) helps to eliminate some of this error. If the capillary blood flow is slow and the finger is squeezed to obtain the sample, error can result from the introduction of tissue juice into the blood sample. If venous blood is not mixed well before measurement, gross errors result.

Salts and solutions of cyanide are poisonous and care should be taken to avoid getting them in the mouth or inhaling their fumes. Drabkin's reagent contains 50 mg of KCN per liter. The smallest dose of potassium cyanide known to kill a human is 300 mg.[7] Nevertheless, Drabkin's reagent must be handled with great care. Many laboratories obtain the reagent commercially, so that handling potassium cyanide is not necessary. The salt is potentially very dangerous and must be locked up if it is used by the laboratory.

Because the Sahli pipets may be less accurate than claimed by the manufacturer, it is wise to set aside several calibrated pipets for use in hemoglobin tests, if possible. Most Sahli pipets supplied by reputable companies should be accurate to 1 percent. These pipets should be cleaned with acid and thoroughly washed with water once a week. They must be washed and dried between measurements.

To eliminate error resulting from poorly calibrated cuvettes or cuvettes that are not matched correctly, most photometric instruments are now supplied with a flow-through cuvette system. The solution to be read is poured directly into the system. After each reading, the solution is emptied into a discard container by means of a valve in the bottom of the cuvette. Since all readings, standards, controls, and unknowns are taken through the same flow-through cuvette, errors caused by imperfectly matched cuvettes are eliminated.

Normal values[8]

For adult male:
   14–17 g/dl
For adult female:
   12.5–15 g/dl
For newborn:
   17–23 g/dl
For three-month-old:
   9–14 g/dl
For ten-year-old:
   12–14.5 g/dl

HEMATOCRIT

The hematocrit is a macroscopic observation by which the percentage volume of the packed red blood cells is measured. This test is relatively simple and reliable. It gives useful information about the red blood cells, which may be correlated with the number of red blood cells and their hemoglobin content (see under Counting Erythrocytes and Leukocytes and under Hemoglobin). These measurements together enable the red cell indexes to be calculated (see under Red Cell Indexes). The hematocrit measurement is more useful and reliable than the red cell count because much less error is associated with it. Most hospital laboratories perform hematocrit determinations along with hemoglobin measurements, and some do the hematocrit even more regularly. A fast quality control check on hemoglobin results is done by comparing them with the hematocrit results, using the following formula:

$$\text{Hemoglobin} \times 3 = \text{hematocrit} \pm 3 \text{ units}$$

The hematocrit is used in evaluating and classifying the various types of anemias according to red cell indexes. There are two widely used manual methods for determining the hematocrit: the Wintrobe method and the microhematocrit method. Most laboratories obtain agreement between these methods. The microhematocrit method has the advantages that it takes less time and labor and requires a smaller blood sample.

When whole blood is centrifuged, the heavier particles fall to the bottom of the tube and the lighter particles sediment on top of the heavier cells. The hematocrit is the percentage of red cells in a volume of whole blood. The value determined in venous blood by the Wintrobe method agrees closely with the value in capillary blood by the microhematocrit method. When reading the hematocrit result, it is important to take the reading *at the top* of the red blood cell layer, particularly when there is an extremely elevated white cell or platelet count. The buffy coat (white blood cells and platelets) should not be included in the measurement of red cell volume for the hematocrit result.

Methods for quantitative measurement

The microhematocrit method is used most commonly. It can be done with either free-flowing capillary blood from a finger puncture or anticoagulated venous blood; a very small amount of blood is needed. The test is also done with a high-speed centrifuge, which means a relatively short centrifugation time. The microhematocrit is therefore a quick test and the results can be ready in a short time.

The Wintrobe method is a macromethod that requires more blood and a longer centrifugation time. Blood must be drawn by venipuncture and properly anticoagulated. This method is not used much today because it is time-consuming.

Both methods provide reliable values and have the same normal values, if the procedures are followed exactly.

An automated hematocrit result is obtained when the model S Coulter counter is used. This result is computed from individual red cell volumes and is not affected by the trapped plasma left in the red cell column for the manual microhematocrit and Wintrobe methods. Therefore, the hematocrit value obtained with the Coulter model S is 2.5 percent lower than the value obtained by the centrifugation methods.[9]

Specimens

Blood for the Wintrobe method must be anticoagulated with EDTA, double oxalate, or heparin, which do not alter the volume of the red blood cells. The blood sample must be well mixed before doing the test.

Capillary blood can be used for the microhematocrit method. Special capillary tubes are filled with the blood directly from the puncture site. These glass tubes are coated with heparin for use with capillary blood and can also be purchased without heparin for use with anticoagulated venous blood. Heparin-lined tubes must always be used with capillary blood but must not be used with anticoagulated venous blood as an excess of anticoagulant can cause cell shrinkage resulting in falsely low values. Free-flowing blood must be used for the microhematocrit measurement.

Properly anticoagulated blood (usually EDTA) is used for automated analysis.

Equipment for manual methods

For the Wintrobe method, a special hematocrit tube called the *Wintrobe* tube is used. This thick-walled glass tube is specially made with a uniform inner diameter and is graduated from 0 to 105 mm. It has a rubber cap, which prevents evaporation during the long period of centrifugation (30–45 minutes). Disposable tubes may be purchased for this method, and this eliminates washing small-bore glass tubes. The Wintrobe tube is filled with blood by using a *Pasteur pipet.* This is a long-stemmed glass capillary pipet and is usually disposable. A standard laboratory centrifuge capable of generating a relative centrifugal force of $2260\,g$ (g is the acceleration due to gravity) is needed to pack the red blood cells sufficiently in the Wintrobe tube.[10]

For the microhematocrit method, special nongraduated glass capillary tubes are used. These tubes are 1 mm in diameter and 7 cm long. They can be purchased lined with dried heparin for use with capillary blood, or plain (without heparin) for use with previously anticoagulated venous blood. Plain capillary tubes may be coated with heparin by filling them with a 1:1000 dilution of heparin and drying in a 56°C oven. Some type of seal is needed for one end of the tube when it contains blood. A special sealing compound (similar to modeling clay) can be used for this purpose, or the end can be heat-sealed with a small gas flame. A special microhematocrit centrifuge is used, capable of producing centrifugal fields up to 10 000 g. The centrifugation time is 5 minutes; this was determined by centrifuging many samples at constant speed for 1–10 minutes and observing when the hematocrit measurement leveled off with maximum packing of red cells. Some centrifuges can reach speeds of 12 500 r/min (revolutions per minute). Because this greater speed leads to a greater relative centrifugal force (RCF), complete cell packing can be reached in 3 minutes with these centrifuges. The head of the microhematocrit centrifuge is made to hold the small capillary tubes. Since the capillary tubes are not graduated, a special reading device is used to measure the percentage of packed red blood cells after centrifugation.

Procedure for microhematocrit determination[11]

1. A puncture from which blood flows freely is made in a finger (or in the heel of an infant).
2. Two microhematocrit capillary tubes are filled to within 2 cm of the end (one-half to two-thirds full).
3. The vacant end of each tube is sealed with Plasticene, a specially manufactured plastic seal for these tubes. The tubes can also be heat-sealed.
4. The sealed tubes are centrifuged in a microhematocrit centrifuge for 4–5 minutes at 10 000 r/min.
5. The microhematocrit result is read with a graphic reading device or some other accurate measuring device. Graphic reading devices give the hematocrit directly as a percentage. Results for duplicate tests should agree within 2 percent.

Procedure for Wintrobe hematocrit determination[12]

1. The Pasteur pipet is used to transfer well-mixed venous blood to a clean, dry Wintrobe hematocrit tube. This is properly done by first placing the pipet in the bottom of the tube and gradually withdrawing it while expelling blood until the tube is filled to the 100-mm mark. Bubbles in the tube must be avoided.
2. The tube is sealed with a cap and centrifuged at full speed in a suitable centrifuge for 30 minutes. During centrifugation, the red cells, which have the highest specific gravity of the blood elements, settle to the bottom. The Wintrobe tube is calibrated from 0 to 105 mm (or 0 to 10.5 cm), and the levels of the various layers may be easily read.
3. After centrifugation, three layers are apparent in the tube. These are, from the bottom: (1) red cells; (2) buffy coat, containing platelets, leukocytes, and other nucleated cells when present; and (3) plasma.
4. The level of the red cell column and the total height of the column of blood are noted. If the tube has been filled to exactly the 100-mm mark, the hematocrit in volume percent is equal to the reading at the top of the layer of packed red blood cells. If the tube is calibrated in centimeters instead of millimeters, the reading is multiplied by 10. When the height of the column of cells and plasma is not exactly 100 mm, a simple calculation can be made to correct for this. The following general formula applies:

$$\text{Hematocrit (\%)} = \frac{\text{packed RBC height}}{\text{total blood height}} \times 100.$$

This is exactly the same as setting up a proportion, as illustrated below:

$$\frac{\text{Reading of packed RBC}}{\text{Reading of plasma level}} = \frac{x}{100}$$

where x = hematocrit (%)

Precautions and technical factors

The blood sample must be properly collected and preserved. If the Wintrobe method is used, EDTA and balanced oxalate are the anticoagulants of choice. The blood must not be clotted or hemolyzed. If clotted blood is used there will be false packing of the red cells, and the true packing in the tube will not be noted (a falsely high result will be observed). In a hemolyzed specimen some of the red cells have been destroyed, so again the packing of the red cells will not be true (a falsely low result will be observed). Centrifugation must be sufficient to yield maximum packing of the red cells. Preferably the centrifugation should be done with the hematocrit tube in an upright position, because it may be difficult to read the level of the packed cells when the tube is on a slant.

The hematocrit value is frequently accompanied by a hemoglobin determination. There should be a correlation between the two results: the hematocrit result should be approximately three times the hemoglobin result.

For the microhematocrit method, the capillary blood collected should be freely flowing. The capillary tubes must be properly sealed so that no leakage occurs. Since these tubes are not calibrated, the level of packed red cells and the total volume of the cells and plasma must be accurately measured by some convenient reading device. The buffy coat layer is not included in the reading for the hematocrit.

The microhematocrit centrifuge provides a greater relative centrifugal force, and less plasma is trapped in the cell layer. The results are therefore more accurate because the plasma does not interfere with the measurement of the red cell layer.

Unique to the hematocrit is the error caused by excess EDTA (inadequate blood for the fixed amount of EDTA in the blood collection tube). The hematocrit will be falsely low because of cell shrinkage.[13] Thus, heparinized capillary tubes must not be used with anticoagulated blood samples. Another error can result if the specimen is overoxalated; again, a falsely low result will occur because of cell shrinkage.

With good technique, the precision of the hematocrit is ±1 percent. Inadequate centrifugation will give falsely high results. If the tubes are not sealed properly, falsely low results will be obtained because more red blood cells will be lost than plasma.

Normal values[14]

For adult male:
  42–52%
For adult female:
  36–46%
For newborn:
  50–62%
For one-year-old:
  31–39%

RED BLOOD CELL INDEXES

In the classification of anemias, quantitative measurements of the average size, hemoglobin content, and hemoglobin concentration of the red blood cells are of substantial aid to the physician (see under Red Cell Alterations). These can be calculated from the total number of red cells, the hemoglobin content per unit volume, and the hematocrit. The calculated values are the mean corpuscular volume (MCV), mean corpuscular hemoglobin (MCH), and mean corpuscular hemoglobin concentration (MCHC). Another quantitative measurement of the red cells, the mean corpuscular diameter (MCD), is made directly.

Determination of these indexes has become routine with the advent of an electronic cell counter, such as the model S Coulter counter. This machine determines the hemoglobin, MCV, and red blood cell count, and then automatically calculates the hematocrit, MCH, and MCHC.

When the indexes are calculated from manually determined values for hemoglobin, hematocrit, and red cell count, the greatest inaccuracy results from errors associated with the red cell count. By electronically counting the number of red blood cells, this error is significantly reduced. Indexes calculated by electronic methods have been found to be more accurate by several investigators.[15],[16] It is important to check all indexes against observations of stained blood films. When the red cell indexes are used in conjunction with an examination of the stained blood film, a clear picture of red cell morphology is obtained.

Since a red blood cell is very small and the amount of hemoglobin in a single cell is minute, the units in which the red cell indexes are measured and recorded are micrometers (10^{-6} m) and picograms (10^{-12} g).

Mean corpuscular volume

The MCV is the average volume of a red blood cell in femtoliters (fl = 10^{-15} L), or cubic micrometers (μm^3). It is calculated by dividing the volume of red cells per liter by the number of red cells per liter, using the formula

$$MCV = \frac{hematocrit \times 10}{RBC \; count \; (10^6/\mu l)}$$

where the factor 10 is introduced to convert the hematocrit reading from volume of packed red cells per 100 ml to volume per liter. For example, if the hematocrit reading is 40 percent and the red cell count is 5 million (5.0×10^6) cells per microliter,

$$MCV = \frac{40 \times 10}{5.0} = 80 \; fl$$

The MCV in normal adults is between 82 and 102 fl.

The MCV indicates whether the red blood cells will appear microcytic, normocytic, or macrocytic. If the MCV is less than 82 fl, the red cells will be microcytic. If it is greater than 102 fl, the red cells will be macrocytic. If it is within the normal range, the red cells will be normocytic. In some macrocytic anemias (for instance, pernicious anemia) the MCV may be as high as 150 fl. In microcytic anemia with marked iron deficiency, it may be 60-70 fl. The chief source of error in the MCV is the considerable error in the manual red cell count.

With the advent of automated cell counters and electronically calculated indexes, the MCV has become increasingly valuable. It is now considered the most reliable automated index and is probably the most effective discriminant for the classification of anemias. Previously, the MCHC was the most reliable index, since it was calculated from the two measurements that could be done most accurately, the hematocrit and the hemoglobin concentration.

Mean corpuscular hemoglobin

The MCH is the average hemoglobin content of a red blood cell in picograms (pg = 10^{-12} g). It is obtained by dividing the hemoglobin content of 1 L of blood by the number of red blood cells. A simple formula can be used to calculate this value:

$$MCH = \frac{hemoglobin \; (g/dl) \times 10}{RBC \; count \; (10^6/\mu l)}$$

For example, if the hemoglobin content is 15 g/dl and the red blood cell count is 5×10^6 cells/μl

$$MCH = \frac{15 \times 10}{5} = 30 \; pg$$

The normal range for the MCH is 27-31 pg. It may be as high as 50 pg in macrocytic anemias or as low as 20 pg or less in hypochromic anemias.

Again, the chief source of error is the red blood cell count, which must be accurate if this calculation is to be of use to the physician. This value is calculated electronically by the model S Coulter counter.

Mean corpuscular hemoglobin concentration

The MCHC is an expression of the average hemoglobin concentration per unit volume of packed red cells, in percent or in grams per deciliter. It may be calculated from the MCV and the MCH or from the hemoglobin and hematocrit values by using the following formula:

$$MCHC = \frac{MCH}{MCV} \times 100$$

or

$$MCHC = \frac{\text{hemoglobin (g/dl)}}{\text{hematocrit}} \times 100$$

For example, if the hemoglobin concentration is 15 g/dl and the hematocrit is 40 percent,

$$MCHC = \frac{15}{40} \times 100 = 37.5\% \text{ (or g/dl)}$$

This measurement tells what percentage of a unit volume (1 dl) of red blood cells is hemoglobin. Normal values range from 33 to 38 percent, and values below 32 percent indicate hypochromia. An MCHC above 40 percent would indicate malfunctioning of the instrument or error in the calculation of the manual measurements used, because only rarely do MCHC values go above 38 percent physiologically. In true hypochromic anemias the hemoglobin concentration is reduced, and values as low as 20-25 percent are not uncommon.

Precautions and technical factors

The red blood cell count, hematocrit, and hemoglobin concentration used must be accurate. It is also essential to check the appearance of the red blood cells in a well-stained blood film against the calculated indexes. The calculations must agree with the appearance of the red cells in the blood film.

Normal values[17]

For MCV:
 82–102 fl
For MCH:
 27.0–31.0 pg
For MCHC:
 33.0–38.0 percent

ERYTHROCYTE SEDIMENTATION RATE

The erythrocyte sedimentation test is another hematologic determination that employs macroscopic observation. If blood is prevented from clotting (by using a suitable anticoagulant) and allowed to settle, sedimentation of the erythrocytes will occur. The rate at which the red cells fall is known as the erythrocyte sedimentation rate (ESR). This rate depends on three main factors: (1) the number and size of erythrocyte particles, (2) plasma factors, and (3) certain technical and mechanical factors.

The most important factor determining the rate of fall of the red blood cells is the size or mass of the falling particle: the larger the particle, the faster it falls. The size of the falling particles depends on the formation of red cell aggregates, which in turn depends on the presence of certain factors in the plasma. The rate of sedimentation appears to be dependent on the amount of fibrinogen or globulin present in the plasma. In normal blood, the red cells tend to remain separate from each other because they are negatively charged and tend to repel each other. In many pathological conditions the phenomenon of erythrocyte aggregation is caused by alteration of the erythrocyte surface charge by plasma proteins. The protein that is most often involved is fibrinogen, although increases in gamma globulins or abnormal proteins also produce this effect. These factors determine the size of the aggregates of erythrocytes. With increased concentrations of large molecules in the plasma, there is a greater tendency for erythrocytes to pile up in rouleau formation (a roll of red cells resembling a roll of coins).

Stages of erythrocyte sedimentation

The sedimentation of the erythrocytes in a sample of blood may be plotted as a curve on graph paper, with the millimeters of fall as the ordinate and the time in minutes as the abscissa. Such a curve shows at first a variable period of gradual fall during which the aggregates of erythrocytes are forming (rouleau formation). Next, very rapid and marked fall of the aggregates occurs, constituting the main portion of the sedimentation of erythrocytes. The last part of the curve represents a more gradual, but relatively slight, falling off of the sedimentation rate as the erythrocyte aggregates are being packed at the bottom of the sedimentation tube. This packing will be more marked in an anemic patient than in an individual with the normal number of erythrocytes. In any event, the effect of anemia on the sedimentation rate will be relatively slight. By far the most important factor in determining the rate of sedimentation is the size of the erythrocyte aggregates, or rouleaux.

Clinical significance of the erythrocyte sedimentation rate

The ESR is a nonspecific screening test for inflammatory activity. In the vast majority of

infections there is at least some increase in the ESR; chorea and undulant fever are two exceptions. The ESR also increases in most cases of carcinoma, leukemia and diseases of the bone marrow, degenerative vascular disease, active rheumatic fever, multiple myeloma, systemic lupus, rheumatoid arthritis, and acute gout. As patients recover from infectious diseases, the sedimentation rate slowly returns to normal. It may still be increased long after other clinical manifestations have disappeared, showing that the defense mechanisms of the body continue to be more active than normal. Increased numbers of erythrocytes, as seen in cases of polycythemia and failure of the right side of the heart, tend to cause a marked slowing of sedimentation. When the hematocrit is greater than 48–50 percent, sedimentation is markedly slowed, regardless of any factors present that might otherwise accelerate it.

A decrease in the ESR will result when the plasma fibrinogen level is decreased, as in cases of severe liver diseases (e.g., acute yellow atrophy). The ESR is not increased in viral diseases, such as infectious mononucleosis and acute hepatitis, probably because fibrinogen production is not increased in these diseases in spite of a pronounced inflammatory reaction. The ESR is also not usually increased in chronic degenerative joint disease (it is increased, however, in inflammatory joint disease).

Methods for determination of the erythrocyte sedimentation rate

There are two methods for determining the sedimentation rate: the Westergren method and the Wintrobe method. Normal values for both methods are 5–20 mm in 1 hour for women and 5–15 mm in 1 hour for men. The normal ESR varies with age, sex, and the specific methodology used.

Both methods use venous blood, which must be properly anticoagulated. EDTA and double oxalate are both satisfactory. Heparin is unsatisfactory and should not be used for the ESR test.

For the Wintrobe method, enough blood is drawn into a Pasteur pipet to fill a *Wintrobe hematocrit tube* to the 100-mm mark. Bubbles must be avoided. The tube is placed in the support rack in an exactly vertical position so that the cells will sediment properly, and the time is noted. At the end of 1 hour, the ESR is read as the length of the plasma column above the cells. This method is simple and requires a small amount of blood.

The Westergren method is the reference method for the ESR.[18,19] For this test, the procedure should be carried out within 2 hours after the blood has been drawn. The blood is mixed well and drawn into a *Westergren tube* to the zero mark. The tube is placed in a rack in an exactly vertical position at room temperature. Direct drafts, sunlight, and vibrations must be avoided. In some Westergren methods, a liquid sodium citrate solution is added to the blood before it is drawn into the tube. A modification of this method eliminates the addition of the citrate solution and still gives satisfactory results. The time when the tube is placed in the rack is noted and readings are taken at 20, 40, and 60 minutes. The length of the plasma level above the red cells is measured in millimeters from the markings on the tube. A larger amount of blood is required for the Westergren method.

Equipment for the Westergren method

The Westergren tube is really an open-ended pipet. It is 300 mm long with an inner diameter of 2.5 mm and is graduated in millimeters from 0 at the top of the tube to 200 at the bottom. The graduated volume of the tube is 1.0 ml. A special rack to hold the Westergren pipets in a vertical position is needed for this test. The Westergren sedimentation rack is constructed so that rubber stoppers attached to springs close the open ends of the tubes when they are placed properly in the rack. Mechanical suction should be used to fill Westergren tubes.

Procedure for the modified Westergren method

1. Five milliliters of venous blood is drawn into EDTA.

2. Two milliliters of well-mixed EDTA blood is diluted with 0.5 ml of 3.8 g/dl sodium citrate or 0.5 ml of 0.85 g/dl NaCl. (The original Westergren method used sodium citrate as the anticoagulant. The modified method employs EDTA blood, but this is diluted to give results consistent with the classic Westergren method.)

3. The diluted blood is mixed by repeated inversions for 3-5 minutes.

4. A Westergren tube is filled to the zero mark by mechanical suction and placed vertically in the Westergren rack.

5. The upper level to which the red cells fall is read in millimeters from the graduation marks on the tube at 20, 40, and 60 minutes. These readings are recorded.

Precautions and technical factors

An anticoagulant that not only prevents clotting but preserves the shape and volume of the red cells must be used. Anticoagulants that prevent erythrocyte sedimentation are unsuitable for this test. Since erythrocyte numbers influence the rate of fall, the specimen must not be hemolyzed. Fibrin clots must not be present. The tube used for the test must be placed vertically in the rack; an angle different from this position can alter the rate of fall significantly. As the blood specimen stands after the venipuncture, the suspension stability of the erythrocytes increases. The test must be set up in a clean Westergren tube within 2 hours after the blood has been drawn to ensure a reliable sedimentation rate. Preferably the test should be set up within 1 hour. Specimens may be refrigerated for up to 6 hours. Temperature and vibrations can affect the sedimentation rate, and these factors should be taken into consideration.

Normal values

For male ESR:
  5-15 mm/hour
For female ESR:
  5-20 mm/hour

COUNTING THE FORMED ELEMENTS OF THE BLOOD (HEMOCYTOMETRY)

Enumeration of the formed elements of the blood is a fundamental measurement in the hematology laboratory. The procedures used for enumeration include manual microscopic observation and the use of electronic counting devices. The cells counted in routine practice are red blood cells, white blood cells, and platelets. Manual techniques, however, lend themselves to enumeration of all small separate bodies in the field of pathology (such as spermatozoa, eosinophils, and cells in cerebrospinal fluid). The main principles for cell enumeration and examination are (1) selection of a diluting fluid that will dilute the cells so that manageable numbers may be counted and will either identify them in some manner or destroy contaminant cellular elements, and (2) use of a *hemocytometer*, or electronic cell counter, that will present the cells to the technician or to an electronic counting device in such a way that the number of cells per unit volume of fluid can be counted. The electronic counting device avoids human error. It is also statistically more accurate because it can count many more cells than can be counted manually by the technician.

Since there are a great many formed elements per unit volume of blood, it is necessary to dilute the blood before attempting to count them. Methods for counting the formed elements of the blood are designed to obtain the number of cells in 1 μl of whole blood. The units formerly used to record cell counts were cells per cubic millimeter. Whether an electronic cell counter or one of the manual methods is used, the steps in the procedure will include diluting the blood sample quantitatively by using special pipets and diluents, determining the number of cells in the diluted sample, and converting the number of cells in the diluted sample to the final result—the number of cells in 1 μl of whole blood.

Blood cell counts are done on minute portions of already small samples of an individual's blood. For this reason, errors are inherent in the best methods, and the steps in the procedure must be performed as carefully as possible to reduce the variation of the final result from the actual or true count.

In most student practice laboratories, a widely used manual method will be employed to provide experience in counting the formed elements. Most of the practice will be done on preserved blood samples. Before using any blood sample, the technician must make certain that it has been preserved with the proper anticoagulant and has been properly labeled, and that its appearance indicates that a good collection technique was used. Each sample should be checked for hemolysis and small clots (known as fibrin clots) as soon as it is received. Clotted blood or samples with fibrin clots are unacceptable for cell counts.

Counting erythrocytes and leukocytes

The leukocyte (white blood cell) count is routinely included in every initial study of a new patient. It is a basic procedure in the hematology laboratory. The erythrocyte (red blood cell) count is not considered a basic laboratory examination, and its limits of significance must be understood thoroughly. Before the advent of automatic cell counting devices, the erythrocyte count had been virtually eliminated from most routine laboratory tests because of the large error (±20 percent) in the manual methods of counting red cells. White cells are still counted manually in many smaller laboratories, and when carefully done, this is an accurate measurement.

Manual cell counting methods are stressed in this chapter. The manufacturers of electronic cell counting devices supply the purchaser with details of the use and care of the instruments. When a new instrument is used by students in a laboratory course, these instructions must be followed explicitly.

Clinical significance of cell counts

The normal leukocyte count varies from 5000 to 10 000 cells/μl. An increase in the leukocyte count above the normal upper limit is termed *leukocytosis*. A decrease below the normal lower limit is termed *leukopenia*. Leukopenia may occur after x-ray therapy; after the administration of certain drugs; in infections with agents such as the typhoid group, certain viruses, and malaria; and in pernicious anemia. Leukocytosis may occur in many acute infections, in severe malaria, after hemorrhage, during pregnancy, postoperatively, in some forms of anemia, in some carcinomas, and in leukemia. Leukemia is a condition of unknown cause and usually of fatal termination, which is characterized by proliferation of the leukocytes and their precursors in the tissues of the body. It is associated with many changes in the circulating cells of the blood. Blood films prepared from leukemia patients should be examined only by qualified persons—a pathologist or an experienced medical technologist. There are two main classifications of leukemia, myelogenous and lymphatic, according to the predominant type of leukocyte seen. Leu-

kemias are further divided into the subclassifications acute and chronic. In the acute condition, the disease progresses rapidly and morphological changes are marked. In the chronic condition, the changes are neither as rapid nor as marked.

The normal leukocyte count varies with age. The white cell count of a newborn baby is 10 000–30 000 cells/μl at birth and drops to about 10 000 cells/μl after the first week of life. By about age 4, the white cell count reaches the normal level.

As mentioned earlier, the leukocyte count is used by the physician to indicate the presence of infection and to follow the progress of certain diseases. It may be elevated in acute bacterial infections, appendicitis, pregnancy, hemolytic disease of the newborn, uremia, and ulcers, and may be decreased in hepatitis, rheumatoid arthritis, cirrhosis of the liver, and lupus erythematosus. A child's leukocyte count usually shows a much greater variation during disease than an adult's. An individual's leukocyte count is subject to some variation during the course of a normal day, being slightly higher in the afternoon than in the morning. There is also an increase in the leukocyte count after strenuous exercise, emotional stress, and anxiety.

Anemia is a term generally applied to a decrease in the number of erythrocytes. There are many types of anemias. It can be caused by excessive blood loss or blood destruction (called hemolytic anemia). Anemias caused by decreased blood cell or hemoglobin formation include pernicious anemia, bone marrow failure anemia, and iron-deficiency anemia. Polycythemia is a condition in which the number of erythrocytes is increased.

Diluents

Because the blood cells are so numerous, they cannot be counted accurately without dilution. When red blood cells are counted, we know from the principles of osmosis that the most important characteristic of the diluent is isotonicity. Two other necessary characteristics of a diluent for red cell counts are that it prevents clumping or clotting of the cells and has the proper specific gravity, so that all the cells will settle as evenly as possible. Hayem's solution is the diluent most commonly used for manual counting of red cells. It contains mercuric chloride ($HgCl_2$) to prevent clumping of the red cells, and sodium sulfate (Na_2SO_4) and sodium chloride (NaCl) to provide the proper specific gravity and isotonicity. Other diluents for red cell counts include 0.85 g/dl saline solution, Gowers' solution, Toison's solution, and Rees-Ecker solution.

In the methods for leukocyte counts, the diluting fluid must meet a very different requirement—it must destroy the more numerous red cells so that the white cells may be counted more readily. (The white cells need not be eliminated when counting red cells.) The principles of osmotic pressure are again employed, but in a different way. The diluent used most commonly for white cell counts is 2 ml/dl acetic acid, which (1) darkens the nuclei of the white cells so that they are easier to see, and (2) hemolyzes the red cells. When the acetic acid hemolyzes the red cells, it converts the hemoglobin released from the red cells into acid hematin, which gives the resulting solution a brown color. The intensity of the brown color is directly related to the amount of hemoglobin present in the red cells. Another diluting fluid used for white cell counts is 0.1 N HCl. The principle is the same with either 2 ml/dl acetic acid or 0.1 N HCl.

Any diluent used must be filtered immediately before use to eliminate foreign particles, which might be confused with the cells to be counted.

Directions for preparation of diluents

1. Hayem's solution for red cell counts. Dissolve 15 g of NaCl, 33 g of anhydrous Na_2SO_4, and 7.5 g of $HgCl_2$, and dilute to 3000 ml with deionized water.
2. Acetic acid for white cell counts (2 ml/dl).

Dilute 60 ml of glacial acetic acid to 3000 ml with deionized water.

Pipets for red and white blood cell counts

To ensure proper dilution of the sample to be used for counting red and white blood cells, the correct diluent is used with pipets manufactured for this purpose. Laboratories employ various brands of diluting pipets, all of which are generally of the same structure. The important differences are determined by the grade of glass used in the manufacture of the pipet and the calibration of the pipet. Precalibration by the manufacturer and calibration checking in the hematology laboratory may appear complex. The procedure is more easily understood if it is compared to a matching process. The pipets can be matched with National Bureau of Standards pipets either by comparing the weight of some substance, such as mercury, contained in the unknown pipet with the weight of the same substance contained in the standard pipet, or by actually counting blood cells in equivalent cell samples. The mark (if any) on the pipet indicating that it has been checked will vary from laboratory to laboratory. It is therefore necessary to identify the calibration check mark and use only pipets that have been properly calibrated. Using matched pipets reduces the error from one source in blood cell counts by increasing the consistency of the dilution.

Several companies manufacture a type of pipet for white and red blood cell counts known as the *Thoma* pipet. Thoma is not a brand name but a type of pipet used for blood cell dilution in most hematology laboratories. Some of the brand names for Thoma diluting pipets are K-exax, Normax, Glasco, Yankee certified, Tri-Lyne, Sargent, and American Optical. It is most important to select only brands of pipets that are reliable and accurate.

Like all cell counting pipets, the Thoma pipet does not measure blood or diluent in definite amounts such as milliliters or millimeters, but instead provides the proper dilution in terms of a certain part of its volume to the total volume. It consists of a graduated capillary tube divided into 10 parts and marked 0.5 at the fifth mark and 1.0 at the tenth, a mixing bulb above the capillary tube containing a glass bead (which facilitates mixing of the blood and diluent), and another short capillary tube above the bulb with an engraved graduation mark (11.0 on the white cell pipet and 101.0 on the red cell pipet) (Fig. 3-6). The marks on the Thoma white cell pipet indicate that there are 11 units of volume in the pipet from the tip to the 11.0 mark above the bulb (Fig. 3-6). The 1.0 mark on the stem means that one of the units of volume for that pipet is contained in the stem from the tip of the pipet to the 1.0 mark. The single unit of volume in the stem is divided into 10 equal portions by measuring from the tip. The bulb is defined as extending from the 1.0 mark on the stem to the 11.0 mark on the short stem above the bulb, and it contains 10 units of volume.

Routinely, the dilution made for the white cell count is 1:20. This is accomplished by measuring whole blood from a well-mixed sample to the 0.5 mark and washing the sample into the bulb with the diluent to the 11.0 mark. The mixture in the bulb will contain 0.5 part of blood and 9.5 parts of diluent in the total of 10 units of volume in the bulb. The one unit in the stem contains diluent only and does not enter into the calculation of the dilution. The dilution factor is calculated by dividing 10 by 0.5, which is the same as determining what the total volume would have to be if one unit of blood were used with the same relative amount of diluent. The dilution is therefore 1:20.

The same procedure is used for the red blood cell dilution, except that the red cell pipet allows a 10 times greater dilution than the white cell pipet. Rather than 11.0 total units of volume, the red cell pipet has 101.0 units of volume (Fig. 3-6). Therefore, when 0.5 unit of blood is measured and diluted to the 101.0 mark, the dilution is 1:200. There are 0.5 unit of blood and 99.5 units of diluent in the mixture contained in the bulb, which holds a total of 100 units. The one unit in the stem of the red cell pipet contains only diluent.

Procedure for dilution with Thoma pipets

1. Filter the appropriate diluting fluid from the stock bottle into a small diluting bottle.

2. Using a properly mixed whole blood sample and the diluting pipet with tubing and mouthpiece attached, draw blood into the capillary bore of the pipet to slightly above the 0.5 mark.

3. Wipe off the *outside* of the pipet with gauze, and adjust the blood level to the 0.5 mark *exactly* by tapping the tip of the pipet with a cot-covered finger or other nonabsorbent material. Do not use gauze for this adjustment, because the liquid portion of the sample inside the stem will be drawn into the gauze, leaving a higher concentration of cells inside the stem. Hold the pipet in a horizontal position.

4. Maintain the blood level at the 0.5 mark by placing the tongue over the plastic mouthpiece on the tubing or by holding the breath. Place the tip of the pipet into the diluting fluid well below the surface of the liquid.

5. Using constant mouth suction, draw the diluent into the pipet while at the same time lightly twirling the pipet between the fingers. Draw the mixture to the top mark above the bulb. While the bulb is being filled, tap the pipet

Fig. 3-6. Red cell and white cell diluting pipets.

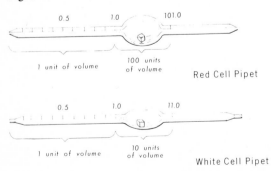

with the finger to knock the bead down below the surface of the solution in the bulb. This will help to prevent bubbles from forming.

6. While removing the pipet from the diluent bottle, maintain the level of the mixture exactly on or slightly (never more than 1 mm) above the top mark by closing the pipet tip with the index finger and holding the breath, or covering the mouthpiece with the tongue. Holding the pipet in a horizontal position is also important. Remove the rubber sucker tubing carefully, continuing to hold the index finger over the pipet tip.

7. As soon as the rubber tubing is removed, hold the pipet horizontally with the thumb and third finger at either end. Shake the pipet vigorously at right angles to its long axis for a few seconds. The glass bead in the pipet should move from one side to the other during the mixing. After shaking, the pipet may be put aside in a horizontal position, preventing any leakage until the cell count is done.

General precautions for pipetting with Thoma pipets

Several precautions can be taken to avoid errors when doing a red or white blood cell count in the hematology laboratory. Pipets must be clean, dry, and without chipped or broken tips. Technique must be practiced until completed pipets are free from bubbles, packing, or clumping of cells. Contaminated diluting fluid must not be used. Periodically check the fluid in the diluting bottle; no blood should be allowed to get into the diluent, because this will affect subsequent cell counts with the same diluent.

The upper dilution mark on the pipets may be exceeded by no more than 1 mm, and the mixture must not be corrected back to the top mark if overdiluted. Adjusting the upper dilution back to the mark forces cells from the bulb into the lower stem of the pipet. The fluid in this stem must be free from cells when dilution has been completed. Absorbent material such as gauze must not be used to adjust the upper blood level to the 0.5 mark. The sample in the stem can be falsely concentrated if gauze or other absorptive materials are used to adjust the blood level.

Preserved blood samples must not be hemolyzed or contain fibrin clots.

Procedure for use of disposable, self-filling pipet systems

The use of disposable, self-filling precalibrated glass capillary pipets for measuring and diluting blood for cell counts has proved extremely helpful. The Unopette system was described previously under Hemoglobin.[20] It consists of a special glass pipet attached to a holder, and a plastic reservoir containing diluent (Fig. 3-5). The pipet fills automatically with blood, either capillary or venous, by means of capillary action, and the blood stops automatically when the correct amount has filled the pipet. This avoids the errors inherent in drawing blood into conventional Thoma pipets. The capillary pipet is inserted into the reservoir containing 3% acetic acid for dilution of white blood cells, emptied carefully, and rinsed, and the resulting solution in the reservoir is mixed well. The manufacturer's directions must be followed carefully. Unopettes are available for hemoglobins, red cell counts, white cell counts, and platelet counts.

Counting chamber for red and white blood cell counts

After proper handling of the blood sample and careful dilution by a known amount to obtain a less concentrated solution, the number of cells in a known volume of the diluted sample is determined. The counting chamber is often called a hemocytometer. Technically, however, a hemocytometer consists of a counting chamber, a cover glass for the counting chamber, and the diluting pipets. In this section the terms counting chamber and hemocytometer are used interchangeably. For a routine count by a hand method, the counting chamber used most often is the Levy-Hausser hemocytometer with Neubauer ruling.

To understand how a counting chamber gives the blood cell count in terms of volume when the chamber is a flat surface, we start with a cube and work backward. Picture a cube 1 mm on each side. The counting chamber allows the cube to be divided into equal units that are $\frac{1}{10}$ mm in depth. When the counting chamber is viewed from the side, one can see that when the cover glass is placed on the chamber, it rests on supports (Fig. 3-7). The space between the bottom of the cover glass and the surface of the counting chamber is $\frac{1}{10}$ mm. Essentially, the chamber provides a series of "slices" of the cube that are 1 mm^2 in area and $\frac{1}{10}$ mm in depth. The only way to be sure the depth is $\frac{1}{10}$ mm is to use plane ground cover glasses that have a constant weight and even surface. The $\frac{1}{10}$-mm slices are arranged so that one may count the cells in one of the slices or in portions of one slice by varying the area of the ruled surface of the chamber. Each counting chamber has two precision-ruled counting areas 3 mm wide and 3 mm long (Fig. 3-8). All hemocytometers used in the hematology laboratory must meet the specifications of the National Bureau of Standards.

When the ruled area of the counting chamber is viewed for the first time under the microscope, it may be difficult to see the nine basic 1-mm squares because each one has been ruled into smaller areas. The 1-mm^2 sections in the four corners are ruled into 16 equal portions (Fig. 3-9). The square in the center of the ruled area is divided into 25 equal portions (Fig. 3-9). In turn, each of the $\frac{1}{25}$-mm squares is divided into 16 parts, providing $\frac{1}{400}$-mm squares (Fig. 3-9). With the surface of the counting chamber ruled in this manner, it is possible to measure aliquots of the diluted blood sample that are contained in 1-mm, $\frac{1}{16}$-mm, $\frac{1}{25}$-mm, $\frac{1}{80}$-mm, and $\frac{1}{400}$-mm squares, all of which are $\frac{1}{10}$ mm in depth. The area to be counted will depend on the type of count to be done.

Other types of counting chambers can also be used to count blood cells. Some of these are the Spencer Brightline with Neubauer ruling and the Levy chamber with Fuchs-Rosenthal ruling.

Mixing and mounting samples in the counting chamber

The diluted blood in the pipet must be mixed before the mixture is placed on the counting chamber. Mixing can be done by hand for a minimum of 5 minutes by holding the pipet so

Fig. 3-7. Counting chamber—Side view.

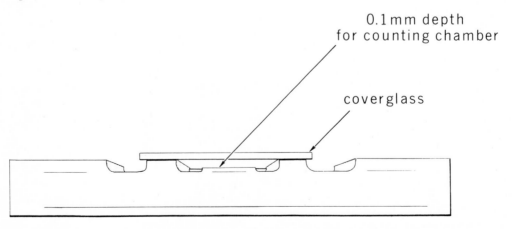

0.1mm depth
for counting chamber

coverglass

(9 square millimeters)

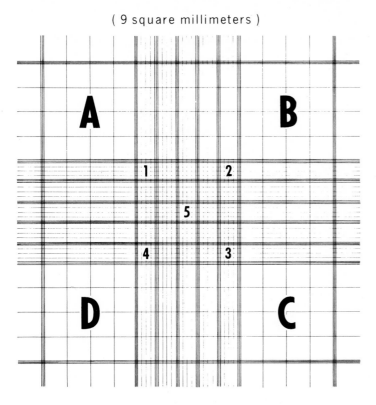

White blood cells are counted in areas A, B, C, and D (4 sq. mm.)
Red blood cells are counted in areas 1, 2, 3, 4, and 5
(80/400 sq. mm.)

Fig. 3-8. Improved Neubauer ruling for one counting chamber area.

that the mixing bead moves freely and the cells are not pushed into the stem. Usually, a mechanical shaker will be available, and the time will vary according to the type of shaker used. Immediately after shaking the pipet and before placing a small portion of the mixture on the chamber, three drops are expelled from the white cell pipet and five drops from the red cell pipet to discard the cell-free diluent. The tip is wiped and the cells are counted in the next drop, which is representative of the well-mixed cell suspension. Pipets may vary in size, so discarding three to five drops may not be adequate. In that case,

approximately one-third of the mixture in the bulb should be expelled before mounting.

While the pipet is held at an angle of about 40°, the chamber between the ruled area and the cover glass is filled with a single drop, which should be drawn rapidly into the chamber by capillarity. Both sides of the hemocytometer must be filled. If the fluid spills into the dividing moats or is otherwise distributed unevenly, mounting must be repeated. Only one drop can be used to fill the chamber. It should not be filled partially with a small drop and filled completely with a second drop; this would result

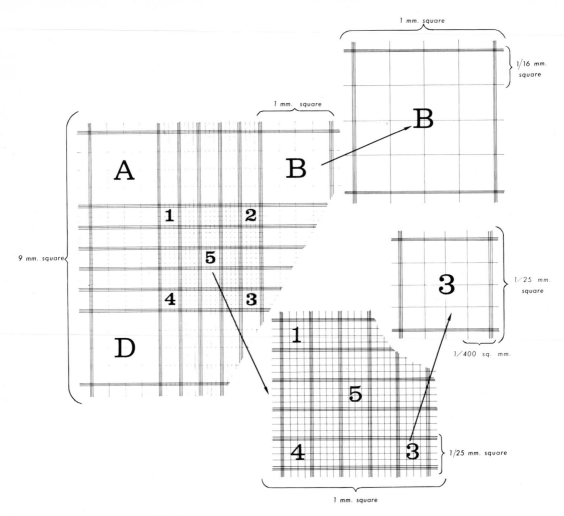

Fig. 3-9. Counting areas of the hemocytometer.

in uneven distribution of the cells. For practice in mounting, however, more of the fluid remaining in the pipet can be used. The counting chamber is filled in the same manner for both red cell and white cell counts.

Shaking the pipet and properly filling the counting chamber are important factors in obtaining a good distribution of cells in the counting areas and in obtaining accurate cell counts.

If the Unopette system has been used, the equipment for the initial blood measurement and dilution can be easily converted to a dropper assembly. In this way, the blood-diluent mixture can be easily mounted on the same kind of counting chamber used for the Thoma pipet method. The dilution of blood is the same as for the Thoma method, so the calculations for both methods are the same when the Levy-Hausser hemocytometer with Neubauer ruling is used.

Before any counting is done, the microscope must be properly adjusted (review The Microscope in Chap. 1). It is necessary to know how to adjust the microscope for proper illumination, and how to focus correctly (avoiding damage to the objectives and the object to be viewed).

Place the filled counting chamber on the stage of the microscope and fasten securely. Place one of the ruled counting areas of the chamber in position over the condenser. Using the low-power objective, turn the coarse-adjustment knob until the objective is about $\frac{1}{4}$ in above the cover glass. Adjust the light, so that the field is evenly illuminated and comfortable to view, by moving the condenser down somewhat and then adjusting the iris diaphragm and rheostat. Turn the coarse-adjustment knob slowly until the ruled area comes into focus, and use the fine-adjustment knob to bring the area into perfect focus. Use the iris diaphragm to adjust the light. If this technique is used, there is little danger of damaging the cover glass with the objective. If the objective touches the cover glass, the cell distribution is altered and a new mounting must be made. After the ruled area is in focus, scan it quickly to identify the various ruled portions. Approximately 1 mm^2 can be seen in each field with the low-power (×10) objective.

When the counting chamber is properly in

place on the microscope and the various ruled areas are identified and understood, cell counting can begin.

Counting and calculating white blood cells by a manual method

White blood cells are counted under low magnification (×10 objective) in the four corner 1-mm squares of the ruled area of the counting chamber. Each square is divided into 16 equal parts. Cells touching the lines on the left side or on the top of the squares are included in the count, but cells touching the lines on the right side or on the bottom of the squares are *not* counted (Fig. 3-10). In this way, every cell is assigned to a square and cells are not counted twice or omitted from the count.

The counts obtained in the 1-mm^2 sections in the four corners are tabulated separately in practice laboratories. These values should not differ by more than 10. Tallying the squares separately provides a check of the distribution of the cells and indicates whether mixing and mounting were adequate. When the values do not agree with 10, another pipet must be used, because remounts

Fig. 3-10. Examples of white blood cells that are counted in a representative area.

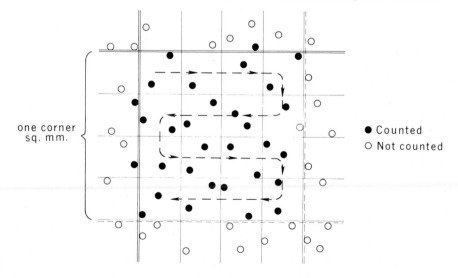

one corner
sq. mm.

● Counted
○ Not counted

from the previously used pipet usually result in progressively higher counts.

In calculating the total count per cubic millimeter of blood, four important facts must be considered: (1) the total number of cells counted in the four 1-mm squares, (2) the dilution of the blood sample, (3) the square area counted, and (4) the depth of the counting chamber. The square area and the depth can be considered together as volume. These four factors are used in the following general formula:

Cells counted in 1-mm^2 areas $\times$ dilution of blood

$\times$ area counted $\times$ depth of chamber

= white cells per microliter of whole blood

For example, the sum of the cells counted in the four 1-mm^2 corner areas is $33 + 32 + 40 + 35 = 140$. In this case, the calculation would be $\frac{140}{1} \times \frac{20}{1} \times \frac{1}{4} \times \frac{1}{0.1} = 7000$ white blood cells/μl. If the square areas and the depth are considered as volume, the general formula is

$$\frac{\text{Cells counted in 4 squares} \times \text{dilution of blood}}{\text{Volume}}$$

$$= \text{white cells}/\mu\text{l}$$

where volume = area $\times$ depth

The count when a total of 140 cells are counted in the four squares would be calculated as

$$\frac{140 \times 20}{4 \times 0.1} = 7000 \text{ white cells}/\mu\text{l}$$

For each white cell count completed in the routine manner, the dilution of the blood and the volume of diluted blood used for counting remain constant. Therefore, the total cells counted may be multiplied by a constant factor to find the final result. Leaving out the number of cells in the last equation, $20/(4 \times 0.1) = 50$. Any total number of cells can be converted to the number of white cells per microliter of blood by multiplying by 50. Thus, 50 is the constant

factor for counting white cells in the routine manner by the manual method presented.

White cells should be counted in duplicate until accuracy is attained, after which duplicate determinations may be done when appropriate (for low counts or counts of grave clinical importance).

The allowable difference[21,22] between duplicate pipets for the same blood sample is 500 cells/μl for counts within the normal range (5000–10 000 cells/μl) and 10 percent of the lowest count when the total count is above or below the normal range. The resulting white cell count is always rounded off to the nearest 50 cells, since the constant in the equation is 50. For example, a white cell count calculated as 8044 would be reported as 8050, and a count calculated as 8022 would be reported as 8000. The general rule for rounding off numbers to the next significant figure is used.

Counting and calculating red blood cells by a manual method

Red blood cells are counted under high-dry magnification ($\times$45 objective). The central 1-mm^2 area of the counting chamber is used. It is best to find this area with the low-power objective and then change to the high-dry objective. The cells in 80 of the $\frac{1}{400}$-mm squares are counted. This is equivalent to counting the cells in $\frac{1}{5}$ of 1 mm^2 ($\frac{80}{400}$). The volume is determined by multiplying the depth ($\frac{1}{10}$ mm) by $\frac{1}{5}$, and is equal to 0.02 μl.

The preferred method for counting the cells in $\frac{1}{5}$ mm^2 is to count the cells in five of the $\frac{1}{25}$-mm squares (Fig. 3-11). Since each $\frac{1}{25}$-mm square contains 16 smaller squares, eighty $\frac{1}{400}$-mm squares will have been counted. The distribution is checked by making duplicate mounts.

The calculation of the red cell count is based on the same principles as those used for the white cell count. The usual blood dilution is 1:200, the area counted is $\frac{1}{5}$ mm^2, and the depth is $\frac{1}{10}$ mm. For example, if 475 red cells are

(Center Square Millimeter)

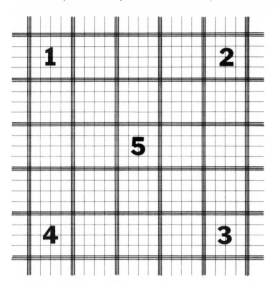

count five 1/25 mm. squares

Fig. 3-11. Red cell counting area.

counted in the proper area, the calculation would be $\frac{475}{1} \times \frac{200}{1} \times \frac{400}{80} \times \frac{10}{1} = 4\,750\,000$ red cells/μl. If the area and depth are converted to volume first, the general equation would be

$$\frac{\text{Cells counted in } \frac{1}{5} \text{ mm}^2 \times \text{dilution}}{\text{Volume}} = \text{red cells}/\mu\text{l}$$

where volume = area $\times$ depth

The constant factor for the red blood cell count is $200(0.2 \times 0.1) = 10\,000$.

The red blood cell count is one of the least accurate procedures done in the hematology laboratory. For this reason, every sample is pipetted in duplicate, and each pipet is mounted on two sides of the counting chamber, giving four possible counting areas. If the counts with the two pipets do not check within 10 percent, the determination is repeated. A generally accepted normal range for red cell counts is 3.7–5.2 million cells/μl for women and 4.5–6.0 million cells/μl for men.

The rules for counting the cells touching the top and left lines of a particular area are the same for red cell counts as for white cell counts.

Precautions and technical factors

Errors in counting white and red blood cells are related to the extremely small size of the sample, the nature of the sample, faulty laboratory equipment, faulty technique, and the inherent error of cell distribution in the counting chamber, which is subject to the laws of chance.[23]

The minute size of the blood sample is illustrated by the fact that a variation of even 1 cell in the red cell count changes the final result by 10 000 cells.

Venous blood must be free of clots and mixed well immediately before it is diluted. Peripheral blood or capillary blood must be obtained freely flowing from a puncture and must be diluted rapidly to prevent coagulation.

Pipets must be checked against National Bureau of Standards pipets, and equivalent samples should agree within 7 percent.[24,25] Pipets must be clean and dry and without chipped tips. The counting chamber must be clean and dry. The usual practice is to clean the chamber and cover glass immediately before each use by flooding them with medicated alcohol and wiping them dry with a piece of gauze. Dirt on the chamber can alter the count.

The blood sample must be measured precisely and diluted properly. The counting chamber must be charged with only one drop of the diluted sample—an excess could raise the cover glass and thus change the depth factor.

Even with excellent technique and equipment, the probable error in red cell counts can be 20 percent, because of the chance error in the distribution of the cells on the counting chamber. The same distribution factor can also affect the white blood cell count, and the error in this count can be 15 percent.

In certain conditions, such as leukemia, the white blood cell count may be extremely high. If it is more than 30 000 cells/μl, a greater dilution of the blood should be used. Using a Thoma red cell diluting pipet, the blood is drawn up to the 1.0 mark and diluted to the 101 mark with the white cell diluting fluid, giving a 1:100 dilution. Other dilutions may be employed when necessary, and are taken into account when the final calculations are made.

When the white cell count drops below 3000 cells/μl, a smaller dilution of the blood should be used to achieve a more accurate count. In this case, the blood is drawn up to the 1.0 mark in the regular white cell diluting pipet, and diluted to the 11 mark for a final dilution of 1:10. The white cell count is determined as usual, using the change in blood dilution in the calculations.

The diluting fluid used for the white blood cell count destroys or hemolyzes all nonnucleated red cells. In certain disease conditions, nucleated red blood cells may be present in the peripheral blood. These cells cannot be distinguished from the white cells and are counted as white cells in the hemocytometer. Therefore, whenever there are five or more nucleated red cells per 100 white cells in a differential done on a stained blood film, the white cell count must be corrected as follows:

$$\frac{\text{Uncorrected WBC count} \times 100}{100 + \text{number of nucleated RBCs per 100 WBCs}}$$

$$= \text{corrected WBC count}$$

The white blood cell count is then reported as the corrected count.

Use of electronic cell counters does not relieve the laboratory worker of the responsibility for being constantly alert for sources of error. Unless equipment is properly calibrated and fundamental aspects such as the quality of the sample are considered carefully, electronic counters are merely tools for producing inadequate results faster.

Automated cell counting methods

A wide range of automated and semiautomated devices are available for measuring different hematologic parameters. The most useful instruments are those for counting cells. Automated cell counters count larger numbers of cells than manual counting methods and thus allow much greater precision. The coefficient of variation (CV), or allowable error, in a manual cell counting method varies from 8 to 15 percent, depending on the type of cell counted. Automated counting methods have been reported as having a CV of 1-3 percent.[26] One of the most commonly used automated systems is the model F Coulter counter for counting red cells, white cells, and platelets; it utilizes a voltage pulse counting mechanism.

Voltage pulse counting method: Coulter counter, model F

In the model F Coulter counter, cells passing through an aperture through which a current is flowing cause changes in electrical resistance that are counted as voltage pulses. An accurately diluted suspension of blood is made in 0.85 g/dl saline or in an isotonic conductive solution such as Isoton (Coulter Diagnostics, Hialeah, Fla.), which preserves the shape of the cells. Both red and white blood cells are diluted in this solution for automated counting. The diluted suspension of cells is poured into a beaker, which is raised until the glass aperture tube and the external electrode of the machine are immersed (Fig. 3-12). A reduced pressure system operated by a vacuum unit draws the suspension through the aperture into a system of tubing following a column of mercury. The Coulter counter system is based in the principle that cells are poor electrical conductors, compared with saline or Isoton, which are good conductors.

The instrument system has a glass aperture tube that can be filled with the conducting fluid (the suspension of diluted cells, for example) and has an electrode (the internal electrode) and an aperture or small orifice that is 100 μm in diameter. Just outside the glass aperture tube is another electrode (the external electrode). The

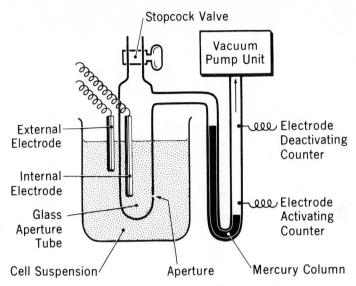

Stopcock Valve

Vacuum Pump Unit

External Electrode

Electrode Deactivating Counter

Internal Electrode

Electrode Activating Counter

Glass Aperture Tube

Cell Suspension

Aperture

Mercury Column

Fig. 3-12. Schematic diagram of a cell counter based on a voltage pulse counting principle.

aperture tube is connected to a U-shaped glass tube that is partly filled with mercury and has two electrical contacts—an activating counter and a deactivating counter. The aperture tube is immersed in the cell suspension, filled with conductive solution, and closed by a stopcock valve. A current now flows through the aperture between the internal and external electrodes. As the vacuum unit draws the mercury up the tube, the cell suspension flows through the aperture into the aperture tube.

Each cell that passes through the aperture displaces an equal volume of conductive solution, increasing the electrical resistance and creating a voltage pulse, because its resistance is much greater than that of the conductive solution. The pulses, which are proportional in height to the volume of cells, are counted. The section of tubing between the activating and deactivating counters is calibrated to contain 0.5 ml (Fig. 3-12). The counting mechanism is started when the mercury reaches the activating counter and is stopped when it reaches the deactivating counter. During this time the cells are counted in a volume of suspension exactly equal to the vol-

ume of glass tubing between the two contact wires in the activating and deactivating electrodes.

If two or more cells enter the aperture at the same time, they will be counted as one cell. This produces a coincidence error for which a correction must be made. The size of the coincidence error may be decreased by decreasing the concentration of the cells and the size of the aperture. However, decreasing the concentration of the cells increases the dilution error and the inherent counting error and makes the error resulting from background "noise" from contaminating particles more critical. When the aperture is decreased, it may become partially or completely plugged with debris. For this reason a compromise is made, and for a count above a certain critical number, a coincidence correction is made by referring to a chart supplied by the manufacturer of the counting instrument.

Variations of the current measured across the aperture make it possible to determine the particle or cell count, cell volume, and particle size. All the cells in 0.5 ml of suspension are counted and the results are displayed. This pulse or count is amplified, numerically registered by the counter, and visualized on an oscilloscope.

Procedure for counting with the model F Coulter counter

1. Turn on the automatic cell counter and allow it to warm up for several minutes.

2. Dilute the blood samples. Separate samples are prepared for counting red cells and white cells. The red cells must be lysed first for the white cells to be counted. This is done by the addition of a saponin solution, Zap Isoton, or a similar solution.

a. Pipet 10 ml of Isoton or saline into vials or beakers. Prepare one vial for a blank and another for a control solution, in addition to the necessary number of vials for unknown samples. Duplicate samples should be prepared until proficiency is attained.

b. Pipet 0.02 ml of oxalated, EDTA, or capillary blood into the Isoton solution, using a Sahli pipet. This gives a 1:500 dilution. The vial can be capped and inverted several times to mix well.

c. From the 1:500 dilution sample, add 0.10 ml to 10 ml of saline or Isoton in another vial, giving a 1:50 000 dilution for the red cell count.

d. To the original 1:500 dilution vial, add 0.1 ml of a special saponin solution, cetrimide-citrate solution, or Zap Isoton (three drops) to lyse the red cells. Lysis of the red cells takes place in seconds, but allow the solution to stand for a few minutes to ensure complete lysis. Normal white cells will remain intact in this solution for 2 hours.

3. Following the manufacturer's instructions, take triplicate readings of a blank with 10 ml of Isoton and three drops of Zap Isoton. This is the background count, and it should be less than 200 cells/μl.

4. Pour the unknown dilution into a small beaker and take triplicate readings. Three consecutive readings should agree within 200 cells/μl.

5. Count the specimen and read the result, rounding it to the nearest 100 for the white cell count. If the white cell count is higher than 10 000, correct it for coincidence loss by using the correction chart supplied with the machine. Correct the reading for the red cell count for coincidence loss, and multiply it by 100 because of the additional dilution of the specimen.

6. Rinse the apertures with Isoton when finished.

Coulter counter, model S

To further minimize laboratory error and increase speed and reliability, the model S Coulter counter is used in many hematology laboratories.[27] The model S uses the voltage pulse counting principle described for the model F Coulter counter, but it also has a totally automatic diluting system. It provides seven hematologic parameters: the white cell count, red cell count, hemoglobin, hematocrit, MCV, MCH, and MCHC. Hemoglobin is determined photometrically by passing a light beam through the mixture in the white cell aperture bath. The light absorbed by the solution at a specific wavelength is proportional to the hemoglobin concentration and is measured by a photosensitive device. The principle is the same as that of the cyanmethemoglobin method (see under Hemoglobin). The model S uses whole blood, which it automatically measures and dilutes.

Normal values[28]

For red blood cell count:

Men:	4.5–6.0 × 10^6 cells/μl
Women:	3.7–5.2 × 10^6 cells/μl
Newborn:	5.0–6.0 × 10^6 cells/μl
Infants:	3.2–4.5 × 10^6 cells/μl
Children:	4.2–5.0 × 10^6 cells/μl

For white blood cell count:

Adults, black:	4000–10 000 cells/μl
Adults, white:	5000–11 000 cells/μl
Newborn:	10 000–20 000 cells/μl
Infants:	6000–15 000 cells/μl
Children:	5000–12 000 cells/μl

Counting platelets

Platelets, or thrombocytes, function in the coagulation of the blood and are therefore associated with the bleeding and clotting, or hemostatic, mechanism of the body. Platelets are formed in the bone marrow from megakaryocytes. They are difficult to count accurately for several reasons: they are small and difficult to discern, they have an adhesive character and become attached readily to glassware or to particles of debris in the diluting fluid, and they clump easily and are probably not evenly distributed in the blood in the first place. Platelets disintegrate easily and are difficult to distinguish from debris. Because of their sticky nature, they also tend to adhere to other platelets in clumps. By using EDTA as an anticoagulant, the clumping tendency of platelets can be decreased.

Specimens

Capillary blood from a finger puncture can be used, but venous blood generally gives more satisfactory results. Platelet counts on capillary blood are generally lower than those on venous blood. EDTA is the anticoagulant of choice for platelet counts.

Methods used to count platelets

With good technique and experience, platelets can be counted accurately by hand. One basic manual method, the Brecher-Cronkite method, utilizes phase-contrast microscopy.[29] The Brecher-Cronkite method uses a blood diluent, 1 g/dl ammonium oxalate, that completely hemolyzes the red cells. The platelets are then counted, generally with a phase hemocytometer and a phase-contrast microscope. An ordinary light microscope may be used to count the platelets, but the differentiation is not as sharp and it causes eyestrain for the technician. Manual methods are time-consuming, cause eyestrain, and are not recommended for large-volume work. A manual platelet count is always done with duplicate pipets.

An automated method with the model F Coulter counter is used in many laboratories.[30] The aperture is $70\,\mu m$ instead of the $100\,\mu m$ used for red and white blood cell counts. It is necessary to correlate the automated count with that estimated from a stained blood film. In the automated counting method, platelet-rich plasma is prepared from the blood specimen before it is used in the counter.

In general, the best results are obtained by using some variation of the direct manual methods. Some hospitals have discontinued platelet counts altogether because the error involved can be very large and a well-prepared blood smear can be used to estimate platelets. With any direct method, the blood used must be freshly obtained from a finger puncture or it must be preserved with EDTA. Balanced oxalate does not preserve the white blood cells or the platelets.

The manual method to be discussed in this chapter is the Rees-Ecker direct method, employing a standard bright-field microscope. In this method, whole blood is diluted with a solution of brilliant cresyl blue, which stains the platelets a light bluish color. The platelets are then counted with a Spencer Brightline hemocytometer. This manual method is also time-consuming.

Clinical significance of the platelet count

The normal number of platelets, depending in part on the method employed for their enumeration, ranges from 140 000 to 400 000 cells per microliter of whole blood. A lower than normal number of platelets may be associated with a generalized bleeding tendency and a prolonged bleeding time. A higher than normal number may be associated with a tendency toward thrombosis.

There are several diseases in which a high or low platelet count can result. Thrombocytopenia, or a decrease in platelets, is found in thrombocytopenic purpura, in some infectious diseases, in some acute leukemias, in some anemias (aplastic and pernicious), and when the patient is undergoing x-ray treatment or chemotherapy (drug treatment). Thrombocytosis, or an increase in platelets, can be found in rheumatic fever, asphyxiation, following surgical treatment, following splenectomy, with acute blood loss, and with some types of drug therapy used in the treatment of leukemia.

Diluents for manual platelet count (Rees-Ecker method)

The diluent used for counting platelets must meet certain requirements. It must (1) provide fixation to reduce the adhesiveness of the platelets, (2) prevent coagulation, (3) prevent hemolysis (unless the method chosen eliminates the red blood cells), and (4) provide a low specific gravity so that the platelets will settle in one plane. A diluent that meets all these requirements is Rees-Ecker solution. Rees-Ecker solution contains sodium citrate, which prevents coagulation, preserves the red blood cells, and provides the necessary low specific gravity; Formalin, which is a fixative; and brilliant cresyl blue, which is a dye used for the identification of the diluent. This dye does not stain the platelets, and it is not essential for the counting procedure. All diluents used, including Rees-Ecker, must be stored in the refrigerator and filtered before each use.

Preparation of Rees-Ecker diluting fluid

In a volumetric flask, 3.8 g of sodium citrate and 0.2 ml of Formalin are diluted to 100 ml with deionized water. A small amount of brilliant cresyl blue is added to color the solution light blue.

Equipment for manual platelet count

The pipets used for platelet dilution must be scrupulously clean; it is preferable to clean them with acid, although a hot detergent appears to give good results. Anything in the pipet to which the platelets could adhere must be removed.

To reduce the error in the initial pipetting and diluting steps, a Unopette system may be used. Unopette pipets and reservoirs are available for counting platelets. Empty reservoirs can be purchased to which the appropriate diluent is added before use.

The Spencer Brightline chamber, in which the lines appear white against a dark background, appears to have definite advantages over other types of counting chambers for platelets. The platelets seem easier to see against the metal-coated surface of the Spencer Brightline chamber. The cell distribution also seems to be better, since the chamber's surface is smoother. However, this type of chamber is more difficult to mount correctly.

Procedure for the Rees-Ecker method[31]

1. The capillary bore of a red cell diluting pipet is rinsed with Rees-Ecker diluting fluid. Any excess fluid is thoroughly expelled from the pipet.
2. Freely flowing blood from a finger puncture or venous blood preserved with EDTA is drawn rapidly into the pipet to the 0.5 mark.
3. The blood is diluted rapidly with Rees-Ecker fluid to the 101 mark on the pipet. Two pipets and two counting chambers are used for each platelet count; each pipet is mounted on both sides of the counting chambers. Blood films are also made at this time in order to check the platelet count.
4. The pipets are shaken immediately after dilution for a minimum of 1 minute.
5. After thorough mixing (for at least 5 minutes), six to eight drops are expelled from each pipet and discarded. The next two drops are mounted, one on each side of one counting chamber. Repeat with the duplicate pipet.
6. The platelets are allowed to settle in the chambers for 10 minutes. The chambers are covered to prevent evaporation—for instance, with a Petri plate containing moistened gauze.

7. The platelets, which appear as small, round, refractile bodies, are counted in the center square millimeter of each of the four counting areas, using the high-power objective ($\times 45$). The counts on the four center squares must agree within 20 000 cells/μl for duplicate mounts and within 40 000 cells/μl for duplicate pipets.

Calculations for manual platelet count

The number of platelets per microliter of whole blood must be calculated. The important factors are: (1) the average number of platelets counted in 1 mm^2; (2) the dilution of the blood (usually 1:200); and (3) the volume of diluted blood counted, which is equal to the depth of the chamber (0.1 mm) times the area in which the cells are counted (1 mm^2); or 0.1 μl. The following general formula applies:

$$\frac{\text{Average no. of platelets in 4 squares} \times 1 \text{ mm}^2 \times 200}{0.1 \text{ mm}}$$

$$= \text{platelets}/\mu\text{l}$$

In this case, a constant factor of 2000 can be used. The normal range for the platelet count with Rees-Ecker diluent is 170 000–400 000 platelets/μl.

Precautions and technical factors

Many of the precautions described for counting erythrocytes and leukocytes also apply to platelet counts. In platelet counts, however, it is imperative that peripheral blood be freely flowing when obtained from a finger puncture. Pipets and counting chambers must be clean and free from lint, since platelets may be confused with dirt and debris. Rapid dilution of the blood is

essential, or the platelets may form clumps and the blood may clot. The pipet must be rinsed with the diluent immediately before the dilution procedure to prevent the platelets from sticking to the walls of the pipet. If clumps of platelets are noted during the platelet count, the procedure should be repeated. Clumping may result from inadequate mixing of the blood with the diluent or from poor technique in obtaining the blood sample.

The range of error for the manual platelet count is 16–25 percent.[32] To minimize the error, duplicate pipets are always prepared and duplicate counts done on both sides of two counting chambers. Duplicate counts of a sample should agree within 10 percent to be acceptable.

For an extremely low platelet count, the original blood specimen can be diluted with a white cell diluting pipet instead of a red cell pipet. The correct dilution factor must be used in the calculations.

Since the erythrocytes and leukocytes are not destroyed by the Rees-Ecker solution, constant focusing of the microscope is necessary to identify the platelets among these larger, more numerous cells. A blood film is made, stained, and viewed microscopically to check each platelet count.

If a platelet count is requested in combination with other counts for the same patient and one wishes to utilize the same finger puncture, it is necessary to take the blood for the platelet count first and then for the remaining counts. The finger must not be squeezed excessively when drawing the blood into the pipet.

Normal values[33]

140 000–400 000 platelets/μl

MICROSCOPIC EXAMINATION OF PERIPHERAL BLOOD

Microscopic examination of the peripheral blood is part of the routine hematologic work-up for most patients seen by a physician and for most new hospital patients. It is most often done by preparing, staining, and examining a thin film of blood on a glass slide. A blood film (also called a blood smear) is part of the complete blood count (CBC) in most hospitals or physicians' offices. The CBC generally includes hemoglobin tests, the white blood cell count, the microhematocrit, and a blood film.

The blood film is the only permanent record of routine hematologic work that can be retained in the laboratory. It may occasionally be necessary to examine a blood film again to check for errors or to evaluate changes in the clinical status of the patient.

More information can be obtained from the examination of a blood film than from any other laboratory test. It is used to study the morphology (form and structure) of the red cells, white cells, and platelets. The various types of white cells are classified and the percentage of each is recorded; this is the white cell differential count. The blood film can also be used to verify the hemoglobin value, the hematocrit, and the red cell count. It is used to check or estimate the white cell, reticulocyte, and platelet counts and the red cell indexes. Because the blood film has so many uses, a well-made smear is essential. Generally, two good films are prepared with each blood count or set of hematologic tests. One of these films is stained and the other is kept in reserve.

Sources of blood for the blood film

The source of blood used for the blood film is an important consideration. Fresh blood from a finger, heel, or big toe puncture is best for morphological examination of the white and red cells. The finger must not be squeezed excessively to obtain the drop of blood, and it must not be touched with the glass slide. If the slide touches the finger, oils or moisture from the finger will lead to a poorly prepared film. The earlobe is sometimes used for making blood films if the finger site is unavailable or for special morphological studies. When the earlobe is used, it must be wiped thoroughly with alcohol and dried well, for it is waxy and wax may lead to bubbles in the film.

If venous blood rather than capillary blood is drawn, EDTA is the anticoagulant of choice. Most of the work in the hematology laboratory is now done on such venous blood. EDTA preserves the morphological features of the white and red cells and gives a more even distribution of the platelets. If blood is collected in EDTA for morphological studies, the film should be prepared as soon as possible, certainly within 2 hours. Balanced oxalate is not an acceptable anticoagulant for morphological studies because it distorts the shape and characteristics of some of the white cells and results in crenation of the red cells.

Preparation of the blood film

Blood is most often examined under the microscope by preparing a thin film or smear of blood on a glass slide or a cover glass, fixing the blood film, and then staining it with a polychromatic stain. Wet films of blood can also be prepared and observed with a phase-contrast microscope or by use of a supravital stain, but these techniques are used less often in the examination of blood.

When a cover glass is used to prepare a blood film, more of the prepared film can be examined, which reduces the sampling error. With a glass slide only a relatively small counting area can be examined. In addition, the leukocytes and platelets are more evenly distributed on a cover glass. The disadvantages of the cover glass method are that it is more time-consuming, more difficult to learn and perform correctly, and requires more care in handling the preparations. Automatic staining devices are available for glass slides, but not for cover glasses. Therefore, although the cover glass method is recommended by many hematologists, the glass slide method is far more commonly used. Only the latter method is described in detail in this text; however, the directions for the examination of the blood film also apply to the cover glass method. In either case, for the correct interpretation of a blood film, (1) the film must be prepared in a technically correct manner, (2) it must be stained correctly, and (3) it must be examined correctly. A film that is not prepared and stained correctly is useless for microscopic examination.

The equipment used for making blood films must be meticulously clean. Precleaned glass slides or slides cleaned with alcohol and wiped dry give the best results. Use of a spreading device is recommended—for example, a margin-free spreader slide with ground-glass edges may be used to spread the film of blood on the clean, lint-free slide. The edges of the spreader slide must be clean and free from chips. Cover glasses can also be used as spreading devices (See Fig. 3-13). The spreading device must be cleaned thoroughly with alcohol and dried between films, and it must be discarded when chipped or broken.

Procedure for making a blood film (slide method)

1. Place a drop of capillary or venous blood preserved with EDTA on one end of a slide, on the midline about 1 cm from the end. The drop should be about 2 mm in diameter (about the size of a match head), as shown in Fig. 3-14. Venous blood must be well mixed for at least 5 minutes on a mechanical rotator or by gentle inversion. If capillary blood is used, touch the top of the drop to the slide, being careful not to let the skin touch the slide. Transfer venous blood to the slide with the aid of two wooden applicator sticks or a capillary pipet.

2. Lay the specimen slide on a flat surface and hold it in position at the left end (these directions are for a right-handed person) with the center finger or the thumb and index finger of the left hand (Fig. 3-14).

3. Place the smooth clean edge of the spreader slide on the specimen slide just in front (to the left of) the drop of blood (Fig. 3-14).

4. Using the right hand, balance the spreader slide on one or two fingers (for example, the middle finger or the index and middle fingers) and draw it backward into the drop of blood at an angle of approximately 45° to the specimen slide.

5. Decrease the spreader slide angle to about 25–35° and allow the blood to flow evenly across the edge of the spreader slide (Fig. 3-14).

6. When the blood has spread evenly across the edge of the spreader slide, quickly push the spreader slide over the entire length of the specimen slide. As the spreader is moved, a thin film of blood will be deposited behind it. The blood film should take up one-half to three-fourths of the slide when properly prepared (Fig. 3-15).

7. Turn the spreader slide over (this gives another clean edge) and prepare a second blood film, using the same procedure. Two films should always be prepared for the same blood specimen.

8. Dry the blood film immediately by waving the slide rapidly through the air or by placing it in front of a fan.

9. Label the film by writing the name of the patient and the date in the blood at the thick end of the film, using a lead pencil (Fig. 3-15).

Fig. 3-13. Spreading devices.

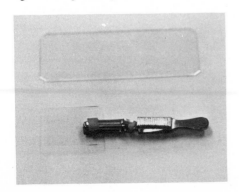

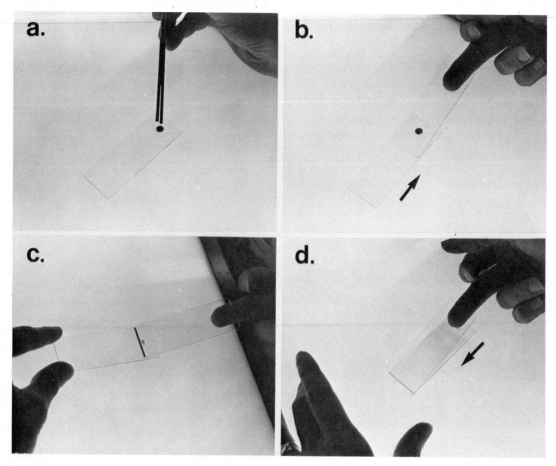

Fig. 3-14. Preparing the blood film.

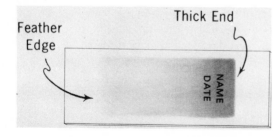

Fig. 3-15. Good blood film.

Feather Edge

Thick End

NAME
DATE

Criteria and precautions for a good blood film

A blood film should satisfy certain criteria when observed macroscopically, as shown in Fig. 3-15. The body of the film should be smooth and not interrupted by ridges, waves, or holes. It should be thickest at the origin and gradually thin out, rather than having alternate thick and thin areas. Pushing the spreader slide with an uneven motion results in thicker and thinner areas in the body of the film.

A good blood film should cover one-half to three-fourths of the length of the slide. All of the initial drop of blood should be incorporated in the film, not just part of it.

The thin end of the smear should have a good feather edge; that is, the film should fade away without a defined border on the end. In some institutions a fairly straight feather edge is sought, while others prefer a more tonguelike edge. We prefer a fairly straight feather edge, especially for doing a white blood cell differential count.

A defined border at the end of a blood film indicates that most of the white cells have piled up at the end. When this occurs, the heavier neutrophils accumulate at the end to a greater extent than the other types of white cells, giving an incorrect distribution of the types of white cells in the body of the smear. Platelets also tend to accumulate at the end of a smear, decreasing the number in the body of the smear.

Chipped or dirty spreader slides will cause abrupt endings, thin streaks in the body of the film, or tails of blood beyond the feather edge. This will also result in inaccurate percentages for the cell types within the body of the film, as the relatively stickier neutrophils and platelets tend to concentrate in such tails. Chips in the spreader slide may be detected by running the index finger lightly over the spreading edge. The spreader slide should be cleaned by rubbing it vigorously with a piece of gauze moistened with medicated alcohol. Be sure all the alcohol is evaporated (the edge is dry) before making the film.

Slides should be made in almost one motion; that is, the drop of blood should be placed on the slide and the smear made immediately. As soon as the blood is placed on the slide it should be spread, because drying of the blood drop will lead to an uneven distribution of cells in the body of the film and the larger white cells will accumulate at the end. Rouleau formation by the red cells and clumping of the platelets will also occur if the blood is not spread immediately. Pressing down on the spreader slide will also lead to an accumulation of white cells and platelets at

the end. This is why it should be balanced on the finger as the blood is spread, rather than held between the finger and thumb.

The degree of thickness or thinness of the blood film is also important. When a film is too thick the cells pile up, which makes them difficult to count and obscures their morphology. A very thin film is satisfactory for morphological studies, but it may be tedious to examine. The thickness of the film is determined by the size of the drop of blood used, the speed of the stroke used to move the spreader slide, and the angle at which the spreader slide is moved. A thick film results when the drop of blood is large, the angle is greater than $45°$, and the spreading motion is fast. A thin film results when the drop of blood is small, the angle is less than $35°$, and the motion is slow.

Blood films with vacuoles or bubbles result from the use of dirty slides or in some cases from an excess of fat in the specimen (as in a specimen obtained after a fatty meal).

Rapid drying of the blood film is essential. When blood films are not dried rapidly, the red cells become crenated, the white cells shrink, and there is an increase in rouleau formation by the red cells.

Only a small part of a blood film is actually examined microscopically. This part is referred to as the examination or counting area, as shown in Fig. 3-16. The counting area must be one where the red and white cells are clearly separated and well distributed. It should be about one cell thick and approximately 6–7 mm ($\frac{1}{4}$ in) long.

Staining the blood film

After a blood film has been prepared, the next step is the staining procedure. The blood film should be stained as soon as possible. If it cannot be stained within a few hours it should be fixed by immersion in absolute methyl alcohol (methanol) for 1 or 2 seconds and air-dried. If

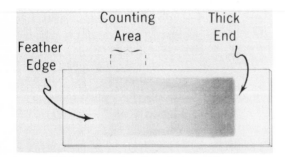

Fig. 3-16. Blood film: Counting area.

this is not done, the slides will stain with a pale blue background of dried plasma.

The stain most often used for the examination of blood films is Wright's stain or a variation of it, Wright-Giemsa stain. Both Wright's stain and Wright-Giemsa stain are adaptations of polychrome Romanovsky stains. Such polychrome stains produce multiple colors when applied to cells, since they are made up of both basic and acidic aniline dyes. Romanovsky stains contain methylene blue (a basic dye), eosin (an acidic dye) and methylene azure (an oxidation product of methylene blue also referred to as polychrome methylene blue). Variations of the Romanovsky stains differ in the way the methylene azure is produced or added to the stains.

Polychrome stains produce multiple colors since they dye both acidic and basic cell components in an acid-base reaction. The acidic cell components such as nuclei (nuclear DNA) and cytoplasmic RNA are stained blue-violet by the basic methylene azure. They are called basophilic (base-loving) as they stain with the basic dye. The more basic cell components such as hemoglobin and eosinophilic granules are stained orange to pink and are called acidophilic (acid-loving) since they stain with the acidic dye. Some structures within cells stain with both components, such as the neutrophilic granules, while the azurophilic granules stain with methylene azure.

The staining method for blood films fixes dead cells, as opposed to supravital staining, which is done with living cells. Fixation is the process by which the blood is made to adhere to the slide and the cellular proteins are coagulated. Wright's stain and Wright-Giemsa stain are used as methanol solutions. The blood cells are fixed by the methanol in the first step of the staining reaction when the Wright-Giemsa dye mixture is added to the blood film. Heat can also be used for fixation, but it is not necessary when the stain contains methanol. The actual polychrome staining of the blood film takes place in the second step of the procedure when an aqueous phosphate buffer solution with a pH of 6.4 is added to the Wright-Giemsa dye.

Wright's stain or Wright-Giemsa stain can be purchased as a dry powder, which is diluted in absolute, anhydrous, acetone-free methyl alcohol (CP), or as a prepared methanol solution. Both powders and solutions are certified by the Commission of Staining.* The preparation of methylene azure by oxidation of methylene blue and addition of eosin is quite complex, so Wright's stain powder may vary slightly from lot to lot.

Preparation of Wright-Giemsa stain and buffer

1. Wright-Giemsa stain. The dye can be purchased as a powder and diluted in methanol.

a. Dissolve 2.0 g of certified Wright's dye and 0.1 g of Giemsa dye in 800 ml of absolute, anhydrous, acetone-free methyl alcohol (CP).

b. Mix the reagents in a tightly stoppered brown bottle.

c. Shake the mixture vigorously at intervals for several days.

d. Allow the stain to age for about 1 month before use. Incubation of the stain at 37°C will hasten the aging process.

e. Filter the stain each day before use.

*H. J. Conn and M. S. Darrow, "Staining Procedures Used by the Biological Stain Commission," 2d ed., Williams & Wilkins Co., Baltimore, 1960.

2. Phosphate buffer (pH 6.4).

a. Dilute 6.63 g of anhydrous monobasic potassium phosphate (KH_2PO_4) and 2.56 g of anhydrous dibasic sodium phosphate (Na_2HPO_4) to 1000 ml with deionized water. (Some authors say that distilled water may be substituted for the buffer if the pH is approximately 6.4. This is not recommended as the pH of water may vary daily.)

b. Check the pH of the prepared phosphate buffer with a pH meter before use. The resulting solution can be made more alkaline by decreasing the amount of monobasic potassium phosphate and increasing the amount of dibasic sodium phosphate.

Procedure for staining blood films

1. Place the air-dried blood film on a level staining rack, with the film side up and the feather edge away from your body.

2. Fix the film by *flooding* the slide with the *filtered* stain. The amount of stain is important. There must be enough to avoid excessive evaporation, which would result in precipitation of stain on the slide.

3. Allow the stain to remain on the slide for 3–5 minutes. This is the fixation period. Determine the exact timing for each batch of stain used.

4. Without removing the Wright-Giemsa stain, add phosphate buffer, using about $1-1\frac{1}{2}$ times as much buffer as stain on the slide so that a layer piles up but none spills off. Add the buffer dropwise, then blow on the surface to mix the stain and buffer. A metallic greenish sheen should form on the surface when the slide is buffered adequately.

5. Allow the stain and buffer mixture to remain on the slide for 10–15 minutes. During this time the staining takes place as a result of the combination of dye and buffer at the correct pH.

6. Wash the slide with a steady stream of deionized water. Precipitation of the metallic scum on the film must be avoided. This is done by first flooding the slide with water, then washing and tipping the slide simultaneously. If this is not done and the dye is poured off the slide before it is washed, the insoluble metallic scum will settle on the blood film.

7. Wipe the dye from the back of the slide when it is still wet by rubbing with a piece of moist gauze.

8. Place the slide in a vertical position to air-dry, with the feather edge (thin edge) up. Never blot a blood film dry. The heaviest part of the film is at the bottom to allow precipitated stain to flow away from the thin edge, which will be used for examination of the blood film.

9. Do not use the slide for microscopic examination until it is dry.

Characteristics of a properly stained blood film

If the blood film has been stained properly, it will appear pink when observed with the naked eye. When examined microscopically with the low-power ($\times$10) objective, the film should be thin enough so that the red and white cells are clearly separated. There should not be an excessive accumulation of white cells and platelets at the edge of the film. In addition, there should be no precipitated stain.

The background or space between the cells should be clear. The red blood cells should appear red-orange through the microscope. Correctly stained leukocytes should have the following colors under the microscope. The lymphocytes and neutrophils should have dark purple nuclei, while the monocyte nuclei should be lighter purple. The granules should be bright orange in the eosinophils and dark blue in the basophils. The appearance of the cytoplasm varies with the different types of leukocytes. In monocytes, the cytoplasm should be blue-gray or have a faint bluish tinge. The neutrophil cytoplasm should be light pink with lilac granules, and the lymphocyte cytoplasm should be a shade of blue, generally clear blue or robin's-egg blue. The platelets should stain violet to purple. If the blood film does not meet these criteria, it should be discarded and a new film should be stained and examined.

Precautions and comments on staining blood films

When staining the blood film, it is important that the staining rack be level so that the stain is uniform throughout the film.

It is important that the stain and buffer be made correctly. The stain should stand for 1 month before it is used, and the pH of the buffer must be correct. With every new batch of stain and buffer, the fixing and staining times should be checked by staining a few slides. If staining of the cells is satisfactory, the times used for fixing and staining should be noted and used with that batch of reagents. If the pH is too acid or too alkaline, the stain will give a false color and appearance to the cells.

Adequate fixing time must be allowed. A minimum of 3 minutes is recommended for the initial reaction of the blood film and Wright-Giemsa stain. Since inadequate fixation allows dissolution of the nuclear chromatin, overfixation is preferable. To achieve the proper staining reactions in the cells, the stain and buffer must be prepared correctly, the correct timing must be determined for each batch of stain and buffer, and the correct staining technique must be used.

Properly applied Wright-Giemsa stain dyes both acidic and basic components of the blood cells. The phosphate buffer controls the pH of the staining system. If the pH is too acid, the parts of the cell taking up acidic dye will be overstained and will appear too red, while the parts of the cells taking up basic dye will appear pale. If the pH of the staining system is too alkaline, the parts of the cells taking up basic dye will be overstained, giving an overall blue effect, with very dark blue to black nuclear chromatin and bluish red cells.

The following situations will indicate *staining errors. A faded or washed out appearance of all the cells* is caused by overwashing, understaining or underfixing, leaving water on the slide, or using improperly made stain. When the slide has an *excessively blue appearance* on gross examination, the red cells will appear blue-red and the white cells will be darker and more granular microscopically. This may result from overfixing or overstaining, inadequate washing, using a stain or buffer that is too alkaline, or using too thick a film. It may be corrected by decreasing the fixation time (the time before the buffer is added to the dye), or increasing the time during which the buffer and stain mixture stands on the slide. Alternatively, the amount of stain used may be decreased and the amount of buffer increased. Finally, the pH of the buffer may be checked with a pH meter and readjusted to 6.4, or a new Wright-Giemsa stain may be tried. When the slide has an *excessively red appearance* to the naked eye, the red cells will appear bright red, the white cells will appear indistinct with pale blue rather than purple nuclei, and brilliant red eosinophilic granules will be seen microscopically. This may be caused by understaining; overwashing; or use of stain, buffer, or wash water that is too acid. To correct this situation the following measures may be tried. The fixation or staining time may be increased. The washing technique may be corrected so that it is adequate but not excessive. The pH of the buffer and water may be checked with a pH meter and adjusted, or a new stain or buffer may be used. *Large amounts of precipitated stain* on the film result from either improper washing (not washing enough to remove the metallic scum) or using an old stain that has started to precipitate. This may be corrected by using the proper washing technique—first flooding the slide with water and then tipping and washing the slide simultaneously—and making sure the stain is filtered daily.

Examination of the blood film

Since accurate examination of the blood film depends on proper use of the microscope, a general review of the procedure to be used is presented for the student viewing a blood film for the first time (see also Use of the Microscope in Chap. 1). The film is first examined with the low-power ($\times$10) objective, moving the slide with the mechanical stage to get different areas into the field of view. The difference in appearance of the various areas results from the technique used in preparing the film: the film is relatively thick at the beginning and gradually thins out to a feather edge. Most of the cells seen under the low-power objective are red blood cells, which appear as small, round, reddish orange bodies.

Scattered among the red-staining cells are the less numerous white blood cells, which are larger and more complex in appearance than the red blood cells. The white cells consist of nuclei surrounded by cytoplasm. The nuclei stain purple, and the cytoplasms stain different colors, depending on their contents. The size of the cell; the shape, size, and chromatin pattern of the nucleus; the presence of nucleoli in the nucleus; and the contents, staining reaction, and relative size of the cytoplasm are used in the identification of white blood cells.

With the low-power objective, an area of the film is found where the red cells are just touching and are not overlapping or piled on top of one another. This area will be found near the feather edge of the film (see Fig. 3-16). The color of the cells should be examined at this magnification. When this area has been found, the oil-immersion ($\times$95–97) objective should be used next. The high-dry ($\times$45) objective is not suitable for examination of blood films, as important morphological changes cannot be seen at this magnification. To change to the oil-immersion lens, the low-power objective is pivoted out of position and a drop of immersion oil is placed on the selected site (where the red cells are just touching each other). The oil-immersion lens is pivoted into the oil while looking at it from the side. The oil must be in direct contact with the lens. If necessary, it can be focused with the fine adjustment. If the slide has been placed upside down on the microscope stage, it will be impossible to bring the blood cells into focus. More light will be needed with the oil-immersion lens. It can be obtained by repositioning the condenser (which should be all the way up for maximum resolution under oil immersion), opening the iris diaphragm, and turning up the rheostat.

Under the oil-immersion objective, red cells appear as round, structureless bodies containing no nuclei, granules, or discrete material. The red color is darker at the edge of the cell than in the center. This variation is caused by the biconcave shape of the red cell, which contains less pigment (hemoglobin) in its thinner center. With oil immersion, most of the red cells in a normal blood film are about the same size, averaging 7.2 μm in diameter. A normal red cell is uniformly round on a dry film, although variations in shape can be produced by poor spreading technique in the preparation of the blood film.

When experience has been gained in using the microscope to view blood films, a more specific technique is used to observe the morphological features of the blood cells.

Certain things must be done whenever peripheral blood films are examined. The blood film must first be evaluated for acceptable gross appearance and staining, as previously described. It must be evaluated for acceptable white cell distribution by observing the feather edge under low power. The numbers of erythrocytes, leukocytes, and platelets should be estimated, and the erythrocyte and platelet morphology should be described. Finally, the percentage of each type of leukocyte should be estimated.

Procedure for examination of the blood film

After the initial manipulations of the microscope and the observations described above, the following steps are taken in the examination of every blood film. These steps will be described in detail; however, in more general terms the blood film will be examined under low power and oil immersion. The *low-power examination* of the blood film should include (1) an evaluation of the quality of the blood film, and (2) an estimate of the red cell count and the leukocyte count, and a scan of the blood film. The *oil-immersion examination* of the blood film should include (1) an examination of the erythrocytes for alterations and variations in morphology, (2) an evaluation of platelet numbers and morphology, and (3) the differential count of the leukocytes and examination of the leukocytes for morphological alterations. Detailed descriptions of these steps follow.

1. *Evaluate the quality of the blood film, using the low-power objective.*

The film should be thin enough that the red and white cells are clearly separated. The space between the cells should be clear. There should be no precipitated dye. The red and white cells should be properly stained, and there should not be a large accumulation of white cells at the feather edge of the blood film. If the blood film does not meet these criteria, it should not be examined further; a new film must be made.

2. *Estimate the red and white cell counts and scan for abnormal cells and clumps of platelets, using the low-power objective.*

A rough estimate of the red cell count can be made by noting the number of cells and the space between them. Normally, fewer and fewer intercellular spaces will be seen as one moves into the thicker portion of the blood film. In the optimal counting area, there should be no agglutination (clumping) or rouleaux (cells stacked like coins).

A blood film should be used to check every white cell count. The number of white cells is estimated in the counting area of the film (the area where the red cells lie side by side with no overlapping) with the low-power objective. With the low-power objective (×10) and the usual

eyepiece (×10)—a total magnification of ×100—approximately 20-30 white cells per field are equivalent to a white cell count of approximately 5000 cells/μl. Under the same magnification, 40-60 white cells per field are equivalent to a white cell count of approximately 10 000 cells/μl. In other words, 5 white blood cells in one low-power field are equal to approximately 1000 cells/μl. Five low-power fields should be counted and the number of white cells averaged to estimate the white cell count.

The slide should also be examined under low power for the presence of immature or abnormal cells. With experience, the cells may be recognizable under low power; however, they are positively identified under oil immersion. If very few such abnormal cells are present they may be overlooked if the slide is examined under oil immersion alone, where the examination area is much smaller. Such abnormal cells should be looked for especially in the feather edge and along the sides of the slide.

The optimal counting area, sides, and feather edge should also be scanned for clumps of platelets. Clumps of platelets should not be seen normally; however, when the platelet count is increased they may be found along the sides and in the feather edge.

3. *Examine red cells for alterations and variations in morphological features under oil immersion.*

The normal red cell is a nonnucleated biconcave disk containing hemoglobin. Most red cells measure 7.2-7.9 μm on a stained blood film.[34] The normal red cell is approximately 2 μm thick; values of 2.14, 2.05, 1.84, and 1.64 μm have been reported as the normal mean thickness.[35] Its mean volume, calculated from the hematocrit and the red cell count, is 87 fl.[35] In estimating the diameters of white blood cells or other structures, it is often advantageous to use the red cell as a 7-μm measuring stick.

When normal red cells are studied on dried and stained blood films, they are nearly uniform in size. Such cells are referred to as *normocytic*. A tool that may be used in evaluating red cell size is a micrometer disk, which is inserted into the microscope; however, this is not necessary with experience. The normal red cell appears as a disk with a rim of hemoglobin and a clear central area, referred to as central pallor. The area of central pallor is normally less than half the diameter of a red cell, although there is some variation within the film. The amount of color in the cell (the staining reaction) and the corresponding amount of central pallor reflect the amount of hemoglobin in the cell. Normal red cells are pink. The staining reaction is referred to in terms of chromasia, and red cells with a normal amount of color are referred to as *normochromic* or, less frequently, *orthochromatic*. Normochromic, normocytic red cells are shown in Fig. 3-17.

It is important to observe red cell morphology only in the optimal counting area. In the thick end of the film the morphological characteristics of the cell are difficult to distinguish, and at the very thin edge of the film the red cells flatten out, appear completely filled with hemoglobin (showing no area of central pallor), and are generally distorted.

When red cells are examined morphologically,

Fig. 3-17. Normal red blood cells (oil-immersion objective).

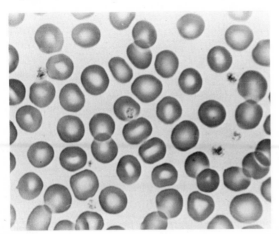

the following characteristics must be observed and noted: (1) variations in color, (2) variations in size, (3) variations in shape, (4) variations in structure and inclusions, (5) the presence of artifacts and abnormal distribution patterns, and (6) the presence of nucleated red cells. These changes will be thoroughly described under Red Cell Alterations. A brief summary follows.

Various terms are used to describe changes in the red cell shape, size, and staining reaction. Alterations in size are described by the terms *anisocytosis*, excessive variation in cell size; *macrocytosis*, predominance of large red cells, with a mean corpuscular diameter (MCD) greater than 9 µm; and *microcytosis*, predominance of small red cells, with an MCD less than 6.5 µm. Alterations in shape are described in terms of *poikilocytes*, red cells with markedly irregular shapes; *sickle cells*, red cells that are sickle-shaped or long and clublike in appearance; *spherocytes*, small, spherical red cells that appear round and completely filled with hemoglobin; and *ovalocytes*, red cells that are oval. Variations in the staining reaction are described by terms such as *hypochromasia*, lack of color (pale-staining cells with very pale central areas); *anochromasia*, concentration of pale-staining hemoglobin around the periphery of the cells, with the center pale; *orthochromasia* or *normochromasia*, the normal amount of hemoglobin and normal staining; and *polychromasia*, mixed staining because of the presence of RNA and hemoglobin (polychromatic "red" cells vary in color from muddy blue to a grayish red-orange and appear as reticulocytes when stained supravitally). The degree of the observed red cell alteration is noted as slight, moderate, or marked.

Several inclusions are also seen under certain conditions in the red cells, and they must be identified. *Basophilic stippling* is seen as pinpoint to granular particles stained blue-green to blue-black. These particles consist of precipitated RNA. Some red cells that show basophilic stippling with Wright's stain will prove to be siderocytes. *Siderocytes* are red cells that contain particulate iron, which stains bright blue-green after treatment with ferric ferrocyanide (Prussian blue). *Howell-Jolly bodies* are spherical particles 1-2 μm in diameter that stain purple to black. These particles are also nuclear remnants, and one or more may be present within a red blood cell.

Rouleau formation by the red cells is also to be noted. It is seen in certain disease conditions, but more often is caused by poor technique in the slide preparation. When the blood film is not dried immediately after it is spread on the slide, rouleaux can result.

4. *Correct white cell count for nucleated red cells, when present.*

When nucleated red cells (*normoblasts*) are seen on the blood film, the number of these cells per 100 white cells is reported. It is necessary to correct the total white cell count when normoblasts are present, since they are not destroyed by the 2% acetic acid used for the white cell count and will be counted along with the white cells. The total white cell count can be corrected in the following way:

Corrected white cell count

$$= \frac{\text{uncorrected white cell count} \times 100}{100 + \text{number of nucleated RBCs per 100 WBCs}}$$

5. *Evaluate the platelet count and morphological changes with the oil-immersion objective.*

The blood film is examined with the oil-immersion objective to estimate the number of platelets and to detect morphological alterations. The platelet count is estimated as adequate, decreased, or increased.

Platelets generally vary from 2 to 5 μm in diameter. They are ovoid structures having a colorless to pale blue background (hyalomere) containing centrally located, reddish to violet granules (chromomere). Platelets are not cells, but portions of cytoplasm pinched off from megakaryocytes, giant cells of the bone marrow. Platelets are often increased in size when the

blood is being actively regenerated; their size is also a function of age, with younger cells being generally larger. Bizarre forms are also noted after splenectomy and in myelofibrosis, hemorrhagic thrombocytosis, and polycythemia vera. Giant platelets are characteristic of platelet disorders associated with thrombocytopenia.

Normally, 6-20 platelets should be seen in each oil-immersion field, representing a normal platelet count of 140 000-400 000/μl. A rough estimate of the platelet count can be made by letting each platelet seen in an oil-immersion field equal approximately 20 000 platelets/μl. Values as low as three to five platelets per oil-immersion field have been considered to represent a normal platelet count. The difference in normal values is probably a result of the use of specimens from different sources: the lower value is more consistent with capillary blood, where some of the platelets are utilized in the clotting mechanism, while the higher value is consistent with anticoagulated venous blood.

One scheme for estimating platelet counts follows. The platelet estimate is reported as adequate if 6-20 platelets are seen per oil-immersion field. Several fields should be checked, and the platelets should be kept in mind while doing the white cell differential. If the average number of platelets is less than six, the estimate should be reported as a *slight*, *moderate*, or *marked decrease*, depending on the magnitude of the decrease. Before this is done, however, the slide should be scanned for clumps of platelets with the low-power objective, especially in the feather edge. If the blood film is well made, without aggregates at the feather edge, and platelets can be found only with great difficulty, the platelet count is below 20 000 platelets/μl. In addition, the tube of blood should be rechecked for the presence of clots, as platelets would be utilized in the clots and the blood film value artificially decreased. If there are more than 20 platelets per oil-immersion field, the estimate should be reported as a *slight*, *moderate*, or *marked increase*, depending on the magnitude of the increase. If there are many masses of platelets at the feather edge and platelets are sufficiently abundant to attract the attention of the observer, it is reasonable to assume almost automatically that the platelet count is increased.

The platelet morphology should be observed and the presence of large, bizarre, or atypical forms should be reported. These should also be observed while doing the white cell differential (Fig. 3-18).

6. *Perform the differential count of white cells and examine for morphological alterations, using the oil-immersion objective.*

The differential count consists of identifying and counting a minimum of 100 white cells. After the red cells and platelets have been examined, the white cells are classified and counted in the optimal counting area of the blood film under oil immersion. The slide should be moved in a way that will allow continuous counting and classification of white cells from margin to margin of the film. When a margin is reached, the slide should be moved toward the thicker end (a distance of one or two microscope

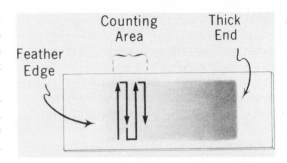

Fig. 3-19. Pathway for differential cell count.

fields) and the white cells counted and classified from margin to margin again (see Fig. 3-19). When exactly 100 white cells have been counted, the numbers of the different types of white cells recorded are estimates of the percentages of these types comprising the total white cell count. For example, if 3 of the 100 cells counted are eosinophils, then 3 percent of the circulating white cells are assumed to be eosinophils.

If any nucleated red cells are encountered in the white cell differential, they should be counted separately; they should not be included in the 100 cells counted. However, the white cell count must be corrected when nucleated red cell forms are noted. This correction was described in step 4 above.

In certain situations it may be necessary to count more or fewer than 100 cells. If the relative numbers of specific types of white cells differ markedly from the accepted normal values, it is advisable to count 200 cells or more before recording percentages. Specifically, 200 cells should be counted if more than 5 percent of the cells are eosinophils, if more than 2 percent are basophils, if more than 10 percent are monocytes, or if the percentage of lymphocytes is greater than that of neutrophils (except in children). If the differential for an adult with a normal white cell count shows fewer than 15 or more than 40 lymphocytes, an additional 100 cells should be counted on another blood film to rule out distribution errors. In cases of leukopenia, if the white cell count is less than 1000

Fig. 3-18. Platelets.

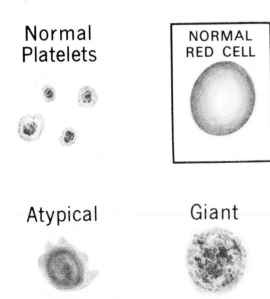

Normal Platelets

NORMAL RED CELL

Atypical

Giant

cells/μl, only 50 cells should be counted in the white cell differential. When such changes are made, the percentages of the different cell types must be calculated, and the number of cells actually counted in the differential must be noted on the report form; for example, 3 percent basophils—200 cells counted. Occasionally, the absolute number of cells of each type is of interest, although values are usually reported as percentages. To calculate the absolute value, multiply the percentage of each cell type, expressed as a decimal, by the total white cell count.

As the cells are being classified and counted, any morphological alterations or abnormalities should be noted, as described later in this section. A white cell cannot be skipped because it cannot be identified. Experience is necessary for morphological studies of white cells, especially when an immature or abnormal cell is seen. Individuals with limited training in hematology should not attempt to identify abnormal white cells. This should be done by a more qualified person, such as a pathologist or a medical technologist with special hematologic training. Persons with limited training should be able to identify and classify the normal white cells, but should be encouraged to seek assistance when a questionable cell is seen.

Normal leukocyte morphology

The five types of white blood cells encountered in normal peripheral blood are shown in Fig. 3-20. Certain characteristics should be kept in mind when cells are to be classified; these are related to size, the nucleus, and the cytoplasm. Whether the cell is small, medium, or large and how it compares to a normal red blood cell, which is approximately 7 μm in diameter, should be noted. Characteristics of the nucleus that should be considered are the shape, the size compared to the rest of the cell, the chromatin

Fig. 3-20. Leukocytes.

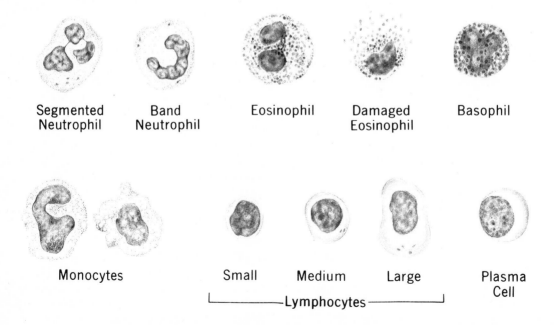

Segmented Neutrophil   Band Neutrophil   Eosinophil   Damaged Eosinophil   Basophil

Monocytes   Small   Medium   Large   Plasma Cell

└──────── Lymphocytes ────────┘

pattern (smooth or coarse), and the presence of nucleoli. Characteristics of the cytoplasm that should be considered include the presence or absence of granules, their staining characteristics, and whether they are specific or nonspecific, as well as the staining properties and relative amount of the cytoplasm. These properties should be noted for all types of cells that may be encountered in the peripheral blood or bone marrow, whether they are of the granulocyte, lymphocyte, erythrocyte, or megakaryocyte series.

Segmented neutrophils

The most numerous of the granulocytes are the polymorphonuclear neutrophilic (PMN) leukocytes or segmented neutrophilic granulocytes. The mean total neutrophil count for adults is 53 percent with a range of 35–71 percent. The mean adult value for segmented neutrophils is 44 percent with a range of 25–63 percent.[36] Infants and children have fewer neutrophils and more lymphocytes (see under Normal Values for Some Hematologic Procedures). Neutrophils vary in diameter from about 9 to 15 μm, and the nucleus forms a relatively small part of the cell. The nucleus can assume various shapes, but its usual configuration is lobular—that is, the elongated nucleus is usually constricted in one to four places, forming a series of bulges or lobes connected by narrow strands of chromatin or narrow filaments; it may have two to five lobes. The chromatin is irregularly arranged in fairly compact masses, and it stains deep reddish purple. These chromatin masses are distinct and clearly distinguishable from the lighter-staining (generally pink-staining) parachromatin (nucleoplasm or karyoplasm). The nuclear membrane is distinct, and no nucleoli are visible. The abundant cytoplasm has a faint pink color and contains a large number of very small, often indiscrete granules distributed throughout it irregularly. These granules are usually light pink or very light violet. A few darker granules may be present. About two-thirds of the granules are specific neutrophilic granules, while the remaining one-third are azurophilic.

Band neutrophils

The band neutrophil is a younger form of the mature neutrophil. Both segmented and band neutrophils should be classified separately in the white cell differential. The mean band neutrophil count for adults is 10 percent with a range of 0–22 percent.[36] Morphologically, band neutrophils are like segmented cells except for the shape of the nucleus. In band neutrophils the nucleus may be rod- or band-shaped, when distinct lobes have not yet formed, or it may have begun to form lobes. In the latter case, the lobes are connected by wide strips or bands rather than narrow threads or filaments as in segmented neutrophils. The College of American Pathologists defines a band as a connecting strip or isthmus that is wide enough to show two distinct margins with nuclear material in between. A filament, on the other hand, is so narrow that there is no visible nuclear material between the two sides. The differentiation between band and segmented neutrophils may be difficult; if there is doubt, the cell should be classified as segmented.[37] (See Fig. 3-20.)

Generally, an increased white cell count (leukocytosis) results from an increase in the absolute number of neutrophils present in the blood; in this case it is called *neutrophilia.* Neutrophilia is found in acute infections; metabolic, chemical, and drug intoxications; acute hemorrhage; postoperative states; certain noninflammatory conditions such as coronary thrombosis; malignant neoplasms; and after acute hemolytic episodes. It is usually accompanied by a "shift to the left," or an increase in the number of immature cells, and by toxic changes in the cytoplasm. An increase in the number of band forms, which may be accompanied by the presence of more immature neutrophils, is significant. The presence of forms more immature than bands is also termed a *leukoblastotic reaction*. Toxic changes in the neutrophil cytoplasm are indicated by the presence of deeply stained basophilic (or toxic) granules, pale blue Döhle bodies, and vacuolization. Toxic changes in the nucleus include hypersegmentation (more than five lobes) and degeneration or pyknosis. The cell size may be increased or decreased.

Eosinophils

Eosinophilic granular leukocytes, or eosinophils, make up 0–8 percent of the total number of leukocytes, with a mean of 3 percent.[38] They are slightly larger than neutrophils, and the nucleus occupies a relatively small part of the cell. The nucleus is also polymorphic, but it usually has fewer lobes than do neutrophil nuclei. Usually two and occasionally three lobes are seen. The nuclear structure is much like that of the neutrophil, but the lobes are plumper and the chromatin often stains lighter purple. The nuclear membrane is distinct, and no nucleoli are visible. The cytoplasm is usually colorless, but it may be faintly basophilic; it is crowded with spherical acidophilic granules, which stain red-orange with eosin and are larger and more distinct than neutrophilic granules. The eosinophilic granules are hard, firm bodies that are not easily damaged; they remain intact when pressed into the nucleus or even when the whole cell is damaged and the cell membrane broken. Eosinophilic granules are also highly refractive, a feature that is often a valuable distinguishing characteristic.

If more than five eosinophils are encountered in the 100-cell differential, 200 cells should be counted. The percentage of each cell type present should then be calculated and the number of cells counted noted on the report form.

Eosinophilia, an increase in the number of eosinophils above normal, is associated with allergic reaction, certain skin disorders, parasitic infections, certain infections such as brucellosis, Hodgkin's disease, and certain leukemias.

Basophils

Basophilic granular leukocytes, or basophils, comprise 0–1.8 percent of the total leukocytes, with a mean of 0.6 percent.[38] They are about the same size as neutrophils, but their nuclei usually occupy a relatively greater portion of the cell. The nucleus is often extremely irregular in shape, varying from a lobular form to a form showing indentations that are not deep enough to divide it into definite lobes. The nuclear pattern is indistinct; there appears to be a mixture of chromatin and parachromatin, and this mixture stains purple or blue and shows little structure. The nuclear membrane is fairly distinct and no nucleoli are visible. The cytoplasm is usually colorless; it contains a variable number of deeply stained, coarse, round or angular basophilic granules. The granules (metachromatic) stain deep purple or black; occasionally a few smaller, brownish granules may be present. Since the granules are soluble in water, occasionally a few or even most of them may be dissolved during the staining procedure. When this occurs, the cell will contain vacuoles in place of granules, and the cytoplasm may appear grayish or brownish in their vicinity. The cytoplasm of a mature basophil is colorless. An immature basophil has a pale blue cytoplasm and is seen only in granulocytic (myelogenous) leukemia.

If more than two basophils are encountered in the 100-cell differential, 200 cells should be counted. *Basophilia*, an increase in the number of basophils, is associated with chronic granulocytic leukemia. It is also seen in allergic reactions, myeloid metaplasia, and polycythemia vera. The basophil number may increase temporarily after irradiation, and basophilia may be present in chronic hemolytic anemia and after splenectomy.

Tissue basophils, also called *mast cells*, are similar but not identical to basophilic granulocytes. They are larger and differ somewhat in their chemical makeup and function.

Monocytes

Monocytes constitute 2-12 percent of the leukocytes in the blood of normal adults, with a mean of 7 percent.[38] They are the largest of the normal leukocytes, measuring 12-20 μm in diameter. The nucleus is fairly large; it may be oval, lobular, notched, or polymorphic, but most frequently it is kidney-shaped. It stains faintly, usually with a very characteristic pattern. Chromatin and parachromatin are sharply segregated, and the chromatin is distributed in a linear arrangement of delicate strands, which gives the nucleus a stringy appearance. (Occasionally the nuclear pattern resembles that of a lymphocyte, and the cytoplasmic differences must be relied on for identification.) The nuclear membrane is delicate but not distinct, and nucleoli usually are not seen. The cytoplasm is abundant, slightly basophilic, and often vacuolated, and has a slate-gray or muddy blue color. Extremely fine and abundant azurophilic granules are present; this granulation is called *azure dust* and is seen only in monocytes. The granules vary in color from light pink to bright purplish red.

Lymphocytes

Lymphocytes constitute 20-53 percent of the leukocytes in the normal adult, with a mean value of 36 percent.[38] Infants and children normally have more lymphocytes and fewer neutrophils than adults. Lymphocytes fall in three size groups: small (8-10 μm), medium (10-12 μm), and large (12-16 μm).[39] There are numerous gradations of size and form from one type to another; some lymphocytes can be as large as monocytes.

The small lymphocyte is composed chiefly of nucleus. The nucleus is round or slightly notched, and the nuclear chromatin is in the form of coarse, dense, deeply staining blocks. There is relatively little parachromatin, and it is not very distinct. Almost the entire nucleus stains deep purple. The nuclear membrane is heavy and distinct, and nucleoli are not usually seen. The cytoplasm appears in the form of a narrow band that stains relatively dark blue, usually free of azure granules.

The medium-sized lymphocyte has a larger nucleus but relatively more cytoplasm than nucleus. The nucleus is round, oval, or slightly notched, and the nuclear chromatin stains dark purple. The chromatin, as in the small lymphocyte, is in the form of heavy blocks, or clumps. Some lighter-staining parachromatin is present, but for the most part it blends in with the chromatin and is not distinct. The nuclear membrane is heavy and distinct, and nucleoli usually are not seen. The cytoplasm may appear smooth and homogeneous or somewhat spongy. It may be almost colorless or may vary from pale blue-green to deeper but somewhat powdery blue. If azure granules are present in the cytoplasm, they are usually spherical and light pink; they vary in size from slightly larger than neutrophil granules to the size of eosinophil granules.

The large lymphocyte shows a further increase in the size of the nucleus and an increase in the relative amount of cytoplasm. The nucleus contains more parachromatin, and so stains more lightly than the nuclei of the smaller forms. However, the chromatin is still present in clumps, without distinct outlines because of the blending of chromatin and parachromatin. The nuclear membrane is distinct and nucleoli usually are not seen. The cytoplasm in this form can be abundant and is most frequently smooth; it may, however, be spongy. It stains in the same way as the cytoplasm of medium-sized lymphocytes, and azure granules are frequently seen. Nucleoli are rarely seen in lymphocytes of normal blood, but they may be seen in cells that have been crushed during the spreading of the film. It is possible that blood lymphocytes contain nucleoli but that they are normally obscured by the coarse nuclear chromatin.

It is sometimes difficult to distinguish between nucleated red cells (normoblasts) and small lymphocytes. The staining reaction of the parachromatin of the two cells is an important diagnostic criterion; the parachromatin of the lymphocyte is pale blue or violet, and that of the normoblast is red or pink. In addition, the cytoplasm of nucleated erythrocytes contains hemoglobin, which stains pink in blood films.

Lymphocytosis, an increase in the number of lymphocytes, is characteristic of certain acute infections (infectious mononucleosis, pertussis, mumps, and rubella, or German measles) and of chronic infections such as tuberculosis, brucellosis, and infectious hepatitis. The toxic changes seen in these diseases are referred to as reactive changes, and are particularly associated with infectious mononucleosis. The cells are called reactive lymphocytes, as the increased amount and apparent activity of the cytoplasm indicate that it may be reacting to some sort of stimulus (see under Leukocyte Alterations).

Plasma cells

In addition to the five types of white cells that normally appear in the peripheral blood, the *plasma cell* (*plasmacyte*) can occur in certain blood specimens. The plasma cell is thought to be a derivative of the lymphocyte or a primitive connective tissue cell. It is large, with a round or oval nucleus that is usually in an eccentric position. The chromatin consists of deeply stained, heavy masses that may be arranged in a radial pattern. The cytoplasm is strongly basophilic. There may be a pale, clear zone in the cytoplasm to one side of the nucleus, referred to as a *hof*. Immature forms may occasionally be seen. Plasma cells function in the synthesis of immunoglobulins. They may be found in the peripheral blood in cases of measles, chickenpox, or scarlet fever and in the malignant conditions multiple myeloma and plasmacytic leukemia.

Blood cell alterations

Morphological changes in the red and white blood cells seen on the stained blood film aid in determining the nature of many blood diseases. Certain diseases produce fairly characteristic alterations of red cells, white cells, and platelets, in addition to other clinical signs. It is most important that the laboratory personnel be well acquainted with the appearance of normal blood cells, so that abnormal or immature cell forms will be recognized immediately. Abnormal or immature cells should be identified by someone experienced in cell morphology. The technician should screen the films and give questionable ones to a pathologist or an experienced medical technologist for final evaluation.

Most abnormalities found in white cells are related to the age of the cell. All white cells in the circulating blood should be mature, and the presence of immature white cells in the blood is considered abnormal. Immature white cells may be differentiated from mature ones by size, the appearance of intracellular structure (e.g., the presence of granules or changes in the nucleoli, chromatin, or nucleus), the staining properties, and the cell function. There is a progressive decrease in cell size with maturity, with the nucleus becoming smaller and the cytoplasmic ratio correspondingly increasing. In granulocytes, granules appear with maturity. In immature white cells the nucleus is round; with age it becomes lobular or indented. Chromatin is fine and lacy in the young cell and eventually becomes coarse and clumped. Nucleoli may be present in young cells and absent in the mature forms. The cytoplasm is basophilic (stains blue) in young granulocytes, and eventually turns pink with maturity. The young nucleus stains reddish violet and becomes strongly basophilic with maturity. The granules in the cytoplasm assume specific staining qualities with increasing cell maturity.

Certain evidence of cell function is observed that is characteristic of specific developmental stages of the white cells. Examples are the presence of nucleoli, which indicate a young cell; mitotic figures, which indicate a young cell; cytoplasmic inclusions, which are characteristic of a mature cell; phagocytosis, which is seen in mature cells; and hemoglobin, which is seen in mature red cells.

The technician should be able to differentiate an immature cell from a mature one. There are many stages of young cells, and it is not necessary for the technician to be able to differentiate among these stages; the trained medical technologist or pathologist makes this evaluation. The medical laboratory technician should be aware of the various developmental stages of the blood cells, and for this reason the following material is presented.

Origin and function of blood cells related to morphological examination and alterations

Final agreement on the origin of all types of blood cells and their relationships to one another has not been reached, and several theories have been put forth. Practically speaking, the origin of blood cells is not important for their identification. Probably the two most popular theories are the *polyphyletic* theory and the *unitarian* theory. According to the polyphyletic theory, all blood cells originate from two or more specific primitive cells. According to the unitarian theory, all blood cells have a common origin in one type of cell, which is given various names, such as the reticuloendothelial cell, the undifferentiated mesenchyme or stem cell, the reticulum cell, and the hemocytoblast.

The original hemopoietic cell has the following properties, which can be considered characteristic of young cells in general. The cell is large, approximately 20–40 μm in diameter on films prepared with Wright's stain. It has abundant cytoplasm, which is slightly basophilic or blue and which may contain a few nonspecific azuro-

philic granules. The margin of the cell is not clearly defined; it is usually indefinite. The nucleus is small in relation to the rest of the cell. The chromatin pattern is fine and open (the term reticular pattern is based on the appearance of this nucleus). The nucleus stains pale rose-purple.

A diagrammatic representation of the unitarian theory, showing the origin and relationships of all blood cell types, is given in Fig. 3-21. It should be remembered that this is theoretical and the actual details are unknown. All stages in the maturation process are gradual, and it is often impossible to identify an exact stage with certainty. The most immature forms in all series (pronormoblast, myeloblast, lymphoblast, and plasmablast) appear very similar morphologically, and their identification is often based on surrounding cell types in various stages of development. The origin of the monocyte is still largely unknown, although it is believed to originate in the bone marrow.

Erythrocyte maturation

Red blood cells are normally produced in the bone marrow. Their maturation takes 3–5 days, and six stages of development have been described. Several systems of nomenclature have been used to describe these stages, two of which will be discussed here. The stages of erythrocyte maturation from the youngest to the mature cell are: pronormoblast (rubriblast), basophilic normoblast (prorubricyte), polychromatic normoblast (rubricyte), orthochromatic normoblast (metarubricyte), reticulocyte (diffusely basophilic erythrocyte), and mature erythrocyte. These stages are diagrammed in Fig. 3-22 (see also Fig. 3-21).

Remember that cells do not jump from one stage to another; there is a gradual progression, and exact classification is often very difficult. Rather than learning the characteristics of the specific stages, one should understand certain statements that are applicable in general to

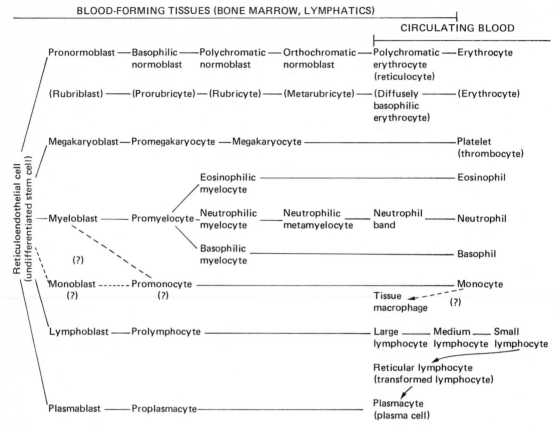

Fig. 3-21. Origin of blood cells. Adapted from Davidsohn and Henry[40] and Diggs et al.[41]

Fig. 3-22. Maturation of the erythrocyte series.

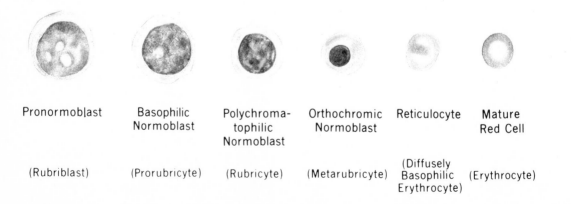

explain the maturation of the erythroblast to a nonnucleated erythrocyte.

Concerning the cell size and cytoplasm, the following statements apply. There is a progressive decrease in size. There is a decrease in the intensity of the blue color because of loss of RNA. There is an increase in red color caused by an increased hemoglobin concentration. Finally, there are no granules in the cytoplasm.

Concerning the nucleus, it is generally round and in the center of the cell. In the early stages the chromatin is fine and lacelike. As the cell matures and the nucleus becomes smaller, the chromatin becomes coarse and more condensed. Finally, the nucleus degenerates into clumps or a solid pyknotic mass, which is eventually released (or extruded) from the cell. At the same time, the color of the nucleus changes from purplish red to dark blue. When the nucleus is extruded, it is phagocytized and digested by marrow macrophages. The reticulocyte, or early nonnucleated erythrocyte, then squeezes through an opening in the endothelial lining of the marrow cavity and thus enters the peripheral circulatory system.

The earliest normoblast (pronormoblast) appears morphologically very much like the myeloblast or lymphoblast, and it may be impossible to distinguish them. It may be necessary to depend on their association with and transition to hemoglobin-containing cells in the same area of the marrow for identification. Cells of the erythrocyte series tend to stain more intensely than myeloblasts or lymphoblasts because of the combination of hemoblogin and RNA in the cytoplasm. The stages are described in terms of the staining reaction of the cytoplasm as it gains in hemoglobin concentration: basophilic cytoplasm is blue, polychromatic cytoplasm shows shades of blue and gray as hemoglobin increases, and orthochromatic cytoplasm is orange-red.

Another erythrocyte developmental series is that of the *megaloblastic erythrocytes*. It is similar to the sequence of maturation of the normoblasts, but the cells are larger, as the name implies. Megaloblasts are found in certain anemias, called megaloblastic anemias, which are the result of vitamin B_{12} or folic acid deficiency. As they develop, cells of the megaloblastic sequence have a more open chromatin pattern in the nucleus. This is referred to as asynchronous maturation or dyssynchronous development of the nucleus and cytoplasm. In megaloblastic anemia these changes are not limited to the erythrocyte series—all types of cells normally produced in the bone marrow are similarly affected, as evidenced by large hypersegmented neutrophils. This increase in size of all the cells makes it difficult to appreciate the increased red cell volume.

Granulocyte maturation and function

Neutrophils normally mature in the bone marrow in the following stages from the youngest to the most mature: myeloblast, promyelocyte (progranulocyte), myelocyte, metamyelocyte, band, and segmented neutrophils. These maturation stages are the same for all granulocytes and are diagrammed in Fig. 3-23. However, since they occur in such small numbers, the stages of eosinophil or basophil development are not identified.

Cells of the neutrophil series are generally round with smooth margins or edges. As the cells mature they become progressively smaller. Most immature cells have cytoplasm that stains dark blue, and becomes light pink as the cells mature. As the cells mature from the myeloblast to the promyelocyte stage, nonspecific granules that stain blue to reddish purple appear in the cytoplasm. Eventually, these nonspecific granules are replaced by specific neutrophilic granules. Both types of granules are not produced at the same time, but they may both be seen in the promyelocyte and myelocyte stages.

Nuclear changes also occur as the cells mature. In the myeloblast the nucleus is round or oval and very large in proportion to the rest of the

| Myeloblast | Promyelocyte | Myelocyte | Metamyelocyte | Band Neutrophil | Mature (Segmented) Neutrophil |

Fig. 3-23. Maturation of granulocytes.

cell. As the cell matures, the nucleus decreases in relative size and begins to contort or form lobes. At the same time, the nuclear chromatin changes from a fine delicate pattern to the more clumped pattern characteristic of the mature cell. The staining of the nucleus also changes from reddish purple to bluish purple as the cell matures. Nucleoli may be apparent in the early forms but gradually disappear as the chromatin thickens and the cell matures.

The term *shift to the left* refers to the release into the peripheral blood of immature cell forms, which are normally present only in the bone marrow. It is derived from the diagrammatic representation of cell maturation, where the more immature forms are shown on the left side (see Fig. 3-21).

Neutrophils exist in the peripheral blood for approximately 10 hours after they are released from the marrow. During this time they move back and forth between the general blood circulation and the walls of the blood vessels, where they accumulate. They also leave the blood and enter the tissues, where they carry out their primary functions. In the tissues, they are utilized to fight bacterial infections and are then destroyed or eliminated from the body by the excretory system (intestinal tract, urine, lungs, or saliva).

Metabolically, neutrophils are very active and can carry out both anaerobic and aerobic glycolysis. The neutrophilic granules contain several digestive enzymes that are able to destroy many kinds of bacteria. The cells are capable of random locomotion and can be directed to an area of infection by the process referred to as *chemotaxis*. Once in the tissues, the neutrophils destroy bacteria by engulfing them and releasing digestive enzymes into the phagocytic vacuole thus formed.

Not as much is known about the other granulocytes—the eosinophils and basophils. Eosinophils are capable of locomotion and phagocytosis; however, they are more active in later stages of inflammation, where they ingest antigen-antibody complexes. The eosinophilic granules contain histamine, peroxidase, and acid hydroxylases and are active in allergic reactions and certain parasitic infections, especially those involving parasitic invasion of the tissues. The basophils are capable of sluggish locomotion. The granules contain histamine, heparin or a heparin-like substance, and 5-hydroxytryptamine. Functionally, little is known about basophils except that they apparently play a role in allergic reactions.

Monocyte maturation and function

Monocytes, like granulocytes, are produced mainly in the bone marrow. The stages of development are monoblast, promonocyte, and monocyte. The monoblast looks very much like the myeloblast or the lymphoblast, and it may be impossible to distinguish them morphologically on films prepared with Wright's stain. In such cases, the term *blast* is used. It may be necessary to classify the type of blast present on the basis of other cell types in the area.

Monocytes remain in the peripheral blood for about 1-3 days after leaving the bone marrow. They are very motile and phagocytic cells. Unlike neutrophils, monocytes do not die after they engage in phagocytic activity. Instead, after 1-3 days in the peripheral blood, they move into the body tissues and are transformed into *macrophages.* Macrophages are thought to be derived from both monocytes and reticuloendothelial (RE) cells. RE cells that have become free are known as *histiocytes*, and a histiocyte that has begun to phagocytize is called a macrophage. Therefore, RE cells, histiocytes, monocytes, and macrophages are considered to be related in terms of function and origin. In addition to phagocytizing bacteria, macrophages appear to make antigens and interact with lymphocytes in the synthesis of antibodies.

Lymphocyte maturation and function

Lymphocytes are normally produced in the lymphoid tissue (nodes, spleen, and thymus) but may also be produced in the bone marrow. The stages of development are: lymphoblast, pro-lymphocyte, and large, medium, and small lymphocyte. The lymphoblast looks very much like the myeloblast, and their morphological differentiation is beyond the scope of this book.

The lymphatic system consists of a network of vessels throughout most of the body tissues. The smaller vessels unite to form larger and larger vessels, which finally come together in two main trunks, the right lymphatic duct and the thoracic duct. The ducts empty into the circulatory system through veins in the neck. Lymph nodes are located all along the lymphatic vessels, and the lymph (fluid within the system) circulates through the nodes as it progresses through the lymphatic system. Many of the lymphocytes are

formed in the lymph nodes and circulate back and forth between the blood, the organs, and the lymphatic tissues. Functionally there are two types of lymphocytes, *T cells*, or *T* lymphocytes, and *B cells*, or *B* lymphocytes.

B lymphocytes function primarily in antibody production or the formation of immunoglobulins. They are related to plasma cells and may transform into plasma cells if appropriately stimulated. B lymphocytes have a short life-span, measured in days, and comprise about 10-30 percent of the blood lymphocytes.

T lymphocytes function in cell-mediated immune responses such as delayed hypersensitivity, graft-versus-host reactions, and homograft rejection. They make up the majority of the lymphocytes circulating in the peripheral blood and have a life-span of months to years as they continually recirculate from blood to lymph.

After antigenic stimulation, small lymphocytes can undergo blast transformation. These transformed cells appear large (15-25 μm) on films prepared with Wright's stain, with a relatively large amount of deep blue cytoplasm. The large nucleus has a reticular appearance, with uniform chromatin and prominent nucleoli. Such cells have various names, including *reactive*, *atypical*, and *reticular* lymphocytes.

Red cell alterations

Clinically, alterations in erythrocyte morphology are associated with many diseases and especially with anemia. Anemia is not a specific disease, but a condition in which there is a decrease in the oxygen-carrying capacity of the blood and therefore in the amount of oxygen reaching the tissues and organs. Its causes are many and varied, and the type of anemia present and its underlying cause must be determined by the physician before treatment can be effectively undertaken. It may or may not be the result of a disorder of the blood or blood-forming tissues.

Classification (types) of anemia

Clinically, all patients with anemia have similar symptoms or complaints regardless of the cause of the anemia. The severity is generally dependent on the hemoglobin concentration of the blood, as most symptoms result from the decreased oxygen-carrying capacity. The primary complaints are tiredness and shortness of breath. Other common complaints are faintness, dizziness, heart palpitation, and headache. All of these symptoms are general and can be present without the clinical condition of anemia. Once the existence of anemia has been demonstrated, usually on the basis of the blood hemoblogin concentration, the physician must determine the underlying cause. Besides the case history and physical examination, the physician will rely on various laboratory procedures, including the appearance of the red cells on the peripheral blood film, in arriving at this diagnosis.

Generally, anemias are classified according to either the appearance of the red cells (morphological classification) or the physiological cause of the anemia (etiologic or pathogenetic classification). We will present a morphological classification, showing some of the more common types of anemia that result in the alterations in red cell morphology observed on the peripheral blood film. Such morphological classifications fail to deal effectively with the hemolytic anemias, and these are described separately. Although they are helpful to the physician, these observations will be transferred into an etiologic system in determining the appropriate therapy for the patient.

Morphologically, anemias are generally classified as (1) normochromic-normocytic, (2) macrocytic, or (3) hypochromic-microcytic. These types will now be discussed in terms of common laboratory changes, especially as reflected by the red blood cell indexes, and common examples of each type will be given. These changes are summarized in Table 3-1.

Normocytic-normochromic anemias

Normocytic-normochromic anemias are characterized by normal-looking red cells on the peripheral blood film and normal red cell index values. The cells produced by the marrow are normal, but the number of cells in circulation is reduced for a variety of reasons. Such anemias may result from acute blood loss resulting from external trauma such as a wound, or internal trauma such as an acute bleeding ulcer or a ruptured organ. Conditions resulting in increased plasma volume, such as pregnancy and overhydration, will also result in normochromic-normocytic anemia. If the bone marrow is suppressed (hypoplastic), as seen in cases of aplastic anemia (the unfortunate result of exposure to various chemicals or drugs), the red cells that remain are normal. Suppressed marrow results in a deficiency of the myeloid series and platelets, seen as decreased leukocyte and platelet counts. Likewise, if the marrow is infiltrated with a neoplasm or malignancy, as in leukemia or multiple myeloma, the remaining red cells appear normal although they are decreased in number. In certain hemolytic diseases and chronic kidney and liver diseases the red cells also appear normal but are reduced in number.

Macrocytic anemias

Macrocytic anemias are primarily represented by the megaloblastic anemias resulting from vitamin B_{12} or folic acid deficiency, or a combination of the two. The deficiency may be nutritional or may result from a malabsorption syndrome such as pernicious anemia, where the patient is unable to absorb vitamin B_{12}. In either case, the deficiency leads to a nuclear maturation defect and megaloblastic anemia. The marrow shows certain changes in the red cell, granulocyte (myeloid), and megakaryocyte (platelet) series. Megaloblastic changes are characterized by larger cells having a more open chromatin pattern in the nucleus

Table 3-1. Morphological classification of anemias

Type of anemia	Changes in red cell indexes			Common red cell alterations[a]	Common examples and causes
	Mean corpuscular volume (MCV)	Mean corpuscular hemoglobin (MCH)	Mean corpuscular hemoglobin concentration (MCHC)		
Normochromic-normocytic	Normal	Normal	Normal	Normal size, shape, and hemoglobin content; decreased cell count	Acute blood loss; aplastic anemia; increased plasma volume; infiltrated bone marrow; some hemolytic diseases; some chronic, renal, and liver diseases
Macrocytic	Increased	Increased	Normal	Macrocytosis, ovalocytes	Megaloblastic anemias from vitamin B_{12} and/or folic acid deficiency; chronic liver disease
Hypochromic-microcytic	Decreased	Decreased	Decreased	Microcytosis (cells may appear large because of decreased hemoglobin content and flattening out on the slide); anisocytosis (slight to marked depending on condition and severity); poikilocytosis (changes characteristic of certain diseases); various inclusions, depending on cause	Iron deficiency (from blood loss, dietary deficiency, or iron metabolism error); globulin synthesis disorders such as thalassemia and porphyria; heme synthesis disorders such as sideroblastic anemias and lead poisoning

[a]Seen on films of peripheral blood stained with Wright's stain.

(asynchronous maturation or dyssynchronous development of nucleus and cytoplasm) and by the presence of larger, hypersegmented neutrophils in the peripheral blood. The enlarged red cells (macrocytes) have mean corpuscular volume (MCV) values of the order of 120–140 fl. Actual hyperchromasia is impossible, but the red cells appear to contain more hemoglobin because of their increased size and therefore thickness. Although the anemia may be severe, the red cell count is decreased more than the hemoglobin concentration, since the cells that are present are large and fairly completely filled with hemoglobin. Other changes seen in the blood film include anisocytosis (erythrocytes varying in size), poikilocytosis (erythrocytes varying in shape), and Howell-Jolly bodies.

Nutritional deficiency of vitamin B_{12} is relatively rare, but nutritional deficiency of folic acid is fairly common. It may be found in chronic alcoholism or other conditions where the diet is not well balanced. Folate deficiency is also observed when the requirement is increased, as in pregnancy, infancy, certain hemolytic anemias, and hyperthyroidism. Celiac disease, tropical sprue, drugs, contraceptives, and liver disease may lead to malabsorption and megaloblastic anemia.

Hypochromic-microcytic anemias

Hypochromic-microcytic anemias are probably the most common types encountered, with iron-deficiency anemia being the one most frequently seen. However, iron deficiency is not a simple classification, as there are several possible causes of this clinical condition. In simplified terms, iron-deficiency anemia may result from decreased iron intake (either from inadequate diet or impaired absorption), increased iron loss (generally from chronic bleeding from a variety of causes), or an error of iron metabolism. In addition, the increased iron requirements in infancy, pregnancy, and lactation may result in iron-deficiency anemia. The physician must determine the cause of the anemia in order to treat it. If it results from a dietary deficiency of iron, a relatively simple and effective treatment is to administer iron, usually orally as ferrous sulfate tablets. However, if it is caused by another condition the administration of iron will do no good, and may do harm either of itself or because it delays the use of appropriate therapy.

If the iron-deficiency anemia results from chronic bleeding, the cause of the bleeding must be determined. The bleeding is most often gastrointestinal, although women with excessive menstrual flow often develop iron-deficiency anemia. Gastrointestinal bleeding leading to iron-deficiency anemia may result from such causes as ulcer, carcinoma or other neoplasms, hemorrhoids, hookworm, or even the ingestion of salicylate (usually as aspirin). The treatment is different for each of these.

All iron-deficiency anemias produce similar changes in red cell morphology. The cells are smaller than normal (microcytic) and the mean corpuscular volume (MCV) is decreased. Unfortunately, the decreased size is not always as apparent on the blood film as it is in the MCV value. In iron-deficiency anemia the amount of hemoglobin within each red cell is significantly decreased; such cells are *hypochromic* (deficient in color). This shows up in the red cell volume,

which is primarily a function of hemoglobin, but may not be evident on the slide because the hypochromic red cell spreads out or flattens and may appear to be of normal size or even larger than normal. The hypochromic cell is extremely pale, showing only a thin rim of color with a significantly increased area of central pallor. The decreased hemoglobin per red cell is measured in the laboratory as decreased mean corpuscular hemoglobin (MCH) and decreased mean corpuscular hemoglobin concentration (MCHC). Other changes that are characteristic of iron-deficiency anemia include anisocytosis and poikilocytosis, which vary in degree with the severity of the disease. Other tests that may be useful in the investigation of iron-deficiency anemias include examination of the stool for occult blood, determination of serum iron and total iron-binding capacity, radiographic study of the gastrointestinal tract, and sometimes bone marrow examination.

Another group of anemias that are microcytic and hypochromic are those that result from disorders in the synthesis of globulin, another component of the hemoglobin molecule. These are the thalassemias, a group of inherited disorders of hemoglobin synthesis. The microscopic appearance of the red cells varies with and within the various types of thalassemias. However, microcytosis, hypochromasia, and basophilic stippling are general observations. Anisocytosis, poikilocytosis, and target cells may also be present, as well as decreased osmotic fragility. Actual differentiation of various forms of thalassemia requires family studies and fairly sophisticated laboratory tests.

The last group of hypochromic-microcytic anemias that will be discussed are those resulting from disorders of porphyrin and heme synthesis. Again, the hemoglobin molecule is malformed. The sideroblastic anemias are a heterogeneous group of disorders that have in common increased storage of iron, especially in the RE system. The bone marrow in these conditions shows sideroblasts, nucleated red cells with granules of iron that can be demonstrated with Prussian blue stain. The granules occur characteristically in a full or partial ring around the nucleus. Besides microcytosis and hypochromasia, the peripheral blood from these patients shows siderocytes, nonnucleated red cells with granules of iron (see also under Alterations in Erythrocyte Structure and Inclusions). As the body is already overloaded with iron that is not being utilized appropriately, iron therapy in these anemias would be harmful to the patient.

A number of chemicals cause sideroblastic anemias by inhibiting heme synthesis. Lead poisoning produces an anemia that is characteristically mildly microcytic and hypochromic and is often characterized by basophilic stippling of the red cells. It is most often seen in children who have ingested lead paint chips and may be seen in adults as the result of industrial exposure to lead.

Hemolytic anemias

One problem with a morphological classification of anemias is that it does not deal conveniently with a broad etiologic class of anemias, namely the hemolytic anemias. The hemolytic anemias are generally classified as congenital or acquired. They are characterized by increased destruction or hemolysis of red cells from a variety of causes, accompanied by increased production of red cells by the bone marrow. This is seen as polychromasia and even nucleated forms of red cells on blood films prepared with Wright's stain, and increased reticulocyte counts. Anisocytosis and poikilocytosis are characteristic of hemolytic anemia in general. An inherited form of spherocytic anemia, hereditary spherocytosis, results from an inherited red cell abnormality and is characterized by the presence of spherocytes in the peripheral blood. This condition is indistinguishable morphologically from certain acquired disorders that result in spherocytic anemia. In such cases a useful laboratory test is the Coombs test, which shows antibodies in the

serum (indirect Coombs test) or coating the red cells (direct Coombs test) of a patient with an acquired (or autoimmune) hemolytic spherocytic anemia. Other changes of shape (poikilocytosis) characteristic of certain hemolytic anemias include the following. Elliptocytes are characteristic of hereditary elliptocytosis, a red cell membrane disorder. Sickle cells are characteristic of sickle-cell anemia, an inherited hemoglobin abnormality. Schistocytes or fragmented cells are characteristic of the microangiopathic hemolytic anemias, and may be produced by mechanical fragmentation caused by some sort of intravascular pathology or intravascular coagulation.

The hemolytic anemias are listed below.

1. Congenital (hereditary) hemolytic anemias
   a. Membrane (shape) abnormalities
      (1) Hereditary spherocytosis
      (2) Hereditary elliptocytosis
   b. Abnormal forms of hemoglobin
      (1) Sickle-cell disease
      (2) Hemoglobin C disease
      (3) Congenital Heinz body hemolytic anemia
      (4) Thalassemias
   c. Abnormal enzyme content (nonspherocytic hemolytic anemias)
      (1) Glucose-6-phosphate dehydrogenase (G6PD) deficiency
      (2) Glycolytic enzyme deficiencies
2. Acquired hemolytic anemias
   a. Environmentally caused
      (1) Hypersplenism (from a variety of causes)
      (2) Intravascular pathology (microangiopathic hemolytic anemias)
      (3) Plasma lipid abnormalities
      (4) Parasites (as in malaria or bartonellosis)
      (5) Chemical toxins
      (6) Antibodies (immune hemolytic anemias)
         (a) Isoantibodies (incompatible transfusions or hemolytic disease of the newborn

(b) Autoantibodies

(c) Drug-induced antibodies

b. Acquired red cell abnormalities

(1) Paroxysmal nocturnal hemoglobinuria

(2) Severe vitamin B_{12}, folate, or iron deficiency

The morphological examination of red cells is very helpful in evaluating and determining the cause of anemia. Therefore, it is important that the medical technician recognize and report changes in red cell morphology so that the physician can effectively evaluate and treat the patient. The following must be observed and noted (see under Examination of the Blood Film): (1) color or staining reaction, (2) size, (3) shape, (4) structure and inclusions, (5) artifacts and abnormal distribution pattern, and (6) nucleated red cells. Alterations or abnormalities that may be observed are listed below.

1. Color (staining reaction)

a. Normochromic

b. Anisochromic

(1) Hypochromic

(2) (Hyperchromic)

(3) Polychromic

2. Size

a. Normocytosis

b. Anisocytosis

(1) Macrocytosis

(2) Microcytosis

3. Shape

a. Poikilocytosis

(1) Ovalocytes

(2) Elliptocytes

(3) Sickle cells (drepanocytes)

(4) Target cells (leptocytes)

(5) Spherocytes

(6) Stomatocytes

(7) Schistocytes (fragmented cells)

(8) Teardrop cells

(9) Echinocytes, burr cells, crenate cells

(10) Acanthocytes

4. Structure and inclusions

a. Basophilic stippling

b. Siderocyte granules (Pappenheimer bodies)

c. Howell-Jolly bodies

d. Ring bodies (Cabot's rings)

e. Parasitized red cells (malarial)

5. Artifacts and distribution pattern

a. Crenation

b. Punched-out red cells

c. Platelets on top of red cells

d. Rouleaux

e. Agglutination

Alterations in erythrocyte color or hemoglobin content (Fig. 3-24)

Normochromic cells

Red cells are described as normochromic when they contain the normal amount of hemoglobin. With Wright's stain the cells show a deep orange-red color in the peripheral area, which gradually diminishes toward the center of the cell. The diameter of the pale central area (central pallor) is less than one-third of that of the normochromic erythrocyte.

Anisochromic cells

These are cells that stain with more than the normal variation in color. They should be described by one of the more specific terms described below.

Hypochromic cells

Red cells that are very pale and show an increased area of central pallor (diameter more than one-third of that of the cell) are termed hypochromic. Hypochromasia is the result of a decrease in the hemoglobin content of the cell and is often accompanied by a decrease in cell size, or microcytosis, evidenced by low MCH and MCHC values. The cells tend to flatten out on the blood film and may appear normal in size. Such cells are particularly characteristic of iron-deficiency anemias.

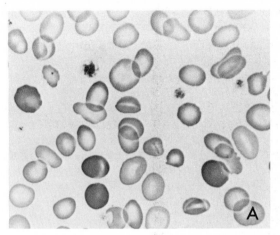 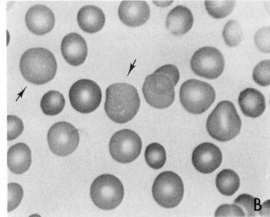

Fig. 3-24. Alterations in erythrocyte color. A. Hypochromic red blood cells. Compare with the four transfused normal cells (oil-immersion objective). B. Polychromatic red cells. These cells are reticulocytes when stained with a supravital dye (oil-immersion objective).

"Hyperchromic" cells

True hyperchromasia cannot exist because normal red cells are filled with hemoglobin and cannot be oversaturated as the cell membrane would burst. However, certain red cells appear to have an increased hemoglobin content. For example, cells that are larger than normal (macrocytes) are also thicker, and therefore the color intensity appears greater on the blood film. Another abnormally shaped red cell, the spherocyte, which is a round cell without a depression in the center, also appears hyperchromic as it is thicker and stains throughout the cell.

Polychromatic cells

These red cells show a faint blue or blue-orange color with Wright's stain. They are young cells that have just extruded their nuclei and stain diffusely basophilic because of the presence of small numbers of ribosomes (or cytoplasmic RNA). When such cells enter the bloodstream they lack 20 percent of their final hemoglobin content and retain the ribosomes for hemoglobin synthesis. Polychromatic red cells are generally larger than mature red cells. With supravital dyes

such as new methylene blue, the RNA reticulum stains blue and the cells are called reticulocytes. The presence of polychromasia (or an increased reticulocyte count) is an indication of increased red cell formation by the marrow.

Alterations in erythrocyte size (Fig. 3-25)

Normocytosis

Red cells are described as normocytic when they are of normal size.

Anisocytosis

This is a general term indicating increased variation in the size of red cells in the blood film. It is often accompanied by variations in hemoglobin concentration.

Macrocytosis

Macrocytes are large red cells. They have a mean cell diameter greater than 9 μm or an MCV greater than 100 fl. They should be differentiated from polychromatic red cells. Macrocytes are

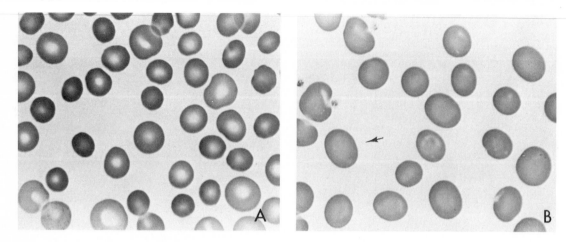

Fig. 3-25. Alterations in erythrocyte size. A. Anisocytosis (oil-immersion objective). B. Macrocytosis. Oval macrocytes are also present (oil-immersion objective).

characteristic of the megaloblastic anemias of folic acid or vitamin B_{12} deficiency.

Microcytosis

Microcytes are small red cells, less than 6.5 μm in diameter with an MCV less than 78 fl. They are often associated with hypochromasia, but their decreased size may not be appreciated on the blood film because they tend to flatten out. Microcytosis is characteristic of iron-deficiency anemia, thalassemia, lead poisoning, sideroblastic anemia, idiopathic pulmonary hemosiderosis, and anemias of chronic diseases.

Alterations in erythrocyte shape (Fig. 3-26)

Poikilocytosis

This is a general term indicating an increased variation in the shape of red cells. Many different variations in shape are seen in blood films, and red cells have been described as appearing pear-, oat-, teardrop-, or helmet-shaped, triangular, fragmented, or having various numbers and types of membrane projections. The size and hemoglobin content can vary greatly within poikilocytes.

They are found in a variety of anemias and hemolytic states, and a particular shape may or may not indicate a specific type of disease.

Ovalocytes

These red cells are oval or egg-shaped. They are wider or fuller than elliptocytes. Large ovalocytes, called macroovalocytes, are characteristic of megaloblastic anemias. Because of their increased size and thickness, these cells may not show an area of central pallor on the blood film.

Elliptocytes

These red cells are similar to but narrower and more elongated than ovalocytes. They may occur in a variety of conditions, the most striking and least pathological being hereditary elliptocytosis.

Sickle cells (drepanocytes)

Sickle cells are most typically narrow, crescent-shaped cells. They have defective membranes and do not function normally. They are the result of a genetic condition in which abnormal hemoglobin is present in the red cells. Sickle cells may

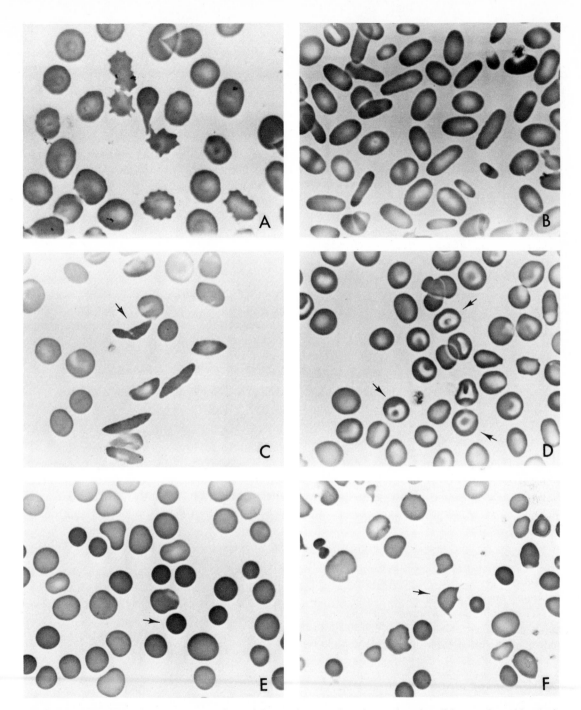

Fig. 3-26. Alterations in erythrocyte shape (photomicrographs taken using the oil-immersion objective). A. Poikilocytosis. Note the variation in shape of the red blood cells, including crenate cells. B. Elliptocytes. C. Sickle cells (drepanocytes). D. Target cells. E. Spherocytes. F. Schistocytes (fragmented cells). The arrow indicates a helmet cell.

be found in sickle-cell disease (Hb S) or sickle-cell trait (Hb SC or Hb S-thalassemia). Sickling of red cells is enhanced by lack of oxygen.

Target cells (leptocytes)

Target cells look like targets, showing a peripheral ring of hemoglobin, an area of pallor or clearing, and then a central area of hemoglobin. They represent another membrane defect. Target cells have excessive cell membrane in relation to the amount of hemoglobin. They are seen in a variety of clinical conditions, especially in various hemoglobin abnormalities and in chronic liver disease.

Spherocytes

Spherocytes are red cells that are not biconcave; instead, they are round or spherical because of the loss of a portion of the cell membrane. As a result, they are small cells, usually less than 6 μm in diameter, and are often called *microspherocytes*. They *appear* hyperchromic, staining a uniform intense orange-red because of the lack of central pallor, a result of the round shape. Spherocytes are characteristic of certain hemolytic anemias, both hereditary (hereditary spherocytosis) and acquired (e.g., drug-induced).

Stomatocytes

Stomatocytes show a slitlike or mouthlike rather than round area of central pallor on the blood film. They are not biconcave, but are bowl-shaped, or concave on only one side. They are often found in chronic liver disease.

Schistocytes (fragmented cells)

Schistocytes have a variety of names and forms, depending on what is left after the cell is fragmented. *Helmet cells*, or keratocytes, are small triangular cells with one or two pointed ends that resemble a helmet. Schistocytosis is a very serious pathological condition. It may be the result of mechanical fracture of cells as they pass through the circulatory system, as on filaments of fibrin resulting from intravascular coagulation or on artificial heart valves. They are also seen in cases of severe burns. The fragmentation may also be the result of toxic or metabolic injury, as seen with certain malignancies. Schistocytes are characteristic of microangiopathic hemolytic anemias and their presence is a danger signal requiring immediate action by the physician.

Teardrop cells

These are pear-shaped or teardrop-shaped red cells with an elongated point or tail at one end. They may be the result of the cell squeezing and subsequently fracturing as it passes through the spleen.

Echinocytes, burr cells, or crenate cells

These are red cells with scalloped, spicular, or spiny projections regularly distributed around the cell membrane. They can usually revert back to normal cells. The term *crenate* is sometimes reserved for artifactual spicular cells, such as artifacts that result when the blood film is not adequately waved dry.

Acanthocytes

Acanthocytes are similar to echinocytes, but their spiny projections are irregularly distributed around the cell membrane. They are not artifacts and cannot revert to normal cells. They are related to and may occur with schistocytes, and represent serious pathological conditions.

Alterations in erythrocyte structure and inclusions (Fig. 3-27)

Basophilic stippling

The presence of dark blue granules evenly distributed throughout the red cell is called baso-

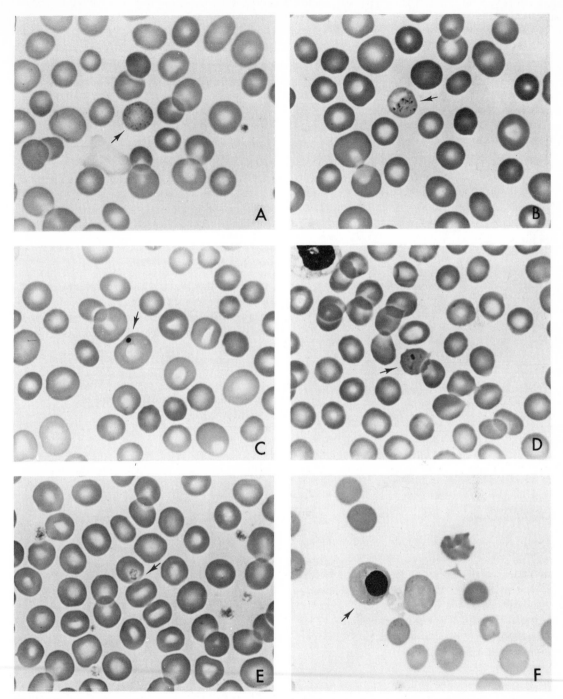

Fig. 3-27. Alterations in erythrocyte structure and inclusions (photomicrographs taken using the oil-immersion objective). A. Basophilic stippling. B. Siderocyte granules (Pappenheimer bodies). C. Howell-Jolly body. D. Parasitized red cell (malarial). Compare this with (E). E. Platelet on top of red cell. F. Nucleated red cell in peripheral blood.

philic stippling. The stippling may be very fine or dotlike, or it may be coarse and larger in size. The stippled cell may resemble the polychromatic red cell; however, these are actual granules, not just an overall blueness. Stippling does not exist in the circulating red cell but results from precipitation of ribosomes and RNA in the staining process. However, the stippling is not an artifact in the clinical sense, as it may indicate abnormal red cell formation in the marrow, as in thalassemia minor, megaloblastic anemia, and lead poisoning.

Siderocyte granules (Pappenheimer bodies)

These are small, dense, blue-purple granules of free iron, uncombined with hemoglobin. Usually only one or two of these granules are present in a cell, and they are located in the cell periphery. They may be confused with Howell-Jolly bodies and can be distinguished and seen better with a specific stain for iron, such as Prussian blue. When siderocyte granules are stained with Wright's stain they are sometimes called Pappenheimer bodies. They are rarely seen in peripheral blood except after removal of the spleen.

Howell-Jolly bodies

Howell-Jolly bodies are round, densely staining purple granules that stain like dense nuclear chromatin. Usually only one or two such bodies are seen in the red cells. They are eccentrically located in the red cell and less than 1 μm in diameter. Howell-Jolly bodies are remnants of the red cell nucleus, and thus are DNA. Under normal conditions they are derived from nuclear fragmentation (*karyorrhexis*) in the later stages of red cell maturation and are thought to be aberrant chromosomes in certain abnormal conditions. These nuclear remnants are normally removed from the peripheral blood by a pitting process in the spleen. Therefore, they are seen after removal of the spleen, and also in cases of

abnormal red cell formation such as megaloblastic anemias and some hemolytic anemias.

Ring bodies (Cabot's rings)

These are threadlike red-violet strands occurring in ring, twisted, or figure 8 shapes. Ring bodies are rare. Their origin is unknown, but they are thought to result from abnormal red cell formation, as in megaloblastic anemias and lead poisoning.

Parasitized red cells (malarial)

In cases of malaria, various stages of the malaria parasites may be seen in the red cells. Depending on the species of malaria organism present, the parasites may appear like and be confused with ring bodies, basophilic stippling, or platelets lying on top of red cells.

Erythrocyte artifacts and abnormal distribution patterns (Fig. 3-28)

Crenation

Crenate cells on the blood film appear like echinocytes, with scalloped, spicular, or spiny projections regularly distributed around the cell surface. In this case they are an artifact resulting from incorrect preparation of the blood film, usually failure to dry it adequately.

Punched-out red cells

Red cells with a punched-out appearance rather than a normal area of central pallor are also drying artifacts. They should not be confused with hypochromic red cells. The remaining cell shows a normal staining reaction with this artifact.

Platelets on top of erythrocytes

When platelets lie on top of red cells in the blood film they may be confused with inclusions,

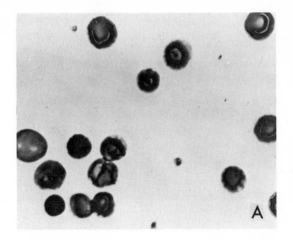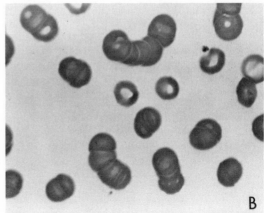

Fig. 3-28. Erythrocyte artifacts and abnormal distribution patterns (photomicrographs taken using the oil-immersion objective). A. Drying artifact in red cells. B. Rouleaux formation, an abnormal distribution pattern.

especially the trophozoite stage of malaria organisms. In such cases, the overlying platelets should be compared with those in the surrounding field.

Rouleaux

Rouleaux represent an abnormal distribution pattern of red cells, which stick together or become aligned in aggregates that look like stacks of coins. This arrangement is a typical artifact in the thick area of blood films. It is clinically significant when found in the normal examination area and associated with elevated plasma fibrinogen or globulin with a corresponding increase in the erythrocyte sedimentation rate, as in multiple myeloma.

Agglutination

Agglutination, irregular or amorphous clumping of red cells in the blood film, represents another alteration in red cell distribution. Clinically, this may be caused by the presence of a cold agglutinin (antibody) in the patient's serum and may indicate an autoimmune hemolytic state or anemia.

Nucleated red cells in the peripheral blood (Fig. 3-27)

Normally, red cells do not enter the blood until the reticulocyte stage of maturation, just after extrusion of the shrunken nucleus. Therefore, the presence of earlier nucleated forms of red cells in the peripheral blood is abnormal. It indicates intense marrow stimulation, such as that seen in acute blood loss, megaloblastic anemias, or pathological conditions associated with various malignancies. The presence of nucleated red cells is termed an *erythroblastotic reaction.*

Cells in the later stages of maturation are most often present, so the cytoplasm is orange-red because the cells contain hemoglobin. However, the nucleus is also present, although shrunken and dark blue in color. Earlier forms may occur and may be difficult to distinguish from small lymphocytes or plasma cells; the presence of pink in the red cell cytoplasm is helpful in such cases. The presence of nucleated red cell forms in the peripheral blood is characteristic of megaloblastic anemias. In these cases the young red cells are larger (macrocytic) and tend to have a more open chromatin pattern than corresponding stages of normocytic red cells (dyssynchrony of nucleus and cytoplasm).

It is important to remember that the white cell count must be corrected when nucleated red cells are observed in the peripheral blood film.

Leukocyte alterations

In the examination of peripheral blood, leukocytes are studied for alterations in both quantity, or number, and quality, or morphology.

Quantitative changes in leukocytes are measured by the white cell count—the actual number of leukocytes in a certain volume of blood. A white cell count above normal is leukocytosis; a count below normal is leukopenia. There can also be increases or decreases in number of any of the five types of white cells that are enumerated collectively in the white cell count, and such changes are measured by the white cell differential. Quantitative changes in any of the cell types are described by the following terms: neutrophilia (increase), neutropenia (decrease); eosinophilia, eosinopenia; basophilia, basopenia; lymphocytosis, lymphopenia; and monocytosis, monocytopenia.

In addition, these increases or decreases may be *relative* or *absolute*. If the change is absolute, the particular cell type shows a numerical increase or decrease from its normal concentration in the blood. If it is relative, there is an alteration (either high or low) of the percentage of the particular cell type as determined in the leukocyte differential, while the numerical concentration is within normal values. Finally, there may be both an absolute and a relative change when both the percentage and the numerical value are above or below normal.

Qualitative or morphological alterations in circulating leukocytes may be described in terms of a shift to the left, referring to the presence of younger or more immature cell forms than are normally found in the peripheral blood. Such changes may be found within any cell line,

including erythrocytes. The presence of younger forms of leukocytes in the blood may be termed a leukoblastotic reaction. Since they often occur along with younger or nucleated red cell forms, the term *leukoerythroblastotic reaction* is also used.

Most alterations in leukocyte morphology can be classified as (1) toxic or reactive changes, (2) anomalous changes, and (3) malignant or leukemic changes.

Toxic or reactive leukocyte alterations

Toxic changes in leukocytes are generally associated with a bacterial infection or a toxic reaction. They are seen on a blood film as toxic granulation, vacuolization, hypersegmentation (hyperlobulation) of neutrophils, a shift to the left, the presence of Döhle bodies, increased or decreased cell size, degeneration or pyknosis of the nucleus, and karyolysis (dissolution of the nucleus).

Reactive leukocyte alterations are particularly characteristic of lymphocytes. Reactive lymphocytes seem to result from viral infections and are often associated with infectious mononucleosis, although many other conditions produce reactive cell forms. Changes generally include increased cytoplasmic basophilia with or without radial or peripheral localization, increased or decreased cytoplasmic volume, increased coarse azurophilic granulation, and alterations in the nuclear chromatin, which becomes either loose, delicate, and reticular, or dark, heavy, and clumped.

Anomalous changes

An anomaly is a deviation from the common rule or an irregularity. Hematologic deviations from normal may be congenital or acquired. Leukocyte anomalies are described later in this section.

Malignant or leukemic changes

Leukemia is a disease of the blood-forming tissues that is generally fatal. It is abnormal, uncontrolled proliferation of one or more of the various leukocyte-producing cells. There are usually, but not always, qualitative changes in the affected cells.

The exact cause of leukemia is not known. There is some evidence to suggest a hereditary predisposition. More recently, environmental causes have been cited, especially exposure to gamma radiation producing genetic mutations or chromosome damage. Various chemicals and drugs have also been implicated, and viruses have been shown to be related to leukemia in mice and other animals, but this has not yet been shown in humans.

Leukemia can occur at any age, but certain forms appear to be age-related. Chronic lymphocytic leukemia (CLL) is generally a disease of later adult years (generally over 50 years of age) and has the best or longest prognosis. Acute lymphocytic leukemia (ALL) is generally a disease of children under 10 (seldom over 20) and peaks between the ages of 2 and 4. Chronic myelogenous leukemia (CML) usually occurs between the ages of 20 and 50, and acute myelogenous leukemia (AML) occurs at all ages but is primarily a disease of middle adult years.

Leukemias are commonly classified according to either (1) the cell type involved, or (2) the number of blasts in the peripheral blood and the corresponding clinical course or prognosis (designated acute, subacute, or chronic). In the first of these systems there are generally two classes of leukemia, *myeloid*, or *myelogenous*, and *lymphoid*, or *lymphocytic*. The youngest cell forms or blasts common to these leukemias are the myeloblast and the lymphoblast, respectively. It may be impossible to distinguish between the myeloblast and the lymphoblast morphologically, especially in the most serious or acute forms of the disease, when only blast forms are seen in the blood. The presence of *Auer bodies* (granules or rods of azurophilic substance) in the cytoplasm is diagnostic of the myeloblast. However, Auer bodies are not seen in all cases of myelogenous leukemia. Other considerations in the dif-

ferentiation of myeloblasts and lymphoblasts are the nucleocytoplasmic ratio, the number of nucleoli, and the nuclear chromatin pattern. However, such differences are often inconclusive and may be misleading. If more mature cells are present they may aid in the identification.

The major symptoms of leukemia are fever, weight loss, and increased sweating, especially night sweats. The liver, spleen, and lymph nodes may be enlarged. There may be a bleeding tendency if the platelet count is decreased (thrombocytopenia).

Leukemias are classified as acute or chronic on the basis of clinical course (prognosis) and the number of blasts present. *Acute leukemias* occur very suddenly. There is usually anemia, which is normocytic and normochromic and which increases as the disease progresses. The platelet count is low to markedly decreased. The leukocyte count varies but is usually moderately to markedly elevated—with 50 000–100 000 cells/μl being not uncommon—although the count may be normal or decreased. Blast cells are present in the peripheral blood film; generally, more than 60 percent blasts indicates an acute leukemic process. The bone marrow is hypercellular and consists predominantly of blast cells. Untreated acute leukemias lead to death within 2–3 months; with treatment the median survival is 12 months for acute myelogenous leukemia and 60 months for acute lymphocytic leukemia. Death is the result of hemorrhage, which increases in severity as the platelet count falls below 20 000 cells/μl, or infection, which results as the granulocyte count falls below 1500 cells/μl. Infection is now the primary cause of death, as bleeding has been reduced with prophylactic platelet transfusions and vigorous transfusion therapy when patients are in a bleeding crisis.

Chronic leukemias begin slowly and insidiously and may exist for a long time without symptoms. Symptoms develop slowly and include fatigue, night sweats, weight loss, and fever. Anemia usually develops late in the disease, but hemolytic anemia may develop as the disease progresses. The platelet count is usually normal and may even increase in chronic myelogenous leukemia; however, in the later stages both thrombocytopenia and anemia usually occur. The white cell count is usually markedly increased, often higher than 100 000 cells/μl, but it can be normal or even decreased. Morphologically, less than 10 percent myeloblasts will be seen in the peripheral blood in chronic myelogenous leukemias, and the blood tends to look like bone marrow as it contains all granulocyte developmental stages. In chronic lymphocytic leukemia, very few to no lymphoblasts are seen in the peripheral blood. The blood characteristically shows a monotonous picture of lymphocytes that are all similar in size and morphology. In addition, many damaged or basket cells may be present, as the lymphocytes tend to be fragile. The average length of survival for patients with chronic myelogenous leukemia is 3–4 years. Chronic lymphocytic leukemia has an average survival of 4–6 years, although prolonged survival for up to 35 years is possible, and about 30 percent of the patients die of causes unrelated to the disease. Infection is the most common cause of death related to chronic lymphocytic leukemia. Chronic myelogenous leukemia tends to proceed to an acute or accelerated stage called a *blast crisis*, and patients eventually die of hemorrhage or infection, as in acute leukemia.

Malignant hematologic conditions other than leukemia include plasma cell dyscrasias (multiple myeloma, primary macroglobulinemia, and Fe fragment or heavy chain disease), Hodgkin's disease (or malignant lymphoma, Hodgkin's type), non-Hodgkin's malignant lymphomas, and some unusual tumors closely resembling hematologic malignancies.

The laboratory has a significant role in the diagnosis and management or treatment of patients with these various hematologic diseases. Many laboratory procedures will be requested by the physician, such as cell and platelet counts, tests to assess the presence of anemia, coagulation studies, white cell differential count, blood film examination, and preparation and selection of appropriate blood components for transfusion therapy.

Again, the actual examination of the blood film in cases of such altered and serious morphology is beyond the scope of the medical technician. However, such changes should be recognized as abnormal and referred to the pathologist or technologist with special training. To identify changes in leukocyte morphology, the cells should be examined for the following features: (1) nuclear chromatin pattern, (2) nuclear shape, (3) size and number of nucleoli, when present, (4) cytoplasmic inclusions, and (5) nucleocytoplasmic ratio. Various alterations in leukocyte morphology are described below and illustrated in Fig. 3-29.

Toxic granulation

Toxic granules are deeply staining basophilic or blue-black granules found in the cytoplasm of neutrophils. Their presence is associated with acute bacterial infections, drug poisoning, and burns.

Döhle bodies

Döhle bodies are small, clear blue staining areas found in the neutrophil cytoplasm. They are remnants of cytoplasmic RNA from an earlier stage of neutrophil development. They are often seen together with toxic granulation in infections, burns, and after administration of toxic agents.

Cytoplasmic vacuolization

Vacuoles are also signs of toxic change and imply the occurrence of phagocytosis. They may be accompanied by irregular depletion of granules or areas of clearing in the neutrophil cytoplasm.

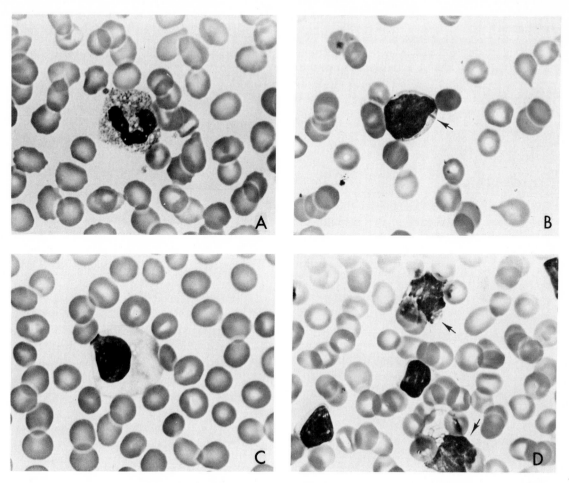

Fig. 3-29. Leukocyte alterations (photomicrographs taken using the oil-immersion objective). A. Neutrophil showing toxic changes (toxic granules, vacuoles, Döhle bodies). B. Auer rod in myeloblast. C. Reactive lymphocyte. D. Smudge or basket cells (arrows). Lymphocytes are also present.

Hypersegmentation of nucleus

Neutrophils that are hypersegmented contain five or more lobes in their nuclei. They are characteristic of the megaloblastic anemias of vitamin B_{12} and folic acid deficiency and are therefore often called pernicious anemia (PA) neutrophils. The megaloblastic neutrophil is larger than the normal neutrophil (all cell types are larger in the megaloblastic process).

Barr bodies

A Barr body is a small knob attached to or projecting from a lobe of the neutrophil nucleus and consisting of the same nuclear chromatin or substance. It is often referred to as the sex chromatin or sex chromosome as it is seen in some of the neutrophils of normal females and is thought to be an inactivated X chromosome.

Auer bodies

Auer bodies are slender, rod-shaped bodies found in the cytoplasm that stain reddish purple (like azurophilic granules). They are found only in the cytoplasm of myeloblasts and promyelocytes and are considered diagnostic in distinguishing myelogenous (myeloblastic granulocytic) from lymphocytic leukemias.

Pelger-Huët anomaly

This anomaly is seen as a failure of the granulocyte nucleus to segment or form lobes normally. The neutrophil nuclei are band-shaped or at most have two lobes in this condition. In addition, the chromatin is quite coarsely clumped. This is a benign anomaly that can be inherited or acquired.

Chédiak-Higashi anomaly

Large blue-green staining masses are observed in the neutrophil cytoplasm, and blue-purple granules are seen in the lymphocyte and monocyte cytoplasm. The disease is inherited and rare. It is found in children and is fatal.

May-Hegglin anomaly

This anomaly is seen in neutrophils and platelets. Döhle bodies are present in neutrophils, and platelets may be decreased in number but some giant forms will be present. The disorder is inherited.

Alder-Reilly anomaly

Heavy azurophilic granulation is observed in neutrophils, eosinophils, basophils, and sometimes lymphocytes and monocytes. This anomaly is inherited.

Reactive or atypical lymphocytes

Reactive or atypical lymphocytes are particularly associated with infectious mononucleosis; however, many other viral infections result in such alterations. In general, the cytoplasm increases in amount and appears to be reacting to a stimulus. Although the cells have been more specifically classified morphologically, they tend to have one or several of the following characteristics.

The cytoplasm tends to become more intensely blue in color (cytoplasmic basophilia). The basophilia tends to be localized, either peripherally, with an increased blue color around the outer edge of the cell, or radially, with areas of blueness radiating from the more central nucleus to the outer edges of the cell like spokes of a wheel. Radial and peripheral basophilia may be combined, in which case the cell is described as resembling a fried egg or a flared skirt. The reactive cell may also show increases or decreases in cytoplasmic volume. Cells with increased cytoplasmic volume, when observed on films prepared with Wright's stain, tend to show indentations by adjacent structures, especially red blood cells. The cytoplasm appears to be flowing around and almost engulfing such structures. The cells also tend to have an increased number of nonspecific azurophilic granules in the cytoplasm.

Reactive or atypical lymphocytes also show nuclear changes. There is generally a sharper separation of chromatin and parachromatin. The nucleus may become loose and delicate, resembling an earlier developmental stage; this is referred to as a reticular appearance, hence the term reticular lymphocyte. In other cases, the nucleus becomes oval or kidney-shaped with heavy clumps of deeply stained chromatin; these are called plasmacytoid changes since the cells resemble plasma cells.

Such atypical lymphocytes have been classified as Downey type I, II, and III lymphocytes. However, in the laboratory it is sufficient to note the presence of reactive lymphocytes, as the three types have similar diagnostic significance. The reactive lymphocyte may resemble the lymphoblast, and it may be necessary to rule out a leukemic process in such cases of reactive lymphocytosis.

Türk cells

These are darkly staining cells having plasmacytoid characteristics. They are classified as atypical lymphocytes[42] or plasma cells[43] by different authors and are associated with viral infections.

Smudge or basket cells

These are damaged white cells. They are cellular fragments consisting of battered or frayed nuclei with no cytoplasmic material. Basket cells are not counted as part of the white cell differential, and a few damaged cells are encountered in most peripheral blood films. They are not significant unless present in large numbers. They may be associated with chronic lymphocytic leukemia, and in some cases of chronic lymphocytic leukemia and acute leukemias the number of basket cells may be greater than the usual lymphocyte count.

COUNTING RETICULOCYTES

Reticulocytes are young red cells that have matured enough to have lost their nuclei but not their cytoplasmic RNA. They do not have the full amount of hemoglobin. The number of reticulocytes is a measure of the regeneration or production of red blood cells. Reticulocytes appear in a blood film stained with Wright's stain as polychromatic red blood cells because of the basophilic cytoplasmic remnant of the immature red cell RNA. Supravital stains may also reveal basophilic stippling and Howell-Jolly bodies. The inclusions seen as basophilic stippling represent precipitation of the RNA as pinpoint particles in the red cells; this precipitation is seen in toxic conditions such as lead or heavy metal poisoning. Basophilic stippling is also visible with Wright's stain. Howell-Jolly bodies are seen in pathological conditions in which one or more larger spherical bodies consisting of nuclear material are found in the red cell (see also under Red Cell Alterations).

In the circulating blood 0.5-1.5 percent of the red cells are usually reticulocytes. This is based on a normal red cell life-span of 120 ± 20 days and a normal red cell count necessitating replacement of approximately 1 percent of the adult circulating red cells each day. The range represents technical or counting errors in the method. A reticulocyte count above this level (reticulocytosis) is clinically significant, indicating that the body is attempting to meet an increased need for red cells. Such an increase in reticulocytes is observed when red cells are being hemolyzed within the body. The bone marrow sends out red cells at an increased rate until only the younger cells are available to be released, although increased red cell production is probably taking place at the same time. The demand may be so great in some instances that nucleated red cells are sent from the bone marrow.

The reticulocyte count is used to follow therapeutic measures for anemias in which the patient is deficient in, or lacking, one of the substances essential for manufacturing red cells. When the deficiency has been diagnosed, therapy is begun. This consists of supplying the missing essential substances to the body and waiting for the body to react by increasing red cell production. New red cells will be released rapidly into the circulating blood, many before they are fully matured, in response to therapy. The corresponding increase in the reticulocyte count indicates a favorable response to therapy. The response to therapy in iron-deficiency anemia (treated with iron) and pernicious anemia (treated with vitamin B_{12}) is followed by reticulocyte counts. As the total red cell count and the hemoglobin concentration reach normal levels, red cell regeneration slows to the normal rate, allowing more time for maturation of the red cells in the bone marrow. This is indicated by the presence of fewer reticulocytes in the circulating blood.

The methods for preparing reticulocyte films

all require supravital staining of the red cells, whether the end result is a dry film or not. In supravital staining the living blood cells are mixed with the stain, as opposed to making a film and staining it. One method consists of spreading the stain on the slide and drying it; the blood is then added to the dried stain and mixed, and the usual blood smear is prepared. Another method uses the same slide preparation, but the stain is mixed with a drop of blood and cover-slipped, and the mixture is sealed on the slide and viewed in the liquid form under the microscope. A third method is to mix blood and stain in a small test tube, allow time for the staining reaction to occur, and then prepare a blood film from the mixture; the prepared blood film is then viewed microscopically. In some procedures the resulting film is counterstained with Wright's stain, using the method previously described. This is not an essential step and it may be omitted, as in the procedure to be described here. Such counterstaining with Wright's stain may be helpful in differentiating basophilic stippling and Howell-Jolly bodies from reticular RNA. The first two methods described employ an alcoholic solution of the dye; the third method uses a saline solution.

Specimen requirements

Anticoagulated whole blood or capillary blood from the finger, toe, or heel may be used. The blood should be anticoagulated with EDTA, as balanced oxalate can interfere with the action of the dye. Heparinized blood should also be avoided as the staining quality is poor. If anticoagulated whole blood is used, the test should be performed within 1 or 2 hours after the specimen is drawn.

Dyes used to stain reticulocytes

Brilliant cresyl blue or new methylene blue is used for the staining of reticulocytes. It has been stated that new methylene blue dye gives more consistent results and sharper blue staining of the reticulum.[44] In addition to the dye, the stain should contain an ingredient to preserve the red cells (provide an isotonic condition). If the third method is used, it is necessary to prevent coagulation. Brilliant cresyl blue contains sodium citrate, which prevents coagulation, and sodium chloride (NaCl), which provides isotonicity. New methylene blue contains sodium oxalate, which prevents coagulation, and sodium chloride. These supravital dyes precipitate the RNA in the reticulocytes, coloring it blue.

Preparation of stains

1. Brilliant cresyl blue. Dilute 1.0 g of brilliant cresyl blue and 0.4 g of sodium citrate to 100 ml with 0.85 g/dl NaCl. Filter before using.
2. New methylene blue. Dilute 0.50 g of new methylene blue N (color index 52030), 0.70 g of NaCl (CP grade), and 0.13 g of sodium oxalate (CP grade) to 100 ml with deionized water. Filter before using.

Procedure for reticulocyte count

1. Two drops of blood (capillary or venous) are added to three drops of reticulocyte dye in a small test tube. If the hemoglobin is low, more blood should be used to ensure proper staining and good films.
2. The blood and dye are thoroughly mixed and allowed to stand for 15 minutes.
3. The cells are resuspended by mixing well, and at least three thin films are made on slides, using small drops of the blood-stain mixture. The usual procedure for making blood films is used. The films must be completely and *rapidly* dried by waving vigorously through the air.
4. When the films are dry, the reticulocytes are counted. A total of 1000 erythrocytes (500 on each of two slides) is counted, using the oil-immersion (X95–97) objective.

5. The count is made in an area of the smear considered to be medium thin, where the erythrocytes are well distributed and not touching (about 100 cells per oil-immersion field).

6. The reticulocytes seen in the count are included in the total 1000 cells counted; however, they are tallied and recorded separately. Separate counts should be recorded for the two slides in order to compare the distribution of reticulocytes.

7. The reticulocytes appear as greenish blue cells with the reticulum showing as a deep blue network of strands or granules within the cells (see Fig. 3-30).

8. If the two slides counted do not agree within 5 cells when the reticulocyte count is 3 percent or less (30 reticulocytes per 1000 cells), another 500 cells must be counted on a third slide. If agreement within five cells cannot be met after counting all three slides, the procedure must be repeated from the beginning with new slides. If the reticulocyte count is greater than 3 percent, a reasonable difference between the counts on the two slides is allowable. This will be determined by the quality control system of the laboratory and is somewhat dependent on the experience of the person performing the procedure.

9. It is essential to focus the microscope carefully and continually when counting reticulocytes. The dye will stain platelet granules and leukocyte granules, and these or precipitated stain may be mistaken for reticulocytes. Inadequate drying will cause the red cells to contain highly refractile areas resembling remnants of RNA. Artifacts in red cells must not be confused with authentic reticulocytes.

10. Reticulocytes are usually reported as a percentage of the total number of erythrocytes counted. However, more meaningful results are attained by correcting the reticulocyte count for the patient's hematocrit and for red cells prematurely released by the marrow, as indicated by the presence of "shift cells" (see under Reticulocyte Count Corrections).

Calculations

The reticulocyte count is reported as the percentage of reticulocytes in the total red cells counted. The following general formula can be used:

$$\frac{\text{Reticulocytes counted}}{\text{Erythrocytes counted}} \times 100$$

$$= \text{percentage of reticulocytes}$$

This formula can be derived from a simple proportion relating the number of reticulocytes counted in a given number of red cells to the number of reticulocytes per 100 red cells, which is the percentage of reticulocytes.

Example

On each of two slides 500 red cells are counted. The first slide shows 16 reticulocytes and the second shows 20 reticulocytes. What is the percentage of reticulocytes in the blood?

$$500 + 500 = 1000 \text{ cells counted}$$

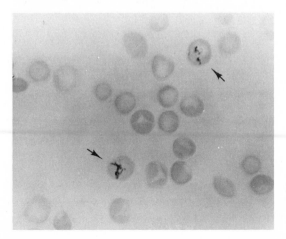

Fig. 3-30. Reticulocytes stained with new methylene blue (oil-immersion objective).

$20 + 16 = 36$ reticulocytes per 1000 cells counted

$$\frac{36 \text{ reticulocytes}}{1000 \text{ cells}} = \frac{x}{100 \text{ cells}}$$

$$x = \frac{36 \times 100}{1000} = 3.6 \text{ reticulocytes per 100 cells}$$

$$= 3.6 \text{ percent reticulocytes}$$

Reticulocyte count corrections[45,46]

Correction for abnormally low hematocrit

There is a relation between the percentage of reticulocytes calculated as shown above and the total erythrocyte count. A meaningful reticulocyte count should indicate the total production of erythrocytes regardless of the concentration of erythrocytes in the blood. The reticulocyte count can be corrected by multiplying the percentage of reticulocytes by the total erythrocyte count. However, red cell counts are not routine in most clinical laboratories, especially when electronic cell counters are not available. In such situations, the patient's hematocrit, which is readily available, can be used in lieu of the red cell count. The patient's hematocrit is compared with a normal hematocrit (considered to be 42 percent for women and 45 percent for men) and then related to the patient's reticulocyte count as shown below:

Corrected reticulocyte count (%)

$$= \text{patient's reticulocyte count (\%)}$$

$$\times \frac{\text{patient's hematocrit}}{\text{normal hematocrit}}$$

Correction for shift cells (reticulocyte production index)

It may also be necessary to correct the reticulocyte count for abnormally early release of red cells from the marrow into the peripheral blood.

Earlier than normal release of cells normally present in the marrow does not necessarily indicate increased marrow production. Abnormally early release of the red cells from the marrow into the peripheral blood is indicated by the presence of nucleated red blood cells and/or polychromatic macrocytes (shift cells) on blood films prepared with Wright's stain. Reticulocytes normally spend approximately 2 days in the bone marrow before being released into the blood, and approximately 1 percent of the circulating red cells are replaced each day. When the hematocrit and rate of marrow release are normal, the apparent reticulocyte percentage may be considered an index of production and set equal to 1.

Normal reticulocyte production index = 1

However, if reticulocytes are being released directly into the blood before maturation in the marrow, as evidenced by the presence of nucleated forms or shift cells on the blood film, the count is corrected by dividing the apparent reticulocyte count by 2 (the usual number of days of maturation). The corrected reticulocyte count is referred to as the reticulocyte production index. If no nucleated cells or shift cells are seen in the blood, the reticulocyte count is divided by 1 (i.e., left unchanged).

When there are both an abnormally low hematocrit and shift cells on the blood film, both corrections should be applied to the apparent reticulocyte count. The following general formula can be used:

Reticulocyte production index

$$= \frac{1}{2} \left[\text{patient's reticulocyte count (\%)} \right.$$

$$\left. \times \frac{\text{patient's hematocrit}}{\text{normal hematocrit}} \right]$$

The factor $\frac{1}{2}$ represents division by a maturation factor of 2. The maturation factor can vary, depending on the severity of the anemia. Marrow can respond to anemia by a two- to fivefold increase in red cell production.[47]

Precautions and technical factors

Careful focusing of the microscope is essential when counting reticulocytes. Stained platelet granules and leukocyte granules must not be mistaken for reticulocytes. Precipitated stain might also be mistaken for reticulum within the erythrocytes; to minimize this possibility the dye must be filtered immediately before use. Immediate drying of the film will prevent the formation of the crystalline-like artifacts that sometimes appear in the red cells and resemble remnants of RNA.

The proportions of dye and blood must be altered if the patient is anemic. More blood must be used. If the procedure is followed carefully, the distribution of reticulocytes on the blood films will be good. With experience, the problem of agreement will be primarily a result of the distribution of reticulocytes on the films and not misidentification of reticulocytes. Reticulocytes have a lower specific gravity than mature red cells and rise to the top of a blood-stain mixture. Therefore, the specimen must be well mixed before the incubation period and immediately before the three slides are made. The slides must be made in a uniform fashion to ensure random sampling.

Procedures employed for reticulocyte counts vary in different clinical laboratories, although the principles are the same. Variations include the manner in which the stain and cells are mixed, the total number of red cells counted and the number of slides observed, the use of a Miller disk in the eyepiece of the microscope to help define the field to be counted, counterstaining of the reticulocyte film with Wright's stain, and the use of corrections for the patient's hematocrit and the presence of shift cells.

Normal values

0.5–1.5 percent reticulocytes[48]

COUNTING EOSINOPHILS

Occasionally it will be necessary to count specific types of leukocytes, such as eosinophils. The eosinophil count is not a routine hematologic test. The relative number of eosinophils can be determined by doing differential studies on a stained blood film, but occasionally it is important to determine the total number of eosinophils in a particular volume of blood. For this purpose a direct method for counting eosinophils has been devised. It is similar in many respects to the counting methods for red and white blood cells.

One direct method is that devised by Randolph.[49] Whole blood is diluted with staining solution. Phloxine, which is present in the diluting fluid, serves to stain the eosinophils red; sodium carbonate and water help to lyse the white cells (except eosinophils), and the red cells are lysed by propylene glycol. If heparin is present in the diluting fluid, it will prevent clumping of the white cells. Sodium carbonate will also enhance the staining of the eosinophil granules. In the modification of the Randolph method described in this section sodium carbonate is omitted.

The normal values for the eosinophil count are 150–300 eosinophils per microliter of blood. A low eosinophil count (eosinopenia) will be found in hyperadrenalism (Cushing's disease) and shock, and after the administration of adrenocorticotropic hormone (ACTH).

It has been shown that the administration of a single 25-mg dose of ACTH intramuscularly to subjects with normal adrenocortical function results in a reduction of the total number of circulating eosinophils.[50,51] This effect has been used as a test of adrenocortical function, but it is not specific, and the value of the test is limited.[52] An inverse relation exists between adrenocortical activity and the number of circulating eosinophils. A modification of the Randolph method is used for random eosinophil counts before and after the administration of ACTH.[53,54]

An increase in the number of eosinophils (eosinophilia) may be seen in cases of trichinosis, widespread metastatic carcinoma, allergies (particularly asthma), skin disease (eczema), and infectious diseases (e.g., scarlet fever).

Diluent for the Randolph method (modified)

The diluent used is a combination of phloxine B and methylene blue in propylene glycol. Another diluent that can be used is a hypotonic solution of eosin.

Preparation of diluent

1. Solution A. Dissolve 0.5 g of phloxine B in 1000 ml of 50 ml/dl propylene glycol in deionized water.
2. Solution B. Dissolve 0.5 g of methylene blue and 1000 ml of 50 ml/dl propylene glycol in deionized water.
3. Mix 1 part of solution B in 9 parts of solution A immediately before use.

Equipment for eosinophil count— Modified Randolph method

The blood for the eosinophil count is diluted in a white blood cell diluting pipet. A special counting chamber is used for this procedure—the Levy chamber with Fuchs-Rosenthal ruling. This chamber usually has a depth of 0.2 mm and has two ruled areas of 16 mm² each.

Procedure for the modified Randolph method

1. Blood (venous blood preserved with EDTA, double oxalate, or heparin or capillary blood is satisfactory) is drawn to the 1.0 mark in a leukocyte pipet (a 1:10 dilution is usually needed for this procedure) and diluted to the 11.0 mark with the propylene glycol-dye diluent. Duplicate pipets should be prepared.
2. The pipets are shaken for 20 minutes and mounted on two sides of a counting chamber.
3. The cells are allowed to settle for 20 minutes, with the chambers covered to prevent evaporation during this waiting period.
4. Eosinophils are counted under low power in each of the four ruled areas (the total area counted is 64 mm²). The eosinophils are identified in the counting chamber by their brightly red-stained granules. The remainder of the leukocytes do not stain, and the erythrocytes are destroyed by the diluent.

Calculations

In calculating the total eosinophil count, the following factors are taken into consideration: (1) the total number of eosinophils counted, (2) the dilution of the blood (usually 1:10), and (3) the volume of the diluted blood, which is equal to the depth of the chamber (0.2 mm) times the area in which the cells are counted (64 mm²), or 12.8 μl. The number of eosinophils per microliter of blood is given by the equation:

$$\frac{\text{Eosinophils counted} \times 10 \; (\text{in } 64 \text{ mm}^2)}{12.8 \, \mu l} = \text{eosinophils}/\mu l$$

By using this formula, a calculation factor of 0.78 is found. The normal value for the eosinophil count is 100–300 cells/μl.

Precautions and technical factors

Venous or capillary blood may be used for this test. The type of blood used should be noted, as simultaneous counts with venous and capillary blood have shown capillary blood to give values 25 percent higher.[54]

The two solutions (A and B) used for the diluting fluid are stable separately, but the final mixture of the two dyes must be used within 4-8 hours. After 8 hours, the dyes will precipitate.[54]

Technical errors should be minimized. The same technical factors apply that were described for other cell counts. To avoid undue rupture of the eosinophil membrane, gentle shaking of the pipets is suggested.

The approximate error in the eosinophil count is ±20 percent when the Fuchs-Rosenthal counting chamber is used. Greater errors are seen when hemocytometers with Neubauer ruling are used.

The direct counting method can be double-checked by use of an indirect counting method. To do this, a white blood cell count is done on the specimen and two blood films are prepared and stained with Wright's stain. The indirect eosinophil count can be calculated as follows:

Eosinophils/μl

= eosinophils in differential (%) X WBC count

If the indirect and direct methods give counts that differ significantly, the procedures should be repeated.

Normal value for eosinophil count

150–300 eosinophils/μl[55]

RED BLOOD CELL OSMOTIC FRAGILITY TEST

The osmotic fragility test is a valuable laboratory procedure that is helpful in the diagnosis of different types of anemia. In simple terms, the osmotic fragility test reflects the shape of the red blood cell and whether or not it tends to be easily hemolyzed. The shape of the red cell is dependent on the volume, surface area, and functional state of the red cell membrane.

When red cells are introduced into a hypotonic solution of sodium chloride, they take up water and swell until a critical volume is reached, and then hemolysis, or rupture, occurs. When the critical volume is reached, the cells are spherical. In this shape the cell has the maximum volume for its surface area, and any further increase in volume would require an increase in the area of the cell membrane. As the cell takes up water it becomes increasingly fragile.

A red cell that is already spherical in shape has an increased osmotic fragility in hypotonic solutions because it can swell only a little before it bursts. Conversely, one that is flat or has a large surface area compared to its volume has a decreased osmotic fragility in hypotonic solutions, because it can swell considerably before it reaches a spherical shape and bursts. The osmotic fragility is thus a measure of the rate of hemolysis of the red cell when exposed to hypotonic solutions of sodium chloride. When the rate of hemolysis of the red cell is increased the osmotic fragility is increased, and when the rate of hemolysis is decreased the osmotic fragility is decreased. An increase in the osmotic fragility of a red cell is sometimes referred to as a decrease in the resistance of the cell to rupture.

Clinical significance

In certain diseases or conditions, the osmotic fragility of the red cell is characteristically increased or decreased. Since the resistance of the red cell membrane corresponds to its geometric configuration, red cell populations comprised of spherocytes demonstrate increased hemolysis, while those comprised of flattened red cells (such as sickle cells, target cells, or hypochromic cells) demonstrate decreased hemolysis.[56] Hypochromic red cells are very thin, contain very little hemoglobin, and therefore swell to a large extent before reaching their critical volume. Diminished fragility is seen in the presence of obstructive jaundice, in iron-deficiency anemias, in thalassemia, in sickle-cell anemia, after splenectomy, and in a variety of anemias where target cells are seen. In conditions where the red cells are already spheroidal, as in congenital hemolytic anemia, hereditary spherocytosis, and wherever spherocytes are found, increased fragility of the cell is demonstrated.

Methods for determination of osmotic fragility

Manual and automated methods are available for estimating the osmotic fragility of the red blood cell. In the manual methods, the test blood and normal ("control") blood are placed in a series of graded-strength sodium chloride solutions and any resultant hemolysis is compared with a 100 percent standard (blood and distilled water). In one such manual method the results can be read after incubation for 1 hour at room temperature (20°); this is called an immediate testing method. In another, incubation for 24 hours at 37°C is required. Incubation at 37°C enhances the changes in red cell fragility. Fragility curves that appear normal in immediate testing methods may appear abnormal when the test is done after incubation of the blood. Thus, the incubation test is helpful in detecting mild cases of spherocytosis and nonspherocytic hemolytic anemia. It is advisable to perform both tests (immediate and incubation) on each sample submitted for investigation.[57]

The osmotic fragility test set up manually to be read immediately (in 1 hour) will be described in this section.[58]

Reagents

1. Buffered sodium chloride stock solution (10 g/dl). Weigh 180.0 g of NaCl (dry for 24 hours in a desiccator before weighing), 27.31 g of dibasic sodium phosphate (Na_2HPO_4), 4.86 g of monobasic sodium phosphate ($NaH_2PO_4 \cdot 2H_2O$). Dilute to 2 L with distilled water. This solution is stable for several months at room temperature if it is kept in a well-stoppered bottle. The pH is important; it must be 7.4.
2. Buffered sodium chloride (1 g/dl) prepared from the stock solution. Mix 20 ml of buffered 10 g/dl NaCl with 180 ml of distilled water.
3. Working sodium chloride solutions. Prepare from the 1 g/dl solution, using distilled water as the diluent, in the following concentrations: 0.85, 0.66, 0.56, 0.52, 0.48, 0.44, 0.40, and 0.32 g/dl. Other concentrations can be included when necessary.

Specimens

A sample of freshly drawn venous blood, anticoagulated with heparin or defibrinated with glass beads, is preferred for the measurement of osmotic fragility. The blood should be drawn with as little physical trauma to the cells as possible. Heparin is the anticoagulant of choice because it causes less distortion of the red cells, but prolonged exposure to heparin will result in distortion of the red cells, so the test should be done as soon as possible. Defibrination with glass beads is another means of preventing clotting. Freshly drawn venous blood is placed in a flask containing small glass beads. The flask is rotated, exposing the blood to the beads. On agitation, the fibrin coats the beads and is removed from the blood.

A normal or control specimen must be drawn at the same time as the sample of the patient's blood. The patient's results are interpreted by comparison with the results for the control specimen. Both specimens are treated in exactly the same way.

Oxalated blood should not be used for this test. The salts present in oxalate anticoagulants may alter the pH of the blood-saline mixture.

Procedure

1. Label nine conical centrifuge tubes for the control specimen and nine for the patient specimen: one tube for each of the eight sodium chloride solutions, plus one tube for distilled water only.

2. Pipet 10 ml of each sodium chloride solution into the appropriately labeled centrifuge tube. Pipet 10 ml of distilled water into the last tube. One set of tubes is prepared for the patient's sample of blood and another for the control sample.

3. Pipet 0.02 ml (using a Sahli pipet) of well-mixed blood into each tube. This must be done very carefully and slowly, as any disturbance of the red cells may alter the results. Carefully rinse the pipet. Do not blow into the solutions to mix them, as this might disturb the red cell membranes. Cover each tube with Parafilm and gently invert it to mix the sample with the sodium chloride solution.

4. Incubate the cell suspensions undisturbed at room temperature for 1 hour.

5. Transfer the tubes carefully to a centrifuge and spin at 2000 r/min for 5 minutes.

6. Carefully decant the supernatant solutions into photometer cuvettes and read in a spectrophotometer at 550 nm (the same wavelength used to read hemoglobin). The absorbance should be set to read 0 for the first tube of the series (the one with 0.85 g/dl of NaCl), as this represents the blank or 0 percent hemolysis. No hemolysis should occur in this tube because the saline solution is isotonic with blood. The tube with only distilled water represents 100 percent hemolysis.

7. Record the absorbance for each cuvette.

8. Calculate the percent hemolysis for each supernatant in the following way:

Percent hemolysis

$$= \frac{\text{absorbance of supernatant}}{\text{absorbance of 100\% hemolysis tube}} \times 100$$

Using linear graph paper, plot the percent hemolysis on the vertical axis and the sodium chloride concentration on the horizontal axis; include the control results.

Interpretation of test and technical factors

The control values should be plotted on the same graph as the patient values. The control results are fundamental for the correct interpretation of the test results. They must fall within the established normal range, for the patient's results to be considered valid. A difference of more than one tube between the patient and the control is significant.[59]

The osmotic fragility test is best reported as a curve on linear graph paper, always including the control results and indicating the saline solution concentrations at which (1) hemolysis begins, (2) hemolysis is complete, and (3) 50 percent hemolysis occurs. The patient's results are interpreted from the appearance of the completed graph line and not from one isolated point on the graph. The tube having the highest concentration of saline in which hemolysis is complete determines complete hemolysis. Normally, hemolysis should be complete in the 0.32 g/dl saline tube. The mean corpuscular fragility (MCF), which is the same as 50 percent hemolysis, is normally seen in the tubes having 0.40-0.44 g/dl NaCl.[60] These results must be obtained at a pH of 7.4 and at 20°C.

Blood films are prepared from both the control and the patient's blood and stained with Wright's stain. The results of the osmotic fragility test should be verified by the red cell morphology observed on the stained film.

Since the ninth tube (distilled water and blood) represents 100 percent hemolysis, it must be clear. If it is not clear for the control specimen, the test must be repeated.

LUPUS ERYTHEMATOSUS CELL TEST

The lupus erythematosus (LE) cell is a neutrophil that has ingested a homogeneous globular mass of altered nuclear material. There is a factor present in the blood of people with systemic lupus erythematosus that has the ability to cause depolymerization of the nuclear chromatin of polymorphonuclear (PMN) leukocytes, and the depolymerized material is subsequently phagocytized, or ingested, by an intact PMN leukocyte, giving rise to the LE cell. The factor is called the LE factor, it is present in the gamma globulin portion of the plasma or serum, and it appears to be an antibody. The transformed nuclear material in the white cell attracts phagocytes, usually segmented neutrophilic granulocytes (PMNs) and occasionally monocytes. The phagocytes with the ingested nuclear material are the LE cells. Formation of LE cells requires the presence of the LE factor, damaged leukocytes, and normal active leukocytes.

Methods for demonstrating lupus erythematosus cells

A variety of tests are used in the laboratory to demonstrate the presence of LE cells and the LE factor. A standard and traditional method is to mash the blood clot, centrifuge the clot fragments, and make buffy coat smears from the resulting cell suspension. This method will be described in this section. In other techniques the blood is defibrinated with glass beads, collected in heparin, or centrifuged in heparinized capillary tubes, and plasma layers are traumatized with a wire. In these methods the plasma LE factor and leukocytes are brought into close contact with each other, and the leukocytes are traumatized— both processes are important in the formation of LE cells. The buffy coat layer obtained in many

of these methods is spread on a slide, stained with Wright's stain, and observed for the presence of LE cells.

Clinical significance of lupus erythematosus cells

Systemic lupus erythematosus (SLE) affects women most commonly and is characterized by skin rash; arthralgia; fever; renal, cardiac, and vascular lesions; anemia; leukopenia; and often thrombocytopenia. In patients suffering from SLE, LE cells are found in the bone marrow and the peripheral blood when the smears are prepared according to a specific procedure.

This phenomenon may also occur in patients with other connective tissue (collagen) disorders, such as rheumatoid arthritis, scleroderma, and hepatitis. A negative test for LE cells does not rule out SLE as a diagnosis.

Certain drugs can also give a positive LE cell test with or without SLE-like symptoms. It is important to be aware of the medications given to the patient. Many drugs can interfere with laboratory results.

Specimens

Whole blood (5-10 ml) is drawn from the patient and allowed to clot in a plain serum tube for 2 hours. The resulting clot is used for the method known as the *mashed clot test* or the *2-hour clot test*.

Procedure for the mashed clot test[61]

1. Leave the blood undisturbed for 2 hours in a plain serum tube after it is drawn.

2. Remove the clot from the tube with applicator sticks and place it in a sieve or mesh.

3. Add approximately 1 ml of the patient's serum to the clot. Using a brass pestle or other pushing device, grind or mash the clot, allowing it to drain through the sieve. Most of the fibrin is removed and trauma is provided so the LE phenomenon can occur.

4. Using a Pasteur pipet, collect the sieved blood and put it in a Wintrobe hematocrit tube.

5. Centrifuge for 10 minutes at 1000 r/min.

6. With a clean Pasteur pipet, carefully remove and discard all but 1 or 2 mm of serum, leaving the cellular layers undisturbed.

7. Transfer the trace of serum together with the buffy coat layer onto a clean glass slide. This should be a large drop of specimen.

8. Using the tip of the Pasteur pipet, mix and transfer a small drop to one end of a microscope slide. Spread quickly as in making a regular blood film and dry rapidly. Repeat this technique, making two or three films.

9. Stain with Wright's stain in the usual manner.

10. Have a pathologist or experienced medical technologist examine the blood film for the presence of LE cells.

Interpretation of test, technical problems, and sources of error

As much of this procedure as possible should be carried out while wearing rubber gloves. This will help to minimize exposure to hepatitis virus.

When using the mashed clot method, if the blood is not allowed to clot for 2 hours a falsely negative result may be obtained. If the clot is allowed to sit for longer than 2 hours cellular autolysis may be extensive.

The blood films made from the LE preparation will not appear as homogeneous as routine finger puncture films or venous blood films. This is primarily caused by the concentration of cellular material.

Under the microscope, the bulk of the LE cell is occupied by a spherical, homogeneous mass that stains purplish brown. The lobes of the PMNs are usually seen at the periphery of the mass. The films, especially their edges (LE cells are most numerous at the edges and the end of the film), are searched and a minimum of 500 PMNs are counted before a negative result is reported. Frequently, dead nuclei will be seen lying free. If these are numerous, the suspicion of SLE is heightened.[62] The presence of dead nuclei is never diagnostic, however.

The presence of one LE cell is not a sufficient basis for reporting a positive result. Several typical LE cells should be seen before a positive report is made.

Certain drugs can give false results in this test.

The LE factor is also termed an antinuclear factor, since it reacts against cell nuclei. The presence of this factor can also be detected by an immunofluorescent method and by a serological method that tests the ability of the serum to agglutinate latex particles.

NORMAL VALUES FOR SOME HEMATOLOGIC PROCEDURES

As explained under What is Normal? in Chap. 1, normal values for any laboratory determination depend on many factors, and probably the most meaningful values are those peculiar to the particular institution and locale. The values presented as normal in this section are from several sources, and it is hoped that they are close to the "true" normal values, if they exist. Table 3-2 shows normal values for adult peripheral blood and Table 3-3 shows normal values for the leukocyte count, leukocyte differential, and hemoglobin concentration at various ages.

Table 3-2. Adult normal values for peripheral blood

Test	Williams[a] Mean ± 1 SD	Wintrobe[b] Mean	Wintrobe[b] 95% range	Coulter counter, model S[c] Mean ± 2 SD
White cell count, × 10^3/μl of blood	♂ 7.25 ± 1.69 ♀ 7.28 ± 1.89	7.0 (median)	4.3–10.0	♂ 7.8 ± 3 ♀ 7.8 ± 3
Red cell count, × 10^6/μl of blood	♂ 5.11 ± 0.38 ♀ 4.51 ± 0.36	♂ 5.4 ♀ 4.8	4.5–6.3 4.2–5.5	♂ 5.4 ± 0.7 ♀ 4.8 ± 0.6
Hemoglobin, g/dl of blood	♂ 15.5 ± 1.1 ♀ 13.7 ± 1.0	♂ 16 ♀ 14	14.0–18.0 12.0–16.0	♂ 16.0 ± 2 ♀ 14.0 ± 2
Volume of packed red cells (hematocrit), %	♂ 46.0 ± 3.1 ♀ 40.9 ± 3.0	♂ 47 ♀ 42	40–54 37–47	♂ 47 ± 5 ♀ 42 ± 5
Mean corpuscular volume (MCV), fl	♂ 90.1 ± 4.8 ♀ 90.4 ± 4.8	91	82–101	♂ 87 ± 7 ♀ 90 ± 9
Mean corpuscular hemoglobin (MCH), pg	♂ 30.2 ± 1.8 ♀ 30.2 ± 1.9	31	27–34	29 ± 2
Mean corpuscular hemoglobin concentration (MCHC), g/dl or %	♂ 33.9 ± 1.2 ♀ 33.6 ± 1.1	34 ± 2	31.5–36	34 ± 2
Platelet count, × 10^3/μl of blood	248 ± 50	140–440		172–392[d]

[a]From Williams et al., "Hematology," McGraw-Hill Book Company, New York, 1972.
[b]From Wintrobe et al., "Clinical Hematology," 7th ed., Lea & Febiger, Philadelphia, 1974.
[c]Manufacturer's values.
[d]Platelet count values determined with the Technicon Auto Counter.

Table 3-3. Normal leukocyte count, leukocyte differential, and hemoglobin concentration at various ages[a]

Age	Total leukocytes/μl	Neutrophils Total	Neutrophils Band	Neutrophils Segmented	Lympho-cytes	Mono-cytes	Eosino-phils	Baso-phils	Hemoglobin (g/dl of blood)
12 mo	11 400 (6000–17 500)[b]	31	3.1	28	61	4.8	2.6	0.4	11.6 (9.0–14.6)
4 yr	9100 (5500–15 500)	42	3.0	39	50	5.0	2.8	0.6	12.6 (9.6–15.5)
6 yr	8500 (5000–14 500)	51	3.0	48	42	4.7	2.7	0.6	12.7 (10.0–15.5)
10 yr	8100 (4500–13 500)	54	3.0	51	38	4.3	2.4	0.5	13.0 (10.7–15.5)
21 yr	7400 (4500–11 000)	59	3.0	56	34	4.0	2.7	0.5	♂15.8 (14.0–18.0) ♀13.9 (11.5–16.0)

Leukocyte differential – average percentages (number per 100 cells counted)

[a]Adapted from Table 2-3, p. 18, Williams et al., "Hematology," McGraw-Hill Book Company, New York, 1972.
[b]Numbers in parentheses give the 95 percent range.

REFERENCES

1. Bong Hak Hyun, John K. Ashton, and Kathleen Dolan, "Practical Hematology," p. 184, W. B. Saunders Company, Philadelphia, 1975.
2. Barbara A. Brown, "Hematology: Principles and Procedures," 2d ed., p. 73, Lea & Febiger, Philadelphia, 1976.
3. *Ibid.*
4. *Ibid.*, p. 71.
5. K. A. Evelyn and N. T. Malloy, Microdetermination of Oxyhemoglobin, Methemoglobin, and Sulfhemoglobin in a Single Sample of Blood, *J. Biol. Chem.*, vol. 126, p. 655, 1938.
6. E. J. King and M. Gilchrist, Determination of Hemoglobin by a CyanHaematin Method, *Lancet*, vol. 2, p. 201, 1947.
7. Israel Davidsohn and John Bernard Henry (eds.), "Clinical Diagnosis by Laboratory Methods," 15th ed., p. 108, W. B. Saunders Company, Philadelphia, 1974.
8. Hyun et al., *op. cit.*, p. 201.
9. J. M. England, D. M. Walford, and D. A. Waters, Re-assessment of the Reliability of the Hematocrit, *Br. J. Haematol.*, vol. 23, p. 247, 1972.
10. M. M. Wintrobe, "Clinical Hematology," 7th ed., pp. 110–111, Lea & Febiger, Philadelphia, 1974.
11. M. M. Strumia, A. B. Sample, and E. D. Hart, An Improved Microhematocrit Method, *Am. J. Clin. Pathol.*, vol. 24, p. 1016, 1954.
12. Wintrobe, *loc. cit.*
13. Davidsohn and Henry, *op. cit.*, p. 116.
14. Hyun et al., *op. cit.*, p. 204.
15. G. Brecher, M. Schneiderman, and G. Z. Williams, Evaluation of Electronic Red Blood Cell Counter, *Am. J. Clin. Pathol.*, vol. 26, p. 1439, 1956.
16. T. B. Magrath and J. Berkson, Electronic Blood Cell Counting, *Am. J. Clin. Pathol.*, vol. 34, p. 203, 1960.
17. Hyun, et al., *op. cit.*, p. 205.
18. International Committee for Standardization in Hematology, Reference Method for the Erythrocyte Sedimentation Rate (ESR) Test on Human Blood, *J. Clin. Pathol.*, vol. 26, p. 301, 1973.
19. A. Westergren, The Technique of the Red Cell Sedimentation Reaction, *Am. Rev. Tuberc. Pulm. Dis.*, vol. 14, p. 94, 1926.
20. "Hematology Manual Using Unopette Disposable Diluting Pipette," Becton, Dickinson & Company, Rutherford, N.J., 1972.
21. J. Berkson, R. B. Magath, and M. Hurn, The Error of Estimate of the Blood Cell Count as Made with the Haemocytometer, *Am. J. Physiol.*, vol. 128, p. 309, 1940.
22. R. Biggs and R. L. Macmillan, The Errors of Some Hematologic Methods as They Are Used in Routine Laboratory, *J. Clin. Pathol.*, vol. 7, p. 269, 1948.
23. Berkson et al., *loc. cit.*
24. Berkson et al., *loc. cit.*
25. Biggs and Macmillan, *loc. cit.*
26. William J. Williams, Ernest Beutler, Allan J. Erslev, and R. Wayne Rundles, "Hematology," p. 12, McGraw-Hill Book Company, New York, 1972.
27. G. M. Brittin, G. Brecher, and C. A. Johnson, Evaluation of the Coulter Counter Model S, *Am. J. Clin. Pathol.*, vol. 52, p. 679, 1969.
28. Hyun et al., *op. cit.*, pp. 200 and 207.
29. G. Brecher and E. P. Cronkite, Morphology and Enumeration of Human Blood Platelets, *J. Appl. Physiol.*, vol. 3, p. 365, 1950.
30. B. S. Bull, N. A. Schneiderman, and G. Brecher, Platelet Count with the Coulter Counter, *Am. J. Clin. Pathol.*, vol. 44, p. 678, 1965.
31. H. M. Rees and E. E. Ecker, An Improved Method for Counting Platelets, *J. Am. Med. Assoc.*, vol. 80, p. 621, 1923.
32. Brown, *op. cit.*, p. 102.
33. Hyun et al., *op. cit.*, p. 223.
34. Wintrobe, *op. cit.*, p. 91.
35. *Ibid.*, p. 92.
36. *Ibid.*, p. 1794.
37. "Manual 76 Surveys Interlaboratory Comparison Programs," p. 17, College of American Pathologists, Skokie, Ill., 1976.
38. Wintrobe, *op. cit.*, p. 1794.
39. Brown, *op. cit.*, p. 60.
40. Davidsohn and Henry, *op. cit.*, pp. 161–164.

41. L. W. Diggs, D. Sturm, and A. Bell, "The Morphology of Human Blood Cells," Abbot Laboratories, North Chicago, Ill., 1970.
42. Wintrobe, *op. cit.*, p. 289.
43. Williams et al., *op. cit.*, pp. 275–276.
44. Wintrobe, *op. cit.*, p. 119.
45. Brown, *op. cit.*, pp. 96–100.
46. Robert S. Hillman and Clement A. Finch, "Red Cell Manual," 4th ed., pp. 56–60, F. A. Davis Company, Philadelphia, 1974.
47. *Ibid.*, p. 60.
48. Davidsohn and Henry, *op. cit.*, p. 178.
49. T. C. Randolph, Differentiation and Enumeration of Eosinophils in the Counting Chamber with a Glycol Stain: A Valuable Technique in Appraising ACTH Dosage," *J. Lab. Clin. Med.*, vol. 34, p. 1696, 1949.
50. A. G. Hills, P. H. Farsham, and C. A. Finch, Changes in Circulating Leukocytes Induced by the Administration of Pituitary Adrenocorticotrophic Hormones (ACTH) in Man, *Blood*, vol. 3, p. 755, 1948.
51. G. W. Thorn, P. H. Farsham, F. T. G. Prunty, and A. G. Hill, Test for Adrenal Cortical Insufficiency: Response to Pituitary Adrenocorticotrophic Hormone, *J. Am. Med. Assoc.*, vol. 137, p. 1005, 1948.
52. D. B. Huntsman, M. C. Dagget, and D. E. Holtkamp, Hinkleman's Solution as a Diluent for Counting Eosinophils, *Am. J. Clin. Pathol.*, vol. 31, p. 91, 1959.
53. T. C. Randolph, Blood Studies in Allergy: Direct Counting Chamber Determination of Eosinophils, *J. Allergy*, vol. 5, p. 96, 1944.
54. M. J. Stephens, Direct Eosinophil Counts, *Minn. Med. Technol.*, vol. 14, p. 3, 1950.
55. Brown, *op. cit.*, p. 105.
56. J. Suess, D. Limentani, W. Dameshek, and M. J. Dolloff, A Quantitative Method for the Determination and Charting of the Erythrocyte Hypotonic Fragility, *Blood*, vol. 3, p. 1209, 1948.
57. Stanley S. Raphael et al., "Lynch's Medical Laboratory Technology," 3d ed., vol. II, p. 1116, W. B. Saunders Company, Philadelphia, 1976.
58. J. V. Dacie and S. M. Lewis, "Practical Hematology," 5th ed., Grune & Stratton, New York, 1975.
59. Davidsohn and Henry, *op. cit.*, p. 132.
60. Raphael et al., *op. cit.*, p. 1115.
61. T. B. Magath and V. Winkle, Technique for Demonstrating L.E. (Lupus Erythematosus) Cells in Blood, *Am. J. Clin. Pathol.*, vol. 22, p. 586, 1952.
62. Raphael et al., *op. cit.*, p. 1104.

BIBLIOGRAPHY

Ackerman, P. G.: "Electronic Instrumentation in the Clinical Laboratory," Little, Brown and Company, Boston, 1972.

Blongren, S. E.: Drug Induced Lupus Erythematosus, *Semin. Hematol.*, vol. 10, 1973.

Brittin, G. M. and G. Brecher: Instrumentation and Automation in Clinical Hematology, *Prog. Hematol.*, vol. 7, 1971.

Brown, Barbara A.: "Hematology: Principles and Procedures," 2d ed., Lea & Febiger, Philadelphia, 1976.

Davidsohn, Israel and John Bernard Henry (eds.): "Clinical Diagnosis by Laboratory Methods," 15th ed., W. B. Saunders Company, Philadelphia, 1974.

Dougherty, William M.: "Introduction to Hematology," C. V. Mosby Company, St. Louis, 1971.

Gagon, T. E., J. W. Athens, D. R. Bogg, and G. E. Cartwright: An Evaluation of the Variance of Leukocyte Counts as Performed with the Hemacytometer, Coulter, and Fisher Instruments, *Am. J. Clin. Pathol.*, vol. 46, 1966.

Hargraves, M. M.: Discovery of the LE Cell and Its Morphology, *Mayo Clin. Proc.*, vol. 44, 1969.

Hargraves, M. M., H. Richmond, and R. Morton: Presentation of Two Bone Marrow Elements: The Tart Cell and the LE Cell, *Proc. Staff Meet. Mayo Clin.*, vol. 23, 1948.

Hillman, Robert S. and Clement A. Finch: "Red

Cell Manual," 4th ed., F. A. Davis Company, Philadelphia, 1974.

Hyun, Bong Hak, John K. Ashton, and Kathleen Dolan: "Practical Hematology," W. B. Saunders Company, Philadelphia, 1975.

"Instruction and Service Manual for the Coulter Counter Model S," 12th ed., Coulter Electronics, Inc., Hialeah, Fla., September 1972.

"Instruction and Service Manual for the Model F Coulter Counter," Coulter Electronics, Inc., Hialeah, Fla., 1967.

Lewis, S. M. and J. F. Coster: Quality Control in Haematology, in "Symposium of the International Committee for Standardization in Haematology," Academic Press, London, 1975.

"Manual 76 Surveys Interlaboratory Comparison Programs," College of American Pathologists, Skokie, Ill., 1976.

"Quality Control in Hematology," Pfizer Diagnostics Company, New York.

Raphael, Stanley S. et al.: "Lynch's Medical Laboratory Technology," 3d ed., vol. II, W. B. Saunders Company, Philadelphia, 1976.

Williams, William J., Ernest Beutler, Allan J. Erslev, and R. Wayne Rundles: "Hematology," McGraw-Hill Book Company, New York, 1972.

Wintrobe, Maxwell M.: "Clinical Hematology," 7th ed., Lea & Febiger, Philadelphia, 1974.

FOUR
COAGULATION AND HEMOSTASIS

Hemostasis is the cessation of blood flow from an injured blood vessel. It is one of the most important natural defense mechanisms of the body. The process of hemostasis involves numerous interdependent factors that are controlled carefully by the body for the purpose of preventing bleeding. When there is an injury to a blood vessel, the hemostatic process is designed to repair the break. Thus, hemostasis is the process whereby the body retains the blood within the vascular system, in spite of the many traumas that injure the blood vessel walls.

The most immediate response of the body to bleeding is *vasoconstriction*. In this process, the damaged blood vessel constricts, decreasing the blood flow through the injured area. A platelet plug can then form, which helps to further inhibit the bleeding. Finally, coagulation factors present in the blood interact, forming a fibrin network or clot, to stop the bleeding completely. Slow lysis of the clot begins, and final repair to the site of the injury thus takes place.

Coagulation and hemostasis are complicated subjects. The discussion in this chapter is simplified, but certain basic concepts must be understood by the technician before coagulation procedures are carried out.

HEMOSTATIC MECHANISM

The hemostatic mechanism is the entire process by which bleeding from an injured blood vessel is controlled and finally stopped. It is a series of physical and biochemical changes that are normally initiated by an injury to the blood vessel and tissues and that culminate in the transformation of fluid blood into a thrombus or clot, which effectively seals the injured vessel. The entire hemostatic mechanism can be divided into three parts: extravascular effects, vascular effects, and intravascular effects.

Extravascular effects consist of (1) the physical effect of the surrounding tissues, such as muscle, skin, and elastic tissue, which tend to close and seal the tear in the vessel that is injured, and (2) the biochemical effects of certain substances that are released from the injured tissues and react with plasma and platelet factors. The latter factors are called the *extrinsic system* of coagulation.

Vascular effects are concerned with the blood vessels themselves, which constrict almost instantaneously when injured. The vasoconstriction phenomenon tends to pass off within a relatively short time, but it may be enhanced and prolonged by local release of a vasoconstricting substance, serotonin.[1] Serotonin is released from the platelets as they adhere to the margins of the injury in the wall of the blood vessel. It promotes local, direct, biochemically stimulated narrowing of the torn blood vessel and of locally intact blood vessels in the same vicinity as the injury.

The intravascular factors take part in an extremely complicated sequence of physiochemical reactions that transform the liquid blood into a firm fibrin clot. This process requires the initiation of a platelet plug. This is followed by reinforcement with fibrin derived from the activation of the *intrinsic system* of coagulation. All the factors necessary for the intrinsic system are contained within the blood. Many natural inhibitors and accelerators are brought into action during this time.

A bleeding tendency can result from a defect in any of the phases of repair; that is, (1) the vascular system itself may be prone to injury; (2) the platelets may be inadequate in number to form the emergency platelet plug; (3) the fibrin clotting mechanism may be inadequate; or (4) the fibroblastic repair may be inadequate. Excessive abnormal bleeding is usually the result of a combination of defects.

COAGULATION STUDIES

Most of the clinical conditions requiring coagulation studies involve the intrinsic system of coagulation. For this reason, the emphasis in this chapter is on laboratory procedures involving this system. The coagulation factors, their nomenclature, and procedures for analyzing some of the more important coagulation factors are discussed.

The blood coagulation mechanism is complicated and involves many factors. Knowing which factor is not performing its proper function is of critical importance to the physician. This knowledge is gained through the use of several different laboratory tests. The proper formation of a blood clot after a scratch or cut depends on healthy functioning of all the factors. In an individual having a weakness or deficiency in one or several of the factors, severe trauma from a serious injury or from surgical treatment can result in collapse of the clotting mechanism. This in turn will result in a most drastic manifestation—severe hemorrhage. This has been dramatically demonstrated in persons whose clotting mechanism is adequate for everyday living but who, during such common surgical procedures as dental extractions or tonsillectomies, erupt into severe bleeding. It is of the utmost importance, therefore, that the laboratory tests in this area be done well. Most of these tests employ macroscopic observations.

The topic of blood coagulation is controversial, and much research is still in progress in this field. It is generally agreed that all the elements necessary for clot formation are normally present in the circulating blood. The fluidity of the blood, therefore, depends on a balance between the coagulant and anticoagulant factors.

The mechanism of coagulation takes place in three major steps: (1) the formation of thromboplastin, (2) the formation of thrombin, and (3) the formation of fibrin. Various clotting factors, or constituents, are involved in this mechanism.

Coagulation factors and their nomenclature

To standardize the complex nomenclature that was used by those involved in coagulation studies, the International Committee on Nomenclature of Blood Clotting Factors was established in 1954.[2] Twelve coagulation factors were described and were designated by Roman numerals

(Table 4-1). It should be noted that no factor VI is recognized at present, and factor III is not a single substance but a variety of substances.

Factor I (fibrinogen)

The term fibrinogen has been in use for many years. Fibrinogen is the soluble precursor of the clot-forming protein, fibrin. It is a plasma protein (globulin) with a molecular weight of 340 000 that is present in normal persons at a concentration of 300–400 mg/dl. A minimum of 60–100 mg/dl is required for normal coagulation.[3]

Fibrinogen is manufactured by the liver. In severe liver disease a moderate lowering of the plasma fibrinogen level may occur, although rarely to the degree where hemorrhage occurs.

By the action of thrombin, peptides are split from the fibrinogen molecule, leaving a fibrin monomer.

Fibrinogen is relatively stable to heat and storage, but may be irreversibly precipitated at 56°C. About 50 percent of transfused fibrinogen disappears from the circulation in 48 hours, and 75 percent disappears within 6 days.

Factor II (prothrombin)

Prothrombin is also a term that has been used for many years. Prothrombin is synthesized by the liver through the action of vitamin K. It is a protein with a molecular weight of about 63 000, and is normally present in the blood in a concentration of approximately 20 mg/dl.

In the presence of calcium ions, prothrombin is converted to thrombin by the enzymatic action of thromboplastins from both extrinsic and intrinsic sources. It is utilized in the clotting mechanism to such a degree that little remains in the serum. In normal plasma, there is an excess of prothrombin relative to the amount of thrombin needed to clot fibrinogen. Nature has provided a wide margin of safety for this important substance.

Factor III (thromboplastin)

Thromboplastin is the name given to any substance capable of converting prothrombin to thrombin. In coagulation, two separate mechanisms utilize thromboplastin, as intrinsic or blood

Table 4-1. Nomenclature of the coagulation factors[a]

Factor	Name	Synonym
I	Fibrinogen	
II	Prothrombin	
III	Thromboplastin	
IV	Calcium	
V	Proaccelerin	Labile factor, accelerator globulin (AcG)
VII	Proconvertin	Stable factor, serum prothrombin conversion accelerator (SPCA)
VIII	Antihemophilic factor (AHF)	Antihemophilic globulin (AHG), antihemophilic factor A
IX	Plasma thromboplastin component (PTC)	Christmas factor, antihemophilic factor B
X	Stuart factor	Prower factor
XI	Plasma thromboplastin antecedent (PTA)	Antihemophilic factor C
XII	Hageman factor	Glass or contact factor
XIII	Fibrinase	Clot or fibrin stabilizing factor (FSF)

[a]Adapted from Raphael et al., "Lynch's Medical Laboratory Technology," 3d ed., vol. II, table 42-2, p. 1202, W. B. Saunders Company, Philadelphia, 1976.

thromboplastin and extrinsic or tissue thromboplastin. All injured tissues yield a complex mixture of as yet unclassified substances that possess potential thromboplastic activity. During clotting of whole blood, platelets appear to be the source of thromboplastin. The clot-accelerating activity of tissues has been assigned the name factor III by the International Committee on Nomenclature of Blood Clotting Factors.

Complete thromboplastins and partial thromboplastins are used in different laboratory diagnostic procedures. The term partial thromboplastin is used to designate thromboplastic reagents that are found to clot hemophilic plasma less rapidly than normal plasma. Complete thromboplastins are able to produce clotting as rapidly with hemophilic plasma as with normal plasma.

Tissue thromboplastin is a high-molecular-weight lipoprotein that is found in almost all body tissues and is concentrated in the lungs and brain.

Factor IV (calcium)

It has been known for many years that calcium is essential for coagulation, and the term factor IV is used for calcium when it participates in this process. The exact mechanism by which calcium acts is not completely known, but the fact that it is essential for clotting makes possible the use of anticoagulants that merely bind up calcium. The calcium concentration is very important in *in vitro* studies of coagulation.

Factor V (proaccelerin)

Factor V is essential for the prompt conversion of prothrombin to thrombin in the clotting of whole blood as well as in the presence of tissue thromboplastins. It is believed to be formed by the liver, and acquired deficiencies have been observed in liver disease. When factor V levels decrease to 30 percent of normal, bleeding occurs. Factor V is a globulin that is labile,

deteriorating rapidly in plasma, especially in oxalated plasma (not so quickly in citrated plasma). The activity of factor V in plasma deteriorates even when the plasma is frozen. It is consumed in the clotting mechanism and is therefore not found in serum. Its activity decreases within a few hours when human blood or plasma is stored at or above room temperature. For this reason, the term labile factor has been used for factor V.

Factor VII (proconvertin)

Factor VII is not destroyed or consumed in the clotting process, so it is present in both plasma and serum. It is a beta globulin with a molecular weight of 60 000. It is synthesized in the liver and requires vitamin K for its production. An acquired deficiency of factor VII results from any disorder that decreases its synthesis in the liver. Factor VII disappears rapidly from the blood when its production is halted, which may occur during drug therapy with coumarin or in a congenitally deficient patient. It remains at a high level in stored blood as well as in serum. There is evidence to suggest that the activity of factor VII actually increases during the clotting process.

Factor VIII (antihemophilic factor)

Hemophilia refers to a sex-linked coagulation disorder. It has been demonstrated that the coagulation defect can be corrected by the use of normal plasma. The terms antihemophilic factor (AHF) and antihemophilic globulin (AHG) have been used to designate the procoagulant present in normal plasma but deficient in the plasma of patients with hemophilia. The term hemophilia A is gradually being adopted to designate the hereditary disease.[4]

Factor VIII is produced by the reticuloendothelial cells and possibly in the spleen. It is a beta globulin with a high molecular weight. Factor VIII is unaffected by vitamin K deficiency and coumarin-type drugs. It is lost rapidly from the bloodstream, having a half-life of 6–10 hours. This rapid clearance occurs in normal persons as well as those with a congenital deficiency.

Factor IX (plasma thromboplastin component)

The disease resulting from a deficiency of this factor is gradually becoming known as hemophilia B. Factor IX is a stable protein factor with a half-life of about 20 hours. It is not consumed during clotting and is not destroyed by aging. It is present in both serum and plasma, and there is probably no significant loss of the factor in blood or plasma stored at 4°C for 2 weeks. Factor IX is an essential component of the intrinsic thromboplastin-generating system. It is synthesized in the liver and requires vitamin K for its production.

Factor X (Stuart factor)

This is a relatively stable factor that is not consumed during the clotting process and therefore is found in both serum and plasma. It is an alpha globulin that requires vitamin K for its synthesis in the liver. Factor X works with other substances to form the thromboplastins that convert prothrombin to thrombin. It helps to form the final common pathway through which products of both the intrinsic and the extrinsic thromboplastin-generating system act. Factor X is stable for several weeks to 2 months when stored at 4°C. It has a half-life of approximately 40 hours.

Factor XI (plasma thromboplastin antecedent)

Factor XI is a beta globulin with a high molecular weight. The exact site of its synthesis is not known. Only part of Factor XI is consumed during the clotting process so it is present in the serum as well as the plasma. It is essential for the intrinsic thromboplastin-generating mechanism.

Factor XII (Hageman factor)

This factor is a stable globulin that is not consumed during the clotting process and is therefore found in both serum and plasma. Factor XII is converted to an active form when it comes in contact with glass. The natural counterpart of glass is not known, but platelets or damaged endothelium may be involved in this primary activation process.

Factor XIII (fibrinase)

Factor XIII is an alpha globulin with a high molecular weight. Its site of production is not known. There is evidence that it is an enzyme (fibrinase) that catalyzes the polymerization of fibrin. This factor is inhibited by ethylenediaminetetraacetic acid (EDTA). Very little factor XIII is present in the serum, the major portion being used up in the polymerization of fibrin.

Mechanism of coagulation

The complex mechanism of coagulation takes place in three major stages.

Stage 1: Generation of thromboplastic activity

The thromboplastic activity necessary to convert prothrombin to thrombin is produced in stage 1 through the interaction of platelets with factors XII, XI, IX, and VIII (the intrinsic pathway), or through the release of tissue thromboplastin from the injured tissues (the extrinsic pathway). Plasma factor VII activates the tissue thromboplastic substances. Various tests will detect stage 1 deficiencies but the one test of choice for screening purposes and for identification of stage 1 deficiencies is the partial thromboplastin time test.

Stage 2: Generation of thrombin

The plasma or tissue thromboplastin plus factor VII produced in stage 1, in the presence of plasma factors V and X, converts prothrombin to the active enzyme thrombin. Laboratory tests are available to detect deficiencies in stage 2. The one-stage prothrombin time test detects deficiencies best in stages 2 and 3. Abnormal formation of a clot results from a deficiency of any of the coagulation factors or the presence of an inhibitor or anticoagulant. The anticoagulants EDTA, oxalate, and citrate remove calcium to prevent clotting *in vitro*. Heparin and Dicumarol prevent the conversion of prothrombin to thrombin, also preventing the clotting mechanism from functioning *in vivo*.

Stage 3: Conversion of fibrinogen to fibrin

Thrombin converts fibrinogen to fibrin, and a fibrin clot is formed that is stabilized by the presence of factor XIII. The thrombin time test measures the concentration and activity of fibrinogen in stage 3.

The presence of calcium ions is necessary in all three stages of the clotting mechanism.

Fibrinolysis

Besides having a system for clot formation, the body also has a means by which the fibrin clot may be removed. The mechanism for clot removal is not completely understood.

As soon as the clotting process has begun, fibrinolysis is initiated to break down the fibrin clot that is formed. Normally, the fibrinolytic system functions to keep the vascular system free of fibrin clots or deposited fibrin. There is evidence that the fibrinolytic system and the coagulation system are in equilibrium in normal persons. As a general rule, fibrinolysis is increased whenever coagulation is increased.

The active enzyme that is responsible for digesting fibrin or fibrinogen is plasmin. Plasmin is not normally found in the circulating blood, but is present in an inactive form, plasminogen. Plasminogen is converted to plasmin by certain proteolytic enzymes. These plasminogen activators are found in small amounts in most body tissues, in very low amounts in most body fluids, and in urine. The decomposition products of fibrin formed during fibrinolysis are removed from the blood by the reticuloendothelial system.

TESTS FOR HEMOSTASIS AND COAGULATION

The tests involved in the study of hemostasis may be divided into three main categories according to the three lines of defense against hemorrhage that were discussed earlier in this section: (1) tests for the vascular factor, (2) tests for the platelets, and (3) tests for the factors involved in coagulation. Tests for the vascular factor include the cuff test (also known as the tourniquet test or capillary resistance test) and tests for bleeding time. Tests for the platelet factor include the platelet count, the bleeding time, and the clot retraction test. There are numerous tests for the plasma factors and whole blood factors involved in coagulation; these include the venous clotting time, the prothrombin time, and the partial thromboplastin time.

Tests for vascular factors

Cuff test

In the cuff test, a blood pressure cuff is placed above the patient's elbow and inflated to a pressure of 100 mmHg. The arm is examined before the pressure is applied to see if any petechiae are present. Petechiae are collections of red blood cells around minute vessels; when these are present, small reddish spots will be seen on the skin. Any petechiae are noted by making a circle around them with ink. The pressure is maintained for 10 minutes, the cuff is removed, and the number of petechiae are counted that have appeared in a circle 5 cm in diameter drawn below the bend of the elbow. A normal value is 0-10 petechiae, and a positive reaction is indicated by more than 10. A positive test result indicates capillary weakness, thrombocytopenia, or both.

Bleeding time tests

Bleeding time tests measure the time required for cessation of bleeding after a stab wound to a capillary bed. The time required will depend on capillary integrity, the number of platelets, and the platelet function.

A number of different bleeding time tests have been devised. Two that are commonly used are the Ivy bleeding time test and the Duke bleeding time test.[5,6] The chief difficulty in performing these tests is in the production of an adequate and standardized skin puncture. An adequate test depends greatly on the skin wound, and therefore on the skill of the technician. Capillary bleeding is tested, and wounds more than 3 mm deep are likely to involve vessels of greater than capillary size, whereas wounds that are shallow are not likely to adequately test the capillaries and the hemostatic factors involved.

A modification of the Ivy bleeding time test devised by Mielke et al. is now considered to be the best bleeding time test.[7] In this test, a plastic or metal sheet or template is manufactured with a slit or slits 1 mm wide and 1 cm long. With a calibrated gauge, a number 11 surgical blade is fitted on the holder so that it protrudes through the bottom of the template exactly 1 mm. The same procedure is employed as for the Ivy method, and a blood pressure cuff is used. Two incisions 9 mm long and 1 mm deep are made. The average of the two bleeding times is reported.

Under the conditions of the test, bleeding is believed to be controlled by capillary retraction and the formation of a platelet plug in the wounds. Tissue factors are also thought to play a role, especially tissue tonus (contraction). Defects in the clotting mechanism have little effect on the bleeding time. The bleeding time is prolonged when there is a combination of poor capillary retraction and platelet deficiency.

The bleeding test is positive (bleeding time is long) in thrombocytopenic purpura and in constitutional capillary inferiority. Normal bleeding times are found in hemophilia and other defects of the clotting mechanism. It is important to realize that the value ascribed to bleeding and capillary clotting tests has undergone a change. With the availability of more specific and sensitive methods, bleeding and clotting tests (especially capillary clotting tests) have very little to offer as diagnostic aids. They may give the physician a false sense of security about the bleeding tendency of the patient. Some hospitals no longer use capillary clotting tests in their battery of coagulation screening tests.

Procedure for Duke bleeding time test[8,9]

1. An earlobe (or heel, in an infant) is cleaned carefully with 70% medicated alcohol. An earlobe on which the patient has been lying is not used.

2. A stab wound 3 mm deep is made in the margin of the earlobe (or heel).

3. Timing is started as soon as bleeding begins.

4. Drops of blood are removed with blotting paper every 10-20 seconds without touching the wound. The patient must remain quiet throughout the test.

5. The time at which bleeding ceases is reported to the nearest 30 seconds.

6. Normal values are 1-6 minutes.

Procedure for Ivy bleeding time test[10,11]

1. A blood pressure cuff is placed on the upper arm, and the forearm is cleaned with 70%

medicated alcohol below the antecubital fossa area and allowed to dry. The area used should be relatively free of veins.

2. The cuff is inflated to 40 mmHg, and this pressure is maintained throughout the test.

3. Three skin punctures 3 mm deep are made in the cleansed area. The punctures should be made in rapid succession, using a number 11 surgical blade.

4. Timing is started as soon as bleeding begins.

5. Blood is removed every 10–20 seconds as it accumulates over the wounds by blotting lightly with the flat side of a piece of blotting paper or other absorbent paper. Care should be taken not to apply any pressure or disturb the lips of the wounds.

6. The time at which bleeding ceases is reported to the nearest 30 seconds.

7. Normal values are 1–7 minutes; values of 7–11 minutes are considered borderline.

Procedure for template bleeding time test[7]

1. A number 11 surgical blade is fitted onto a holder so that the blade protrudes through the bottom of the template exactly 1 mm. The entire apparatus is wrapped and autoclaved before use.

2. A site on the forearm is selected away from obvious blood vessels.

3. A blood pressure cuff is placed on the arm and inflated to 40 mmHg.

4. The skin is cleaned with alcohol and allowed to dry.

5. Two cuts are made. This device gives cuts exactly 9 mm long and 1 mm deep. With such shallow cuts, venules are virtually never cut.

6. After 5–15 seconds of no bleeding (venospasm occurs during the first 5–15 seconds after the cuts have been made), bleeding usually starts. Timing starts when the bleeding begins.

7. While the cuts are bleeding, the blood is blotted as necessary from the sides of the cuts to avoid disturbing the clot as it is formed.

8. Normal values are 4–6 minutes; the upper limit of normal is about 8 minutes.

Precautions in bleeding time tests

Bleeding time tests are not always significant because normal bleeding times are found in patients who have defects in the clotting mechanism. Bleeding time is prolonged in conditions where there is a combination of poor muscle contraction in the blood vessels and platelet deficiency. Obtaining an adequate bleeding time depends greatly on the depth of the skin puncture. When the Duke method is used, the ear must not be congested and the patient's head must not move. In the Ivy method, the blood pressure cuff must be maintained at 40 mmHg throughout the test.

When prolonged bleeding times (over 7 minutes) or shortened bleeding times (under 1 minute) are obtained, the test must be repeated on the other arm or ear. The Duke method is not used to check the Ivy method.

The template method is considered the best bleeding time test because the skin punctures are uniformly deep.

Tests for platelet factors

Tests for the platelet factors involved in hemostasis include the platelet count (see under Counting Platelets, Chap. 3), the bleeding time tests described above (Duke, template, and Ivy methods), the prothrombin consumption test, and the clot retraction test. The bleeding time tests are especially concerned with platelets—the number of platelets present and their ability to form a plug. Prolonged bleeding times will generally be found when the platelet count is below 50 000 platelets/μl and where there is platelet dysfunction. A bleeding time test should not be done unless a platelet count has been done shortly before.

Clot retraction tests

Normal blood will clot completely and the clot will begin to retract within 1 hour. At the end of 18–24 hours, the clot should have retracted completely and serum should be expressed. The clot should be tough and elastic and not easily broken with an applicator stick. Retraction is primarily dependent on normal platelet function. The extent of the retraction is influenced by the amount of fibrin formed, the presence of intact platelets within the fibrin network, and physical interference from trapped red blood cells. When the platelet count is less than 100 000 cells/μl, poor clot retractility is usually seen.

Prothrombin consumption test

This test is done to determine the amount of prothrombin remaining in the serum after clotting has occurred. Normally, prothrombin is used up as it is converted to thrombin. Increased serum prothrombin results from a quantitative or qualitative platelet deficiency.

Tests for plasma coagulation factors

Common screening tests of the plasma coagulation system are the one-stage prothrombin time, the partial thromboplastin time, and the thrombin time. Other satisfactory tests for coagulation are bleeding time, platelet counts, and clot retraction tests. Once it has been determined by the coagulation screening tests that the patient has a coagulation disorder, the exact factor, deficiency, or abnormality should be identified.

In monitoring anticoagulant therapy, the prothrombin time is most generally employed when the patient is receiving coumarin drugs. Heparin therapy is usually followed by determining the whole blood coagulation time (Lee-White method) or the activated partial thromboplastin time.

The manual methods for doing coagulation tests have been replaced in many laboratories by automated and semiautomated equipment. Several machines are available that can do coagulation tests such as prothrombin times and partial thromboplastin times. Some of these machines can detect the formation of the clot photoelectrically, thus eliminating the error associated with visual timing of clot formation.

Two manual techniques for performing plasma clotting tests are discussed in this section: the prothrombin time and the partial thromboplastin time.

Specimens for plasma clotting tests

For coagulation tests, it is conventional to mix nine volumes of blood with one volume of anticoagulant. All tests are done on plasma. Variations in the hematocrit will alter the ratio of plasma to anticoagulant. Because it is impractical to adjust the ratio of anticoagulant to blood, the 9:1 ratio is used unless the hematocrit is very abnormal.

It is very important when drawing blood for coagulation studies that a clean entry into the vein be made. The blood should come smoothly and promptly into a *plastic syringe.* As soon as the blood has been drawn, the needle should be removed and the blood allowed to flow down the side of the specimen tube to the appropriate mark. The tube should be quickly stoppered and inverted *without foaming* several times. There must be no contamination of the specimen with tissue juice as a result of a poor vein entry, as this will alter the results. One anticoagulant of choice for coagulation studies is sodium citrate. Sodium oxalate can be used if the test is performed promptly after collection of blood.

Prothrombin time (Quick's one-stage method)[12]

This test was devised on the assumption that when an optimal amount of calcium and an excess of thromboplastin are added to decalcified plasma, the rate of coagulation depends on the concentration of prothrombin in the plasma. The prothrombin time is therefore the time required for the plasma to clot after an excess of thromboplastin and an optimal concentration of calcium have been added. It is a test of stages 2 and 3 of the clotting mechanism.

Specimens for the prothrombin time test must be anticoagulated with either sodium citrate or sodium oxalate. Oxalated plasma is not recommended unless the test is performed within 1 hour after the blood has been collected. A ratio of one part of citrate or oxalate to nine parts of blood must be maintained. The blood must be free of clots when visually examined before the test. If more than 4 hours elapse before the prothrombin time is measured, there will be progressive inactivation of some of the factors.

The normal values for the prothrombin time range from 11.2 to 14.5 seconds. A normal prothrombin time shows that the elements of stages 2 and 3 of the coagulation mechanism are probably not disturbed. This finding, coupled with a prolonged venous clotting time, places the abnormality within stage 1. The prothrombin time is used to follow the progress of patients treated with Dicumarol (a therapeutic coumarin anticoagulant drug used to inhibit clotting, especially for preventing postoperative thrombosis and pulmonary embolism) and to screen for factor deficiencies in hemorrhagic diseases. Antithrombotic drugs are being used increasingly and they present some very real hazards to the patient. If the degree of anticoagulation is insufficient, rethrombosis or embolism can occur. If there is too much anticoagulation, fatal hemorrhage can take place. The laboratory tests for coagulation can provide information whereby therapeutic balance is maintained. The laboratory is responsible for advising the physician about the level of anticoagulation achieved. Two categories of antithrombotic drugs are the coumarins, which act as vitamin K antagonists, and heparin. Coumarin drugs, such as Dicumarol, are moni-

tored by use of the one-stage prothrombin time test.

The reagents necessary for the prothrombin time test are primarily calcium chloride and thromboplastin. These reagents must be prepared in specific concentrations or purchased commercially. A commercial control is tested with each batch of prothrombins. Each prothrombin control must be prepared before use according to the manufacturer's directions. Control values and limits will vary with the brand of control used. Proper use of the control can detect deterioration of the thromboplastin, use of a calcium solution of the wrong concentration, or use of the wrong incubation temperature.

Procedure for prothrombin time[12]

1. As soon as possible, centrifuge the collected blood at 3000 r/min for at least 10 minutes. Remove the plasma after centrifugation.

2. Pipet 0.2-ml portions of the thromboplastin-calcium chloride mixture into small test tubes (8 by 75 mm is suitable).

3. Incubate the tubes containing the thromboplastin-calcium chloride mixture and the tubes containing portions of the plasma at 37°C. Allow 1 minute for the thromboplastin and plasma to reach 37°C.

4. Pipet (using 0.1-ml pipets) 0.1-ml samples of plasma and blow them into the tubes containing the thromboplastin-calcium chloride mixture. Start the stopwatch simultaneously.

5. Shake the tubes and leave them in the water bath (37°C) for a minimum of 7-8 seconds. Then remove them and tip them gently until a clot is formed.

6. Stop the stopwatch immediately when a clot is observed, and record the time.

All plasma samples are tested at least in duplicate and usually in triplicate. Determinations must agree within certain limits; the allowable difference between the results of duplicate or triplicate tests varies with the prothrombin time. According to one study, for prothrombin times up to 30 seconds, agreement should be within 1 second for duplicates and 2 seconds for triplicates; for times between 30 and 60 seconds, agreement should be within 2 seconds for duplicates and 3 seconds for triplicates; and for times over 60 seconds, the result is reported as "over 60 seconds." The test must be repeated if the allowable error is exceeded.

Precautions and technical factors

The prothrombin time should be performed within 1 or 2 hours of blood collection when sodium oxalate is used as the anticoagulant. If sodium citrate is used, the test should be done within 4 hours. The plasma may be frozen and stored up to 1 week without appreciably affecting the result of the prothrombin time test.

When using the thromboplastin-calcium mixture, it is important to mix the suspension very well.

The sample of venous blood must be preserved properly, using sodium oxalate as the anticoagulant. The blood must be free of clots; if any clots are present, a new specimen must be drawn. The ratio of anticoagulant to blood specimen must be 1:10 (0.5 ml of anticoagulant and 4.5 ml of whole blood). The prothrombin time test must be done within 4 hours after the blood is drawn, because of progressive inactivation of certain factors. If a prothrombin time of more than 1 minute is obtained, the test should be repeated on a new sample. All plasma samples are tested at least in duplicate (often in triplicate). A control specimen must be used to detect deterioration of the thromboplastin, inaccurately prepared reagents, or an incorrect incubation temperature, all of which could result in inaccurate test values.

Partial thromboplastin time

The activated partial thromboplastin time (PTT) is the single most useful procedure available for routine screening of coagulation disorders. It measures deficiencies mainly in factors VIII, IX, XI, and XII, but can detect deficiencies of all factors except VII and XIII. The test is based on the observation that when whole thromboplastin is used, as for the prothrombin time test, the times obtained for hemophilic plasma are about the same as those for normal plasma. With a partial thromboplastin solution or platelet substitute, the times obtained for hemophilic plasma are much longer than those for normal plasma. One important use of the PTT test is in the control of patients on heparin therapy. The sensitivity of the thromboplastin reagent must be evaluated before this test is used as a heparin control. The platelet substitute acts as a partial thromboplastin, and it is more sensitive to the absence of factors involved in intrinsic thromboplastin formation than are the more complete tissue thromboplastins used in the prothrombin time tests. An unsensitized test may be used, or sensitization (that is, activation) may be obtained by separate addition of a kaolin suspension.[13] Kaolin ensures maximal activation of the coagulation factors.

The normal values for the activated PTT test, using manual methods, are 35–45 seconds. Values of 45–50 seconds are considered borderline, and results over 50 seconds are considered abnormal.[14]

Specimens for the PTT test are best collected by using sodium citrate as the anticoagulant, with nine parts of whole blood to one part of anticoagulant. Oxalated plasma is not recommended unless the test is done promptly after blood collection. The specimen should be collected carefully and preserved on ice until it reaches the laboratory.

The principle of this test relies on the assumption that during anticoagulation, the calcium present in the blood is bound to the anticoagulant. After centrifugation, the plasma contains all the intrinsic coagulation factors except calcium (removed during anticoagulation) and platelets (removed during centrifugation). Under carefully controlled conditions and with properly prepared reagents, calcium, a phospholipid platelet substitute (the partial thromboplastin), and kaolin are added to the plasma to be tested. The time required for the plasma to clot is the activated partial thromboplastin time. If commercial reagents are used, and they are in many laboratories, the normal times proposed by the manufacturer should be followed.

Control specimens are always run along with the patient's specimen. Normal control results must always fall within the normal control range; if they do not, something is wrong with the reagents, equipment, or technique being used. When the control is out of range, the entire test must be repeated.

Procedure for partial thromboplastin time with kaolin[13]

1. As soon as possible after the blood has been collected, centrifuge the anticoagulated specimen at 2500 r/min for at least 10 minutes.

2. Remove the plasma from the cells immediately and place on ice.

3. Warm the calcium reagents at 37°C.

4. Pipet 0.1 ml of activated platelet substitute suspension (kaolin plus partial thromboplastin) into the desired number of tubes (duplicates for patient and control samples) and incubate at 37°C for a minimum of 1 minute.

5. Add 0.1 ml of plasma (unknown or control) to the activated thromboplastin mixture already incubating in the tubes. Mix well and allow to incubate for at least 2 minutes. The minimum incubation time for this mixture is 2 minutes. Incubation times over 5 minutes may cause loss of certain factors in the plasma coagulation system being measured.

6. Blow in 0.1 ml of the calcium solution and start the stopwatch immediately.

7. Mix the tube once, immediately after adding the calcium reagent. Allow the tube to remain in the water bath, gently tilting the tube every 5 seconds.

8. After 30 seconds, remove the tube from the water bath. Wipe off the outside of the tube so that the contents can be clearly seen. Gently tilt the tube back and forth. The end point is the appearance of fibrin strands and is usually sharp.

9. At the appearance of fibrin strands, stop the stopwatch and note the time.

10. Control and patient plasmas must always be tested in duplicate and the two results averaged to obtain the final result. The duplicate results should agree within 1.5 seconds. If they do not, another test should be done. When the clotting time is longer, duplication of results is more difficult and the allowable range of variation is wider. If formation of the clot has not started by the end of 2 minutes, the test may be stopped and the results reported as greater than 2 minutes.

Precautions and technical factors

The PTT test may be done without the addition of kaolin. In this case the normal results range from 40 to 100 seconds, with 120 seconds or longer being considered abnormal. Use of kaolin gives maximal activation of the coagulation factors and therefore more consistent and reproducible results.

If there are enough stopwatches, more than one test can be done at a time by starting the separate incubations at intervals to allow time for the manipulations and observations of the clots.

When sodium oxalate is used as the anticoagulant, the test must be performed within 1 hour of blood collection. Citrated blood should be centrifuged within 30 minutes of collection and may be stored on ice for up to $1\frac{1}{2}$ hours. Plasma allowed to sit longer than the recommended time will give abnormal results.

When kaolin suspensions are used, it is necessary to mix the solutions vigorously before any pipetting is done, as kaolin in suspension settles out very quickly.

Tests for whole blood clotting time (Lee-White method)

This test is not very reliable for the detection of mild or moderate procoagulant defects. In gross defects it gives an abnormal result. It is not recommended as a single screening test of procoagulant function, but it is used to monitor heparin therapy, although it has been largely replaced by more convenient methods.

The Lee-White method for determining venous blood coagulation time is still in general use in some laboratories. Capillary blood clotting tests are unreliable because the sample is contaminated with thromboplastin from the tissue juice. The Lee-White test measures the time required for freely flowing blood to clot after it has been removed from the body. The results are influenced by the nature of the surface of the test tube used and by the diameter of the tube. Temperature and agitation of the blood sample also influence the test results; vigorous agitation of the tubes shortens the clotting time. Only when these factors are carefully controlled and there is no mixture of tissue fluid with the blood sample can the venous clotting time be regarded as representing the *intrinsic coagulative power* of the blood. Contamination with tissue thromboplastin because of a poor venipuncture will shorten the clotting time. This test in no way differentiates between deficiencies in the clotting factors and the presence of anticoagulants, both of which can prolong the clotting time.

Procedure for Lee-White venous clotting time test[15]

1. Make a clean venipuncture. It is important that the vein be penetrated without excessive probing. Start a stopwatch as soon as the blood enters the syringe, and draw 5 ml of blood.
2. Place 1 ml of blood carefully into each of three small serological tubes (inner diameter, 8 mm).

3. Allow the tubes to stand undisturbed at room temperature for 10 minutes.
4. After the 10-minute waiting period, tip the first tube gently at 1-minute intervals until the blood is completely clotted.
5. After the blood in the first tube has clotted, tip the second tube in a similar fashion at 1-minute intervals until clotting is observed.
6. After the blood in the second tube has clotted, tip the third tube every 30 seconds until clotting is observed.
7. Report the clotting time of the third tube to the nearest 30 seconds. The normal range is 15-25 minutes.

Precautions and technical factors

In doing the venipuncture to obtain the blood specimen, the vein should be penetrated cleanly with as little probing as possible. Any excessive probing could introduce tissue juices into the specimen, which would contaminate it with thromboplastin and thus shorten the clotting time.

If the tubes containing the blood are clotted at the end of the initial 10-minute waiting period, the test is unsatisfactory and must be repeated. One cause of such early clotting could be contamination with tissue thromboplastin.

Vigorous agitation of the tubes can also shorten the clotting time. Some methods for this test require that the three tubes used for the blood specimen be rinsed out with saline solution before their use. The surface of the tubes and their inner diameter influence the clotting time.

The venous clotting time test, when properly performed, may be considered a screening test for abnormalities of the clotting mechanism. When there is a deficiency of any of the factors required for clotting, the venous clotting time will be abnormal. This is also true when an abnormal inhibitor is present in the blood. This test cannot differentiate between an inhibitor or a plasma factor deficiency; other more specific tests must be performed.

Other tests for coagulation

Several other tests for specific coagulation factors are done in a coagulation laboratory. These include the prothrombin consumption test, thromboplastin generation test, plasma recalcification time (plasma clotting time), thrombin time, fibrinogen titer, and quantitative tests for fibrinogen.

REFERENCES

1. Stanley S. Raphael et al., "Lynch's Medical Laboratory Technology," 3d ed., vol. II, p. 1199, W. B. Saunders Company, Philadelphia, 1976.
2. I. S. Wright, The Nomenclature of Blood Clotting Factors, *J. Am. Med. Assoc.*, vol. 180, p. 733, 1962.
3. Barbara A. Brown, "Hematology: Principles and Procedures," 2d ed., p. 115, Lea & Febiger, Philadelphia, 1976.
4. Israel Davidsohn and John Bernard Henry (eds.), "Clinical Diagnosis by Laboratory Methods," 15th ed., p. 425, W. B. Saunders Company, Philadelphia, 1974.
5. A. C. Ivy, P. F. Shapiro, and P. Melnick, The Bleeding Tendency in Jaundice, *Surg. Gynecol. Obstet.*, vol. 60, p. 781, 1935.
6. W. W. Duke, The Relation of Blood Platelets to Hemorrhagic Disease: Description of a Method for Determining the Bleeding Time and Coagulation Time and Report of Three Cases of Hemorrhagic Disease Relieved by Transfusion, *J. Am. Med. Assoc.*, vol. 14, p. 1185, 1910.
7. C. H. Mielke, I. A. Kaneshiro, J. M. Maher, J. M. Weiner, and S. I. Rapaport, The Standardized Normal Ivy Bleeding Time and Its Prolongation by Aspirin, *Blood*, vol. 34, p. 204, 1969.
8. Duke, *loc. cit.*
9. R. Biggs and R. G. Marfarlane, *Human Blood Coagulation*, p. 401, Blackwell Scientific Publications, Ltd., Oxford, 1962.
10. Ivy et al., *loc. cit.*
11. J. V. Dacie and S. M. Lewis, "Practical Hematology," p. 264, Grune & Stratton, New York, 1968.
12. A. J. Quick, "Bleeding Problems in Clinical Medicine," p. 43, W. B. Saunders Company, Philadelphia, 1970.
13. R. R. Proctor and S. I. Rapaport, The Partial Thromboplastin Time with Kaolin, *Am. J. Clin. Pathol.*, vol. 36, p. 212, 1961.
14. Brown, *op. cit.*, pp. 128–129.
15. R. I. Lee and P. D. White, A Clinical Study of the Coagulation Time of Blood, *Am. J. Med. Sci.*, vol. 145, p. 495, 1913.

BIBLIOGRAPHY

Brown, Barbara A.: "Hematology: Principles and Procedures," 2d ed., Lea & Febiger, Philadelphia, 1976.

Davidsohn, Israel and John Bernard Henry (eds.): "Clinical Diagnosis by Laboratory Methods," 15th ed., W. B. Saunders Company, Philadelphia, 1974.

Edson, J. Roger: "Hemostasis Handout," Department of Laboratory Medicine and Pathology, Coagulation Laboratory, University of Minnesota, January 1976.

Graham, J. B., D. A. Barrett, B. Blomback, H. M. Cann, R. M. Hardisty, M. J. Larriew, and J. H. Renwick: A Genetic Nomenclature for Human Blood Coagulation, *Thromb. Diath. Haemorrh.*, vol. 30, 1973.

Hyun, Bong Hak, John K. Ashton, and Kathleen Dolan: "Practical Hematology," W. B. Saunders Company, Philadelphia, 1975.

Lewis, S. M. and J. F. Coster (eds.): "Quality Control in Haematology, Symposium of the International Committee for Standardization in

Haematology," Academic Press, London, 1975.

Quick, A. J.: "Hemorrhagic Diseases," Lea & Febiger, Philadelphia, 1957.

Quick, A. J., M. Stanley-Brown, and F. W. Bancroft: Determination of Prothrombin, *Am. J. Med. Sci.*, vol. 190, 1935.

Raphael, Stanley S. et al.: "Lynch's Medical Laboratory Technology," 3d ed., vol. II, W. B. Saunders Company, Philadelphia, 1976.

Williams, William H., Ernest Beutler, Allan J. Erslev, and R. Wayne Rundles: "Hematology," McGraw-Hill Book Company, New York, 1972.

Wintrobe, Maxwell M.: "Clinical Hematology," 7th ed., Lea & Febiger, Philadelphia, 1974.

FIVE
URINALYSIS

Of all the diagnostic procedures performed in the laboratory, the analysis of the urine is perhaps the oldest and most important. Urine samples are readily available, and many of the routine tests are relatively simple to perform. The simplicity of the tests in no way means that they are unimportant or should be performed sloppily or in haste. The physician relies heavily on the laboratory findings of the urinalysis in diagnosing and treating many diseases. It cannot be overemphasized that it is extremely important in the urinalysis department, as well as in the other departments of the laboratory, to do careful, accurate work at all times. The life of the patient is often dependent on the accuracy of the laboratory personnel.

In general, urine can be considered a fluid composed of the waste materials of the blood. It is formed in the kidney and excreted from the body by way of the urinary system.

The urinary system consists of two kidneys and ureters, the bladder, and the urethra. The urine is formed in the nephron (working unit of the kidney), passed on to the bladder for temporary storage by way of the ureters, and then eliminated from the body by way of the urethra (see Fig. 5-1).

KIDNEY AND URINE

Kidney function

The kidney functions as a means of eliminating waste materials from the body, but a better definition of this important organ is that it is a regulator of the extracellular fluid. The extracellular fluid is a water solution containing numerous dissolved substances; it consists of all the liquid in the body, outside the individual tissue cells. It includes the liquid part of the blood plasma, the lymph, and the interstitial fluid, which is the fluid in the space between the cells of the body. The kidney regulates the extracellular fluid in such a way as to keep its composition constant. This is very important, for the extracellular fluid is actually the environment of the individual body cells, and even slight changes in its composition may result in death. The kidney protects the extracellular fluid against changes in volume, acidity, composition, and osmotic pressure.

In maintaining the extracellular fluid, the kid-

287

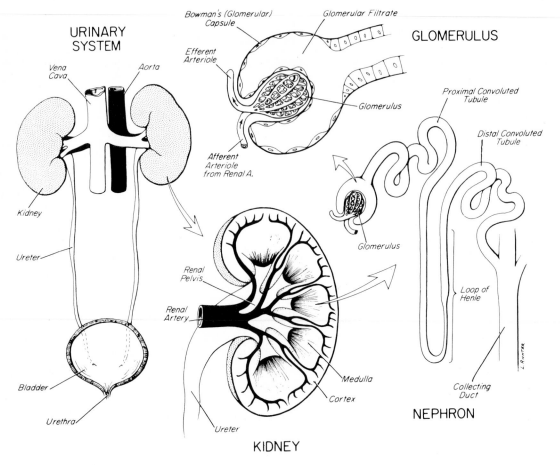

Fig. 5-1. The urinary system.

ney does the following.[1] It acts to eliminate excess water from the body and thus to maintain the volume of the extracellular fluid. This is clear from the relationship between the amount of water or fluid that is ingested daily and the amount of urine that is eliminated from the body. Waste products of metabolism such as urea and creatinine are eliminated from the body through the urine, maintaining the composition of the extracellular fluid. Foreign substances such as drugs or excess substances from the diet are also eliminated in the urine. Composition is also maintained by the retention of substances neces-sary for normal body function such as proteins, amino acids, and glucose. For instance, larger particles are retained in the blood because they are unable to be filtered or cross into Bowman's capsule (a function of particle size), and certain substances such as glucose are actively reabsorbed from the renal tubules back into the blood. Finally, the acidity and osmotic pressure of the extracellular fluid are maintained by various mechanisms, such as filtration, reabsorption, and secretion, which have the net effect of regulating the electrolyte balance and osmotic pressure of body fluids.

Formation of urine[2]

Urine is formed in the nephron, which is the working unit of the kidney (Fig. 5-1). Each kidney contains about 1.2 million nephrons. Each nephron consists of two main parts: the glomerulus, or renal corpuscle, and the renal tubules. The formation of urine involves three processes, namely filtration, reabsorption, and secretion.

The glomerulus is the portion of the nephron made up of blood vessels. All of the blood in the body circulates through the kidney (one-quarter of the heart's output at a time), eventually going to a glomerulus. The glomerulus is a small structure, consisting of a knot or tuft of blood capillaries. Blood enters the glomerulus from the renal circulation through the afferent arteriole and leaves through the efferent arteriole. Urine formation begins with the glomerulus, the structure that delivers the blood, with its waste products and essential constituents, to the working portion of the kidney.

The renal tubular portion of the nephron begins with *Bowman's capsule,* also called the glomerular capsule. Bowman's capsule is a cup-shaped structure or sac that encircles the glomerulus (Fig. 5-1). As blood circulates through the glomerulus, it is filtered into Bowman's capsule. The function of the glomerulus is filtration. The glomerular capillaries are covered by the inner layer of Bowman's capsule, forming a semipermeable membrane. This membrane passes all substances with molecular weights less than about 70 000. This is basically the blood plasma without proteins and fats, as these molecules are too large to pass through the glomerular membrane. The filtrate is an ultrafiltrate of blood and is referred to as the *glomerular* filtrate. This is the first step in urine formation. However, the glomerular filtrate is significantly altered by reabsorption of some materials and secretion of others before it becomes urine.

The remainder of the nephron after the glomerulus consists of a series of renal tubules, which have certain functions. Beginning with Bowman's capsule, the tubules (which are only one cell layer thick) are as follows: the proximal convoluted tubule, the loop of Henle, and the distal convoluted tubule. The total length of these tubules in each nephron is 30–40 mm. The nephron ends with the distal convoluted tubule (Fig. 5-1).

All of the nephrons of each kidney eventually come together into progressively larger and larger tubules. These are the collecting tubules, and they combine to form the ureter, which delivers the urine to the bladder for temporary storage and then elimination from the body through the urethra. The fluid in the collecting tubule is urine.

Anatomically, the kidney is arranged in two portions: an outer, highly vascular area called the cortex, and a central area called the medulla (Fig. 5-1).

Blood enters the kidney through the renal artery, which branches into smaller and smaller units, finally forming the afferent arterioles going to the glomeruli. The efferent arterioles, which leave the glomerulus, run close to the corresponding renal tubules of the nephron, facilitating reabsorption and secretion between the blood and glomerular filtrate. The efferent arterioles eventually join to form the renal vein.

An extremely large amount of blood is filtered through the kidney each day. In fact, about 180 L of glomerular filtrate is produced daily, while only 1 or 2 L of urine is eliminated from the body. Clearly, much of the glomerular filtrate must be reabsorbed into the body. The majority of the water in the glomerular filtrate (87.5 percent) is reabsorbed into the body in the proximal convoluted tubule, the first portion of the nephron after the glomerular capsule. The water is actually passively reabsorbed along with sodium ions (Na^+), 87.5 percent of which are actively reabsorbed by the sodium pump mechanism. Along with the water, chloride and bicarbonate ions (Cl^- and HCO_3^-) and 40–50 percent of the urea in the filtrate are also passively reabsorbed at this point.

All threshold substances such as glucose, amino acids, creatine, pyruvate, lactate, and ascorbic acid, which normally are present in the blood and not in the urine, are actively transported across the cell membrane of the proximal tubule and reabsorbed into the blood. Phosphate is reabsorbed in the proximal convoluted tubule under hormonal control and depending on the body's tissue and fluid electrolyte balance. In addition, 90 percent of the uric acid and most of the protein passing through the glomerulus are reabsorbed in the proximal tubule. Creatine is not reabsorbed and may be excreted in the proximal tubule as are sulfates, glycuronides, and hippurates.

As the modified glomerular filtrate passes through the loop of Henle, it loses both water and sodium in the descending portion and then sodium without water in the ascending portion.

In the distal tubule the remainder of the sodium is reabsorbed. This is influenced by the hormone aldosterone. The pH of the urine is determined in the distal tubule, especially through excretion of hydrogen and ammonium ions (H^+ and NH_4^+) in exchange for Na^+. Potassium is also excreted and exchanged for sodium in the distal tubules. The remainder of water is reabsorbed in the distal tubules under the influence of antidiuretic hormone (ADH).

The body's electrolyte balance is controlled by the kidney, with the result that the urinary pH differs from the blood pH. Urine is generally more acid than blood, because acid substances are produced as end products of metabolism. These substances are buffered in blood by a bicarbonate-carbonic acid buffer system. They pass into the glomerular filtrate as salts, but sodium must be returned to the blood to conserve its concentration of base and maintain its pH within narrow limits. This is done by exchanging Na^+ for H^+, resulting in elimination of acid from the blood and in acidification of the urine. Urine has a normal pH of 5 or 6, while blood is slightly basic at about pH 7.4. Potassium ions (K^+) are also exchanged for Na^+ in compe-

tition with H^+. When it is necessary to retain more Na^+, ammonia (NH_3) is formed from glutamine and combines with H^+ to form NH_4^+, allowing for greater exchange of H^+ for Na^+. The osmotic pressure is controlled in the distal tubules through the secretion of ADH, which is controlled by the osmotic pressure of blood. Urea, the major waste product of nitrogen (protein) metabolism, is eliminated from the body through the urine. Urea is not actively reabsorbed or secreted by the kidney; instead, it moves passively into and out of the nephron with water. With average rates of urine flow, about 60 percent of the urea is reabsorbed and 40 percent is excreted in the urine.

In summary, in the adult more than 1 L of blood flows through the kidney each minute. The blood is filtered through the glomerulus into Bowman's capsule, producing the glomerular filtrate, which is an ultrafiltrate of plasma. The glomerular filtrate has a pH of 7.4 and an osmolality (measure of the concentration of solutes) similar to that of plasma, about 285 milliosmoles (mosmol) per kilogram of water, with a specific gravity of about 1.008. The filtrate is modified by reabsorption and some secretion in the proximal tubules. In the distal tubules more water is absorbed and the urine is acidified. The rate of flow of the filtrate is reduced as it passes through the tubules and water is reabsorbed into the blood. The rate of flow is 130 ml/min in the proximal tubules; 16 ml/min in the loop of Henle, and 1 ml/min as the urine enters the collecting tubules. The filtrate is concentrated and acidified as it passes through the tubules; by the time it reaches the collecting tubules the resulting substance, urine, has a pH of approximately 6 and an osmolality of 800–1200 mosmol/kg.[3]

Composition of urine

The composition of urine varies a great deal, depending on such factors as diet and nutritional status, metabolic rate, the general state of the body, and the state of the kidney or its ability to function normally. Urine is a complex aqueous mixture consisting of 96 percent water and 4 percent dissolved substances, most of which either are derived from the food eaten or are waste products of metabolism. The dissolved substances consists primarily of urea (the principal end product of protein metabolism), sodium chloride (NaCl), sulfates, and phosphates. The substances present in normal urine may be divided into organic and inorganic compounds. The major ones are:

Normal organic substances
    Urea
    Uric acid
    Creatinine

Normal inorganic substances
    As cations:
        Sodium (Na^+)
        Potassium (K^+)
        Ammonium (NH_4^+)

    As anions:
        Chloride (Cl^-)
        Phosphate (PO_4^{3-})
        Sulfate (SO_4^{2-})

Many other substances are normally present in urine in lesser amounts. Other products of nitrogen metabolism include amino acids, ammonia, traces of proteins, glycoproteins, enzymes, and purines. Excretion of urea and these substances is related to protein intake.

The amount of creatinine excreted is not related to dietary factors, but to the amount or mass of muscle in the body. Each individual excretes a uniform amount of creatinine every day, and this may be used to determine the completeness of timed urine collections. Since creatinine is normally filtered through the glomerulus and none is reabsorbed into the blood, increased concentrations of blood creatinine

imply impaired glomerular filtration, and therefore blood creatinine may be used as an indicator of renal function.

Other constituents found in small amounts in normal urine include calcium, intermediary metabolic products such as oxalate, hormonal metabolites, biogenic amines (catecholamines), enzymes, and small or trace amounts of sugars, proteins, cholesterol, fatty acids, vitamins, and metals.

Normal but concentrated urine will commonly crystallize certain chemicals out of solution at room or refrigerator temperature. Therefore, a routine urinalysis will commonly show crystals of uric acid or its salts, the urates, at an acid pH, while phosphates will commonly crystallize out of solution in concentrated urine of an alkaline pH. Such crystallization will show grossly as cloudiness or turbidity of the urine, and the crystals are identified morphologically by microscopic examination. Although they are the primary constituents of urine, urea and sodium chloride do not crystallize out of urine specimens.

Normal urine specimens also contain certain formed elements, which are observable in the microscopic examination of the urinary sediment. These include red blood cells, white blood cells, renal tubular epithelial cells, transitional epithelial cells, squamous epithelial cells, histiocytes, and a few hyalin casts. All of these formed elements are found in very small numbers in normal urine, and increased numbers represent an abnormal (and even seriously pathological) situation.

Many abnormal substances occur in urine in various conditions. It is important to know the relative amounts of these substances, because some of them are present in small amounts in normal urine. These abnormal substances may exist as dissolved substances or as solids, which are seen in the microscopic examination of the urinary sediment. Some of the more important substances that are considered abnormal in the urine are:

Acetone and aceto-acetic acid	Casts	Fat	Spermatozoa
	Cystine	Glucose	Sulfanilamides
Bile (or bilirubin)	Epithelial cells (renal type)	Hemoglobin	Urobilinogen
Blood (red blood cells)		Protein	White blood cells (or pus)

ROUTINE URINALYSIS

The chemical or microscopic analysis of the urine is known as *urinalysis*. Several gross observations are also part of the urinalysis. The urinalysis is an important part of the initial examination of patients in all branches of medicine. It is made up of a number of different tests and observations. Some of these tests are chemical and others are not. When the urinalysis is performed in an orderly fashion and the results are recorded accurately, the combination of observations and test results will provide the physician with a valuable picture of the patient's general health pattern. Many disorders are diagnosed with the help of test results showing common abnormalities in the urine. The urinalysis is made up of three general parts: observations of physical properties (such as urinary volume, color, transparency, odor, foam, pH, and specific gravity); simple chemical tests for abnormal constituents (such as sugar, protein, acetone, acetoacetic acid, bilirubin, blood, and urobilinogen); and the microscopic examination of the urinary sediment.

A urinalysis can give valuable information about the physiology or function of the kidney in general, an indication of renal infection at any point along the urinary tract, and information about the state of the body in general.

A typical routine urinalysis has traditionally included tests for, or observations of, the following:

Color	pH
Transparency	Sugar
Odor and foam	Protein
Specific gravity	Sediment (microscopic analysis)

These tests have long been part of the routine urinalysis. As early as 1821, William Prout's set of routine urine tests included observations of the daily urinary volume, color, specific gravity, and pH (estimated by the reaction of litmus paper to urine). The presence of protein and sugar were also determined—protein by heat, and sugar by taste or high specific gravity (over 1.030).[4] Analysis of the urinary sediment has also been traditional since the development of medical microscopy, with the pioneering course taught by Alfred Donne in Paris in 1837.[4] Early microscopists differentiated pus cells from crystals and amorphous deposits in cloudy urine, while casts of coagulated albumin were found to be associated with Bright's disease.

Certain other tests have traditionally been done when necessary, either when indicated by the results obtained from the routine tests or when called for by the laboratory director. These special tests include the following:

Test for ketone bodies (acetone and acetoacetic acid)
Bilirubin test
Urobilinogen test
Hemoglobin (occult blood) test
Nitrite test

With the development of commercial chemical tests for urinary constituents (in particular, multiple-reagent strips), the tests listed above have become part of the routine urinalysis in many institutions. Additional tests are added to the routine as the manufacturers modify and add to their products. Most of the commercial tests that are available are adaptations of older procedures. Many commercial tests can be purchased either individually or as a combination test or multiple-reagent strip. In this book, the tests are described individually in terms of the particular constituent being tested for.

When a test is to be employed, certain factors must be kept in mind and understood by the worker. These include the *basic principle* on which the test is based, the *sensitivity* or lowest concentration of the substance that can be detected by the method, the *range* of concentrations of the substance over which changes in the concentration can be detected, and the *specificity* of the test for the substance being measured. In addition, the medical laboratory personnel should have a general idea of the clinical application of the substance being tested for, and should be able to correlate the test results for the substance with other changes in the urine specimen—for instance, correlate a cloudy red color of the urine with a positive chemical test for blood and the presence of red blood cells in the urinary sediment. It is also important to understand when confirmatory tests are necessary after initial screening tests show the presence of certain constituents. This will be discussed in detail later in this section.

Depending on various factors, additional tests will be required after the routine urinalysis. These include quantitative tests for urinary sugar and protein and further procedures such as thin-layer chromatography to identify reducing sugars other than glucose (e.g., galactose) that may be present in the urine.

Collection and preservation of urine specimens

The collection and preservation of urine specimens and the relative advantages of random versus 24-hour collections were discussed in Chap. 1. Important considerations in the proper collection and handling of urine for routine examination include the container used, the collection procedure, and the conditions of storage and/or preservation from the time of collection until the specimen is tested. Some aspects of the collection procedure may be out of the hands of the laboratory. A good working relationship and good avenues of communication are necessary among all members of the medical team to ensure that a suitable specimen is collected and delivered to the laboratory for examination.

For routine urinalysis, a freely voided specimen, rather than one obtained by catheterization, is usually suitable. If the specimen is likely to be contaminated by vaginal discharge or hemorrhage, a clean-voided midstream specimen as required for bacteriologic examination (described in Chap. 10) may be necessary. It may be necessary to pack the vagina or use a tampon to avoid vaginal contamination. Although any random urine specimen voided during the day may be used for routine urinalysis, a fairly concentrated specimen is preferable to a dilute one. The first specimen voided in the morning is usually the most concentrated one, as fluids are not taken while the patient is asleep but dissolved substances are still excreted by the kidneys. A concentrated specimen is especially desirable when examining for protein and the contents of the urinary sediment. When testing for the presence of sugar, the best specimen to use is one voided 2 or 3 hours after a meal. This is the major exception to the recommended use of the first morning specimen for routine tests.

It is of primary importance that the containers used to collect the urine specimen be clean and dry. Although several types of containers are suitable for this purpose, disposable containers, either coated paper or plastic, are gradually replacing the traditional glass jars.

Probably the most important consideration is that the urine specimen be fresh or suitably preserved, usually by refrigeration. Ideally, the urine should be examined within $\frac{1}{2}$ hour of collection, as decomposition begins within this time, urine being an excellent culture medium, for bacterial growth. If this is impossible, the urine must be preserved in some way. The most common and simple method preservation is to refrigerate the specimen. It can be kept in this way for

6-8 hours with no gross alterations, and such a refrigerated specimen should be examined within this time period. Chemical preservatives are usually reserved for 24-hour urine collections, as they may interfere with parts of the routine urinalysis.

Decomposition of urine primarily involves the growth of bacteria. At room temperature, bacteria reproduce rapidly. This bacterial growth results in a cloudy-looking specimen. Changes in pH also occur as a result of bacterial growth. These changes interfere markedly with other tests. Other substances, namely phosphates and urates, may precipitate out of solution, adding to the turbidity of the urine specimen.

Some of the other changes that occur on prolonged standing at room temperature are the following: the pH becomes alkaline because of the breakdown of urea by the bacteria to form ammonia; red blood cells, white blood cells, and casts disintegrate; sugar decomposes, acetone evaporates, acetoacetic acid is converted to acetone; bilirubin is oxidized to biliverdin; and urobilinogen is oxidized to urobilin. It can be seen from these many changes that it is most important that only fresh urine specimens be used in performing a urinalysis.

In summary, for routine urinalysis the urine specimen must be collected in a suitable clean, dry container. In most cases the first specimen freely voided in the morning is preferred, although a specimen collected 2-3 hours after eating is preferable when testing for sugar. The specimen must be examined when fresh, ideally within 30 minutes, or suitably preserved, such as by refrigeration for up to 6-8 hours.

Classification of urinalysis tests

There are three general categories of urinalysis tests, grouped according to their degree of accuracy: *screening* tests, *qualitative* tests, and *quantitative* tests. Most of the tests performed in the urinalysis laboratory are in either the screening or the qualitative category. It is important to know the category in which a given test belongs so that results are reported meaningfully.

Screening tests tell only whether a substance is present or absent, and the results are reported as *positive* or *negative*. For most screening tests, any random sample of urine can be used, but the first morning specimen is recommended. A specimen obtained 2-3 hours after a meal is preferred for the urine sugar test.

Qualitative tests give a rough estimate of the amount of substance present. They are also called semiquantitative. Results of qualitative or semiquantitative tests are usually graded as negative, trace, 1+, 2+, 3+, or 4+. For most qualitative tests, an early morning specimen is preferred, the exception again being tests for sugar.

Quantitative tests determine accurately the amount of the substance that they detect. These tests are much more time-consuming than screening or qualitative tests, and for this reason they are not done routinely in the laboratory. The two most common quantitative tests performed in the urinalysis laboratory are those for sugar and for protein. The results of a quantitative test are usually reported in milligrams per deciliter, grams per deciliter, milliequivalents per liter, milligrams per 24 hours, grams per 24 hours, or milliequivalents per 24 hours. For quantitative tests a complete 24-hour urine specimen is needed. An appropriate preservative should be added to the container, and the specimen should be stored in the refrigerator until the test is done. The total volume of the 24-hour specimen is measured and recorded; the urine is thoroughly mixed before a measured aliquot is withdrawn for analysis.

PHYSICAL PROPERTIES OF URINE

The first part of a routine urinalysis usually involves an assessment of physical properties, such as volume, color, transparency, odor, and foam. Another physical property, specific gravity, is discussed later in this chapter. Observation of physical properties is probably the easiest part of a urinalysis. However, these simple observations are extremely useful both for the eventual diagnosis of the patient and for the laboratory personnel who perform the complete urinalysis. Such tests often give clues leading to findings in subsequent portions of the urinalysis. For example, if a urine specimen is cloudy and red, the presence of red blood cells will probably be revealed by microscopic analysis of the urinary sediment. If red cells are not found, all parts of the urinalysis must be carefully rechecked for accuracy. Chemical tests for hemoglobin might be falsely negative when ascorbic acid is present in urine; however, the presence of blood might be indicated by an abnormal red color and confirmed by the presence of red cells in the urinary sediment. If hemoglobin is present without red cells, the only indication of ascorbic acid interference might be the abnormal color of the urine.

Certain tests are performed when abnormal physical properties are observed. For example, a chemical test for the pigment bilirubin is necessary when it is suspected on the basis of abnormal color of the urine. These are only two examples of several situations in which the complete urinalysis may be evaluated by the laboratory for reliability before results are reported to the physician, or abnormal constituents are found in subsequent tests because abnormal physical properties were noted.

The final evaluation of urinalysis results will be described more completely after all parts of the routine urinalysis have been discussed. Physical properties are summarized in Table 5-1.

Volume

Although it is a physical property, the volume of the urine is not measured as part of a routine urinalysis. However, in certain conditions the volume of urine excreted in 24 hours is a valuable aid to clinical diagnosis. In normal adults with normal fluid intake, the average 24-hour urine volume is 600–1600 ml.[5] The total volume of urine excreted in 24 hours must be measured when quantitative tests are performed, since it enters into the calculation of results in these tests. The volume is usually measured in a graduated cylinder.

Under normal conditions, there is a direct relation between urine volume and water intake. That is, if water intake is increased, the kidney will protect the body from excessive retention of water by eliminating a larger volume of urine than normal. Conversely, if water intake is decreased, the kidney will protect the body against dehydration by eliminating a smaller amount of urine. There are various situations that result in abnormal urine volumes. The term *polyuria* refers to the consistent elimination of an abnormally large volume of urine, over 2000 ml in 24 hours. *Diuresis* refers to any increase in urine volume, even if the increase is only temporary. *Oliguria* refers to the excretion of an abnormally small amount of urine, less than 500 ml in 24 hours. The complete absence of urine formation is *anuria*. Finally, the excretion of urine at night is called *nocturia*. These terms merely describe abnormalities in urine volume. Each abnormality has several possible causes, reflecting various abnormal conditions. It is the responsibility of the physician, with the aid of the routine urinalysis and other clinical or laboratory findings, to determine the actual cause and significance of volume changes.

Color

The color of normal urine varies considerably, even in one person in a single day. Numerous words have been used to describe the range of normal color (few institutions agree on exact terms). In general, it can be said that normal urine is some shade of yellow. The exact name that is attached is not as important as the recognition that the color is normal. It is advisable for each institution to use precise terms to

Table 5-1. Physical properties of urine

Physical property	Report description	Possible cause	Procedure
Normal color	Light straw Straw Dark straw Light amber Amber Dark amber	Urochrome, the chief pigment in normal urine with uroerythrin and urobilin	Mix urine and note color.
Abnormal color	Pale	Dilute urine	Mix urine and note color.
	Dark yellow or brown-red	Concentrated urine	
	Yellow-brown or "beer-brown"	Bilirubin	
	Orange-red or red-brown	Urobilin (excreted colorless as urobilinogen)	
	Bright orange	Pyridium (aminopyrine drugs)	
	Clear red	Hemoglobin	
	Cloudy red	Red blood cells	
	Dark red or "port wine"	Porphyrins	
	Clear dark reddish brown or "cola"	Myoglobin or myohemoglobin	
	Dark brown and black	Melanin, homogentisic acid, phenol poisoning	
	Milky white	Pus, phosphates, some urates, fat	
	Green, blue, orange	Drugs, medications, foodstuffs	
Transparency	Clear Hazy Cloudy Very cloudy Turbid	Mucin, phosphates, bacteria, urates, pus, blood, fat	Mix urine, hold up to light, and note transparency. Confirm cause under microscope.
Odor	Aromatic	Normal, volatile acids	Smell.
	Ammoniacal	Breakdown of urea by bacteria on standing	
	Putrid or foul	Urinary tract infection	
	Sweet or "fruity"	Ketone bodies	
Foam	White, small amount	Normal	On dark urine, stopper and shake. Note color and foam.
	Yellow, large amount	Bilirubin or bile pigments	

define normal color. One such system is to describe the color as varying from straw to amber, straw indicating the lighter color and amber the darker. In this system all normal urine could be classified as being light straw, straw, dark straw, light amber, amber, or dark amber. Any other terms would indicate abnormal color. Another system commonly used is to make a notation only if the color is abnormal.

Urine that is more highly colored has a greater concentration of normal waste products because its volume is diminished. Color, however, is not an adequate measure of concentration. Specific gravity or osmolality values are preferred.

The color of normal urine seems to result from the presence of three pigments: urochrome, uroerythrin, and urobilin. Urochrome is a yellow pigment and is present in larger concentrations than the other two. Uroerythrin is a red pigment, and urobilin is an orange-yellow pigment.

The ability to recognize normal color is, of course, necessary to ensure the recognition of abnormal color. Several abnormal colors require special attention.

Pale

Pale urine suggests that the urine is dilute. The paleness results from a large volume with correspondingly low concentrations of normal constituents, as in polyuria. Pale urine is often associated with diabetes mellitus or diabetes insipidus. In cases of diabetes mellitus, a pale greenish urine is characteristic. However, the large sugar content in diabetes mellitus results in a high specific gravity, whereas dilute urine is characterized by low specific gravity. Pale, foamy urine specimens are seen, along with large amounts of protein, in the nephrotic syndrome.

Dark yellow or brown-red

Highly colored dark yellow or brown-red urine is indicative of very concentrated constituents and a correspondingly low volume. It is often seen in conditions associated with fever, where water is eliminated through sweat rather than the kidney. When such concentrated and acid urine is excreted, a pink or red precipitate of urates or uric acid, also referred to as brick dust, is often seen.

Yellow-brown or "beer-brown"

This is a very characteristic and alarming color to the experienced observer. It indicates the presence of bilirubin, a highly colored bile pigment, which is related to the clinical condition jaundice if it is also present in the blood. Urine specimens containing bilirubin will foam considerably when shaken, and the foam will have a vivid yellow color. This is not true of other highly colored urine specimens. Whenever bilirubin is suspected, it is the responsibility of the laboratory worker to perform a chemical test to detect it. This is extremely important, for bilirubin may appear in the urine before clinical jaundice develops and detection will lead to early treatment of the condition, whatever its cause. On standing, urine containing bilirubin may become green as a result of the oxidation of bilirubin to biliverdin, a green pigment.

Orange-red or orange-brown

This color is very similar to that of urine containing bilirubin and results from a related pigment, urobilin. In fact, urines that are tested for bilirubin on the basis of color should also be tested for urobilinogen. When freshly voided, the pigment urobilin is present in a colorless form, urobilinogen. The urine slowly takes on color on standing because of oxidation of urobilin to urobilinogen. If shaken, urine containing urobilin will not produce a colored foam.

Bright orange (orange-red, orange-brown, or red)

This is very similar to the color of urine containing bilirubin or urobilinogen, although it is somewhat more vivid. In this case the color is caused by the presence of phenazopyridine (Pyridium) or other aminopyrine drugs, which have been given to the patient as a urinary analgesic. The presence of this substance presents a problem as it interferes with or masks several tests such as tests for bilirubin, urobilinogen, protein, and ketone bodies.

Clear red

Urine that is clear and red characteristically contains hemoglobin, the color pigment of red blood cells. The hemoglobin results from increased red cell destruction in the body (intravascular hemolysis), which has several causes such as incompatible blood transfusion reaction, autoimmune hemolytic anemia, paroxysmal noctural hemoglobinuria, march hemoglobinuria, glucose-6-phosphate dehydrogenase deficiency, and certain infections and drugs. The urine may be bright red, red-brown, or even black as a result of the conversion of hemoglobin to methemoglobin. Urine with this color should be tested chemically for the presence of hemoglobin.

Cloudy red

This is similar to the clear red color. However, it is caused by the presence of red blood cells, rather than merely hemoglobin; hence the cloudy appearance. It is important to differentiate hematuria (red cells in urine) from hemoglobinuria (hemoglobin in urine). This may be most easily done by observation under the microscope. However, if the urine is very dilute, red blood cells will lyse, resulting in hemoglobinuria. For this reason the specific gravity is important to the physician in determining whether the cause of red urine is hematuria or hemoglobinuria. The intensity of the red will depend on the number of red cells present; the urine ranges from smoky red or reddish brown to a highly colored cloudy specimen.

Dark red or "port wine"

This is characteristic of the presence of porphyrins in the urine.

Dark reddish brown or "cola"

This is characteristic of myoglobin or myohemoglobin, the form of hemoglobin contained in muscles. It is especially associated with cases of extensive muscle injury.

Dark brown or black

This color may result from melanin or homogentisic acid. In both cases the urine is colorless when voided and becomes black on standing. Both are the result of serious conditions, and the color must not be overlooked. Melanin is associated with melanoma, a type of tumor. Homogentisic acid is associated with alkaptonuria, a result of an inborn error in the metabolism of tyrosine. Phenol poisoning may also result in an olive-green to black urine. Specific chemical tests for all these possible causes of black urine must be performed, since immediate diagnosis and treatment is imperative in each case. These conditions are rarely encountered.

Miscellaneous colors

Various bizarre urine colors such as yellow, orange, red, pink, blue, green, and brown may result from such causes as vitamins, vegetables, fruits, certain chemicals, and dyes. These have very little clinical significance. However, they are important to the laboratory from a technical standpoint. Certain drugs interfere with other chemical tests that are performed as part of a routine urinalysis, and such interference may be suspected when the urine shows an unusual color. Each laboratory should have on hand reference materials to help determine the cause of possible interference. Some useful references include the following:

1. Philip D. Hansten, "Drug Interactions," Lea & Febiger, Philadelphia, 1973.
2. D. S. Young, L. C. Pestaner, and Val Gibberman, Effects of Drugs on Clinical Laboratory Tests, *Clin. Chem.*, vol. 21, no. 5, 1975.
3. "Factors Affecting Urine Chemistry Tests, False Positive and False Negative Reactions with Various Ames Tests For," Ames Company, Elkhart, Ind., 1977.

Transparency

When voided, urine is normally clear; most urines, however, will become cloudy when allowed to stand. Cloudiness of a specimen when voided is usually of clinical significance and should not be disregarded.

The degree of cloudiness is observed in a well-mixed urine specimen at the time of urinalysis. When cloudiness is noted, it must be accounted for in the microscopic analysis of the urinary sediment, since it is caused by solid materials that will be visible under the microscope.

As with color, numerous words have been used in attempts to describe the degree of transparency of a urine specimen. Again, it is advisable that a particular institution use only one system of nomenclature. For example, the transparency may be said to vary from clear to hazy, cloudy, very cloudy, and turbid.

The cloudiness that develops in most urine specimens on standing may result from the presence of *mucin*, or *mucous shreds,* in the urine. Mucous shreds are especially likely to solidify in urine stored under refrigeration and are of little clinical significance, although they are increased in inflammatory states of the lower urinary or genital tract. Other substances commonly responsible for the development of cloudiness in urine are *amorphous phosphates* and occasionally *carbonates.* These are especially likely to form in alkaline urine on standing and are of no diagnostic significance. *Bacteria* are another common cause of cloudiness in urine specimens that have been allowed to stand. In this case, bacteria are not clinically significant. However, if the specimen is fresh or was collected under conditions suitable for bacteriologic examination, bacteria indicate a urinary tract infection. *Spermatozoa* or *prostatic fluid* may also cause clouding of the urine, as may contamination with *powders* or certain *antiseptics.*

There are other causes of turbidity in urine specimens that may have pathological significance. *Amorphous urates,* like amorphous phosphates, are often responsible for normal cloudiness in urine specimens. They appear as a white or pink cloud of material, which settles out as the urine stands, especially if it is refrigerated. Unlike amorphous phosphates, the urates are characteristic of acid urines. The characteristic appearance is often referred to as brick dust, seen as a pink to red precipitate usually in highly colored, concentrated urine. This precipitate is visible under the microscope. Amorphous urates may have pathological significance when present in large numbers in various febrile conditions associated with highly concentrated urine, and also in some cases of gout and leukemia.

The occurrence of *white blood cells,* or *pus,* in urine is another abnormal cause of cloudiness. The white blood cells will be seen as white cloudiness in the urine and, when present in large numbers, will give the urine a milky appearance. Along with the white cells, bacteria will often be present, giving the urine a particularly foul odor.

Both bacteria and white blood cells should be confirmed in the microscopic analysis of the urinary sediments. Another cause of cloudiness, already mentioned under Color, is the presence of *red blood cells.* These are especially pathological, unless they are the result of vaginal contamination, and give the urine a characteristic smoky red or reddish brown appearance. They should be confirmed in the microscopic analysis of the sediment, and if present in very small numbers they will be noted only on examination under the microscope. Finally, fat, although only rarely present, may be a pathological cause of cloudiness in the urine specimen. In this case the urine has an opalescent appearance. Fat may even be found floating on top of the urine specimen in cases of fat embolism or phosphorus poisoning.

Again, it is stressed that most urine specimens show some cloudiness, and the cause of the cloudiness should be accounted for in the microscopic analysis of the urinary sediment.

Odor

Normal urine has a characteristic, faintly aromatic odor because of the presence of certain volatile acids. However, if allowed to stand, urine acquires a strong *ammoniacal* odor. This is caused by the breakdown of urea by bacteria (which are invariably present in the urine specimen), resulting in the formation of ammonia. This odor is important as an indication that the urine specimen is probably too old for the urinalysis to have clinical significance. Along with

the breakdown of urea, various other decomposition reactions will have occurred, altering or destroying other components that were present at the time the urine was voided. Urine heavily infected with bacteria may have a particularly unpleasant odor, which may be described as *foul* or *putrid.* This is also caused by the action of bacteria on urea, forming ammonia, plus the decay of proteins that are also present in infection. Practically, it cannot be distinguished from the smell of old urine. Therefore, foul-smelling urine will indicate urinary infection only if the specimen is known to be fresh.

Another characteristic odor that is significant clinically is a so-called *fruity,* or *sweet,* odor. This results from the presence of acetone and acetoacetic acid, especially in cases of diabetic ketosis.

Finally, the ingestion of certain foodstuffs will result in a characteristic urine odor. Probably the most obvious is the odor of asparagus. This is of no clinical significance.

Foam

Normal urine will foam slightly when stoppered and shaken, and the foam will be white. When certain bile pigments are present, especially bilirubin, the urine will foam significantly and show a vivid yellow color. This is a simple test for the detection of bilirubin, which should be performed on abnormally dark, or beer-brown, urine specimens. However, it is not a confirmatory test, and all urine specimens suspected of containing bilirubin should be tested chemically whether the foam test is positive or negative.

pH

One function of the kidney is to regulate the acidity of the extracellular fluid. Some information about this function, and other information as well, may be obtained by testing the urinary pH.

The pH is the unit that describes the acidity or alkalinity of a solution. In ordinary terms, acidity refers to the sourness of a solution, while alkalinity refers to its bitterness. Lemon juice is an example of a sour, or acidic, solution; baking soda (sodium bicarbonate) is a bitter, or alkaline, substance in solution. In chemical terms, acidity refers to the hydronium ion (H_3O^+) concentration of a solution and alkalinity refers to its hydroxyl ion (OH^-) concentration. These concentrations are usually expressed in terms of pH.

All solutions can be placed somewhere on a scale of pH values from 0 to 14. There are some solutions that are neither acidic nor basic. These solutions are neutral and are placed at 7 on the pH scale. Water is an example of a neutral solution; its pH is 7. Water is neutral because the concentration of hydronium ions is equal to the concentration of hydroxyl ions.

A solution with more hydronium ions than hydroxyl ions is an acidic solution. On the pH scale an acidic solution has a value ranging from 0 to 7. The farther it is from 7, the greater the acidity. For instance, solutions of pH 2 and pH 5 are both acidic; however, a solution of pH 2 is more acidic than a solution of pH 5. In simpler terms, a solution of pH 2 is more sour than a solution with a higher pH value. For example, lemon juice has a pH of about 2.3, while orange juice has about pH 3.5.

An alkaline solution has a pH value greater than 7. It can be anything from 7 to 14; the farther it is from 7, the greater the alkalinity, or the more bitter the solution.

Clinical importance

Regulation of the pH of the extracellular fluid is an extremely important function of the kidney. Normally, the pH of blood is about 7.4 and varies no more than ±0.05 pH unit. If the blood pH is 6.8-7.3, marked acidosis will be seen clinically; if it is 7.5-7.8, marked alkalosis will be observed. A pH less than 6.8 or greater than 7.8 will result in death. The carbon dioxide produced in normal metabolism results in a tremendous amount of acid, which must be eliminated from the blood and extracellular fluid, or death will

result. This acid is normally eliminated from the body by the lungs and the kidneys.

Because the kidney is generally working to eliminate excess acid, the pH of urine is normally between 5 and 7, with a mean of 6. The kidney is capable of producing urine ranging in pH from 4.5 to 8.0. The urine is normally acidified through an exchange of hydrogen ions for sodium ions in the distal convoluted tubules. In the disease renal tubular acidosis this exchange and the ability to form ammonia are impaired, resulting in a relatively alkaline urine with a pH of 6-6.5. Certain metabolic acid-base disturbances may also be reflected in measurements of urinary pH as the kidney attempts to compensate for changes in blood pH. Such acid-base disturbances are classified as metabolic or respiratory acidosis and alkalosis, and measurements of titratable acidity, ammonium ion concentration, and bicarbonate excretion are used in these distinctions. Although the kidney is essential in controlling the pH of blood and extracellular fluid, measurements of urinary pH are not necessarily used to obtain information about this role. The routine urinalysis includes a measurement of urinary pH for the following reasons:

1. Freshly voided urine usually has a pH of 5 or 6. However, on standing at room temperature, urea is converted to ammonia by bacterial action. The production of ammonia raises the hydroxyl ion concentration, resulting in an alkaline urine specimen. Therefore, unless it is known that a urine specimen is fresh, an alkaline pH probably indicates an old urine specimen.

2. Alkalinity of freshly voided urine may indicate a urinary tract infection with large numbers of bacteria present. In addition, white cells are probably present.

3. The urinary pH gives a clue to the chemical constituents that will be found in the microscopic analysis of the urinary sediment.

4. If the urine specimen is dilute and alkaline, various formed elements, such as casts and red blood cells, will rapidly dissolve.

5. Persistently acidic urine may be seen in a

variety of metabolic disorders, especially diabetic acidosis resulting from an accumulation of ketone bodies in the blood.

6. Persistently alkaline urine may be seen in some infections, in metabolic disorders, and with the administration of certain drugs.

7. It is sometimes necessary to control the urinary pH in the management of kidney infections, in cases of renal calculi (stones), and during the administration of certain drugs. This is done by regulating the diet; meat diets generally result in acidic urine and vegetable diets in alkaline urine.

Methods of measuring urinary pH

In most instances a precise measure of the urinary pH is not necessary. A rough estimate obtained with an indicator is sufficient. Such indicators include litmus paper, nitrazine paper, and the methyl red and bromthymol blue indicator systems. Litmus paper is not sensitive enough for routine urinalysis. Commercial reagent strip tests for urinary constituents, marketed as single- or multiple-reagent strip tests by the Ames Co., Elkhart, Ind., and Bio-Dynamics/bmc, Indianapolis, Ind., make use of a methyl red and bromthymol blue indicator system. If a more precise measurement of urinary pH is clinically necessary, a closed glass electrode and a pH meter may be employed. In some instances the titratable acidity of urine may be determined by titration with 0.1 N sodium hydroxide (NaOH) to an end point of pH 7.4.

Blue and red litmus paper

Blue and red litmus paper will indicate only whether a solution is acidic or basic. Blue litmus will turn red in an acidic solution, and red litmus will turn blue in a basic solution. However, this test is not sensitive enough to be of use in a routine urinalysis.

Reagent strip tests for pH

These tests utilize a methyl red and bromthymol blue indicator system. They are generally available in combination with other tests for urinary constitutents. Examples include Combistix, Labstix, Bili-Labstix, and N-Multistix produced by the Ames Co., and Chemstrip produced by Bio-Dynamics/bmc. The methyl red and bromthymol blue system shows a range of pH from 5 to 9 and gives an estimated value that can be reported to $\frac{1}{2}$ pH unit within this range. The pH value is not affected by the buffer concentration of the urine. However, the specimen must be tested when fresh, since bacterial growth may result in a significant shift to an alkaline pH, giving falsely alkaline values.

Procedure

The procedure and report protocol depend on the commercial products used. The manufacturer's color charts and directions should be followed. In general, the procedure is as follows:

1. Dip the test area of the reagent strip into fresh, well-mixed urine. Remove immediately.

2. Tap the edge of the strip against the container to remove excess urine.

3. At the appropriate time, compare the test area closely with the color chart provided by the manufacturer.

4. Tests for pH can usually be read immediately after wetting the strip, although the time is not critical. The manufacturer's directions should be followed.

Precautions

Note on reagent strips in general: Certain precautions must be followed with all commercial reagent strips. These are stated by the manufacturer and are supplied with each product. For example, store reagent strips in a cool, dry place to prevent deterioration. Do not use strips if they are discolored. Do not touch the test areas. Keep the test areas away from detergents or other contaminating substances that are present in the work area. Dip the test areas into the urine specimen completely, but briefly, to avoid dissolving the reagents out of the test areas. Remove only the number of reagent strips required at a particular time, and keep the container tightly covered at all times to prevent deterioration. Read the test results carefully, at the time specified by the manufacturer, in a good light and with the test area held near the appropriate color chart on the bottle label.

Nitrazine paper

Nitrazine paper such as pHdrion paper (Micro Essentials Laboratory, Brooklyn, N.Y.) makes use of a universal pH indicator, sodium dinitrophenolazo-naphthol disulfonate, which has a pH range from 4.5 to 7.5. There is a color change from yellow to blue as the pH value increases. The color is easily matched against reference color charts.

Procedure with nitrazine paper

1. Tear off 1 in of nitrazine paper.
2. Dip the paper in urine briefly.
3. Compare the paper with a permanent color scale as soon as the color stabilizes. This will take only a few seconds.

Note: Most nitrazine paper is manufactured with color charts ranging from pH 3 or 4 to pH 9. However, nitrazine paper has an accurate range of only 4.5-7.5. For this reason, only results that compare with colors 5, 6, and 7 are accurate. If the moistened paper compares with a color below 5, the result should be reported as acidic. If the moistened paper compares with a color greater than 7, the result should be reported as alkaline.

pH meter

The most accurate measurement of pH is made with a pH meter. Such accuracy is only rarely necessary in urinalysis; however, the principles of use of the pH meter will be discussed at this time. The pH meter is more commonly used in the clinical laboratory to measure the pH of blood and to check the pH of certain reagents such as buffers that are prepared for use in the laboratory. In principle, the pH meter is similar to the chloridometer described in Chap. 2.

The pH meter consists of three basic parts: (1) a glass-bulb electrode; (2) a reference electrode, which is usually a calomel electrode; and (3) a sensitive meter or measuring device. The glass-bulb electrode contains a solution of a certain fixed pH or hydrogen ion concentration. When the electrodes are placed in a solution of unknown pH, an electrical potential is produced between them that depends on the hydrogen ion concentration of the solution compared to the fixed concentration of the solution in the glass bulb. This potential, which is proportional to the hydrogen ion concentration of the test solution, is measured with the aid of the reference electrode. The potential of the reference electrode is compared to the potential of the pH electrode (the glass-bulb electrode) and is measured by means of the meter. The meter is an electronic voltmeter (potentiometer) that measures millivolts (mV). Results are read from an arbitrary pH scale of 0-14 pH units or from a millivolt scale. A reading of 0 mV is equivalent to a pH of 7.0.

Procedure

The procedure will vary with different pH meters and the manufacturer's instructions should be followed. However, certain considerations and precautions, such as standardization, apply to all instruments.

1. Before the pH meter can be used to test the pH of unknown solutions, it must be standard-

ized or calibrated. This is done by immersing the electrodes in a buffer solution of known pH at a particular temperature and then adjusting the instrument with the calibration knob to the correct value. The buffer that is chosen for standardization should be close to the expected pH of the test sample, and a second buffer with a different known pH should be tested, and the instrument adjusted accordingly, to ensure that the pH meter is accurate over a range of values. For example, the buffers used for calibration might have pH values of 7.0 and 4.0. Standard buffer solutions or powders from which they may be prepared are commercially available; directions for preparing standard buffers are available from the National Bureau of Standards. The pH meter should be standardized each time it is used.

2. The pH electrodes are fragile and should be treated accordingly. The manufacturer's directions about storage and activation should be followed carefully. In some cases the electrodes are stored in water, in other cases in saline or buffer.

3. The unknown solution is placed in a clean, dry glass beaker. The electrodes are then immersed in the solution, and a reading is taken from the pH scale.

4. Before and after use the electrodes should be sprayed clean with deionized or distilled water and carefully dried with an appropriate tissue.

5. Since the pH varies with temperature, the buffer used and the urine sample to be tested must be within $5°C$ of each other.

SPECIFIC GRAVITY (AND REFRACTIVE INDEX)

The kidney is a regulator of the volume, acidity, composition, and osmotic pressure of the extracellular fluid. A measurement of the specific gravity of urine is one means of assessing the ability of the kidney to regulate the composition and osmotic pressure of the extracellular fluid.

Urine is a mixture of substances dissolved and suspended in water. In normal urine, these dissolved substances are primarily urea and sodium chloride. A determination of the specific gravity of urine is a measure of the amount of dissolved substances present.

More technically, specific gravity describes the weight of a solution compared to the weight of an equal volume of water. It is the ratio of the density of the solution to the density of pure water. Density is the mass or weight of a substance per unit volume. Since the density of a solution varies with temperature, the temperature must be specified when specific gravity is determined. The specific gravity of a solution may be defined as the weight of one volume of the solution at a specific temperature divided by the weight of an equal volume of water at the same temperature.

From this definition, it is clear that the specific gravity of water is always 1.000. (Since specific gravity is a ratio, it has no units.) The specific gravity of urine should always be reported to the third decimal place.

For example, assume that 1 L of pure water at room temperature is found to weigh 996.5 g. To calculate the specific gravity of a solution, divide the weight of that solution by the weight of an equal volume of water. In this case, 996.5 g divided by 996.5 g equals 1.000, which is the specific gravity of water.

It has been stated that the specific gravity of a solution is a measure of the dissolved substances present in the solution. Assume that 20 g of NaCl is added to the 1 L of water weighed in the preceding example. Assume that there is no change in volume, although this is not strictly true. The weight of the solution of sodium chloride in water will be 996.5 g plus 20 g, or 1016.5 g. To calculate the specific gravity of this sodium chloride solution, divide its weight by the weight of an equal volume of water: 1016.5 g divided by 996.5 g equals 1.020, which is the specific gravity of this particular sodium chloride solution.

It is now possible to apply this information to the specific gravity of urine. Remember that urine is a water solution of various substances, primarily urea and sodium chloride. However, several other dissolved substances are normally present in urine, and several abnormal substances will increase the specific gravity of urine when they are present. To determine the specific gravity of a urine specimen, assume that 1 L of urine weighs 1008.5 g. In addition, assume that 1 L of water at the same temperature weighs 996.5 g. The specific gravity of the urine specimen should then be 1008.5 g divided by 996.5 g, or 1.012.

Of course, it would be extremely time-consuming to determine the specific gravity of each urine specimen in this way, especially since the number of specific gravity determinations in a single day will vary from 1 to 100 or more, depending on the laboratory, and specific gravity determinations are only part of a routine urinalysis. Fortunately, a less time-consuming method is available. One method used to measure specific gravity involves a device called a urinometer. A urinometer is a type of hydrometer, which is a floating instrument devised to determine the specific gravity of liquids. This floating device is weighted with mercury on the bottom and has an air bulb and a graduated stem above. The device is weighted with sufficient mercury to float at the 1.000 graduation when placed in deionized water (see under The Urinometer).

Although specific gravity is the most convenient measure of the urine solute concentration, it is not the only one available. Two other measures of solute concentration are osmolality and the refractive index. The measurement of osmolality is actually preferred as a means of determining the solute concentration; however, it is not practical in routine urinalysis. Osmolality may be determined by measuring the freezing point of a solution, since the freezing point is depressed in proportion to the amount of dissolved solids present. In normal persons having a normal diet and fluid intake, the urine will contain about 500–850 mosmol per kilogram of water.

The refractive index of a solution is the ratio of the velocity of light in air to its velocity in the solution. This ratio varies directly with the number of dissolved particles in solution, and as such, the refractive index varies, and corresponds with, although it is not identical to, the specific gravity of a urine specimen. Measurement of the refractive index of urine has become extremely convenient with the development of the clinical refractometer (see under The Refractometer). This device requires only a few drops of urine (compared to a minimum of 15 ml with the urinometer), and the results agree well with urinometer readings. Although the device measures the refractive index, its scale is calibrated in specific gravity, refractive index, and total solid content. Probably the major obstacle to universal use of this instrument is its cost compared to that of a urinometer. However, it is rapidly gaining in popularity because of its ease of operation and smaller sample requirement.

Clinical application

Clinically, the specific gravity of urine may be used to obtain information about two general functions: the state of the renal epithelium, and the state of hydration of the patient. If the kidney is performing adequately, it is capable of producing urine with a specific gravity ranging from 1.003 to 1.030 or higher.[6] However, if the renal epithelium is not functioning adequately, it will gradually lose the ability to concentrate and dilute the urine. The specific gravity of the protein-free glomerular filtrate is 1.007. Without any active work on the part of the kidney, this will increase to 1.010 as a result of simple diffusion as the filtrate passes through the kidney tubules. Thus, if the kidney has completely lost its ability to concentrate and dilute the urine, the specific gravity will remain at 1.010. If it is known that the kidney is functioning adequately, the state of hydration may be reflected by the specific gravity. For example, if the urine is consistently very concentrated, dehydration is implied.

The normal urinary specific gravity in healthy individuals having a normal fluid intake should range between 1.016 and 1.022 in a 24-hour period.[7] Normal specific gravity may range from 1.005 to 1.030, but is usually between 1.010 and 1.025.[8] Since the specific gravity is a reflection of the amount of dissolved substances present in solution, it varies inversely with the volume of urine (this is because a fairly constant amount of waste is produced each day). Therefore, if the urinary volume increases because of increased water intake, and the amount of waste produced remains constant, the specific gravity of the urine decreases. In other words, if the urinary volume is high the specific gravity is low, and vice versa, assuming the kidney is functioning normally. With an individual on a restricted fluid diet for 12 hours, the normal kidney is capable of concentrating urine to a specific gravity of about 1.022 or more. A specific gravity of 1.023 or more on a random urine specimen represents normal concentrating ability.[7] If the individual is placed on a very high fluid diet, the normal kidney is capable of diluting the urine to a specific gravity of about 1.003. The concentrated first urine specimen passed in the morning should have a specific gravity greater than 1.020 if the kidney is functioning normally.[8]

Two frequently observed cases where specific gravity does not vary inversely with urinary volume are diabetes mellitus and certain types of renal disease. With diabetes mellitus an abnormally large urinary volume associated with an abnormally high specific gravity is observed. This is caused by the presence of large amounts of dissolved sugar, which raises the specific gravity of the urine. In certain types of renal disease such as glomerulonephritis, pyelonephritis, and various anomalies, there is a combination of low specific gravity and low urinary volume. This probably results from the inability of the renal epithelium either to excrete normal amounts of water or to concentrate the waste products. The specific gravity in these cases may eventually be fixed at about 1.010.

Abnormally high specific gravity values, usually greater than 1.035 and up to 1.050 or more, may also be encountered after certain diagnostic x-ray procedures in which a radiographic dye such as Renografin or Hypaque is injected intravenously to obtain a pyelogram of the kidney. Such high specific gravity readings will be accompanied by delayed falsely positive reactions for protein with the sulfosalicylic acid procedure, and the dye may crystallize out of the urine as an abnormal colorless crystal resembling plates of cholesterol.

The urinometer

The specific gravity of a urine specimen is often measured with a urinometer. The urinometer is a glass float weighted with mercury, with an air bulb above the weight and a graduated stem on the top (Fig. 5-2). It is weighted to float at the 1.000 graduation in deionized water when placed in a glass urinometer cylinder or appropriate-sized test tube. It is important that the cylinder, or test tube, be of the correct size so that the urinometer can float freely. The specific gravity of the urine is read directly from the graduated scale in the urinometer stem.

Calibration

To obtain correct specific gravity readings in urine, the urinometer must be weighted to read exactly 1.000 in deionized water. Two methods may be used to test the urinometer calibration: the specific gravity value may be read from the scale in deionized or distilled water, or it may be read in a solution of known specific gravity.

1. Calibration in deionized or distilled water. Exactly the same procedure is followed as for

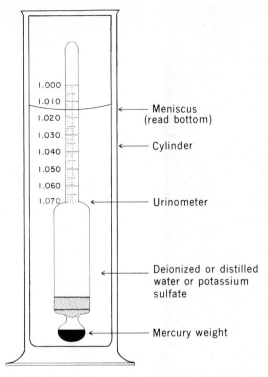

Fig. 5-2. Urinometer and urinometer cylinder.

urine. The reading on the urinometer scale should be exactly 1.000. If it is not, a correction must be applied to all values obtained for urine specimens with the urinometer. For example, suppose the urinometer reads 1.002 in deionized water. The specific gravity of water is 1.000. Therefore the urinometer correction is 0.002. In this case, the apparent reading is greater than it should be, and 0.002 must be subtracted from subsequent specific gravity readings. If a urine specimen has an apparent specific gravity of 1.037, this value minus 0.002 results in the corrected specific gravity of 1.035 for the urine specimen.

2. Calibration in potassium sulfate (K_2SO_4) of specific gravity 1.015. Any solution of a known specific gravity can be used to check the urinometer. However, the solution most commonly used is one of potassium sulfate with a specific gravity of 1.015. This solution may be prepared by diluting 20.29 g of K_2SO_4 to 1 L in deionized water. A reading is obtained in the known solution following exactly the same procedure as in urine or water. The reading on the urinometer scale should be exactly 1.015. If it is not, a correction must be applied to all urine specimen readings obtained with that urinometer. For example, if the urinometer reads 1.012 in the potassium sulfate solution, the correction is 1.015 minus 1.012, or 0.003. In this case, the reading is less than it should be. Therefore, 0.003 must be added to all specific gravity readings. For the urine specimen in the preceding example, the apparent reading in this case would be 1.032. The corrected specific gravity is 1.035.

Few urinometers read exactly 1.000 or 1.015 in water or potassium sulfate, respectively. Therefore, it is necessary to calibrate each urinometer before it can be used with accuracy. In addition, the correction can change from day to day, so it is necessary to calibrate the urinometer each day before urine specific gravity readings are determined.

Temperature correction

By definition, the specific gravity of a solution is dependent on temperature. Urinometers are calibrated to read 1.000 in water at a particular temperature. If the urine specimen is either warmer or cooler than the urinometer calibration temperature, the result will be inaccurate. For precise work 0.001 should be added to the urinometer reading for each 3°C that the urine specimen is above the calibration temperature, and 0.001 should be subtracted from the urinometer reading for each 3°C below the calibration temperature.

Most urinometers are calibrated at 60°F, which is 16°C. The calibration temperature is stated on each urinometer. Since room temperature is approximately 18-22°C, it is acceptable to report the specific gravity reading directly from the scale if the reading is made when the urine specimen is at room temperature. However, a significant error will result if the reading is taken on a urine specimen that has been refrigerated. The temperature of a refrigerated urine specimen is 4°C, which is 12° less than 16°C. The temperature correction in this case is $(12°/3°) \times 0.001 = 0.004$. Assuming that the specimen reads 1.015 at 4°C, its actual specific gravity is $0.015 - 0.004 = 0.011$. Instead of applying this correction, the urine specimen should be allowed to warm up to room temperature before its specific gravity is determined.

Correction for abnormal dissolved substances

The specific gravity represents the amount of dissolved substances present in urine. In determining the specific gravity of a urine specimen, the clinician is interested in assessing the kidneys' ability to concentrate and dilute normal waste products. In certain instances the specific gravity of a urine specimen is elevated because of the presence of abnormal constituents such as glucose, which may give the impression that the kidney is adequately concentrating the urine when in reality it is not. For this reason it is important to know how to correct for the presence of abnormal substances such as glucose.

Each gram of glucose present per 100 ml of urine will raise the specific gravity 0.003. Urine specimens of persons with diabetes mellitus often contain as much as 3 or 4 g of glucose per 100 ml of urine. This would represent a considerable error in the apparent specific gravity, as seen in the following example.

Assume that the apparent specific gravity of a urine specimen is 1.020. However, it is determined that this urine contains 4 g of glucose per 100 ml of urine. Therefore, the specific gravity is elevated 4×0.003, or 0.012, because of the presence of glucose. The actual specific gravity of this specimen in terms of normal urine constituents is $1.020 - 0.012$, or 1.008.

In this example the urinary specific gravity was lower than normal. However, in diabetes, urinary function is often normal in spite of the large sugar content. For this reason, it is common to find diabetic urine specimens with specific gravity values well above 1.030, even up to 1.060. When values above 1.030 are discovered, diabetes is often suspected, and the technician should expect to find indications of large amounts of sugar in the urine. This is not to say, however, that all specimens with abnormally high specific gravity readings contain sugar.

It is not usual for the laboratory to correct specific gravity readings for the presence of sugar when laboratory results are reported. Instead, the clinician will be aware that the specific gravity is elevated because of the presence of sugar and take this into account in the assessment of kidney function. If the results are corrected by the laboratory, this must be noted on the report form and the values both before and after correction must be reported.

Another abnormal substance that raises the specific gravity of a urine specimen is protein. Protein also raises the specific gravity 0.003 for every gram per 100 ml of urine. However, unlike glucose, 1 g per 100 ml represents an extremely large amount of protein and is seldom seen. Therefore, it is generally unnecessary to correct the urinary specific gravity when protein is present unless the amounts of protein present are extremely large.

Procedure

1. Check the cleanliness of the urinometer cylinder. Clean the urinometer cylinder at the end of each day or laboratory period, following the standard procedure for chemically clean glassware. A dirty cylinder will result in a thin, hard-to-read meniscus.

2. Calibrate the urinometer in deionized water or potassium sulfate before use each day. Follow the same procedure as with urine (see steps 3–8).

3. Fill the test tube to about 1 in from the top with well-mixed urine. (Be sure the test tube is the correct size for the urinometer—that is,

that the urinometer is able to float freely. All tubes should be of the same size and filled to the same level with urine.)

4. Remove any bubbles from the top of the urine with gauze or filter paper.

5. Grasp the urinometer stem at the top and insert slowly. Avoid wetting the stem above the water line, as excessive wetting of the stem will cause the urinometer to be depressed, and this will result in an inaccurate reading. Twirl the urinometer slightly as it is inserted, and note the reading as soon as it comes to rest. Be sure the urinometer floats freely away from the sides of the container while reading results.

6. See that the following requirements are met when reading the specific gravity:

a. Use a clean urinometer.
b. Make sure there are no bubbles around the urinometer.
c. Avoid wetting the stem above the water line.
d. Have the urinometer float freely about 1 in off the bottom of the container.
e. Read on a flat level surface.
f. Read at the bottom of the thick meniscus.
g. Keep the eye at the same level in relation to the urinometer for each reading.
h. Recalibrate the urinometer each day in deionized water or standard potassium sulfate.

7. Apply the appropriate correction to the results when necessary, and report the corrected specific gravity.

8. Rinse the urinometer in fresh water and dry the stem before proceeding to the next specimen.

9. When all determinations are complete, clean the urinometer and cylinder. Store the clean urinometer floating in fresh deionized water in the cylinder.

The refractometer[9,10]

The refractive index of urine is closely correlated with the specific gravity. Since the development of the Goldberg refractometer, a temperature-compensated small hand-held instrument called a

TS Meter (American Optical Co., Buffalo, N.Y.), measurements of the refractive index have become common in routine urinalysis (Fig. 5-3). They have the advantage that they require only a drop of urine, while the urinometer requires at least 15 ml of specimen. In addition, the refractometer is simple to operate and rapidly gives reliable results. Its major disadvantage is its cost.

Although the refractometer actually measures the refractive index, the scales of the instrument are calibrated in terms of total solids (grams per 100 grams) for plasma or serum, or in terms of specific gravity for urine. Up to a value of 1.035, the urinary refractive index and specific gravity agree. Few normal urines have values greater than 1.035; higher values suggest the presence of unusual solutes in the specimen such as glucose, protein, or radiopaque compounds. Beyond a value of 1.035, the refractive index is poorly correlated with the specific gravity and should be reported only as greater than 1.035, rather than extrapolated to a higher value.

The refractive index changes with temperature, but the Goldberg refractometer compensates for temperature. Its main prism contains a liquid whose index of refraction varies with temperature, changing the deflection of the light beams traveling through it and thus compensating for changes in the refractive index of the sample. Corrections for glucose and protein apply as for the urinometer.

Calibration

The refractometer should be calibrated each day with distilled water and two standard sodium chloride (NaCl) solutions of known refractive index. The sodium chloride solutions may be the same standards that are used in the determination of osmolality. The distilled water should read 1.000. One sodium chloride standard, with an osmolality of 750 mosmol/kg, should read 1.011. It is prepared by weighing 24.03 g of oven-dried sodium chloride and adding it to 1000 ml of distilled water in a volumetric flask.

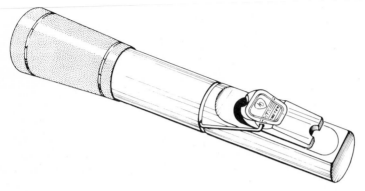

Fig. 5-3. Refractometer.

The second sodium chloride standard, corresponding to 1600 mosmol/kg, should read 1.023. This solution is prepared by weighing 51.37 g of oven-dried sodium chloride and adding it to 1000 ml of distilled water in a volumetric flask.

Procedure

1. Clean the surface of the instrument prism and cover by rinsing with water. Dry with a soft cloth or tissue.

2. Close the cover of the plate of the instrument.

3. Apply a drop of urine to the exposed portion of the measuring prism, at the notched bottom of the cover, using a disposable pipet or dropper. The liquid will be drawn into the space between the prisms by capillary action.

4. Hold the instrument up to a light source.

5. Looking through the eyepiece, make the reading on the appropriate scale at the point where the dividing line between the bright and dark fields crosses the scale.

6. Rinse the prism and cover with water and dry with a soft cloth or tissue.

SUGAR

Although a test for sugar in the urine should be included in every routine urinalysis, determinations of urinary sugar are not necessarily included to obtain information about the state of the kidney or urinary tract. The occurrence of sugar in the urine indicates that diabetes mellitus should be suspected, and tests for urinary sugar are commonly used for the diagnosis and management of this disease.

The type of sugar that is present in the urine in cases of diabetes mellitus is *glucose,* which is also called *dextrose.* Any condition in which glucose is found in the urine is termed *glycosuria (or glucosuria)*, which comes from the Latin words for glucose and urine. Although diabetes

mellitus is suspected in cases of glycosuria, the occurrence of glycosuria is not diagnostic of the condition, since there are many other causes. For example, glycosuria may be observed after large amounts of sugar or foods containing sugar are eaten, in cases of acute emotional strain where glucose is liberated by the liver for energy, and after exercise. It may also be associated with pregnancy, certain types of meningitis, hypothyroidism, certain tumors of the adrenal medulla, and some brain injuries (see also Glucose in Chap. 2).

In addition, certain abnormal conditions are characterized by the presence of sugars other than glucose in the urine. *Galactosuria* is the presence of the sugar *galactose* in the urine. It results from a metabolic error and must be diagnosed early in life to prevent permanent physical and mental deterioration. For this reason, it is often desirable to include in the routine urinalysis methods that test for sugar in general, rather than those specific for glucose, especially when screening urine specimens from pediatric patients.

The occurrence of glucose in the urine is not normal. The blood glucose concentration normally varies between 65 and 100 mg/dl (Nelson-Somogyi method). After a meal it may increase to 120-160 mg/dl. Normally, all the glucose in the blood is filtered by the glomerulus and reabsorbed into the blood. However, if the blood glucose concentration becomes too high (usually greater than 170-180 mg/dl), the excess glucose will not be reabsorbed into the blood and will be eliminated from the body in the urine.

The lowest blood glucose concentration that will result in glycosuria is termed the *renal threshold*, and it varies somewhat from person to person. The most common condition in which the renal threshold for glucose is exceeded is diabetes mellitus. In simplified terms, diabetes mellitus is a deficiency of the hormone insulin, which has the effect of lowering the blood glucose concentration. As a result of the deficiency of insulin, the blood glucose concentration exceeds the renal threshold, and glucose is spilled over into the urine. Tests for diabetes mellitus include tests for blood glucose (see under Glucose in Chap. 2) in addition to tests for urinary glucose.

Virtually all tests for urinary sugar may be classified as one of two types: (1) nonspecific tests for sugars in general, which are based on the ability of glucose to act as a reducing substance, and (2) specific tests for glucose, which are based on the use of the enzyme glucose oxidase.

Tests that are based on the reducing ability of glucose are not specific for glucose. In these tests, the glucose is merely acting as a reducing agent, and any compound with a free aldehyde or ketone group will give the same reaction. Glucose is not the only reducing substance that may be found in urine. The nonglucose reducing substances (NGRS) include uric acid, creatine, galactose, fructose, lactose, pentose, homogentisic acid, ascorbic acid, chloroform, and formaldehyde. All these substances and glucose have the ability to reduce a heavy metal from a higher to a lower oxidation state. Usually copper(II) ions are reduced to copper(I) ions. Since this is an oxidation-reduction reaction, the reducing substance is oxidized to a higher oxidation state. When glucose is the reducing agent, it is oxidized to gluconic acid. A positive reaction is indicated by a color change, which varies in intensity in proportion to the amount of reducing substance present in the urine specimen. These are qualitative tests, and the results may be graded as negative, trace, 1+, 2+, 3+, and 4+, depending on the intensity of color formation, giving a rough estimate of the amount of reducing substance in the specimen.

Commonly used nonspecific tests for urinary sugar that will be described in detail are Benedict's qualitative test and the Clinitest tablet test (Ames Co.). Although these nonspecific tests are often thought of as testing for glucose, it must be remembered that they will give the same reaction with any reducing substance that may be present in the urine, either naturally or as a contaminant. In cases where the presence of a reducing sugar other than glucose—for instance, galactose—is suspected in the urine, a nonspecific test must be performed. Although specific tests for glucose are commonly used as screening tests for the presence of glucose, all specimens obtained from pediatric patients should be tested by a nonspecific method as well.

If the presence of a nonglucose reducing substance is indicated by a negative test specific for glucose coupled with a positive nonspecific test for reducing substances, the nonglucose reducing substance must eventually be identified. The method that should be used to identify the nonglucose reducing substance may be determined by referring to a standard textbook of laboratory procedures. The methods that are used include the mucic acid test, the osazone test, Seliwanoff's test, Tauber's test, and thin-layer or paper chromatography.

Tests that are specific for glucose are all based on the enzyme glucose oxidase. An enzyme is often described as a biological catalyst, a substance that must be present before a chemical reaction will occur. Glucose oxidase, like most enzymes, is absolutely specific. It will react only in the presence of glucose and it will not react with any other substance. The basic reaction in tests with glucose oxidase is diagrammed below:

Step 1:

$$\text{Glucose (in urine)} + O_2 \text{ (from air)} \xrightarrow{\text{glucose oxidase}} \text{gluconic acid} + H_2O_2$$

Step 2:

$$H_2O_2 + \text{reduced form of dye} \xrightarrow{\text{peroxidase}} \text{oxidized form of dye} + H_2O$$

where the change from the reduced to the oxidized form of the dye is indicated by the color change of an oxidation-reduction indicator. The glucose oxidase, peroxidase, and reduced form of the oxidation-reduction indicator are all impregnated on a reagent dip strip or paper strip. The products that are commercially available differ in the chromogen used as the oxidation-reduction indicator and the substance that is impregnated with the reactants.

Although glucose oxidase tests are specific for glucose, large urinary concentrations of ascorbic acid, from the therapeutic doses of vitamin C or from drugs such as tetracyclines in which it is a reducing agent, pose a problem, as they may inhibit or delay color development. Contamination of the urine container with strongly oxidizing cleaning agents such as bleach or hydrogen peroxide may cause a falsely positive reaction for glucose.

Specific tests for urinary glucose that will be described in detail are Clinistix and Diastix (Ames Co.), Chemstrip (Bio-Dynamics/bmc), and Tes-Tape (Eli Lilly & Co., Indianapolis, Ind.). The Ames and Chemstrip tests for urinary glucose are available as either single-reagent strips or multiple-reagent strips. These products are sold under various names, depending on the particular combination, and tests for pH, protein, ketones, blood, substances that react with Ehrlich's reagent, and nitrite may be impregnated on the same reagent strip.

The original formulations of glucose oxidase tests for glucose, such as Clinistix and Tes-Tape, were useful merely as screening tests, and the results were to be reported only as positive or negative for glucose even though the intensity of color formation was said to be related to the amount of glucose present in the specimen. Specimens that show positive reactions with Clinistix or Tes-Tape should be retested with one of the qualitative tests for urine sugar to give an estimate of the amount of glucose present. However, the chromogen system in the reagent strips has been refined in Diastix and Chemstrip, and these strips can be used both for initial screening of the urine specimen and to obtain a qualitative estimate of the amount of glucose present in specimens from adult patients. However, it must be remembered that nonglucose reducing substances will not be detected by tests that are specific for glucose; therefore, specimens from infants and pediatric patients and specimens in which NGRS are suspected should always be subjected to nonspecific tests for reducing substances in addition to the specific tests for glucose.

Since the specific tests with glucose oxidase are generally more sensitive to the presence of glucose, they may give a positive reaction in the presence of very small amounts of glucose, while a less sensitive nonspecific test for urinary sugar will give a negative reaction. The earlier Clinistix screening test, which is specific for glucose, is being replaced by Diastix, which is also specific for glucose but may be used as both a screening and a qualitative test.

Occasionally it is necessary to determine exactly how much sugar is present in a urine specimen. In this case, the qualitative result is not sufficient, and a quantitative result is required. Results of quantitative urinary sugar determinations are typically reported in terms of grams per 24 hours of urine excretion. For these tests a complete 24-hour urine collection is required. The total volume of the specimen must be measured and the specimen preserved with a suitable chemical preservative that will not interfere with the reaction employed to test the specimen. Two methods that are often used are Benedict's quantitative method and the Somogyi method for quantitative urinary sugar. The exact procedure may be found in one of the many textbooks of clinical laboratory procedures. Both these methods are based on the reducing ability of glucose and make use of the reduction of copper(II) to copper(I).

Benedict's qualitative test[11,12]

Principle

This is a nonspecific test for urinary sugar based on the reducing ability of glucose or any non-glucose reducing substance that may be present in the urine specimen. It is a qualitative test in which the degree of color formation is proportional to the amount of reducing substance present in the specimen, and the results are graded as negative, trace, 1+, 2+, 3+, and 4+. Benedict's test has been virtually replaced by the commercial analog Clinitest. It is included here to illustrate the basis from which the modified tests were developed.

The test is based on the ability of glucose or any nonglucose reducing substance to reduce the blue copper(II) hydroxide [$Cu(OH)_2$] in Benedict's qualitative reagent in the presence of heat to copper(I) oxide (Cu_2O), which is yellow or

red. A positive reaction is graded as a change in color ranging from blue to green, yellow, orange, and finally red. The overall reaction is:

$$CuSO_4 + 2NaOH \rightarrow Cu(OH)_2 + Na_2SO_4$$
(Bluish)

Rapid reaction (occurs as if one step):
$\xrightarrow{heat}$ CuO (Black) $\xrightarrow{reducing\ substance\ (e.g.,\ glucose)}$ Cu_2O (Yellow to red) + oxidized form of reducing substance (e.g., gluconic acid)

This reaction may be shortened to:

$$2Cu^{2+} + \text{reducing sugar (e.g., glucose)} \xrightarrow[heat]{alkali}$$
$$Cu_2O + \text{oxidized sugar (e.g., gluconic acid)}$$

The copper(II) ions are supplied in Benedict's qualitative reagent in the form of copper sulfate ($CuSO_4$). In the presence of a strong alkali this is converted to copper(II) hydroxide. The heat is supplied by means of a boiling-water (100°C) bath. The reaction may be stopped by removing the source of heat. This is done by cooling the test tubes in a cold-water bath after exactly 5 minutes of boiling. The time of boiling is critical (since the reaction has not necessarily reached completion after 5 minutes) if the results are to be graded accurately. However, the time of cooling is not critical. The tubes are merely brought back to room temperature and the results are read when convenient.

Benedict's qualitative reagent

Dissolve 17.3 g of $CuSO_4 \cdot 5H_2O$ in 100 ml of deionized water. Dissolve 173 g of sodium citrate ($Na_3C_6H_5O_7 \cdot 2H_2O$) and 100 g of anhydrous sodium carbonate (Na_2CO_3) in 700 ml of deionized water. Add these reagents to the water slowly with constant swirling. It may be necessary to apply heat to dissolve the reagents completely. When cool, combine the two solutions, and dilute volumetrically to 1 L with deionized water. This reagent keeps indefinitely.

Procedure

1. Measure exactly eight drops of well-mixed urine into a test tube.

2. Add 5 ml of Benedict's qualitative reagent.

3. Place in a boiling-water bath for exactly 5 minutes. Both the time and temperature of the water bath are critical.

4. Remove from the boiling-water bath and immediately cool to room temperature in a cold-water bath for approximately 10 minutes.

5. A positive reaction depends on the presence of a fine yellow, orange, or brick-red precipitate. The test is then graded on the basis of the color of the *mixed* solution.

6. Grade results according to the following criteria:

Negative: either no change in the blue color of the reagent or the occurrence of a white or green precipitate from phosphates in the urine; also, an alteration of the color of the reagent without any precipitate formation.

Trace: slight amount of yellow precipitate with a greenish blue to bluish green mixed solution. (This represents less than 0.5 g/dl of sugar.)

1+: moderate amount of yellow precipitate with green, often referred to as apple green, mixed solution. (Approximately 0.5 g/dl of sugar.)

2+: large amount of yellow precipitate with a yellowish green, often called muddy green, mixed solution. (Approximately 0.75g/dl of sugar.)

3+: large amount of yellow precipitate with greenish yellow, or muddy orange, mixed solution. Some blue color remains in the supernatant. (Approximately 1.0 g/dl of sugar.)

4+: large amount of yellow to red precipitate with reddish yellow to red mixed solution. More importantly, no blue remains in the supernatant. (Approximately 2.0 g/dl sugar or more.)

Note: Tests for ketone bodies should routinely be performed on all 3+ and 4+ Benedict's qualitative reactions. In addition, tests for ketone bodies should be performed routinely on all urine specimens from pediatric patients.

Clinitest tablet test[13,14,15]

Principle

This is a qualitative, nonspecific test for urinary sugar. The principle of Clinitest is essentially the same as that of Benedict's qualitative test: the ability of glucose to reduce copper(II) to copper(I) in the presence of heat and alkali. The Clinitest tablet may be thought of as a solid form of Benedict's qualitative reagent. In addition, the Clinitest tablet contains anhydrous sodium hydroxide, which results in moderate boiling when added to dilute urine in addition to giving off heat in its reaction with citric acid. In other words, the heat for the reaction is also supplied in the tablet, making a boiling-water bath unnecessary. Aside from this, the reaction of Clinitest is analogous to Benedict's reaction. Results are also graded as negative, trace, 1+, 2+, 3+, or 4+ by comparison with a permanent color chart supplied with the tablets. Colors are comparable to those described for Benedict's qualitative test.

Clinitest tablets, like Benedict's qualitative reagent, will react with sufficient quantities of any reducing substances in the urine, including other reducing sugars such as lactose, fructose, galactose, maltose, and pentoses. Commercial reagent strips with test areas specific for glucose may be used to confirm the presence or absence of glucose. Sugars other than glucose are best identified by thin-layer chromatography. Since it is a reducing substance, large amounts of ascorbic acid may cause falsely positive results. It has been reported that urine specimens that have a low specific gravity and contain glucose may give slightly elevated results with Clinitest.

Both a five-drop and a two-drop Clinitest method have been described by the manufacturer and color charts are available for both. The two-drop method was developed in response to a "pass-through" phenomenon that may occur if more than 2 g/dl of sugar is present in the urine. Such concentrations of urinary glucose are possible in patients with diabetes mellitus. In the pass-through phenomenon, after the addition of the Clinitest tablet the solution goes through the entire range of colors and back to a dark greenish brown because of caramelization of the large amount of sugar in the urine by heat. The final color does not compare with any section of the color chart; however, it corresponds most closely to a color indicating a significantly lower result. Thus it is extremely important to observe the entire Clinitest reaction and wait an additional 15 seconds so that this pass-through to a lower color is not missed and a falsely low result is not reported.

Contents of the tablet

The Clinitest tablet contains copper sulfate, citric acid, sodium carbonate, and anhydrous sodium hydroxide.

Precautions

Observe the precautions in the literature supplied with Clinitest tablets. The bottle must be kept tightly closed at all times to prevent absorption of moisture and must be kept in a cool, dry place, away from direct heat and sunlight. The tablets normally have a spotted bluish white color. If not stored properly they absorb moisture or deteriorate from heat, turning dark blue or blackish. In this condition they will not give reliable results. They are also available individually packaged in aluminum foil to help prevent absorption of moisture. Although they are more expensive in this form it is useful when a limited number of tests are performed.

Procedure

Five-drop method

Follow the directions supplied with the Clinitest tablets.

1. Place 5 drops of urine in a test tube and add 10 drops of water.

2. Add one Clinitest tablet.

3. Watch while boiling takes place, but do not shake.

4. Wait 15 seconds after boiling stops, then shake the tube gently, and compare the color of the solution with the color scale.

5. Grade the results as negative, trace, 1+, 2+, 3+, or 4+. These results correspond to the following concentrations (g/dl): trace, 0.25; 1+, 0.5; 2+, 0.75; 3+, 1.0; and 4+, 2.0.

6. Watch the solution carefully while it is boiling. If it passes through orange to a dark shade of greenish brown, the sugar concentration is more than 2.0 g/dl and the result should be recorded as 4+ without reference to the color scale. Urines showing this pass-through phenomenon should be retested with the two-drop method.

Two-drop method

Follow the directions supplied with the Clinitest tablets.

1. Place 2 drops of urine in a test tube and add 10 drops of water.

2. Add one Clinitest tablet.

3. Watch while boiling takes place, but do not shake.

4. Wait 15 seconds after boiling stops, then shake the tube gently, and compare the color of the solution with the color scale supplied for the two-drop method.

5. Watch the test throughout the entire reaction and waiting period, as the pass-through phenomenon may also occur with the two-drop test with concentrations of sugar over 10 g/dl.

6. Report the results as negative, trace, 0.5

g/dl, 1 g/dl, 2 g/dl, 3 g/dl, 5 g/dl, and over 10 g/dl if a pass-through reaction occurs. Note the use of a two-drop method on the report slip.

Sensitivity

Clinitest reagent tablets will detect as little as 0.25 g of sugar in 100 ml of urine.

Clinistix reagent strip test for glucose[16,17,18]

Principle

This is a specific test for glucose based on the use of the enzyme glucose oxidase, which is impregnated on a dip strip. Glucose oxidase will oxidize glucose to gluconic acid and at the same time reduce atmospheric oxygen to hydrogen peroxide. The hydrogen peroxide formed will, in the presence of the enzyme peroxidase, oxidize the reduced form of o-tolidine to the oxidized form of the indicator. A positive reaction is seen as a change of color from red to blue. Although there will be some gradation in the intensity of the blue color, this is merely a screening test and the results should be reported as positive or negative. The overall reaction is:

$$\text{Glucose} + O_2 \xrightarrow[\text{oxidase}]{\text{glucose}} \text{gluconic acid} + H_2O_2$$

$$H_2O_2 + \underset{\text{(Red)}}{\text{reduced } o\text{-tolidine}} \xrightarrow{\text{peroxidase}}$$

$$\underset{\text{(Blue)}}{\text{oxidized } o\text{-tolidine}} + H_2O$$

Clinistix is more sensitive to the presence of glucose than either Benedict's test or the Clinitest tablets and will detect 0.1 g/dl of glucose or less in the urine. For this reason, some urine specimens react positively with Clinistix and negatively in the Benedict or Clinitest methods. Since Clinistix is specific for glucose while Benedict's test and Clinitest are nonspecific, a urine specimen containing a nonglucose reducing substance will give a negative Clinistix reaction and positive Benedict's and Clinitest reactions.

Clinistix was the original reagent strip test produced by the Ames Co. specifically for glucose and was incorporated as the glucose portion of various other multiple-reagent strips by the manufacturer. However, Clinistix is now being replaced by Diastix, which is based on the same principle and chemical reactions. Diastix has a different chromogen indicator system that is equal in sensitivity to the Clinistix system but also gives a rough estimate of the amount of glucose present in the specimen. It therefore eliminates the need for a confirmatory test on specimens from adults when the glucose screening test is positive.

Contents of the reagent strip

The Clinistix reagent strip contains glucose oxidase, peroxidase, and o-tolidine.

Precautions

Observe the precautions in the literature supplied with the Clinistix strips. The reagent strips must be properly moistened. The test area must be completely moistened, but excessive contact with the specimen will dissolve the reagents from the strip. The results must be read within 10 seconds or falsely positive results may be obtained.

Large concentrations of ascorbic acid (vitamin C) cause falsely negative results or results that are delayed for 2 minutes or so, while bleach or peroxide may cause falsely positive reactions. The color reaction is influenced by specific gravity, temperature, and the pH of the urine. A very high specific gravity may depress the color development, and a low one may intensify it.

Procedure

Follow the directions supplied with the strips.

1. Rapidly dip the test end of the strip in the urine.

2. Read the results after exactly 10 seconds, looking for the presence of a purple color.

3. Record the results as positive or negative. If the test area remains red, the result is negative. A positive result is indicated by the appearance of a purple color in the test area.

Sensitivity

Clinistix reagent strips detect as little as 100 mg of glucose in 100 ml of urine.

Tes-Tape test for glucose[19]

Principle

Tes-Tape is also a screening test specific for glucose. The principle of the test and the reaction are virtually identical to those of Clinistix; the tests differ in the oxidation-reduction indicator employed and the material the reagents are impregnated on. In Tes-Tape the reagents are impregnated on a tear strip of special paper, and the indicator is yellow in its reduced form and green to blue in its oxidized form. Therefore, a positive reaction is the appearance of a green to blue color. Like Clinistix, Tes-Tape is more sensitive to the presence of glucose than are the Benedict's and Clinitest methods and will detect 0.1 g/dl of glucose or less.

Contents of the tear strip

Tes-Tape is impregnated with glucose oxidase, peroxidase, and an oxidation-reduction indicator in its reduced form.

Precautions

Observe the precautions in the literature supplied with the product.

Procedure

Follow the manufacturer's directions.
1. Tear off approximately $1\frac{1}{2}$ in of tape.

2. Dip part of the tape into the urine specimen; remove it immediately.

3. Wait for 30 seconds; then observe for the appearance of any green color.

4. Record the results as positive or negative. If the test area remains yellow after 30 seconds, the result is negative. If any green color is present at this time, the result is positive.

Diastix reagent strip for glucose[20]

Principle

Diastix is a specific test for glucose based on the use of glucose oxidase, which is impregnated on the reagent strip. The chemical reaction is the same as for Clinistix, the difference being the chromogen system used to indicate the presence of glucose. The reagent area contains glucose oxidase, peroxidase, a blue background dye, and potassium iodide as the chromogen. In a positive reaction oxidation of potassium iodide results in the formation of free iodine, which blends with the background dye to give shades of green through brown. The reactivity of the strips may be influenced by the specific gravity and temperature of the urine, but not by the pH of the sample over the pH range 4–9. Large amounts of ketone bodies may decrease the color development of Diastix. For this reason, it is suggested that diabetic patients screen their urine with a combination strip, Keto-Diastix, rather than test for glucose only, so that they will not record a falsely low result for glucose when large amounts of ketone bodies are present in their urine. As with Clinistix, large amounts of ascorbic acid may give falsely negative or delayed results for glucose. This suppression is not as great as with Clinistix, but it may cause problems. Bleach and peroxidase may cause falsely positive reactions, as with Clinistix.

Diastix has the advantage of being suitable as a screening test for the presence of glucose in the urine, and giving a rough estimate of the amount of glucose present. Thus, only one test is necessary for the screening and semiquantitation of glucose in urine from adult patients. It is as effective a screening test as Clinistix, as it also detects as little as 100 mg of glucose in 100 ml of urine. However, urine specimens from pediatric patients must be subjected to a nonspecific test for urinary sugar (Clinitest or Benedict's test) in addition to the specific glucose screening test in order to detect the presence of sugars other than glucose.

Diastix is incorporated in the glucose test area in various other multiple-reagent strips produced by the manufacturer, Ames Co. These other tests include: Combistix, Hema-Combistix, Keto-Diastix, Labstix, Multistix, N-Multistix, N-Uristix, and Uristix.

Procedure

Follow the directions supplied with the reagent strips.

1. Dip the reagent area of the strip briefly into the specimen.

2. Compare the test area with the color chart after *10 seconds* to see whether the reaction is positive or negative for glucose.

3. Compare the test area with the color chart at *30 seconds*, for a semiquantitative result, and report the results as indicated on the chart.

Sensitivity

Diastix reagent strips detect as little as 100 mg of glucose in 100 ml urine.

Chemstrip reagent strip for glucose

Principle

Chemstrip is also a specific test for glucose based on the use of glucose oxidase. The chemical reaction is the same as for Clinistix and Diastix, the difference being the chromogen system used as the indicator. The test area for glucose on the various Chemstrip products contains glucose oxidase, peroxidase, a yellow background dye, and *o*-tolidine as the chromogen. A positive reaction is indicated by a color change from yellow to shades of green as the yellow background dye combines with the blue oxidized *o*-tolidine. Test results are said to be unaffected by variations in the pH or temperature of the urine.

Like Diastix, Chemstrip may be used on specimens from adult patients both as an initial screen-test for the presence of glucose, and as a semiquantitative test for the amount of glucose present in the urine. However, urine specimens from pediatric patients should be routinely subjected to a nonspecific test for urinary sugar as well.

Procedure

Follow the directions supplied by the manufacturer.

1. Dip the test area of the strip briefly into the specimen.

2. Read the results between 30 seconds and 2 minutes after wetting the reagent strip.

3. Compare the test area with the color chart and report the results as indicated on the chart.

Sensitivity

Chemstrip detects 40 mg of glucose in 100 ml of urine.

PROTEIN

One of the most important and indispensable portions of the routine urinalysis is a test for urinary protein. In the detection and diagnosis of renal disease, probably the most significant single finding is that of urinary protein. The presence of protein will also be correlated with certain findings in the urinary sediment, as part of the eventual diagnosis. In cases of renal disease, it is essential that the diagnosis be made and treatment started as soon as possible to prevent extensive and permanent renal damage.

The occurrence of protein in the urine is an abnormal conditon, probably the most important pathological condition found in a routine urinalysis. It is referred to as *proteinuria*. Previously it was referred to as "albuminuria"; however, this is a poor term, since the protein that may be present in the urine is derived from the plasma proteins, mainly albumin and globulin.

Normally, the glomerular filtrate, the initial stage in the formation of urine, is an ultrafiltrate of blood plasma without the larger protein molecules and certain fatty substances. If the glomerular capsule is damaged, protein molecules can pass through and end up in the urine. Thus, one cause of protein in the urine is increased permeability of the glomerulus. However, a very small amount of protein normally does not find its way into the glomerular filtrate. In normal situations, all of this protein is reabsorbed back into the blood through the renal convoluted tubules. Although the concentration of protein that normally filters into the glomerular filtrate is extremely small and only 1/180 of the glomerular filtrate is eliminated from the body as urine (the rest is reabsorbed), failure to reabsorb any protein from this large volume of glomerular filtrate will result in fairly large amounts of protein in the urine. In other words, another cause of proteinuria might be termed decreased reabsorption of protein by the renal tubular cells. It is usually impossible to say which mechanism is responsible for the occurrence of proteinuria; it is most likely a combination of the two. The important consideration is that there is proteinuria and that it indicates the presence of some sort of renal disease.

Although proteinuria is indicative of renal disease, additional tests will be needed for the final diagnosis by the physician. These will include observations of the urinary sediment, especially for the presence and type of casts, and determination of the amount of protein excreted per day by quantitative tests. The results of a microscopic analysis of the urinary sediment and the patient's case history will also be considered.

There are situations in which small amounts of urinary protein may occur transiently in normal persons. In particular, they may be found in young adults after excessive exercise or exposure to cold, or in so-called orthostatic proteinuria, which occurs in persons engaged in normal activity but disappears when they are lying down. In general, the proteinuria associated with renal disease is consistent, while that found in normal persons is transient.[21] To determine the cause of the proteinuria, it is often necessary to quantitatively determine the amount of protein in a 24-hour urine collection. Tests for orthostatic proteinuria are made on urine collections obtained both when the patient is at rest and after the patient has been walking and standing, but not sitting. The methods used will be determined by the physician or the particular laboratory.

There is a correlation between the presence of casts in the urinary sediment and proteinuria, since casts are made of precipitated protein. The occurrence of casts with proteinuria distinguishes an upper urinary tract (kidney) disorder from a disorder of the lower urinary tract. Bacterial infections of the kidney are often indicated by the presence of white blood cells and bacteria in the urinary sediment in addition to protein in the urine. In these cases the amount of protein excreted is usually fairly small. White blood cells and bacteria in the urinary sediment in the absence of urinary protein probably indicate a lower urinary tract infection without renal involvement.[22,23]

The implications of protein in the urine are extremely serious. Extensive renal destruction is incompatible with life, and any renal destruction is permanent. Therefore, prompt diagnosis and treatment are vitally important. In addition, the loss of protein from the blood plasma will result in severe water balance problems, since the osmotic pressure of the blood is largely dependent on the concentration of plasma proteins. This is readily seen in the edema that is often associated with kidney disorders.

Tests for urinary protein

Tests for urinary protein are of two major types: (1) turbidimetric tests, which are based on the precipitation of protein by chemicals or coagulation by heat, and (2) colorimetric tests, which are based on the use of the "protein error" of pH indicators. Many equally acceptable tests fit into these two categories, and the test that is used will depend on the individual laboratory situation and volume of work. It is important to learn the general principle, which can then be applied to the particular test that is used in practice.

In the turbidimetric tests, the protein is either precipitated out of the urine specimens by means of a chemical, which is usually a strong acid, or it is coagulated out of solution with heat. The results are read in terms of the amount of precipitate or turbidity that is formed in a test tube or in terms of the size of a ring of contact between reagents. The amount of turbidity or precipitation is roughly proportional to the amount of protein present in the urine specimen, and these results are generally graded as negative, trace, 1+, 2+, 3+, or 4+. Coagulation tests depend on the fact that protein is most insoluble at the isoelectric point (a particular pH) of the protein molecule. At the isoelectric point, protein will readily precipitate out when heat is applied. For the proteins found in urine the isoelectric point is approximately pH 5; therefore in these tests the pH of the test solution and urine is adjusted in some way to 5.

Since the results in turbidimetric tests are determined by the presence of either turbidity or a precipitate, it is important that the urine be free from particles before the test is performed. For this reason, the tests include a step to clear the urine specimen. This is usually done by filtering the specimen and then testing the clear filtrate, or by centrifuging the specimen and testing the clear supernatant for the presence of protein. If the urine is centrifuged, the solid material left after collecting the supernatant is the urinary sediment, which is observed under the microscope.

A normal constituent of urine that may give falsely positive results in precipitation tests for urinary protein is mucin. Interference by mucin may be avoided by acidifying the urine with acetic acid to precipitate the mucin, then filtering to remove the precipitated mucin, and finally testing the clear filtrate. However, interference may be avoided simply by adding sufficient sodium chloride or other salt to raise the specific gravity to a level that will keep the mucin in solution.

The turbidimetric tests for urinary protein include Roberts' test and Heller's test, which are ring, or contact, tests; Exton's sulfosalicylic acid test and the analogous commercial product, Bumintest (Ames Co.); and many tests that make use of acetic acid, salt, and heat, which are variously called the heat and acetic acid test, the salt and acetic acid test, and Purdy's test.

Colorimetric tests for urinary protein involve the use of pH indicators—substances that have characteristic colors at specific pH values. At a fixed pH, certain pH indicators will show one color in the presence of protein and another color in its absence. This phenomenon is referred to as the *protein error of indicators* because it is often a problem in the laboratory, but it is put to use in testing for urinary protein. In this case the pH of the urine is held constant by means of a buffer, so that any change of color of the indicator will indicate the presence of protein.

The tests for urinary protein that make use of the protein error of indicators are all commercial ones. They are available as reagent strip tests, either alone or in combination with other tests. Although they are useful primarily as screening tests for protein, these strip tests can be read semiquantitatively as negative, trace, 1+, 2+, 3+, or 4+ to give a rough estimate of the amount of protein present. To do this, the resulting color must be matched closely with the color chart, which may be technically difficult. This difficulty is overcome by automated instruments that have been developed to read commercial reagent strip tests. An additional problem with reagent strips is that if the urine is exposed to the reagent strip for too long, the buffer may be washed out of the strip, resulting in the formation of a blue color whether protein is present or not. Therefore, a positive colorimetric reagent strip test for protein should be confirmed by a protein precipitation test to give a better estimate of the amount of protein present in the urine specimen.

Sources of error

There are several sources of error in the tests for urinary protein in addition to the two just described. Colorimetric reagent strip tests for protein are more sensitive to the presence of albumin than they are to globulin, hemoglobin, Bence Jones protein, and mucoprotein. If these proteins are present in the urine without albumin, falsely negative results may result. Turbidimetric tests are equally sensitive to all of these proteins. Therefore, urine containing proteins other than albumin would give a negative reagent strip test for protein and a positive turbidimetric test.

If a urine specimen is exceptionally alkaline or highly buffered, colorimetric reagent strip tests for urinary protein may give a positive result in the absence of protein. However, a very strongly alkaline urine may completely neutralize an acid precipitating agent, resulting in a falsely negative test for protein.

Other sources of error in the precipitation tests include the presence in the specimen of x-ray contrast media and of the metabolites of drugs such as tolbutamide. X-ray contrast media will precipitate in the acid test solution, giving a delayed positive reaction. This interference is suspected when very high specific gravity values, greater than 1.035, are obtained and the colorimetric reagent strip test for protein is negative. Unusual crystals of the x-ray media may also be found in the urinary sediment in such cases. Metabolites of drugs such as tolbutamide (an oral drug used to treat diabetes), which are excreted in urine, are insoluble in acid and give falsely positive results in the protein precipitation methods. These substances do not affect colorimetric reagent strip tests.

Turbidity in the urine specimen itself also poses a problem in the precipitation tests. Some urines are turbid when they are voided and many become turbid as they are cooled. Such urines must be clarified before they are tested by a turbidimetric procedure, and in some cases this is quite difficult. Such turbidity does not interfere with the colorimetric reagent strip tests.

Not all the numerous tests that have been developed for the detection of urinary protein will be described in this book. The procedures that are described here were chosen because they show methods that involve slightly different principles and have been found workable in teaching fairly large groups of students.

Heat and acetic acid test[24]

Principle

There are several variations of the heat and acetic acid test. The one discussed here differs from most in that is uses a boiling-water bath rather than a burner flame as a source of heat. The boiling-water bath facilitates testing large numbers of urine specimens at one time.

The test is based on the precipitation of protein with acetic acid and heat. The acetic acid is present to adjust the pH to the isoelectric point of proteins, so that they will readily precipitate when heat is applied. Salt is present to prevent the precipitation of mucin by raising the specific gravity. Precipitated mucin would be indistinguishable from protein and would give falsely positive results.

The amount of protein that is precipitated is roughly proportional to the amount of protein in the urine specimen. Therefore, results should be graded and reported as negative, trace, 1+, 2+, 3+, or 4+.

Reagent

Dissolve 150 g of NaCl in water. Add 50 ml of glacial acetic acid. Dilute to 1 L with water.

Procedure

1. Centrifuge an aliquot of urine. (Use exactly 10 ml of urine if the sediment is to be used for microscopic analysis.)

2. Decant the supernatant into a second test tube with one motion. (Leave exactly 1 ml for microscopic analysis.)

3. Check the supernatant for clarity. If centrifuging did not clear the urine, make a note of this, or set up a blank for comparison in reading the final results.

4. To the supernatant add approximately one-third volume of the salt and acetic acid reagent. Mix.

5. Place the mixture in a boling-water bath for 5 minutes.

6. Cool to room temperature in a cold-water bath, and allow the precipitate to settle for a short time.

7. Grade and report the results as follows:

Negative: clear solution or, if turbid before boiling, no increase in turbidity (less than 0.01 g/dl of protein)

Trace: faint turbidity throughout the solution (0.05 g/dl)

1+: small amount of precipitate filling less than one-fourth of the solution (0.25 g/dl)

2+: moderate amount of precipitate filling one-fourth to one-half of the solution (0.5 g/dl)

3+: heavy precipitate filling one-half to three-fourths of the solution (1 g/dl)

4+: coagulation of the entire solution or precipitate filling more than three-fourths of the solution (2–3 g/dl)

Bumintest tablet test and sulfosalicylic acid test[25]

Principle

These analogous tests are based on the precipitation of protein with sulfosalicylic acid. In the case of Bumintest (Ames Co.), the reagent is supplied in the form of a tablet that contains sulfosalicylic acid and sodium bicarbonate. The sodium bicarbonate causes rapid dissolution of the tablet by its effervescent interaction with water. Various concentrations of sulfosalicylic acid have been described for use in tests for urinary protein, although a 5 g/dl solution is probably the most common. In the procedure described here, a 6 g/dl solution is employed so that 9 ml of cleared urine, resulting from the routine 1:10 concentration of the urinary sediment, can be used. If 5 g/dl sulfosalicylic acid is used, the procedure is identical to that described for Bumintest. In all cases, the free sulfosalicylic acid in the working reagent serves to precipitate any protein in the specimen. It is specific for albumin, globulins, glycoproteins, and Bence Jones protein. Since the test does not rely on heat for precipitation, Bence Jones protein will precipitate like any other protein (it is soluble below 40° (and above 60°C).

Sulfosalicylic acid procedures may give falsely positive results with compounds used for diagnostic x-ray procedures. The reaction in this case is delayed somewhat and the precipitate is rather fluffy, unlike the normal protein precipitate. Such interference is suggested by specific gravity values greater than 1.035 and may be confirmed by checking the patient's history for the use of x-ray diagnostic procedures. When it occurs, the colorimetric reagent strip results for protein should be used.

In both cases, a positive reaction is the presence of turbidity. The amount of turbidity that is formed is roughly proportional to the amount of protein in the specimen. The results are graded as negative, trace, 1+, 2+, 3+, or 4+. Since the results depend on the degree of turbidity, it is important to begin with a urine specimen that is free of turbidity. A filtered or centrifuged specimen should be used.

Working Bumintest reagent

Dissolve four Bumintest tablets in 30 ml of deionized water. This produces a 5 g/dl solution of sulfosalicylic acid. It is ready for use when effervescence subsides, and it is stable indefinitely.

Sulfosalicylic acid reagent (6 g/dl)

Weigh 60 g of 5-sulfosalicylic acid ($C_7H_6O_6S \cdot 2H_2O$) and dilute to exactly 1000 ml with deionized water in a volumetric flask.

Procedure—Bumintest or 5 g/dl sulfosalicylic acid

1. Place equal parts of the reagent solution and cleared urine in a test tube. (Use at least 10 drops of each.)
2. Shake the test tube gently, and note the degree of turbidity by looking at the illuminated tube against a dark background.
3. Grade and report the results as outlined after the following procedure.

Procedure—6 g/dl sulfosalicylic acid

1. Centrifuge an aliquot of urine. Note the clarity of the centrifuged urine.
2. Pour 9 ml of the supernatant urine into a test tube.
3. Add 3 ml of 6 g/dl sulfosalicylic acid reagent.

4. Stopper the tube.
5. Mix by inverting the tube twice.
6. Let stand exactly 10 minutes.
7. Invert *twice.*
8. Observe the degree of precipitation and grade the results according to the following descriptions. To avoid making the test too sensitive, examine negative and trace reactions in ordinary room light, avoiding a Tyndall effect (scattering of light by colloidal particles), which might result from examination in too bright a light. If an agglutination viewer is available, use it to grade results higher than trace.

Results

Negative: no turbidity or no increase in turbidity (0.005 g/dl or less)
Trace: barely perceptible turbidity in ordinary room light (0.010 g/dl)
1+: distinct turbidity but no granulation (0.050 g/dl)
2+: turbidity with granulation but no flocculation (0.20 g/dl)
3+: turbidity with granulation and flocculation (0.50 g/dl)
4+: clumps of precipitate or tube of solid precipitate (1.0 g/dl or more)

Sensitivity

Sulfosalicylic acid tests for urine protein detect 5-10 mg of protein in 100 ml of urine.

Colorimetric reagent strip tests for protein (Albustix and Chemstrip)[26,27,28]

Principle

Commercial colorimetric reagent strip tests for urinary protein are based on the protein error of indicators. The reagent strips contain a buffer so that any color change in the test area is caused by the presence of protein, rather than a change of pH. The commercial reagent strips that are available differ in the buffer and pH indicator system impregnated on them; otherwise they are analogous. In Albustix (Ames Co.) and Chemstrip (Bio-Dynamics/bmc), urinary protein tests are supplied either individually, or in combination with other chemical tests in multiple-reagent strips.

Albustix and other multiple-reagent strips produced by the Ames Co. are plastic strips with protein test areas impregnated with a citrate buffer and tetrabromphenol blue. The citrate buffer provides a pH of approximately 3. At this pH tetrabromphenol is yellow in the absence of protein and yellow-green, green, or blue in its presence. The shade of the color is dependent on the amount of protein present.

Chemstrip products use tetrabromphenolphthalein ethyl ester as the indicator. This gives essentially the same color change in the presence of protein.

The test area in both products is more sensitive to albumin than to globulin, hemoglobin, Bence Jones protein, or mucoprotein. Therefore, these products may give negative reactions for specimens that test positive with precipitation methods.

Falsely positive reactions may occur when protein is absent if the urine is exceptionally alkaline or highly buffered. Contamination of the urine container with residues of disinfectants containing quaternary ammonium compounds or chlorhexidine may also cause falsely positive results. The tests are not affected by turbidity, x-ray contrast media, most drugs and their metabolites, and urine preservatives, which occasionally affect other protein tests.

Procedure

Observe the precautions and follow the instructions supplied by the manufacturer.

1. Dip the reagent area of the strip briefly into the specimen. Overwetting may wash out the buffer, resulting in falsely positive results.

2. Remove excess urine by tapping or drawing the edge of the strip along the rim of the urine container.

3. Compare the color that develops with the color chart supplied by the manufacturer and report as indicated on the chart. Albustix may be read immediately, although the time is not critical. Chemstrip should be read 30–120 seconds after dipping.

4. If it is the policy of the institution, confirm positive results by doing a turbidimetric test.

Sensitivity

Commercial reagent strip tests for protein detect 5–20 mg of albumin in 100 ml of urine.

KETONE BODIES

In the past, tests for ketone bodies were not part of the routine urinalysis. They were performed when ketone bodies were indicated by other findings in the urinalysis or when specifically requested. However, a test area for ketone bodies is included on most commercial multiple-reagent strips for the routine screening of urine and are now included in most routine urinalyses.

Ketone bodies (also called *acetone bodies*) are a group of three related substances: acetone, acetoacetic acid (or diacetic acid), and β-hydroxybutyric acid. Their structural similarity is illustrated in Fig. 5-4. They are normal products of fat metabolism and are not normally detectable in the blood or urine.

In fat catabolism (the phase of metabolism in which fats are broken down for energy), acetoacetic acid is produced first. It is converted to either β-hydroxybutyric acid or acetone. All three ketone bodies are utilized by muscle tissue

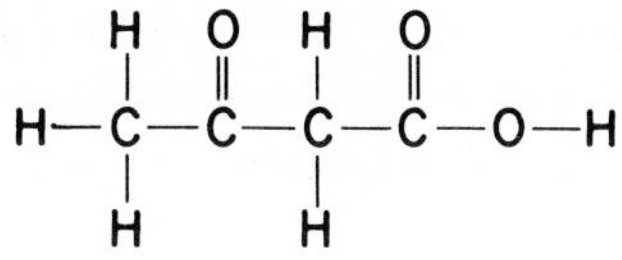

H   O   H   O
| || | ||
H—C—C—C—C—O—H
| |
H   H

Acetoacetic Acid

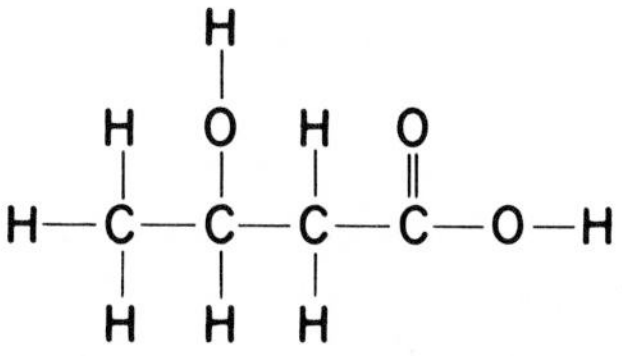

H
|
H   O   H   O
| | | ||
H—C—C—C—C—O—H
| | |
H   H   H

β-hydroxybutyric Acid

H   O   H
| || |
H—C—C—C—H
| |
H   H

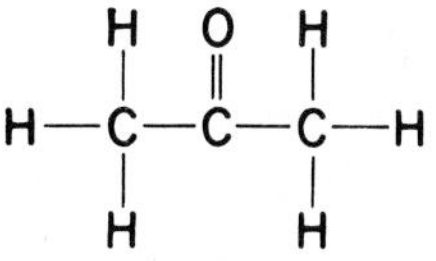

Acetone

Fig. 5-4. The ketone bodies.

as a source of energy and are eventually con-verted to carbon dioxide and water. When nor-mal amounts of fat are utilized by the body, the muscles are able to use the entire ketone produc-tion as an energy source. However, if more fat than normal is metabolized, the muscles are unable to utilize all the ketone bodies. The clinical result is an increased concentration of ketones in the blood (*ketosis*) and in the urine (*ketonuria*).

Whenever fat (rather than carbohydrate) is used as the major source of energy, ketosis and ketonuria may result. The two outstanding causes of ketone accumulation are diabetes mellitus and starvation. In diabetes mellitus, the body is un-able to use carbohydrate as an energy source and attempts to compensate by resorting to fat cata-bolism, which results in accumulation of the ketones. In starvation, the body is depleted of stored carbohydrate and must resort to fat as an

energy source. The same situation may occur in cases of severe liver damage. Most carbohydrate is stored as liver glycogen. In liver damage, there is no stored glycogen, hence the body must again resort to fat for energy. Finally, a ketogenic diet will result in ketone accumulation. A ketogenic diet is one that is high in fat and low in carbohydrates—specifically, a diet containing more than 1.5 g of fat per 1.0 g of carbohydrate. Low-carbohydrate diets used for weight reduc-tion may be ketogenic diets.

The physiological effects of ketone accumula-tion (ketosis and ketonuria) are serious. Aceto-acetic acid and β-hydroxybutyric acid contribute excess hydrogen ions to the blood, resulting in acidosis. As mentioned under pH, acidosis is an extremely serious condition and results in death if allowed to continue. Therefore, the body attempts to compensate for excess acid in the blood by eliminating acid through the urine. The kidney is capable of producing urine with a pH as low as 4.5. Thus, the occurrence of ketones in the urine is associated with a low urinary pH. Before insulin was used in the treatment of diabetes mellitus, acidosis was the cause of death in two-thirds of all cases. In the treatment of diabetes mellitus, it is important to control the amount of insulin so that ketosis and acidosis do not occur. A typical urine specimen from an uncontrolled diabetic is pale and greenish, con-tains a large amount of sugar, has a high specific gravity and a low pH, and contains ketone bodies.

Another physiological effect of ketosis con-cerns the substances acetone and acetoacetic acid. Both have been found to be toxic to brain tissue when present in increased concentrations in the blood. Of the two, acetoacetic acid is the most toxic. Hence, ketosis can result in perma-nent brain damage.

When ketones accumulate in the blood and urine, they do not occur in equal concentrations. Acetone is present in the smallest concentration, and there is 5–15 times more acetoacetic acid than acetone. β-Hydroxybutyric acid is present in the greatest concentration; usually there is two to four times more β-hydroxybutyric acid than acetoacetic acid.[29] However, most of the tests for ketosis and ketonuria are most sensitive to the presence of acetoacetic acid. There are no simple laboratory tests for β-hydroxybutyric acid. Most tests react with acetone, acetoacetic acid, or both. The most commonly used test is Rothera's or commercial modifications of it. These tests use the reagent nitroprusside. They are often referred to as tests for acetone, but they are all significantly more sensitive to the presence of acetoacetic acid than to acetone. There is one test that is specific for acetoacetic acid—Gerhardt's test. However, this test is positive only in the presence of large amounts of acetoacetic acid, indicating severe ketonuria. It is now seldom used because of the availability of improved commercial tests for ketone bodies.

It was mentioned above that in the normal formation of ketone bodies, acetoacetic acid is produced first and β-hydroxybutyric acid and acetone are produced from it. Similarly, if a urine specimen containing all three ketone bodies is allowed to stand after it is voided, the β-hydroxybutyric acid and acetoacetic acid will be converted to acetone. Since it is volatile, acetone will eventually disappear from the urine specimen. This means that urine should be tested for ketone bodies when fresh, or a falsely negative result may be obtained. Heat accelerates this conversion; therefore, refrigeration should be used to preserve the urine if it cannot be tested immediately.

Tests for ketone bodies should be included in the routine urinalysis whenever urine specimens are found to contain over 2+ sugar, on urine specimens from patients under 16 years of age, and when requested by the physician. Some tests for ketone bodies in urine specimens as described below.[30,31,32]

urine samples suspected of containing ketone bodies. It has now been virtually replaced by commercial tablet and reagent strip tests for these substances. We include it here as an example of the principle on which the commercial tests are based. Although it is often thought of as a test for acetone, it is more sensitive to acetoacetic acid. It will detect acetoacetic acid at a dilution of 1:125 000 and acetone at a dilution of 1:10 000. The test is based on the reaction of acetoacetic acid or acetone with sodium nitroprusside in an alkaline solution, with the formation of a reddish purple color.

Reagents

1. Rothera's reagent. Pulverize 7.5 g of sodium nitroprusside and mix with 200 g of ammonium sulfate.
2. Concentrated ammonium hydroxide.

Procedure

1. Place 1 g of Rothera's reagent in a test tube.
2. Add 5 ml of well-mixed urine. Mix thoroughly.
3. Carefully overlay the solution with 1 ml of concentrated ammonium hydroxide.
4. Observe the interface for the presence of a reddish purple ring within 1 or 2 minutes. (A brown color is of no significance.)
5. Grade and report the results as follows:

Negative: a brown ring at the interface or no color formation
Trace: delayed appearance of a faint pinkish purple ring
2+: a narrow dark purple ring
4+: a wide dark purple ring appearing rapidly

Rothera's test[33]

Rothera's test is a qualitative test for acetone and acetoacetic acid that has long been used for

Acetest tablet test

Acetest (Ames Co.) is another qualitative test for acetone and acetoacetic acid based on a color reaction with sodium nitroprusside. The principle is virtually identical to that of Rothera's method. In addition, it can be used to test whole blood, plasma, serum, or urine. Urine specimens must meet the same requirements for analysis as with Rothera's test.

Contents of the tablet

The Acetest tablet contains sodium nitroprusside (nitroferricyanide), glycine, and a strongly alkaline buffer.

Precautions

Observe the precautions in the literature supplied with the product. Do not use black or discolored tablets.

Procedure

Follow the manufacturer's directions.
1. Place the tablet on a clean surface, preferably a piece of white paper.
2. Place one drop of urine, serum, plasma, or whole blood on the tablet.
3. For testing urine, compare the color of the tablet with the color chart 30 seconds after application of the specimen.

For testing serum or plasma, compare the color of the tablet with the color chart 2 minutes after application of the specimen.

For testing whole blood, 10 minutes after the application of the specimen remove the clotted blood from the tablet and compare the color of the tablet with the color chart.

If acetone and acetoacetic acid are present, the tablet will show a color varying from lavender to deep purple. Report the results as negative, small, moderate, or large, as the manufacturer directs.

Sensitivity

Acetest detects 5–10 mg of acetoacetic acid in 100 ml of urine and 20–25 mg of acetone in 100 ml of urine.

Reagent strip tests for ketone bodies (Ketostix and Chemstrip)

The reagent strip tests for acetoacetic acid and acetone are based on a color reaction with sodium nitroprusside, analogous to the reaction in Rothera's test and the Acetest tablet test. The reagents are the same as for Acetest in both Ketostix (Ames Co.) and Chemstrip, but are impregnated on a reagent strip rather than in tablet form. The reagent strips may be used to test urine, serum, or plasma. They are more sensitive to acetoacetic acid than to acetone. Urine specimens must meet the same requirements for analysis as with Rothera's test; the main requirement is that the specimen be fresh to prevent conversion to acetone, which may be lost by evaporation. Preservatives do not prevent deterioration of urine ketones.

Urine specimens containing Bromsulphalein, very large amounts of phenylketones, or the preservative 8-hydroxyquinoline may give color reactions similar to that produced by acetoacetic acid and acetone. This is true of all tests using a reaction with nitroprusside.

When large amounts of ketone bodies are present in the urine it is advisable to use a reagent strip with a combined test for glucose and ketone bodies. This is especially true of patients with diabetes mellitus who monitor their own urine specimens for glucose content, as significant amounts of glucose might be overlooked without a concurrent test for ketone bodies.

Contents of reagent strip and chemical principle

The reagent areas in the strip tests for ketone bodies contain sodium nitroprusside (nitroferricyanide), glycine, and a strongly alkaline buffer. In an alkaline medium, acetoacetic acid and acetone react with nitroprusside in the presence of glycine to form a purple complex.

Procedure

Follow the manufacturer's directions.

1. Dip the reagent area of the strip briefly into urine, serum, or plasma, or pass the reagent end of the strip through the urine stream.

2. Remove excess urine by tapping or drawing the edge of the strip along the rim of the urine container.

3. Compare the color in the test area of the strip with the color chart supplied by the manufacturer at the time specified. Ketostix and other Ames products must be read exactly 15 seconds after dipping. Chemstrip products may be read 60-120 seconds after dipping.

4. Report the results as negative, small, moderate, or large, as the manufacturer directs.

Procedure for large amounts of ketones (dilution)

When a patient is monitored with repeated determinations of acetone and acetoacetic acid in plasma or urine, the concentrations of these compounds may start at very high levels and fall, but still give results that correspond to large on the color chart. Repeated reports of large do not reflect the changes as they occur. In such instances, semiquantitative results can be obtained by doing the analyses on several dilutions of each specimen until a large result is no longer seen. The report on this analysis should show that such dilutions have been done and when a reading of large is no longer obtained. An example of such a report would be: undiluted, large; 1:2 dilution, large; 1:4 dilution, moderate. This applies with both tablet and reagent strip tests.

Sensitivity

Reagent strip tests for ketone bodies detect 5-10 mg of acetoacetic acid in 100 ml of urine and 100 mg of acetone in 100 ml of urine.

Gerhardt's test[33]

Gerhardt's test is specific for acetoacetic acid; however, it is capable of detecting only large amounts of acetoacetic acid. Therefore any specimen giving a positive result in Gerhardt's test must also give a positive result in the various nitroprusside tests.

Gerhardt's test has been used as a means of determining the severity of ketosis. A positive result indicates severe ketosis, and treatment must be started immediately. For this reason, Gerhardt's test was performed whenever a positive reaction occurred with Rothera's test.

Rather than performing Gerhardt's test, a measure of the severity of ketosis may be obtained with reagent strip or tablet tests by diluting the original, concentrated specimen until a moderate result is obtained, as described above. For example, if the specimen required a 1:3 dilution for a moderate reaction, the result would be reported as: undiluted, large; 1:3 dilution, moderate. This method has virtually eliminated the need for Gerhardt's test in routine urinalysis. Gerhardt's test is included in this section as it is a simple test for salicylates in the urine and therefore can be used as an emergency test in case of aspirin overdose or poisoning. For this purpose, however, it is also being replaced by a commercial test, the Phenistix (Ames Co.) reagent strip test for phenylpyruvic acid, which also reacts with metabolites of aspirin or other salicylates.

Principle

Both acetoacetic acid and salicylates react with a 10 g/dl solution of ferric chloride ($FeCl_3$), forming a Bordeaux red color. For this reason, whenever a Bordeaux red color develops when ferric chloride is added to urine, the presence of acetoacetic acid or salicylates must be confirmed. As mentioned previously, acetoacetic acid is converted to acetone in the presence of heat. Gerhardt's test is specific for acetoacetic acid and does not detect acetone. Therefore, to confirm the presence of acetoacetic acid, the test solution is heated by boiling. After boiling, the Bordeaux color will not be present if acetoacetic acid was present in the urine. Since salicylates are unaffected by heat, the color will remain after boiling if the original specimen contained salicylates.

Reagent

The reagent used is a 10 g/dl FeCl$_3$ solution.

Procedure

1. Place 5 ml of urine in a test tube. Add ferric chloride reagent dropwise until any precipi-

tate of ferric phosphate dissolves. This generally takes only 5-10 drops of ferric chloride, and ferric phosphate does not always precipitate.

2. Observe the color of the solution. If acetoacetic acid or salicylates are present, a red-brown to Bordeaux red color will develop.

3. To confirm the presence of acetoacetic acid, divide the test solution in half and boil one portion for 5 minutes. If the color disappears or becomes lighter after boiling, acetoacetic acid was present. If the color remains unchanged after boiling, salicylates are present.

4. Report the results as positive or negative for acetoacetic acid or salicylates.

TWO BY-PRODUCTS OF RED BLOOD CELL DESTRUCTION: BILIRUBIN AND UROBILINOGEN

As described under Liver Function in Chap. 2, individual red blood cells do not exist indefinitely in the body; they are degraded after approximately 120 days. As part of red cell degradation, the heme portion of the hemoglobin molecule is converted to the bile pigment bilirubin by the reticuloendothelial (RE) cells. Bilirubin is a vivid yellow pigment. An increase in its concentration in the blood indicates jaundice. Although it is useful in the bile, bilirubin is a waste product that must eventually be eliminated from the body. When formed by the RE cells, bilirubin is not soluble in water and is normally carried through the bloodstream linked to plasma protein, primarily albumin. This water-insoluble form of bilirubin is often referred to as free bilirubin or unconjugated bilirubin.

Bilirubin is normally excreted from the body by the liver, through the intestine. It cannot be excreted by the kidney because free bilirubin linked to protein cannot pass through the glomerular capsule. When free bilirubin reaches the liver, it is converted to a water-soluble product by the Kupffer cells of the liver. It is made soluble by conjugation with glucuronic acid and some other hydrophilic substances to form bili-

rubin glucuronide. The water-soluble form is often referred to as conjugated bilirubin. Being water-soluble, conjugated bilirubin can be eliminated from the body by way of the kidney or the intestine. Normally, it is excreted by the liver into the bile and eliminated from the body through the intestine.

In the intestine, most of the bilirubin is converted to urobilinogen by the action of certain bacteria that make up the intestinal flora. Urobilinogen is actually a group of colorless chromogens. Approximately half of the urobilinogen formed in the intestine is absorbed into the portal blood circulation and returned to the liver. In the liver, most of the urobilinogen is excreted into the bile once again and returned to the intestine.

A very small amount of urobilinogen—about 1 percent of that formed in 1 day—escapes this liver clearance and is excreted from the body in the urine. Urobilinogen in the intestine is either eliminated from the body unchanged or oxidized to the colored compound urobilin, which gives the feces its normal color. The net effect is that, in normal circumstances, 99 percent of the urobilinogen formed from bilirubin is eliminated in the feces.

Thus, urine normally contains only a very small amount of urobilinogen and no bilirubin. Both are abnormal urinary constituents. However, there are several serious conditions in which either or both of these substances are found in the urine.

Tests for urinary bilirubin and urobilinogen were formerly performed only when indicated by abnormal color of the urine or when liver disease or a hemolytic condition was suspected from the patient's history. Because they are part of commercial multiple-reagent strips they are now included in the routine urinalysis. The presence of bilirubin in the urine is an early sign of liver cell disease (hepatocellular disease) and obstruction of the bile flow from the liver. It is especially useful in the early detection and monitoring of hepatitis, a highly infectious disease of particular importance to laboratory workers.

The presence of urobilinogen in the urine is increased in any condition that causes an increase in the production of bilirubin and any disease that prevents the liver from its normal function of returning urobilinogen to the intestine via the bile. The physician usually needs information about urinary bilirubin and urobilinogen in addition to serum bilirubin levels to determine the liver disorder or cause of jaundice. The clinical significance of these substances and laboratory tests for them are described in the following sections.

BILIRUBIN

Jaundice is a condition that occurs when the serum bilirubin concentration becomes greater than normal and there is an abnormal accumulation of bilirubin in the body tissues. Since bilirubin is a vivid yellow pigment, its accumulation in the tissues results in yellow pigmentation of the skin, the sclera or white of the eyes, and the mucous membranes. The causes of jaundice are numerous and must be discovered as soon as possible so that treatment may be started. There are several classifications of the various types of jaundice; one of them describes three types: prehepatic, hepatic, and posthepatic or obstructive (see also under Liver Function in Chap. 2).

Prehepatic jaundice is also known as *hemolytic* jaundice. It occurs in conditions where there is increased destruction of red cells—for instance, in infants with blood group incompatibilities, in neonatal physiological jaundice, and in hemolytic anemias. The liver is basically normal, so there is an increased formation of conjugated bilirubin and subsequently of urobilinogen. While there is an increased concentration of urobilinogen in the stool, the liver cannot pick up or reexcrete the large amount of urobilinogen returned to it via the portal circulation. Therefore, more urobilinogen goes into the general blood circulation and is eliminated in the urine. In summary, prehepatic, or hemolytic, jaundice is characterized by increased free bilirubin in the blood and increased urobilinogen in the stool and urine. However, all the bilirubin that is conjugated by the liver goes into the intestine, where it is converted to urobilinogen, and no bilirubin is found in the urine.

Hepatic jaundice results from conditions that involve the liver cells directly, preventing normal excretion. It can be caused by specific damage such as conjugation failure in neonatal physiological jaundice, where there is an enzyme deficiency. Diseases of conjugation failure result in increased concentrations of unconjugated bilirubin in the blood and then in the urine. Disturbances of the transport mechanisms by which conjugated bilirubin is passed into the bile canaliculi also occur in hepatic jaundice. There is diffuse or overall hepatic cell involvement in such conditions as viral hepatitis, toxic hepatitis from heavy metal or drug poisoning, and cirrhosis. In these cases the ability of the liver cells to remove and conjugate free bilirubin is diminished and increased amounts of free bilirubin are found in the blood. In addition, bilirubin that is conjugated by the liver is not excreted into the bile and is found in increased amounts in the blood; this conjugated bilirubin can now be eliminated by the kidney and is therefore found in the urine. Urobilinogen that is formed and goes into the portal circulation cannot be removed by the liver cells, and will also appear in the urine. Urinary urobilinogen is useful in the early detection of hepatitis, but as the disease progresses the liver is unable to form and pass conjugated bilirubin into the bile, so that the amount of urobilinogen in the urine is also decreased.

Posthepatic, or *obstructive,* jaundice occurs when the common bile duct is obstructed by stones, tumors, spasms, or stricture. As a result, the conjugated bilirubin is regurgitated back into the liver sinusoids and the blood. If the blockage is sufficiently extensive, liver cell function may be impaired so that both free and conjugated bilirubin are found in the blood. The conjugated bilirubin will be excreted by the kidney and therefore found in the urine. Since conjugated bilirubin is unable to reach the intestine, no urobilinogen is formed and it is absent in the blood and urine. Since urobilinogen is not formed, urobilin is absent and the stools have a characteristic chalky white to light brown color.

A chemical test for bilirubin should be included in the urinalysis when indicated on the basis of urine color or when requested by the physician. Urine containing bilirubin will typically have a beer-brown color and produce a yellow foam when shaken. If only small amounts of bilirubin are present these signs may be lacking, or the urine may appear only slightly darker than normal. In addition, bilirubin is not stable in solution but will be oxidized to biliverdin, which is a green pigment. Thus, urine containing bilirubin will typically be beer-brown when voided and will turn green on standing, especially if exposed to light. Tests for bilirubin will not be positive in the presence of biliverdin, so the urine must be examined when fresh. Small amounts of

urinary bilirubin may be undetectable if the urine is tested 1-4 hours after it is voided.

Several methods are available to test for bilirubin in urine. One of the oldest laboratory methods is the foam test for bilirubin. It was used by the early Greeks to help determine the cause of jaundice. However, this method of simply shaking the urine and looking for the presence of a yellow foam is not sufficient today. Several chemical tests for bilirubin are available. Smith's test involves the use of tincture of iodine diluted with nine times its volume of alcohol. This reagent is overlaid on the urine, and the interface is observed for the presence of an emerald green ring. Gmelin's test makes use of fuming nitric acid, which may be combined with the urine in a number of ways. The results involve a play of colors; green and violet are associated with the presence of bilirubin. The tests that will be discussed in detail here are Harrison's test and commercial diazotization tests.

Harrison's test[34]

Principle

This test depends on precipitation of bilirubin with barium chloride and subsequent oxidation of the bilirubin to biliverdin with Fouchet's reagent. The formation of biliverdin gives the barium chloride a green color, which constitutes a positive reaction. The barium chloride may be provided in several ways. In the modification of Harrison's test described here, it is supplied on thick filter paper that has been soaked in a saturated solution of barium chloride. Barium chloride tablets are available commercially. The same procedure is performed directly on the surface of the commercial tablet.

Certain substances may interfere with Harrison's test. Since Fouchet's reagent contains ferric chloride, salicylates in the urine will produce a purple color that may mask the normal positive color. In addition, the presence in the urine of other pigments, such as metabolites of the drugs Pyridium and Serenium, may give atypical color reactions that obscure the normal positive color.

Reagents

1. Fouchet's reagent. Dissolve 25 g of trichloro-acetic acid in 100 ml of distilled water. Add 10 ml of 10 g/dl $FeCl_3$.
2. Barium chloride paper. Soak thick filter paper (Schleicher and Schuell number 470) in saturated barium chloride. Dry and cut into small strips.

Procedure

1. Hold a strip of barium chloride paper perpendicularly in the urine for a few seconds.
2. Place one or two drops of Fouchet's reagent on the saturated area.
3. Look for the appearance of a green color, which constitutes a positive reaction.
4. Report the results as positive (formation of a green color) or negative (formation of any color except green, or no color formation).

Sensitivity

Harrison's test detects 0.1–0.2 mg of bilirubin in 100 ml of urine.

Diazotization tests[35,36,37]

The tablet and reagent strip tests for bilirubin are based on the coupling of bilirubin with a diazonium salt in an acid medium to form azobilirubin, which gives a blue or purple color. The tablet test is more sensitive to small amounts of bilirubin, and several institutions routinely test certain specimens—those that are negative with the reagent strips, but are expected to contain bilirubin from the case history or urine color—

with the more sensitive tablet test before reporting the result as negative.

Falsely positive tests for bilirubin may occur with urine specimens from patients who have received large doses of phenothiazine or chlorpromazine. In addition, metabolites of drugs such as Pyridium and Serenium give a red-orange color at a low urinary pH. This vivid red-orange color might be mistaken for that of bilirubin in the gross urine specimen, and might mask the reaction of small amounts of bilirubin or give atypical color reactions.

Ictotest tablet test

Principle

Ictotest (Ames Co.) is typical of various tests that use diazo compounds with sulfanilic acid, naphthylamines, and other substances to demonstrate the presence of bilirubin as azobilirubin. The tablets are supplied with a special mat. Urine is placed on the mat, the liquid portion is absorbed, and the bilirubin remains on the outer surface of the mat. The tablet contains the reactive ingredients. When bilirubin is present, it reacts with p-nitrobenzenediazonium p-toluenesulfonate, resulting in a blue or purple color. Other ingredients in the tablet provide the proper pH and ensure solution of the tablet when water is added, so that the reaction can take place.

Contents of the Ictotest tablet and mat

The Ictotest tablet contains p-nitrobenzenediazonium p-toluenesulfonate (bilazo), sulfosalicylic acid, and sodium bicarbonate. The mats are absorbent asbestos cellulose.

Precautions

Observe the precautions in the literature supplied by the manufacturer. Be sure to use the special mat provided. Either side may be used. Observe the results within 30 seconds, since a confusing pink color may appear after 30 seconds.

Procedure

1. Place five drops of urine on either side of the special test mat supplied with the reagent tablets.

2. Place the tablet in the center of the moistened area.

3. Flow two drops of water on the tablet.

4. Observe the mat around the tablet for the appearance of a blue to purple color within 30 seconds.

5. Report the results as positive or negative according to the following criteria:

Negative: the mat shows no blue or purple within 30 seconds. Ignore any color that forms after 30 seconds or a slight pink or red that may appear.

Positive: the mat around the tablet turns blue or purple within 30 seconds. Ignore any color change on the tablet itself.

Sensitivity

Ictotest detects 0.1 mg of bilirubin in 100 ml of urine.

Reagent strip tests for bilirubin (Multistix and Chemstrip)

Principle

These tests for bilirubin are available only on multiple-reagent strips in conjunction with other tests. They are both diazotization tests and are analogous to the Ictotest tablet test. The test area for bilirubin on Multistix and other Ames Co. reagent strip products is impregnated with 2,4-dichloroaniline diazonium salt. On Chemstrip and other Bio-Dynamics/bmc products the test area for bilirubin contains 2,6-dichlorobenzenediazoniumfluoroborate.

The reagent strip tests for bilirubin are difficult to read and the color formed after reaction with urine must be carefully compared with the color chart supplied by the manufacturer. Proficiency in reading these results comes with experience and is essential for reliable results. Many negative urine specimens as well as specimens containing varying amounts of bilirubin should be tested to gain experience and proficiency. In addition, control specimens that are positive for bilirubin should be tested daily to maintain proficiency.

Since both of these tests are less sensitive for bilirubin than the tablet test or oxidation methods such as Harrison's test, it may be necessary to routinely test all urine specimens suspected of containing bilirubin, yet negative with the reagent strip tests, with a more sensitive method. The reagent strips are subject to interference from the same substances that interfere with Ictotest.

Precautions

Observe the precautions and follow the directions in the literature supplied by the manufacturer.

Procedure

1. Dip the reagent strip briefly into the urine specimen.

2. Remove excess urine by tapping the edge of the strip against the rim of the urine container. Hold the strip in a horizontal position to prevent mixing of chemicals from adjacent reagent areas.

3. Compare the test area for bilirubin closely with the color chart supplied by the manufacturer. Multistix should be read 20 seconds after dipping. Chemstrip products may be read 30–120 seconds after dipping.

4. Report the results as positive or negative for bilirubin.

Sensitivity

Multistix detects 0.2–0.4 mg of bilirubin in 100 ml of urine. Chemstrip products detect 0.5 mg of bilirubin in 100 ml of urine; large amounts of ascorbic acid lower the sensitivity of this test.

UROBILINOGEN

Urobilinogen is a by-product of red blood cell degradation and results from intestinal reduction of bilirubin. Increased destruction of red cells may be accompanied by large amounts of urobilinogen in the urine. Therefore, urobilinogen will be seen in hemolytic anemias, pernicious anemia, and malaria. In the absence of increased red cell destruction, the tests may be considered liver function tests. One of the first effects of liver damage is impairment of the mechanism for removing urobilinogen from the blood circulation and excreting it through the intestine. This results in removal of urobilinogen by the kidney and its presence in the urine. Tests for urinary urobilinogen are thus useful for the early detection of liver damage. Urobilinogen is found in the urine in conditions such as infectious hepatitis, toxic hepatitis, portal cirrhosis, congestive heart failure, and infectious mononucleosis.

Normally, 1 percent of all the urobilinogen produced is excreted in the urine and 99 percent is excreted in the feces. However, under certain conditions urobilinogen is completely absent from the urine and the feces. When the normal intestinal bacterial flora are destroyed, as by antibiotic therapy, urobilinogen cannot be produced. Urobilinogen is also absent if the liver does not conjugate bilirubin, or if there is biliary tract obstruction such as from gallstones, resulting in failure of conjugated bilirubin to reach the intestinal tract.

Tests for urobilinogen have become routine only since their inclusion in multiple-reagent strips. Urine should certainly be tested for urobilinogen when requested by the physician or whenever its presence is suspected on the basis of abnormal urine color. Urine containing urobilinogen will often show a characteristic orange-red or orange-brown color because of the presence of urobilin. Whenever a test for bilirubin is performed, a test for urobilinogen should also be done.

It is particularly necessary to use a fresh urine specimen when testing for urobilinogen, since it is unusually unstable and is rapidly oxidized to urobilin. This oxidation takes place so readily that most urine specimens that contain urobilinogen will show an abnormal color caused by partial oxidation to urobilin. The presence of urobilinogen and that of urobilin have the same clinical significance; however, they take part in different chemical reactions, and urine is more frequently tested for urobilinogen. Normally, 1–4 mg of urobilinogen is excreted in the urine each day. This is less than 1 Ehrlich unit* in each 2-hour urine collection period.

Another substance that is related to urobilinogen is porphobilinogen. The porphyrins are a group of compounds that are utilized in the synthesis of hemoglobin. The heme portion of hemoglobin is a type of porphyrin, namely ferroprotoporphyrin 9. In normal individuals porphyrins are eliminated from the body in the urine and feces, mainly as coproporphyrin I with a small amount of coproporphyrin III. However, certain errors of porphyrin metabolism lead to increased excretion of other porphyrins in the urine. These conditions are collectively called porphyrias, and in some of them porphobilinogen is present in the urine. The Watson-Schwartz test, which is described here as a test for urobilinogen, will also detect porphobilinogen. Although urine specimens can be screened for the presence of substances that react in Ehrlich's test (urobilinogen and porphobilinogen) with commercial reagent strip tests, all positive results should be confirmed and further identified with the Watson-Schwartz test for Ehrlich-reactive substances.

*The Ehrlich unit is a traditional measure of urobilinogen activity; 1 Ehrlich unit is equivalent to 1 mg of urobilinogen per 100 ml.

Ehrlich's qualitative aldehyde reaction for urobilinogen and porphobilinogen (Watson-Schwartz test)[38,39,40,41,42,43]

Principle

Ehrlich's aldehyde reaction occurs with urobilinogen but not with urobilin. Therefore, absolutely fresh urine is necessary for this test. In the presence of Ehrlich's reagent, urobilinogen gives a characteristic cherry red color. This color is the result of the reaction of p-dimethylaminobenzaldehyde in concentrated hydrochloric acid with urobilinogen and porphobilinogen to form a colored aldehyde. The color is enhanced in the presence of saturated sodium acetate, which also inhibits color formation by skatoles and indoles, which might be present in the urine. However, porphobilinogen and certain intermediate Ehrlich-reactive compounds give the same cherry red color with Ehrlich's reagent and sodium acetate and must be distinguished from urobilinogen. To do this, the test solution is extracted with the organic solvents chloroform and butanol. Urobilinogen is soluble in both solvents, porphobilinogen is not soluble in either, and intermediate Ehrlich-reactive compounds are soluble in butanol but not in chloroform (Table 5-2).

In addition, fresh urine should be cooled to room temperature before the test is carried out to prevent the "warm aldehyde" reaction. This is a weak Ehrlich reaction that takes place at body temperature with a chromogen (probably indoxyl) that is present in normal urine. Sulfonamides, procaine, 5-hydroxyindoleacetic acid, and other compounds react with Ehrlich's reagent and may interfere with the test.

Reagents

1. Ehrlich's reagent. Combine 0.7 g of p-dimethylaminobenzaldehyde, 150 ml of concentrated hydrochloric acid, and 100 ml of deionized water.
2. Saturated sodium acetate in deionized water.
3. Chloroform.
4. Butanol.

Procedure

1. Place 1 volume (approximately 3 ml) of urine in a test tube. Add an equal volume of Ehrlich's reagent. Mix well by inversion.

2. Add 2 volumes of saturated sodium acetate and mix. A red or deep pink (cherry red) color is a positive result and indicates the presence of urobilinogen, porphobilinogen, or other Ehrlich-reactive compounds. If the test is positive at this stage, split the colored solution into two parts, and continue with step 3.

3. Add a few milliliters of chloroform to one portion of the colored solution and shake vigorously. Observe whether the color is completely extracted into the lower chloroform layer. Extract the colored solution with chloroform as many times as is necessary. If the color is caused by urobilinogen, it will be extracted into the chloroform layer. Color caused by porphobilinogen or intermediate Ehrlich-reactive compound will not be extracted into chloroform.

4. If the color is not extracted by chloroform, extract the other portion of the colored solution with a few milliliters of butanol to distinguish porphobilinogen from intermediate Ehrlich-reactive compounds. Color caused by urobilinogen or intermediate Ehrlich-reactive compounds will be extracted into the butanol.

5. Report the results as positive or negative for urobilinogen, positive for porphobilinogen, or positive for both urobilinogen and porphobilinogen (very rare). Do not report the finding of intermediate Ehrlich-reactive compounds.

Table 5-2. Results of Watson-Schwartz test

Result	Ehrlich's reagent plus sodium acetate	Chloroform extract	Butanol extract
Negative	No pink color		
Urobilinogen	Pink	Pink	Pink
Porphobilinogen	Pink	Colorless	Colorless
Intermediate Ehrlich-reactive compounds	Pink	Colorless	Pink

Reagent strip tests for urobilinogen[44,45,46]

The inclusion of a test area for urobilinogen in commercial multiple-reagent strips has made testing for the presence of urobilinogen (or Ehrlich-reactive substances) part of the routine urinalysis. However, positive reactions with the reagent strip tests should be confirmed, and urobilinogen should be distinguished from porphobilinogen and intermediate Ehrlich-reactive substances, by the Watson-Schwartz test. The reagent strips available for the detection of urobilinogen in the urine include Urobilistix and other multiple-reagent strips produced by Ames Co. and various Chemstrip products produced by Bio-Dynamics/bmc.

The specimen requirements are the same as for the Watson-Schwartz test. The tests detect only urobilinogen and give negative results if only urobilin is present. Therefore, a fresh urine specimen must be used.

Since the body normally eliminates 1–4 Ehrlich units of urobilinogen through the urine each day, random normal urine specimens contain up to 1 Ehrlich unit per 100 ml (equivalent to 1 mg of urobilinogen per 100 ml). The *absence* of urobilinogen cannot be determined with these reagent strip tests, although it may be of clinical significance.

Metabolites of drugs such as Pyridium (phenazopyridine) that color the urine red, or that turn red in an acidic medium, may mask the reaction or give falsely positive results with both reagent strip tests for urobilinogen.

Urobilistix

The reagent strips manufactured by Ames Co. that have test areas for urobilinogen are based on the Ehrlich reaction in which p-dimethylaminobenzaldehyde reacts with urobilinogen in a strongly acidic medium to form a colored aldehyde. The reddish brown color that is formed varies with the amount of urobilinogen present.

After a timed interval, the color is compared with a graded color chart. The results are given in terms of Ehrlich units per 100 ml. However, the test is not specific for urobilinogen and reacts with substances known to react with Ehrlich's reagent. These substances include porphobilinogen, sulfisoxazole (Gantrisin), p-aminosalicylic acid, sulfonamides, procaine, and 5-hydroxyindoleacetic acid. Therefore, urines that give a positive reaction in this test should be checked and the presence of urobilinogen, porphobilinogen, or intermediate Ehrlich-reactive substances should be determined by the Watson-Schwartz test.

Chemstrip

The test area for urobilinogen is impregnated with p-methoxybenzenediazonium fluoroborate which reacts with urobilinogen in an acidic medium to form a red azo dye. Values are read in milligrams per deciliter by comparing the color formed within a certain time interval with a graded color chart. The test is specific for urobilinogen; porphobilinogen or other Ehrlich-reactive substances are not detected with this procedure.

Procedure (Urobilistix and Chemstrip)

1. Dip the reagent strip briefly into the specimen.
2. Remove excess urine by tapping the edge of the strip against the rim of the urine container.
3. Read the results as follows. With Urobilistix, compare the color of the test area after 60 seconds with the color chart supplied by the manufacturer and report as indicated on the chart. With Chemstrip, compare the test area 10-120 seconds after dipping with the color chart and report as indicated on the chart.

Sensitivity

Urobilistix detects 0.1 Ehrlich units in 100 ml of

urine (or 0.1 mg in 100 ml). Chemstrip detects 0.4 mg of urobilinogen in 100 ml of urine.

Schlesinger's test for urinary urobilin[47]

Principle

Urobilin is an oxidation product of urobilinogen. Urobilin is colored and urobilinogen is colorless. Both compounds have the same clinical significance when present in urine; however, they undergo different chemical reactions.

Reagent

The reagent used in this test is a saturated alcohol solution of zinc acetate.

Procedure

1. Mix equal parts of urine and alcohol-zinc acetate in a test tube. Filter the mixture.
2. Examine the filtrate for green fluorescence by viewing the tube from above as it is passed through the direct rays of a fairly strong light (e.g., Wood's light).
3. Report as positive or negative.

Quantitative determination of urinary urobilinogen

Quantitative determinations of urinary urobilinogen are very similar to Ehrlich's qualitative aldehyde reaction. In the quantitative determination the reagents are measured volumetrically and the degree of color formation is measured with a photometer. One difference between this and other quantitative tests is related to the freshness of the specimen. Because urobilinogen is so rapidly oxidized to urobilin, it is impossible to employ a complete 24-hour urine collection. Instead, a complete 2-hour collection is used. A specimen collected between 1 and 3 p.m. is preferred, since excretion of urobilinogen is highest during this period. The test must be performed within $\frac{1}{2}$ hour of collection because of the instability of urobilinogen. In addition, specimens must be protected from sunlight and other sources of intense heat. Therefore, they are collected in brown bottles and stored under refrigeration.

HEMOGLOBIN AND BLOOD IN URINE

Chemical tests for hemoglobin in urine also react with myoglobin (which is muscle hemoglobin) and red cells.[48,49,50,51,52] Such tests are included in the routine urinalysis with a multiple-reagent strip. The physician is interested in detecting the presence of all three of these substances and in knowing which is present. Although the chemical tests are more sensitive to the presence of hemoglobin and myoglobin than to intact red cells, most positive reactions are actually caused by the presence of red cells. Before reagent strip tests were available, the detection of blood in the urine was based on gross observation of blood through a change in the appearance (color) of the urine and the presence of red cells in the microscopic examination of the urinary sediment. Without a chemical test for hemoglobin, its presence would be missed.

It is clinically significant to differentiate between red cells and hemoglobin in the urine. Since tests for hemoglobin are positive in the presence of both free hemoglobin and red cells, it would seem that this differentiation is made mainly by the finding of red cells in the microscopic analysis of the urinary sediment. However, the presence of hemoglobin and the absence of red cells in the urine does not necessarily mean that the hemoglobin was originally free urinary hemoglobin. Red cells rapidly lyse in urine, especially when it has a specific gravity of 1.006 or less or is alkaline. For this reason urine should be absolutely fresh when examined for the presence of red cells. In addition, the specific gravity and pH of the urine will be useful in differentiating between red cells and free hemoglobin in the urine.

Hemoglobinuria, or the presence of free hemoglobin in the urine, results from a variety of conditions and disease states. It may be the result of hemolysis in the bloodstream, in a particular organ, in the kidney or lower urinary tract, or in the urine sample itself. Hematologic disease states resulting in hemoglobinuria include hemolytic anemia, hemolytic transfusion reactions, paroxysmal nocturnal hemoglobinuria, paroxysmal cold hemoglobinuria, and favism. Severe infectious diseases such as yellow fever, smallpox, and malaria also result in hemoglobinuria, as do poisonings with strong acids or mushrooms, severe burns, and renal infarction. Finally, significant amounts of free hemoglobin occur whenever excessive numbers of red cells are present as a result of various renal disorders, infectious or neoplastic diseases, or trauma in any part of the urinary tract.

Hematuria is the presence of red blood cells in the urine. It results from a great variety of renal diseases, including both lesions of the kidney itself and bleeding at any other point in the urinary tract. Hematuria is a sensitive, early indicator of renal disease, and usually is accompanied by the presence of hemoglobin. Although blood will not be present in every voided specimen in every case of renal disease, occult blood (i.e., blood that is not grossly visible but is found by laboratory tests) may be present in almost every renal disorder. There may be little correlation between the amount of blood and the severity of the disorder, but its presence may be the only indication of renal disease. Other laboratory findings besides the presence of occult blood indicate the presence of renal disease. Protein is usually present along with blood, although available chemical tests are more sensitive to the presence of occult blood than of protein. In addition, findings in the microscopic analysis of the urinary sediment, such as the presence of casts, especially red cell casts, are particularly useful in detecting renal disorders.

Myoglobinuria is the presence of myoglobin in the urine. It is a rare finding. Chemical tests for occult blood are equally sensitive to the presence of hemoglobin and myoglobin. Myoglobinuria results from traumatic muscle injury (such as from traffic accidents), excessive unaccustomed exercise, beating or other crush injury, or bullet wounds.

Numerous tests are available for the detection of hemoglobin (or blood) in both urine and feces. Most of these tests are based on the same general principles and reaction. They all make use of peroxidase activity in the heme portion of the hemoglobin molecule. The reagents most commonly used have been gum guaiac, benzidine, or *o*-tolidine. Benzidine is no longer used as it is a carcinogen. They all involve the presence of hydrogen peroxide (H_2O_2) or a suitable precursor. Peroxidase activity of the hemoglobin molecule liberates oxygen from hydrogen peroxide. This oxygen will cause the oxidation of the chromogen (gum guaiac or *o*-tolidine) to colored oxidation products, which are usually blue or green. These reactions are summarized below:

$$\text{Hemoglobin} + H_2O_2 \xrightarrow{\text{peroxidase}} \text{oxygen}$$

$$\text{Oxygen} + \text{chromogen} \longrightarrow$$
$$\text{blue or green oxidation products}$$

The reagents that have been used in testing for hemoglobin have varying degrees of sensitivity. Of the three, *o*-tolidine is the most sensitive to the presence of hemoglobin, benzidine is less sensitive, and gum guaiac is least sensitive. However, the sensitivity of the tests is reported to be dependent on the amount and order of the reagents rather than the type of indicator.[53]

Since all these tests are based on the peroxidase activity of heme, other substances with peroxidase activity also give positive reactions in the tests for occult blood. In urine such peroxidase activity may be present in white blood cells and bacteria. Large doses of vitamin C (ascorbic acid), which is popularly used as a cold remedy or which may be present with parenteral drugs (such as tetracycline) in which it is a reducing agent, may inhibit or delay the color reaction. This results from reaction of the released hydrogen peroxide with ascorbic acid (a strong reducing agent) instead of the color indicator. Such interference can be confirmed with a reagent strip test specific for ascorbic acid, such as C-Stix (Ames Co.). The sensitivity of the reagent strips is reduced in urines with high specific gravity. Falsely positive results can be produced by residues of strongly oxidizing cleaning agents in the urine container. Finally, microbial peroxidase, associated with urinary tract infections, may cause a falsely positive reaction.

The gum guaiac filter paper test for occult blood in feces (see Chap. 7) may also be used to test urine for the presence of hemoglobin. The urine should be centrifuged to remove white blood cells, so that only free hemoglobin in the urine will be measured. Commercial reagent strip tests for the detection of occult blood use o-tolidine as the color indicator.

Reagent strip tests for hemoglobin and blood (Hemastix and Chemstrip)

Principle

The reagent strips are used to test for hemoglobin, red cells, and myoglobin in the urine. The tests are based on the oxidation of o-tolidine resulting from the peroxidase activity of hemoglobin. The tests areas are impregnated with a buffered mixture of organic peroxide and o-tolidine. These tests are more sensitive to free hemoglobin than to intact red cells and may not react when only a few intact red cells are present with no free hemoglobin. To detect red cells, uncentrifuged urine must be used, as the result

would be negative if all the red cells were intact and no hemoglobin was present in the supernanant. The color that results from the reaction varies with the amount of hemoglobin present. After a timed interval, the color is compared with a graded color chart and reported as directed by the manufacturer.

Procedure

1. Dip the test area of the strip briefly into the specimen.
2. Remove excess urine by tapping the edge of the strip along the rim of the urine container.
3. Compare the color that develops with the color chart supplied by the manufacturer and report as indicated on the chart. With Hemastix, read 30 seconds after dipping. With Chemstrip, read 60–120 seconds after dipping.

Sensitivity

Hemastix detects 0.015 mg of hemoglobin in 100 ml of urine or 5 intact red blood cells per microliter. Sensitivity is reduced in urines with high specific gravity. Chemstrip detects hemoglobin content corresponding to 10 red blood cells per microliter or 5 intact red blood cells per microliter.

Qualitative test for free hemoglobin in urine

Since it may be of clinical significance to differentiate between hemoglobin and red cells in the urine, the following procedure may be used in addition to the microscopic analysis of urinary sediment.

Procedure

1. Screen the uncentrifuged urine with the reagent strip and C-Stix, which is specific for ascorbic acid.

2. If both C-Stix and the reagent strip for blood are negative, report hemoglobin as negative.

3. If C-Stix is positive, the specimen is unsatisfactory and a new specimen should be requested following abstinence from vitamin C for 24 hours.

4. If the reagent strip for blood is positive, centrifuge the specimen and retest the supernatant with Hemastix.

5. If the reagent strip for blood in the supernatant urine is negative, report hemoglobin as negative. If positive, report hemoglobin results as small, moderate, or large.

NITRITE

Reagent strip tests for nitrite (N-Multistix and Chemstrip)

Tests for nitrite have not been part of the routine urinalysis. However, they have recently been included on commercial multiple-reagent strips such as N-Multistix and on the various Chemstrip products.

Principle

The presence of urinary nitrite indicates the existence of a urinary tract infection. Detection of such infections is particularly important in pregnant women and young girls to prevent permanent renal damage. Traditionally, urinary tract infections are diagnosed through quantitative urine culture, where the organism that causes the infection is cultured and identified. Nitrite tests are merely screening tests that aid, but in no way replace, quantitative urine cultures. The existence of urinary tract infections is suggested by certain findings in the routine urinalysis. These include the presence of white blood cells, bacteria, and sometimes casts in the microscopic examination of the urinary sediment; chemical tests might show protein and a more alkaline urinary pH.

Chemical tests for nitrite included on reagent strips are based on the Griess test.[54] They are not very sensitive and have stringent specimen requirements. To show a positive reaction the urine must be present in the bladder for at least 4 hours, and preferably overnight, so that certain species of bacteria can convert nitrates, which are normally present in urine, to nitrites, which are normally absent. The reagent strips contain an aromatic amine that reacts with nitrite to give a diazonium salt. This salt reacts with another compound on the strip to give a red-violet (pink) azo dye. The pink color is therefore related to the presence of bacteria in the urinary tract. However, the amount of color produced cannot be related to the number of bacteria present, and the results should be reported only as positive or negative.

Limitations

The test is primarily useful if positive. If the nitrite test area shows a negative reaction, urinary infection cannot be ruled out. The urine must be retained in the bladder for 4 hours or more for adequate conversion of nitrate to the nitrite that is detected in the test. Therefore, a first morning urine specimen should be used. Some urinary tract infections are caused by organisms that do not contain the reductase necessary to convert nitrate to nitrite. In addition, the test is less sensitive in urines having a high specific gravity and high ascorbic acid content. Falsely positive reactions may also occur. They may be caused by bacterial growth in "old" urine specimens or by medication such as phenazopyridine that colors the urine red or that turns red in an acidic medium.

Procedure

Follow the manufacturer's directions and precautions.

1. Dip the test area of the strip briefly into the specimen.

2. Remove excess urine by tapping the edge of the strip along the rim of the urine container.

3. Compare the color that develops with the color chart supplied by the manufacturer. Report as positive or negative within the time specified by the manufacturer.

Sensitivity

N-Multistix detects 0.075 mg of sodium nitrite in 100 ml of urine. Chemstrip detects 0.05 mg of nitrite in 100 ml of urine.

ASCORBIC ACID

Background and significance

Although ascorbic acid is not a normal constituent of urine, it is sometimes present. It is different from the constituents that are commonly tested for and have been described up to now. Most of the substances tested for in urine are either abnormal constituents or constituents that are present in abnormal concentrations and are the result of metabolic processes within the body. These substances must be detected because their presence in the urine reflects conditions that are unhealthy. Ascorbic acid is not such a substance (although its presence in urine may result in a tendency to kidney stone formation in some persons). Its presence in the urine is important because of the interfering effect it has on other chemical tests, especially the reagent strip tests for glucose and blood that depend on the release of hydrogen peroxide by peroxidase. Although the manufacturers of these products continue to make modifications to reduce the inhibitory effect of ascorbic acid, it remains a problem.

Inhibiting quantities of ascorbic acid are found in the urine of patients who have ingested large quantities of vitamin C. Quantities of vitamin C in excess of those required by the body for normal function are quickly eliminated through the urine.

The interfering effect of ascorbic acid results from its action as a strong reducing agent. In reagent strip tests for glucose and blood, hydrogen peroxide is used to oxidize a chromogen from a reduced form to a colored oxidized form. Ascorbic acid interferes by reducing the released hydrogen peroxide to water, preventing or delaying the desired oxidation of the chromogen indicator. These reactions are summarized below:

Desired reaction with peroxidase:

$$H_2O_2 \text{ (Released through peroxidase activity)} + \text{reduced chromogen} \longrightarrow$$

$$\text{oxidized chromogen} + H_2O \text{ (Colored)}$$

Effect of ascorbic acid:

$$H_2O_2 + \text{ascorbic acid (Reduced form)} \longrightarrow$$

$$\text{dehydroascorbic acid} + H_2O \text{ (Oxidized form)}$$

The presence of ascorbic acid in the urine may be suspected when a reagent strip test for blood is negative although the urinary sediment shows the presence of red cells (over 1+). It may also be suspected when strip tests for glucose on urine specimens from diabetic patients give inconsistent results, showing negative reactions even though the tests for ketones and the copper reduction tests for sugar are positive. In such cases ascorbic acid may be confirmed by a reagent strip test specific for ascorbic acid. If this is not available, a clinical history of ingestion of large doses of ascorbic acid may suffice.

Reagent strip test for ascorbic acid (C-Stix)

The reagent strip test for ascorbic acid makes use of its reducing properties. The strips have a test area impregnated with phosphomolybdates buffered in an acidic medium. Phosphomolybdates are reduced by ascorbic acid to a colored compound, molybdenum blue. The reagent strips may give a falsely positive reaction with gentisic acid and L-dopa. They will not do so with urates, salicylates, or creatinine, however.

Procedure

Follow the directions supplied by the manufacturer. Dip the test end of the strip into the specimen. Ten seconds later compare the color of the reagent area of the strip with the color chart supplied by the manufacturer, and report the results as indicated on the chart.

Sensitivity

C-Stix detects 5 mg of ascorbic acid in 100 ml of urine.

URINARY SEDIMENT

Urinary sediment refers to all solid materials suspended in the urine specimen. Very few urine specimens are absolutely clear, and even those that appear clear to the naked eye have some solid material suspended in them. In addition, many urine specimens obviously contain solid material, as evidenced by their cloudiness. Any amount of cloudiness that is visible to the naked eye must be accounted for in a microscopic analysis of the urinary sediment. The solid material present in urine specimens may be identified only under the microscope, and a microscopic examination of the urinary sediment is essential in any routine urinalysis. It may be the most important part of the urinalysis.

When the urinary sediment is to be examined, a concentrated portion of the urine is used rather than a well-mixed specimen. The sediment is concentrated before examination to ensure detection of less abundant constituents. To concentrate the sediment, a well-mixed, measured portion of urine is centrifuged. The clear supernatant is decanted and the solid material, which settles to the bottom during centrifugation, is examined under the microscope (the supernatant may be further tested for chemical constituents, such as urinary protein). The various parts of the sediment are identified and counted to give semi-quantitative results. For these results to have any meaning, a constant amount of urine must be centrifuged and a constant volume of supernatant removed. Urine is therefore centrifuged in a graduated centrifuge tube. Results in this section are based on centrifuging exactly 10 ml of urine and removing exactly 9 ml of supernatant, leaving 1 ml of sediment for examination under the microscope. The actual volume used may be different, but it must be consistent within each laboratory.

The urinary sediment consists of a great variety of material. Some of the constituents are normal, while others are abnormal and represent serious conditions. It is important to learn to identify both the normal and abnormal constituents. In general, the normal constituents are more easily seen under the microscope, and must be recognized so that they do not obscure the presence of the less obvious but more serious abnormal constituents. Recognition of the abnormal constituents is extremely important in the diagnosis and treatment of various renal diseases. They often give information about the state of the kidney and the urinary tract. In addition, the microscopic analysis of the sediment will help to confirm and account for findings in other portions of the routine urinalysis. For example, protein in the urine is often associated with the presence of casts in the sediment.

Urine specimen requirements

The ideal specimen for microscopic analysis of the urinary sediment is a fresh, voided, first morning specimen. A first morning specimen is preferable since it is the most concentrated, and therefore small amounts of abnormal constituents are more likely to be detected. In addition, the formed elements are less likely to disintegrate in more concentrated urine.

A fresh urine specimen is particularly important for reliable results. If the urine cannot be examined shortly after it is voided, it should be refrigerated. If it must be kept in the refrigerator for more than a few hours, a chemical preservative should be added. Formalin may be used as a preservative that will fix the various formed elements. However, it interferes with chemical tests. Other preservatives, such as toluene, may be used to prevent bacterial contamination. None of the preservatives is completely satisfactory, and fresh collections are definitely preferred.

Changes that may occur as the urine stands include the following. Red blood cells become distorted because of the lack of an isotonic solution. They either swell or become crenate which makes them difficult to recognize, and they finally disintegrate. White blood cells also disintegrate in hypotonic solutions. Casts disintegrate, especially as the urine becomes alkaline, since they must have sufficient acidity and solute concentration to exist. Other components that are found only in acidic urine will disappear as the urine becomes alkaline. The increase in alkalinity results from the growth of bacteria and production of ammonia. Finally, bacteria multiply rapidly, obscuring various components.

In addition to being a fresh first morning collection, the urine specimen should be clean and free of external contamination. This is sometimes a problem with female patients, since vaginal contamination will result in the presence of epithelial cells, red cells, and white cells. In such cases it may be necessary to use a clean-voided midstream specimen, which is also required for quantitative urine culture. It may also be necessary to pack the vagina or use a tampon in some cases to avoid vaginal contamination.

Special aids to examination of the urinary sediment

Traditionally, the urinary sediment has been examined microscopically by placing a drop of urine on a microscope slide, cover slipping, and observing the preparation with the low-power objective ($\times 100$ total magnification) and high-power objective ($\times 400$–450 total magnification) of a bright-field microscope. Since the preparation is a wet mount, oil immersion cannot be used in this examination. When the sediment is examined under the bright-field microscope, correct light adjustment is essential. The light must be sufficiently reduced, by correct positioning of the condenser and the iris diaphragm, to give contrast between the unstained structures and the background liquid. The correct light adjustment requires care and experience.

Contrast may also be achieved with structures such as leukocytes and other cells by using special stains or by flowing a drop of acetic acid under the cover glass. Acetic acid may be used to stain the cell nucleus, as in the routine hematologic white cell count, but red cells are lysed by the addition of acetic acid. Also, certain crystals that are sometimes present in urine will be dissolved or converted to other forms by acetic acid.

The microscopic examination of urinary sediment may also be facilitated by the use of special stains, a green filter, phase-contrast microscopy, differential interference microscopy, dark-field microscopy, and polarized light microscopy.

Several stains have been used to help observe cellular detail and recognize structures in the urinary sediment. Methylene blue (Loeffler's) solution may be added to the sediment to aid in the recognition of cellular structures and bacteria. A crystal violet safranine stain as described by Sternheimer and Malbin is useful in the identification of cellular elements.[55] This is available commercially as Sedi-Stain (Clay Adams Division of Becton, Dickinson & Co., Parsippany, N.J.). Another stain that is commercially available and useful in the identification of cellular elements is Cyto-Diachrome (Regis Chemical Co., Morton Grove, Ill.). This is a supravital stain. The staining reactions of various components of the urinary sediment are supplied by the manufacturers. When such stains are used, it is recommended that both stained and unstained sediment be mounted and observed, as the stain may cause precipitation of some constituents. This is especially a problem with alkaline urine specimens. In these cases the precipitated background material may obscure important pathological constituents, while in other cases, such as when crystals are to be identified, a stain is not useful.

Filters can also aid the examination of the urinary sediment. A colored filter placed over the microscope light source can help bring out details in various structures in the unstained sediment. The filter used should be of a color complementary to the detail being studied. A green filter is especially useful for the observation of cells and casts.

Illumination techniques other than those of the bright-field microscope may be useful (see also under The Microscope in Chap. 1). Phase-contrast illumination is useful in the examination of unstained urinary sediment, particularly for delineating translucent elements such as hyalin casts and mucous threads, which have a refractive index similar to that of the urine in which they are suspended. Some laboratories use a phase-

contrast microscope for routine examination of the urinary sediment.

Differential interference illumination is also useful in the examination of unstained urinary sediment. Since it gives an apparently three-dimensional view of the object being observed, inclusions such as granules or vacuoles within a cell or cast can be more correctly visualized. Besides increasing color contrast, the geometric shape is observable.

Polarized light, with or without a first-order red filter, may be used to study substances that polarize (bend or rotate) light when viewed with polarizing filters. Such birefringent bodies include various crystals and fat globules. Polarizing filters show the typical Maltese cross appearance (light cross against a dark background) of anisotropic, doubly refractive fat globules, whether as free-floating fat in the urine, within oval fat bodies, or in fatty casts.

General comments—Constituents of the urinary sediment*

In general, the constituents of the urinary sediment are of a biological or chemical nature. The biological part (also called the organized sediment) includes the red blood cells, white blood cells, epithelial cells, fat of biological origin, casts, bacteria, yeast, fungi, parasites, and spermatozoa. (Casts are long cylindrical structures that result from the solidification of material within the lumen of the kidney tubules.) The biological portion is the more important part of the sediment, the cells and casts being of primary importance (unfortunately, they are also the most difficult to detect).

The chemical portion (also called the unorganized sediment) consists of crystals of chemi-

*Photomicrographs used in this section are printed by the courtesy of Dr. Ellis S. Benson and Dr. G. Mary Bradley, Department of Laboratory Medicine and Pathology, University of Minnesota, and Dr. Patrick Ward, Mt. Sinai Hospital, Minneapolis, Minnesota, with permission from the University of Minnesota Medical School.

cals and amorphous chemical material. In general, it is less important than the biological portion. However, some abnormal crystals do have pathological significance. In addition, the crystalline or chemical portion is sometimes so large that it tends to obscure the more important parts, which must be searched for with great care.

Constituents of the urinary sediment that may be encountered on microscopic examination will now be described. Unless otherwise specified, the staining reactions that are described are those of Sternheimer-Malbin crystal violet safranine stain (Sedi-Stain).

Cellular constituents

Red blood cells

Red blood cells are abnormal urinary constituents, and the presence of more than one or possibly two per high-power field is always of pathological significance. The condition in which red cells are found in the urine is termed hematuria. Often, the clinician will want to distinguish between hematuria and hemoglobinuria (free hemoglobin in the urine). This may be done by observing red cells under the microscope. However, red cells lyse so easily in urine that the specimen must be absolutely fresh when this distinction is attempted. In addition, lysis may occur within the urinary tract, yet not be intravascular.

The degree of hematuria may vary from a frankly bloody specimen on gross examination to a specimen that shows no change in color. Blood may be seen as merely a tiny red button in the bottom of the centrifuge tube after spinning. The amount of blood detected in the chemical reagent strip test for hemoglobin should be quantitated in the microscopic analysis of the sediment. Hematuria may be the result of bleeding at any point along the urogenital tract and may be seen with almost any disease of the urinary tract. It is a sensitive early indicator of renal disease,

and is usually accompanied by the presence of hemoglobin. To determine the cause of hematuria, the clinician will try to determine the site of bleeding. This involves various types of information, both laboratory and clinical. Part of this information will depend on other findings in the microscopic examination and other portions of the routine urinalysis. For example, bleeding through the glomerulus will often be accompanied by red cell casts, as seen in acute glomerulonephritis or disease of the glomerulus. This is an extremely serious situation, and red cell casts must be looked for carefully when red cells occur. There may be little correlation between the amount of blood and the severity of the disorder, yet the hematuria may be the only indication of renal disease. The occurrence of hematuria without accompanying protein and casts usually indicates that the bleeding is in the lower urogenital tract.

Red cells are not easy to find under the microscope. Their detection requires careful examination. The high-power objective is used, and the light must be reduced by proper adjustment of the condenser and iris diaphragm or they will be missed. Their detection also requires continual refocusing with the fine adjustment of the microscope.

In absolutely fresh urine, red cells will be unaltered or intact and appear much as they do in diluted whole blood. They have a characteristic bluish green sheen, are intact biconcave disks that are especially apparent as they roll over, have a generally smooth appearance as opposed to the granular appearance of white cells, and are about 7 μm in diameter (Fig. 5-5). However, they rapidly undergo morphological changes in urine specimens and are rarely observed as described. This is because urine is rarely an isotonic solution with red cells (the solute concentration within the red cell is rarely the same as the solute concentration of urine). The urine may be more or less concentrated than the blood, and the changes described below result.

When the urine is hypotonic or dilute, as evidenced by low specific gravity, the red cells

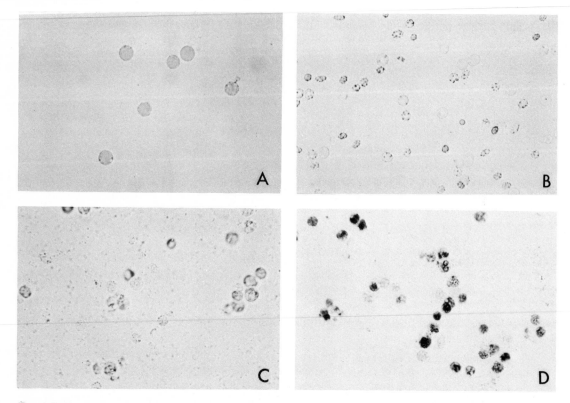

Fig. 5-5. Red cells and leukocytes in the urinary sediment. A. Intact red cells, unstained. B. Variety of red cell types: intact, crenate, and of various sizes, unstained. C. Leukocytes and many bacteria, unstained. D. Leukocytes and bacteria, stained. Photomicrographs taken using the high-dry objective.

appear *swollen* and *rounded* because of diffusion of fluid into them. If the urine is hypertonic or concentrated (high specific gravity), the red cells appear *crenate* and *shrunken* (Fig. 5-5) because they lose fluid to the urine. When crenate, the red cells have little spicules, or projections, that cause them to be confused with white cells. However, a crenate red cell is significantly smaller than a white cell and has a generally smooth, rather than granular, appearance. Finally, when the urine is dilute and alkaline, the red cells will often appear as *shadow* or *ghost cells* (Fig. 5-5). In this situation the red cells have burst and released their hemoglobin; all that remains is the faint colorless cell membrane, a ghost or shadow of the original cell. This form is

often seen in old urine specimens. Eventually, even the ghosts will disappear as the cell completely disintegrates.

Red cells are not only difficult to detect in a urine specimen, they are often confused with other structures that are found in the urinary sediment. For instance, red cells are often confused with leukocytes; however, the leukocyte is larger and has a generally granular appearance plus a nucleus (Fig. 5-5). If morphological differentiation is impossible, a drop of 2% acetic acid may be added to a new preparation or introduced under the cover glass. Acetic acid will lyse the red cells and at the same time stain (or accentuate) the nuclei of leukocytes. With a Sternheimer-Malbin stain, red cells in acidic urine may stain slightly purple or not at all. If the urine is alkaline, the alkaline hematin that is formed stains dark purple.

Yeast may also be confused with red cells in urine. However, yeast cells are generally smaller than red cells, are spherical rather than flattened, and vary considerably in size within one specimen (Fig. 5-6). In addition, since yeast reproduces by budding, the occurrence of buds or little outgrowths should identify yeast.

Fig. 5-6. Other cell forms in the urinary sediment. A. Intact red cells and one squamous epithelial cell, stained. B. Bladder epithelium with leukocytes, stained. C. Oval fat body, unstained. D. Oval fat body (or possibly a small piece of fatty cast), unstained. E. Yeast, unstained. F. Bacteria and four leukocytes, unstained. Photomicrographs taken using the high-dry objective.

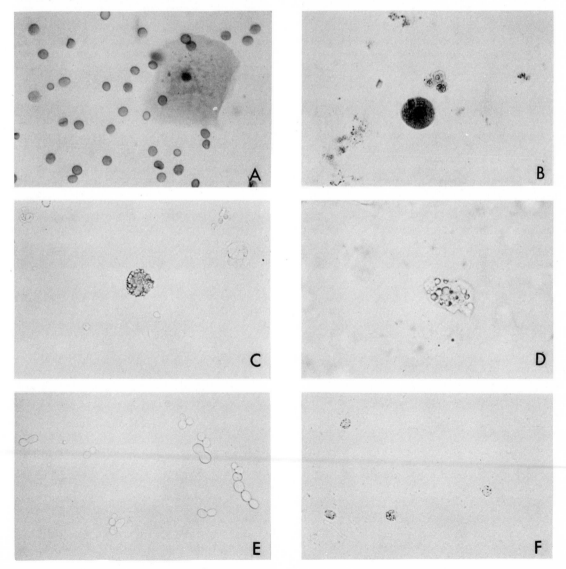

Bubbles or *oil droplets* are also confused with red cells, especially by the inexperienced. These vary considerably in size, are extremely refractive or reflective, and are obvious under the microscope.

The identification of red cells in urinary sediment may be aided by the use of a chemical test for hemoglobin. Red blood cells in the sediment should be correlated with a positive reagent strip test for blood and hemoglobin. However, since chemical tests are more sensitive to hemoglobin than to intact red cells, it is possible to have a negative reagent strip test when only a few intact red cells are present and no hemolysis has occurred. Such a situation is quite rare, although it is possible. The tests are sensitive to 5-10 red cells per microliter, but the sensitivity of the reagent strips is reduced in urine with high specific gravity. Falsely negative or delayed reagent strip tests for hemoglobin are possible when large amounts of vitamin C are present. In this case, the sediment result can be confirmed by the use of a reagent strip test for ascorbic acid, such as C-Stix. Another clue would be the gross appearance of the urinary sediment, or a red button of cells in the bottom of the centrifuge tube.

Falsely positive reagent strip tests for blood are also possible. Unless hemoglobin or myoglobin is present without red cells (both are rare situations), the chemical test should be confirmed by the presence of red cells in the sediment. Falsely positive chemical tests (positive reagent strip with no hemoglobin, myoglobin, or red cells in the sediment) can be produced by residues of strongly oxidizing cleaning agents such as bleach in the urine container, or by peroxidase in microorganisms associated with urinary tract infections.

Red cells that are present in the urinary sediment should be reported by grading them as occasional, 1+, 2+, 3+, or 4+. The criteria for grading will be given under Laboratory Procedure: Microscopic Examination of the Urinary Sediment.

Leukocytes

The presence of a few leukocytes in urine is normal. More than an occasional cell (1-5 per high-power field) is considered abnormal. The presence of large numbers of leukocytes in the sediment indicates inflammation at some point along the urogenital tract. The inflammation may result from a bacterial infection or other causes. The presence of leukocytes is thus often associated with bacteria, but bacteria or white cells can be present without each other. In bacterial infections, ingested bacteria are often seen within the cell. If the leukocytes originate in the kidney, rather than lower in the urinary tract (such as in the bladder), they may form cellular casts. Therefore, the presence of casts (usually cellular or granular) along with leukocytes and bacteria would help distinguish an upper (kidney) from a lower (bladder) urinary tract infection. Protein is usually present along with casts, and may or may not be present in a lower urinary tract infection.

The condition in which increased numbers of leukocytes are found in urine is termed *pyuria*. Pyuria may cause clouding of the urine, and when this is severe enough the urine will have a characteristic milky white appearance. Under the microscope the white cells may appear singly or in clumps. They may be mononuclear or polynuclear, although they are most commonly polymorphonuclear leukocytes.

Leukocytes must be searched for with the high-power objective, reduced light, and continual refocusing with fine adjustment. Typically, they are about 10-12 μm in diameter (about twice the size of red cells); however, this size difference may not be obvious. Leukocytes have thin cytoplasmic granulation and a nucleus. Even if the nucleus is not distinct, the center of the cell appears granular (Fig. 5-5). White cells are not nearly as fragile as red cells, but they will disintegrate in old alkaline urine specimens. Various stages of disintegration may be observed in a single urine specimen. Neutrophil leukocytes are especially vulnerable in dilute alkaline urine specimens, and about 50 percent can be lost within 2–3 hours if the urine is kept at room temperature.[56]

Identification of white cells is also aided by the use of a Sternheimer-Malbin stain, but precipitation of the stain in the highly alkaline urines associated with leukocytes and bacteria may pose a problem. When stained, neutrophilic leukocytes show a red-purple nucleus and violet or blue cytoplasm, although the same urine specimen may have a variety of staining reactions. *Glitter cells* may also be present. These are larger, swollen neutrophilic leukocytes that appear in hypotonic urine; their cytoplasmic granules are in constant random motion (Brownian motion). When stained, glitter cells have a light blue or almost colorless cytoplasm and the Brownian motion of the granules may or may not be observed. Although glitter cells may be found in chronic pyelonephritis, they are also seen in dilute urine specimens from patients with lower urinary tract infections.[57] In the latter case their significance is uncertain.

Other structures may be mistaken for leukocytes. Most often this occurs with red cells and epithelial cells. White cells are generally larger than red cells, appear granular, and have a nucleus. A 2% acetic acid solution may be used to aid in their identification. There are several very different morphological types of epithelial cells, but in general they are larger than white cells and have smaller nuclei. The nuclei are generally more distinct and are surrounded by more cytoplasm (Fig. 5-6).

White cells should be reported by grading the number present as occasional, 1+, 2+, 3+, or 4+. Criteria for grading will be given under Laboratory Procedure: Microscopic Examination of the Urinary Sediment.

Epithelial cells

The structures that make up the urinary system consist of several layers of epithelial cells, except for the single-layered tubules of the nephron.

The epithelial cells of organs such as the urethra and bladder (besides contaminating cells of the male and female genital tracts) are continually sloughed off into the urine and replaced by cells originating from deeper layers. Therefore, urine always contains some epithelial cells.

The outer layer of cells, which are normally replaced, consists of *squamous epithelial* cells. These are very large flat cells made up of a thin layer of cytoplasm and a single distinct nucleus (Fig. 5-6). They are large enough to be seen easily under low power and sometimes roll into cigar shapes, which are mistaken for casts. When stained, these cells show a purple nucleus and abundant pink or violet cytoplasm. This type of epithelial cell is of little significance and should be reported only if present in large numbers. Squamous epithelial cells are seen especially in urine specimens from female patients as a result of contamination from the vagina or vulva. Such contamination is minimized in a clean-voided midstream collection of urine.

As the epithelial cell layers become deeper, the cells become thicker and rounder looking, more and more like leukocytes. *Bladder epithelial* cells are such forms. Their size varies with the depth of origin in the transitional epithelium, which lines the bladder. They are generally larger than renal tubular cells and have a round nucleus (sometimes two nuclei) as opposed to the lobular nucleus of the leukocytes. The more superficial bladder epithelial cells are large flat cells of a squamous nature. The cells become smaller and rounder as the layers become deeper. Bladder epithelial cells stain with a dark blue nucleus and varying amounts of pale blue cytoplasm, which may have occasional inclusions. Some of these cells have tails and are indistinguishable from the *caudate* cells of the renal pelvis (Fig. 5-6).

Renal epithelial cells line the nephron tubules. Their occurrence in urine is most important, for it implies serious pathology and destruction of renal tubules, as does the presence of epithelial casts. They cannot be identified on the basis of microscopic evidence alone, since they resemble both white blood cells and cells from deeper layers lining the urinary system. Morphologically, renal epithelial cells closely resemble leukocytes, especially degenerating ones, but they are typically larger and have a single distinct nucleus (Fig. 5-6). When stained, renal epithelial cells have a dark purple nucleus and a small rim of orange-purple cytoplasm. Renal cells are often found in association with casts. The presence of epithelial or granular casts will help confirm their identification, and when renal cells are suspected, casts should be searched for with great care. The phase-contrast microscope is particularly useful in such situations.

Oval fat bodies

These are cells that are filled with fat droplets. They indicate a serious pathological condition and must not be overlooked when present in the urinary sediment. The fat droplets are generally contained within degenerating or necrotic renal epithelial cells, although some oval fat bodies may be macrophages that have filled with fat. The fat droplets contained within these cells are highly refractive, coarse droplets that vary greatly in size (Fig. 5-6). Although they are considered cells filled with fat, the cell nucleus is generally not visible. Certain aids to the identification of oval fat bodies are available. When stained with Sternheimer-Malbin stain, fat globules do not become colored but appear highly refractive in a blue-purple background. With Sudan III stain, fat globules appear orange or red. Polarized light is useful for indicating the presence of cholesterol esters in the fat. Cholesterol esters are anisotropic or doubly refractive and show a typical Maltese cross pattern when viewed with polarizing filters (Fig. 5-6). However, triglycerides, or neutral fat, do not show this pattern with polarized light. The appearance of a Maltese cross pattern alone cannot be used to determine whether fat is present in urine, as many crystals, and urine contaminated with starch, give the same pattern. Fat should be conformed by care-

ful microscopic examination or specific staining.

Oval fat bodies are often seen along with fat droplets and fatty casts in the urinary sediment, and the other two components should be searched for carefully when one is present. Oval fat bodies resulting from tubular epithelial degeneration of the nephron are associated with large amounts of protein in the urine, as in the nephrotic syndrome. The fatty material in the tubular cells may be the lipoprotein that passes through the damaged glomerulus in this syndrome. The lipoprotein may be ingested by the renal tubular cell, which metabolizes it into cholesterol.[58]

Fat globules

Fat globules may be found in the urinary sediment as highly refractive droplets of various sizes (Fig. 5-6). When their source is biological (rather than contamination), a serious pathological condition implying severe renal dysfunction exists. Such *lipuria* is also associated with the nephrotic syndrome and its various causes, diabetes mellitus, and conditions that result in severe damage of renal tubular epithelial cells such as ethylene glycol or mercury poisoning.[59] Fat globules are found in association with oval fat bodies and fatty casts. Fat stains orange or red with Sudan III stains. The identification may be aided by the use of polarized light, as cholesterol will show a Maltese cross pattern when so viewed. Fat in urine may also come from extraneous sources such as unclean collection utensils or oiled catheters. This is less common with the use of disposable urine collection containers.

Other cellular constituents

Bacteria

Under normal conditions the urinary tract is free of bacteria. However, most urine specimens contain at least a few bacteria because of contamination when the urine is voided. Bacteria multiply rapidly when urine stands at room temperature. In specimens that are obtained in a manner suitable for urine culture and kept under sterile conditions, the presence of bacteria may indicate a urinary tract infection. In this case, they are likely to be associated with the presence of white blood cells, although this is not always true. Bacterial infection should be confirmed by quantitative urine culture.

Bacteria are easily recognized morphologically. They are extremely small, only a few micrometers long. They may be either rods or cocci and may occur singly or in chains (Fig. 5-5). They are often motile, which helps in their identification. Bacteria are most often seen in alkaline urine and may be confused with amorphous material at first, but this will not be a problem as experience in observation is gained. In lower urinary tract (bladder) infections, bacteria are generally, but not always, associated with the presence of neutrophilic leukocytes. Mild proteinuria and a positive reagent strip test for nitrites may also be seen. With upper urinary tract (kidney) infections, bacteria may be seen along with leukocytes and leukocyte or granular casts. Mild proteinuria is also typical in such cases and a positive nitrite reagent strip reaction may be seen.

Yeast

Yeast cells are occasionally seen in urine, especially from females and diabetic patients. They are often present as the result of contamination of the urine from a vaginal yeast infection. They are associated with the presence of sugar in the urine. Sugar is the energy source for yeast cells, which grow and multiply rapidly when it is present. For this reason yeast cells are often discovered in the urine of diabetics, along with a high sugar content, low pH, and ketones. However, yeast cells are also common contaminants from skin and air.

Yeast cells are often mistaken for red blood cells. They are generally smaller than red cells and show considerable size variation, even within a specimen. They have a typically ovoid shape, lack color, and have a smooth and refractive appearance. The most distinguishing characteristic is the presence of little buds, or projections, because of their manner of reproduction (Fig. 5-6). Pseudomycelial forms of *Candida* sp. (the type of yeast usually present) may also be seen as hyphae (filaments). These should not be mistaken for casts.

Trichomonas vaginalis

Trichomonas vaginalis is the parasite most frequently seen in urine specimens. It may be present as the result of vaginal contamination. The organism is motile, which is an aid to its identification. When a urethral or bladder infection is suspected, the organism must be searched for immediately after the urine is voided. *Trichomonas* is a unicellular organism—a protozoan. It has a characteristic appearance with anterior flagella and an undulating membrane, the motility of which is helpful in identification as it appears to swim through the urinary sediment. The organisms are larger than typical leukocytes and may resemble flattened epithelial cells.

Other parasites

Various other parasites may be seen in urine as the result of fecal or vaginal contamination and may be common to particular geographic areas. Examples are *Schistosoma haematobium* and amebas such as *Entamoeba histolytica*.

Spermatozoa

Spermatozoa may also be present as urinary contaminants. They are easily recognized, having oval bodies with long delicate tails, and they may be motile or stationary.

Tumor cells

Tumor cells and other cell forms with altered cytological features may be found in the urinary sediment. However, these cell forms cannot be diagnosed from the usual urinary sediment preparation but require special collection and stains and examination by qualified personnel. If their presence is suspected from the examination of the sediment, the specimen should be referred to such qualified individuals.

Casts

Formation and significance

Casts are at once the most difficult portion of the urinary sediment to discover and the most important. Their importance and their name derive from the manner in which they are produced. Casts are formed in the lumen of the tubules of the nephrons (the working units of the kidney) by solidification of material in the tubules. They are important because anything that is contained within the tubule is flushed out in the cast. Thus a cast represents a biopsy of an individual tubule and is a means of examining the contents of the nephron. It is believed that casts may be formed at any point along the nephron, either by precipitation of protein or by grouping together (conglutination) of material within the tubular lumen.

Before casts can form within the renal tubules, certain conditions must exist. Since the cast is made of protein, there must be a sufficient concentration of protein within the tubule. In addition, the pH must be low enough to favor precipitation and there must be a sufficient concentration of solutes.[60] Since these conditions most likely exist in the distal tubules, it is felt that cast formation is more likely in the distal than in the proximal convoluted tubules. For the same reasons, casts are not likely to be found in dilute alkaline urine, since these conditions do not favor their formation. This also means that the urine must be examined when fresh, for as it becomes alkaline with aging the casts will disintegrate.

Since casts represent a biopsy of the kidney,

they are extremely important clinically. They often contain red blood cells, leukocytes, epithelial cells, fat globules, and bacteria (Fig. 5-7). These inclusions are not normally present within the renal tubule; they represent an abnormal situation. The formation of casts implies that there was at least a temporary blocking of the renal tubules. Although a few hyalin casts (made of precipitated protein only) are normal, increased numbers of casts indicate renal disease rather than lower urinary tract disease. The number of hyalin casts may increase in mild irritations of the kidney associated with fever. The presence of other types of casts represents a serious situation.

Casts are extremely difficult to see and must be searched for carefully with reduced light and the low-power objective ($\times 100$ total magnification). They are found and graded under low power, but must be identified as to type by means of the high-power objective. The refractive index of the cast is nearly the same as that of glass, which means that the image is very difficult to see under the microscope. It is for this reason that phase-contrast and differential interference microscopy are so useful in the examination of the urinary sediment. Phase-contrast microscopy gives sufficient contrast that structures are not overlooked, while differential interference microscopy gives an appreciation of the shape and inclusions within these structures. Stains such as the Sternheimer-Malbin stain are also particularly useful for the discovery of casts in the urinary sediment. Casts that might otherwise be overlooked in bright-field examination, especially by the inexperienced observer, become obvious when so stained, although the presence of mucus strands in the sediment might be confusing, especially when searching for hyalin casts.

As might be imagined from the shape of the tubular lumen, casts are cylindrical bodies and have rounded ends. To be identified as a cast, a structure should have an even and definite outline, parallel sides, and two rounded ends. Al-

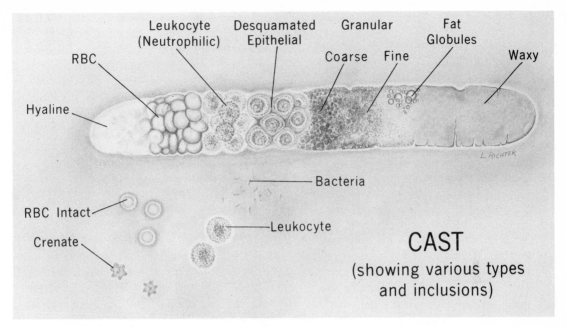

Fig. 5-7. Archetypal cast (showing various types and inclusions).

though they vary somewhat in size, casts should have a uniform diameter (about seven or eight times a red cell diameter) and be several times longer than wide (see Fig. 5-7). Structures that resemble hyalin casts and are seen in the urinary sediment are *cylindroids*. They are similar to casts in every respect except that they have one end that tapers to a point or tail. The mechanism of formation and site of origin of cylindroids are not known, but they seem to occur in conjunction with hyalin casts and are considered to have the same significance clinically. Cylindroids are often confused with strands of mucus, and care must be taken to avoid this mistake.

Classification of casts is not always simple. In the laboratory it is done mainly on the basis of morphological groupings: hyalin, finely granular, coarsely granular, waxy, cellular, or fatty. However, a urine specimen may contain more than one morphological type, and a particular cast may be of mixed morphology—for instance, one end may be hyalin and the other cellular. This is shown in the extreme in Fig. 5-7. A classification

on the basis of composition and origin has been described by Lippman.[61] This system recognizes only three main types of casts: hyalin, epithelial, and blood. The system is especially useful for understanding cast formation, but it is not completely practical for use in the laboratory, where only morphological classification is possible.

Casts are felt to arise either by precipitation of protein within the renal tubule or by conglutination of material within the tubular lumen. Both types of casts may contain inclusions. Casts formed by protein precipitation may trap any other substance, such as leukocytes, fat, bacteria, red cells, or desquamated renal tubular epithelium, that may be present. Casts formed by either mechanism may appear coarsely or finely granular or waxy, as cells disintegrate when the cast is retained in the tubule before being flushed out of the kidney. Structures will also disintegrate if the urine specimen stands.

In any case, casts have a protein matrix, and the presence of casts in the urine is virtually always accompanied by proteinuria. Tamm-

Horsfall protein is a specific mucoprotein that has been identified immunologically and found to be present in all casts.[62] Other immunoproteins such as immunoglobulins G and M have been identified in certain casts, although they are not found exclusively in any particular type of cast or disease state.[63]

The following morphological classification is based on appearance, physical properties, and existence of cellular components. The appearance of a cast when it is seen in the urine may not be the same as when it was originally formed in the renal tubule. If the cast is retained in the kidney (as happens in oliguric patients), cells present in it change in appearance. As the cells degenerate in the cast, their cytoplasm becomes granular. This is followed by loss of cell membranes, resulting in large or coarse granules. As these granules further degenerate, the cast shows smaller or fine granules. The final step in this degeneration is complete lack of structure, with the protein changed or coagulated into a thick, very refractive, opaque substance with a waxlike appearance. It is therefore thought that waxy casts originated from cellular casts. These are the most serious casts pathologically, as the formation of the waxy material implies a greatly lengthened transit time, or shutdown of the portion of the kidney where the structure evolved.

The width or diameter of a cast is important clinically. Since casts are generally formed within the distal convoluted tubules of the nephron, which have a fairly constant diameter, there is normally little variation in cast diameter, although casts from small children are narrower than those from adults. *Narrow* casts probably result from swelling of the tubular epithelium, as in an inflammatory process, with narrowing of the tubular lumen. They are not particularly important and tend to be of a hyalin type. *Broad* casts are much more serious. Their diameter is several times greater than normal. This is felt to result from their formation in dilated renal tubules or in collecting tubules (several nephrons

empty into a common collecting tubule, which has a greater diameter than the renal tubule). Severe chronic renal disease or obstruction (stasis) will often result in dilation and destruction of renal tubules. Cast formation in the collecting tubules must result from urinary stasis in the group of nephrons feeding a single collecting tubule. If not, the fluid pressure would be far too great for cast formation to occur. This represents serious stasis, and the presence of a significant number of broad casts in the urine sediment is considered to be a bad sign. Broad casts can be of almost any type, but because of the degree of stasis necessary for their formation, most tend to be waxy.

The types of casts that are encountered in the microscopic analysis of the urinary sediment will now be described in a morphological classification. Staining reactions that are described pertain to the Sternheimer-Malbin crystal violet safranine stain (Sedi-Stain).

Hyalin casts

Hyalin casts are colorless, homogeneous, nonrefractive, semitransparent structures (Fig. 5-8). They are the most difficult casts to discover under the microscope. They require careful adjustment of light with the bright-field microscope; the light must be sufficiently reduced to give contrast by properly positioning (lowering) the condenser and closing the iris diaphragm. Phase-contrast and interference microscopy are especially valuable tools in the search for hyalin casts. Stain is also useful; hyalin casts stain a uniform pale pink or pale blue. Hyalin casts may be difficult to distinguish from mucus threads when they are present in the urine, both when stained and when observed by phase-contrast microscopy.

Hyalin casts result from precipitation of Tamm-Horsfall protein within the lumen of kidney tubules. Since the casts are believed to result from gel formation, they include any material that may be present, such as cells or cellular debris.

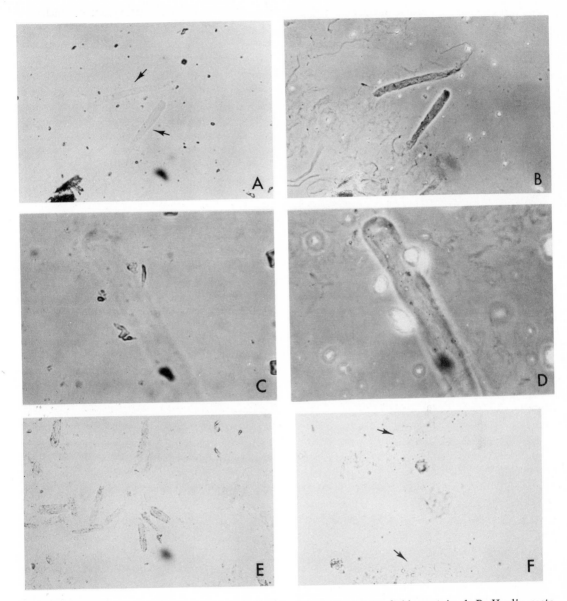

Fig. 5-8. Casts in the urinary sediment. A. Two hyalin casts; bright field, unstained. B. Hyalin casts, same field as (A); phase contrast. C. Hyalin cast; bright field, unstained. D. Hyalin cast, same as (C); phase contrast. E. Mixture of hyalin finely granular casts; bright field, unstained. F. Two hyalin fatty casts, with oval fat bodies also present; bright field, unstained. Low-power objective: A, B, E; high-dry objective: C, D, F.

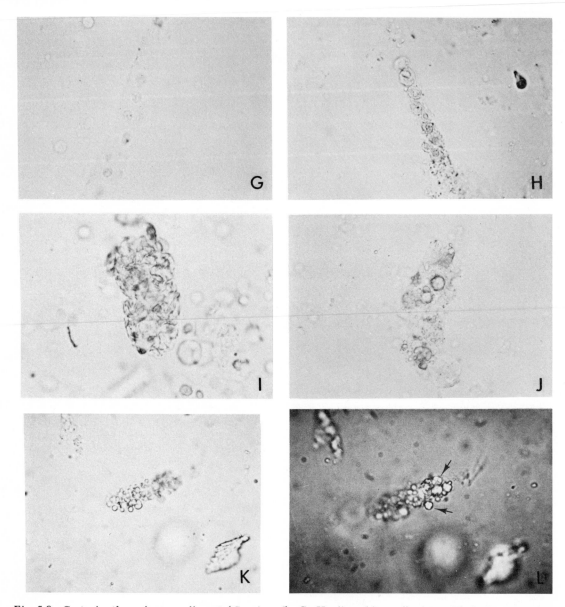

Fig. 5-8. Casts in the urinary sediment (*Continued*). G. Hyalin white cell cast, with leukocytes also present; bright field, unstained. H. Cellular cast, probably desquamated epithelial cells; bright field, unstained. I. Red blood cell cast; bright field, unstained. J. Fatty cast; bright field, unstained. K. Fatty cast; bright field, unstained. L. Fatty cast, same field as (K) with polarized light showing Maltese cross. High-dry objective: G, H, J, K, L; oil-immersion objective: I.

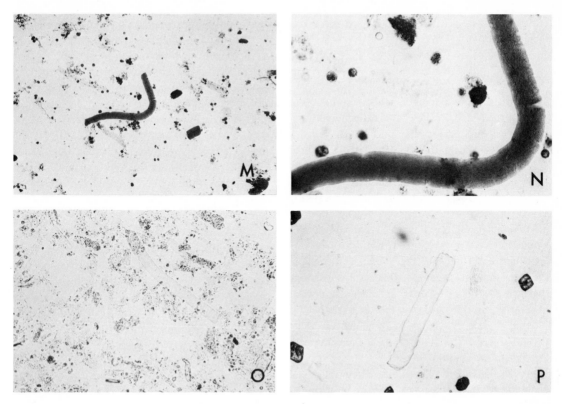

Fig. 5-8. Casts in the urinary sediment (*Continued*). M. Stained sediment showing mixture of casts, waxy and granular; bright field, N. Enlarged view of the cast in (M), a broad cast in transition from granular to waxy. Red cells, leukocytes, and hyalin finely granular casts are also present. O. Mixture of casts as seen in telescoped sediment; waxy, granular, possibly red cell casts, from the same patient as (M) and (N). Bright field, unstained. P. Broad waxy cast; note broken ends. Uric acid crystals are also present. Bright field, unstained. Low-power objective: M, O, P; high-dry objective: N.

Although they are generally of the classical shape for identification as a cast (i.e., parallel sides, uniform diameter, definite borders, and rounded ends), very interesting modifications, representing molds of the tubular lumen where they are formed, may be observed. Some hyalin casts are broad, while others are thin and elongated; serpentine and folded forms are not unusual. Cylindroids are most likely hyalin casts with one end that has not rounded off.

Hyalin casts are soluble in water and even more soluble in slightly alkaline solution. They are therefore more likely to be found in concentrated, acidic urine and may not form in advanced renal failure because of the inability to concentrate the urine or maintain the normal acid pH.[64] In addition, hyalin casts dissolve if the urine stands and becomes alkaline. Hyalin casts may be further classified according to their inclusions as hyalin cellular (name type of cell present), hyalin coarsely granular, hyalin finely granular, and hyalin fatty casts.

Simple hyalin casts are the least important clinically, and a few (less than one per low-power field) may be seen in urine from normal individuals. They may be seen in large numbers (20 or

30 per low-power field) in moderate or severe renal disease.[65]

Cellular casts

These casts contain intact leukocytes, red cells, or epithelial cells. They are called leukocyte (white cell or pus) casts, red blood cell (or blood) casts, and epithelial casts. A truly cellular cast appears to result from clumping, or conglutination, of cells rather than simply precipitation of protein, although they are still incorporated in a protein matrix. Alternatively, smaller numbers of the same cell types may be embedded in a hyalin cast.

Cellular casts indicate the presence of cells in the renal tubules. Whenever this occurs, although there are a variety of causes and different degrees of severity, a serious situation exists.

Cellular casts are more easily detected under the microscope than hyalin casts, since the cells give them a definite structure compared with homogeneous solidified protein. They must still be searched for with care, however, and proper illumination of the bright-field microscope is essential. Phase-contrast or interference microscopy and stains are useful tools in the examination of the urinary sediment for cellular casts. The various types of cellular casts are described in the following sections.

Leukocyte casts

These casts are also referred to as white cell casts, or pus casts when neutrophilic leukocytes are present. When leukocytes are present in a cast, it is obvious that the cells originated in the kidney. The leukocytes may enter the nephron from the blood by passing through the glomerulus into the glomerular capsule in glomerular diseases. More commonly, they probably enter the nephron from the blood by squeezing through the cells making up the renal tubules, often in response to a bacterial infection within the nephron. Such phagocytic neutrophils are typically seen in pyelonephritis, a renal infection. In such cases leukocytes and bacteria are also present in the urinary sediment. The presence of casts (particularly leukocyte casts) along with leukocytes and bacteria is used to distinguish an upper from a lower urinary tract infection.

Leukocyte casts are seen fairly easily in the urinary sediment with the bright-field microscope (Fig. 5-8). The cells are fairly prominent, and the characteristic multilobular nucleus can usually be seen. Small leukocytes stain purple to violet, while large ones may be pale blue, in a pink matrix. As the cells disintegrate within the cast, their cytoplasm becomes granular, cell borders merge, and nuclei become indistinct, resulting in a granular cast when the cells are no longer distinguishable. The number of cells in a cast varies—some casts are packed with cells while others show only a few cells in a hyalin matrix. Leukocyte casts packed with cells still have a protein matrix, and should have parallel sides and rounded ends. It is sometimes difficult to distinguish such a leukocyte cast from a clump of leukocytes (pseudoleukocyte cast), which may originate lower in the urinary tract. The distinction is of clinical significance. It may also be difficult, if not impossible, to distinguish a leukocyte cast from an epithelial cast, especially when cells begin to deteriorate. Here, the best indicator is probably the nature of other constituents in the urinary sediment. Leukocytes and bacteria in the sediment would be associated with leukocyte casts, while epithelial casts are more likely to be accompanied by cells appearing to be renal epithelium. Glitter cells are often seen when phagocytic neutrophils are present. When a morphological distinction is impossible, the cast should be reported merely as a cellular cast, rather than misidentifying it. The physician will use information about other constituents in the sediment, the results of other urinalysis and laboratory tests, and the patient's case history in arriving at a diagnosis.

Epithelial casts

Epithelial casts represent a most serious situation, although they are very infrequently seen in the urine, as renal tubular disease (nephrosis) is relatively rare. They may be seen in cases of exposure to nephrotoxic substances such as mercury or ethylene glycol (antifreeze), or in infections with viruses such as cytomegalovirus or hepatitis virus. They result from destruction or desquamation of the cells that line the renal tubules. These cells are responsible for the work done by the kidney. The damage may be irreversible, depending on the severity of the disease process. The time needed to replace renal epithelial cells, if the basement membrane is left intact, is unknown; however, cells do not show maximum concentrating ability for up to 6 months after severe loss of tubular epithelium.[66]

The epithelial cast often appears to consist of two rows of renal epithelial cells, implying tubular desquamation (Fig. 5-8). However, the cells may also vary in size, shape, and distribution, showing a varying amount of protein matrix. When the cells are haphazardly arranged in the cast in varying stages of degeneration, cellular damage and desquamation from different and separate portions of the renal tubule is implied.[67] The epithelial cast does not remain constant once formed, but undergoes a series of changes. These changes result from cellular disintegration as the cast remains within the kidney, as a result of decreased urine flow (statis). Therefore, a range of epithelial casts from cellular to coarsely granular, finely granular, and finally waxy may be seen. The waxy type represents the most serious situation, as prolonged blockage of renal flow is required for them to form. All of these types of casts are often seen in the same specimen; such specimens are referred to as "telescoped" urinary sediments (Fig. 5-8).

Epithelial casts may be difficult to distinguish from leukocyte casts, as previously discussed. When stained, the cells have a blue-purple nucleus and lighter blue-purple cytoplasm in a pink matrix. Phase-contrast and interference microscopy are also helpful in this examination.

Red blood cell casts

The observation of red blood cell casts in the urinary sediment is probably the most significant diagnostic finding and indicates a serious renal condition. Their presence must not be missed. The red cells enter the nephron by leakage through the glomerular capsule. It is possible that they bleed into the renal tubules at a point beyond the glomerular capsule; however, this would be a far less common path, as red cell casts are almost always associated with diseases that affect the glomerulus, such as acute glomerulonephritis and lupus nephritis. Once red cells are present in the lumen of the nephron, they clump together to form red cell casts. Red cell casts are probably the most fragile ones in the urinary sediment, which may be why they are rarely observed and why fragments are more often found. When physical conditions indicate that red cell casts may be present, it is imperative that the urine specimen be absolutely fresh and gently treated. The casts may be so fragile that they disintegrate under the microscope as the observer watches.

Red cell casts have a characteristic orange-yellow color caused by hemoglobin, which makes them unlike anything else seen in the urinary sediment (Fig. 5-8). Stain is not very useful in the identification of blood casts; however, they may have intact red cells, which stain colorless or lavender in a pink matrix. Phase-contrast and interference microscopy are both very useful in detecting red cell casts.

The number of cells present in the red cell cast is variable. Often only a few intact cells are seen in a hyalin matrix. Such casts are probably less fragile than those made up primarily of clumped red cells. If many cells are clumped together to form the cast, the matrix is often not visible. These casts are more fragile and, unfortunately, more serious from the patient's standpoint.

There is disagreement concerning the composition and origin of blood casts. They are often divided into two types: red blood cell casts and "true" blood casts. The red blood cell cast may be composed of a solid mass of conglutinated red cells with no matrix visible between the packed cells. The true blood cast shows a completely homogeneous matrix with no cell margins. Both types of casts have a characteristic orange-yellow color. Red blood cell casts may be formed by the clumping of red blood cells, which disintegrate, like the cells in epithelial casts, to form true blood casts. The true blood casts would then be analogous to waxy casts. In any case, the occurrence of red cells within a cast, regardless of the number of cells, represents a serious situation. When red blood cells are found in the urinary sediment, in conjunction with red cell casts of any sort, renal (usually glomerular) involvement is indicated.

Granular casts

The granules seen in granular casts are felt to be the result of the breakdown of cells within the cast or the renal tubule. Once all the cells have become granules, it is impossible to say for sure what sort of cell was originally present in the renal tubule. Such a distinction is useful, as red cell casts indicate glomerular injury, epithelial cell casts indicate renal tubular damage, and leukocyte casts indicate interstitial inflammation or infection. Often casts are seen that are basically granular but show some cells in transition to granules. When cells are present they should be identified if possible. Once again, phase-contrast and interference microscopy are helpful in this distinction. The end product of this disintegration is the waxy cast, a finding that represents serious pathology.

The size of the granules within the granular cast varies; they become progressively smaller as the cells disintegrate. The number of granules also varies, and casts range from those that are completely filled with granules to those that are basically hyalin and contain only a few granules.

Such granules may have been present in the renal tubule and trapped in a protein matrix as the cast was formed. Although granular casts are generally reported as coarsely or finely granular, such a distinction is not clinically significant; the term granular is sufficient. The distinction between coarsely and finely granular is subjective, but relatively easily made. If the cast has a definite hyalin matrix with only a few granules, it is usually reported as hyalin coarsely or hyalin finely granular. When large numbers of granules are present, it is described as coarsely or finely granular.

Coarsely granular casts

These casts appear to contain degenerated cells in the form of large granules. They tend to be darker, shorter, and more irregular in outline than finely granular casts (Fig. 5-8). The darker color and larger granules make them easier to find than either hyalin or finely granular casts. They stain with dark purple granules in a purple matrix. Fat may be present in these casts showing as refractive globules that do not stain.

Finely granular casts

These casts look much like hyalin casts; however, the presence of fine granules makes them more distinctive and easier to find. They are usually grayish or pale yellow in the unstained sediment and stain with fine dark purple granules in a pale pink or pale purple matrix (Fig. 5-8). Fat globules may also be found, appearing as highly refractive globules that do not stain.

Waxy casts

Waxy casts resemble hyalin casts and may be mistaken for them. They are much more significant clinically. The waxy cast is homogeneous, like the hyalin cast, but it is yellowish and more refractive with sharper outlines. It appears hard whereas the hyalin cast has a delicate appearance.

Waxy casts tend to be wider than hyalin casts (they are described as broad casts or broad waxy casts) and usually have irregular broken ends and fissures or cracks in their sides. Fairly long forms are also seen (Fig. 5-8). Phase-contrast and interference microscopy and staining are useful in the examination of waxy casts. They stain pale pink or light to darker purple with Sternheimer-Malbin stain.

Waxy casts are felt to be the final step in the disintegration of cellular casts and are especially serious since they imply renal stasis. They are associated with severe chronic renal disease and renal amyloidosis, and are seen only rarely and in small numbers in acute renal diseases.[68]

Fatty casts

The importance and probable mechanism of formation of fatty casts have been discussed along with oval fat bodies and fat globules. These three structures are often seen together in the same urine specimen, along with extremely large amounts of protein (3+ or 4+) and the pale foamy appearance of the specimen associated with the nephrotic syndrome. They are serious because they represent fatty degeneration and desquamation of the renal tubular epithelium. They are also seen in diabetes mellitus with renal degeneration and in toxic renal poisoning as from ethylene glycol or mercury.

Fatty casts, as the name implies, contain droplets of fat. These droplets are highly refractive under the microscope (Fig. 5-8). They stain bright orange with Sudan III stain and show a Maltese cross under polarized light if cholesterol esters are present (Fig. 5-8). When stained with Sternheimer-Malbin stain, fatty casts show a pink matrix with unstained refractive fat globules. Fatty casts may be seen as a protein matrix almost completely filled with fat globules, or as fat globules contained within a hyalin, cellular, or granular cast.

Structures confused with casts

Mucus threads may be confused with casts. Their refractive index is similar to that of hyalin casts; however, they are long ribbonlike strands with undefined edges and pointed or split ends. They also appear to have longitudinal striations.

Rolled squamous epithelial cells may also be mistaken for casts when they have rolled into a cigar shape. However, they have pointed ends rather than rounded ones and are shorter, and a single round nucleus may be discovered with careful focusing.

Bits of *hair* or *threads* of material fibers are also mistaken for casts by the beginner. However, these are extremely refractive structures that have nothing in common with the appearance of protein microscopically. Likewise, *scratches* on the glass slide or cover glass may be mistaken for casts at first. Again, they are much too definite and obvious to be important. Finally, *hyphae of molds* are sometimes mistaken for hyalin casts. This is similar to mistaking yeast for red cells. Hyphae are much more refractive and are jointed and branching, which can be observed on closer examination.

Crystals and amorphous material

Significance

Crystals and amorphous precipitates of certain chemicals make up what has been called the unorganized urinary sediment. These materials are obvious under the microscope. Because they are so striking, there is a natural tendency to pay considerable attention to them, but they are the most insignificant part of the urinary sediment and deserve little attention. In the past, great emphasis was placed on the identification of these materials. However, it is generally preferable to search carefully for more pathological constituents and note only briefly the occurrence of crystals.

Most urine specimens contain some crystalline material when voided. As urine specimens stand, especially when refrigerated, most become cloudy because of the precipitation of amorphous material and crystals. The student should learn to identify normal crystals and amorphous materials, however, for the following reasons: First, if they are abundant they will obscure such important structures as red blood cells, white blood cells, and casts. The more important structures must be searched for with extreme care when crystals and amorphous materials are present. The use of a stain, such as the Sternheimer-Malbin stain or a supravital stain, may be especially useful in this case. Second, the precipitation of certain crystals will accompany kidney stone formation (lithiasis). This is one reason for the attention that was formerly given to urinary crystals. Finally, substances such as cystine, leucine, and tyrosine may crystallize in urine and indicate serious metabolic disorders. Administration of sulfonamide drugs may cause the formation of sulfonamide crystals, especially in acidic urine. The formation of sulfonamide crystals within the kidney may result in blockage of renal output and severe renal damage. This problem was greater when sulfonamide drugs were first introduced, and the identification of such crystals is now losing importance.

Normal crystals should be identified and reported merely as a few or many per low-power field ($\times 100$). Microscopic examination is sufficient; they do not require chemical tests. Abnormal crystals should be reported by grading the number according to the criteria given under Laboratory Procedure: Microscopic Examination of the Urinary Sediment. They cannot be reported on the basis of microscopic evidence alone, but require confirmatory chemical tests. The identification of normal urinary crystals and amorphous material is further simplified by the fact that they occur in either acidic or alkaline urine. Therefore the pH of the urine should always be known when the microscopic examination is made. It must be remembered that it is

the shape, rather than the size, that is characteristic of crystals.

Normal crystals of acidic urine

Amorphous urates

This is the amorphous material found in acidic urine. Chemically, amorphous urates are the sodium salts of uric acid. *Amorphous* means without shape or form. The urates show a characteristic yellowish red shapeless granulation (Fig. 5-9). When present in sufficient numbers, they form a characteristic fluffy pink precipitate often called brick dust. Amorphous urates tend to precipitate out of urine that is highly concentrated, as in cases of fever. Such urine specimens are typically highly colored (dark amber) and show large amounts of fluffy pink precipitate. Although of an alarming appearance to the patient, such specimens are of little concern clinically.

Uric acid

These crystals have a variety of shapes and colors. Typically they are yellow or reddish brown, much like the chemically related amorphous urates. The most typical shape is the whetstone. Other shapes include rhombic plates or prisms, somewhat oval forms with pointed ends ("lemon-shaped"), wedges, rosettes, and irregular plates (Fig. 5-9). They are usually recognized by color, but some, especially the rhombic plates, may appear colorless.

Uric acid crystals are commonly seen in urine specimens, especially after the specimen has been standing. Amorphous urates and uric acid may be associated with gout or stone formation, besides chronic renal disease and certain leukemias, especially after chemotherapy. However, their presence in urine is not diagnostic of these conditions. A hexagonal form of uric acid may be mistaken for cystine crystals, which are abnormal and important to detect.

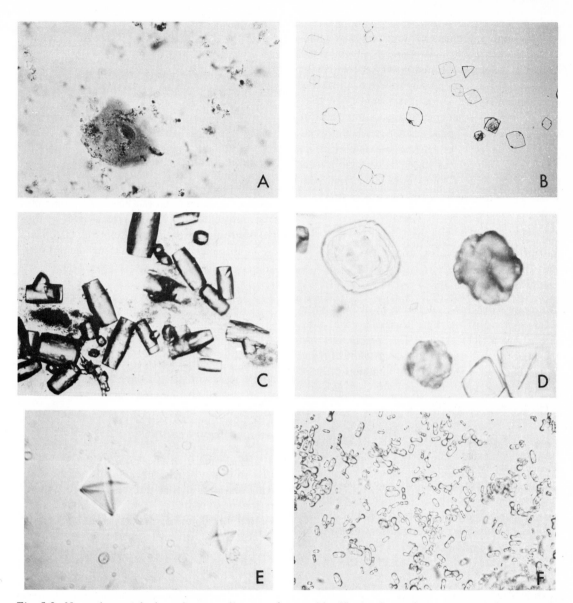

Fig. 5-9. Normal crystals in urinary sediment of an acid pH. A. Amorphous urates and squamous epithelial cell, stained. B. Typical lemon-shaped uric acid crystals, unstained. C. Barrel-shaped uric acid with amorphous urates in background. D. Laminated form of uric acid crystals. E. Typical envelope-shaped (tetrahedral) calcium oxalate crystals; red cells are also present. F. Rare form of dumbbell calcium oxalate. Low-power objective: B, C, F; high-dry objective: A, D, E.

Calcium oxalate

Calcium oxalate crystals have a characteristic "envelope" appearance. They vary somewhat in size but are typically small, colorless, glistening octahedralons (Fig. 5-9). Less frequently they may appear in a dumbbell shape. Although most common in acidic urine, calcium oxalate crystals may also be seen in neutral or alkaline urine specimens. They are of little clinical significance, although they may be present in association with stone formation, as calcium oxalate occurs in a large percentage of stones.

Normal crystals of alkaline urine

Amorphous phosphates

The amorphous material found in alkaline urine is amorphous phosphates. Generally, the phosphates give a finer or more lacy precipitate than the amorphous urates and are colorless (Fig. 5-10). Phosphates are the most common cause of turbidity in alkaline urine and are seen as a fine white precipitate microscopically.

Triple phosphates

Triple phosphates are colorless crystals and commonly show great variation in size, from tiny to relatively huge crystals. They have a characteristic "coffin-lid" shape that is impossible to miss. Less commonly, they occur in a fern-like form as they go into solution (Fig. 5-10).

Ammonium biurate

This ammonium salt is the alkaline counterpart of uric acid and amorphous urates in urine. The crystals are spherical with radial or concentric striations and long prismatic spicules, resembling thorn apples (Fig. 5-10). They are yellow and may be mistaken for some forms of the sulfonamide drugs that may precipitate out of urine.

Sulfa crystals are usually seen in acidic urine, however. Ammonium biurates are often present in old urine specimens, especially those that contain unusual sediment constituents and have been retained for teaching purposes. They are much less frequently seen in fresh urine collections.

Calcium phosphate

Calcium phosphate crystals are colorless. They may appear as flat plates (which are often mistaken for epithelial cells) or as slender wedges that occur singly or in rosettes (Fig. 5-10) and may be mistaken for certain sulfonamide crystals.

Calcium carbonate

Calcium carbonate crystals are tiny, colorless granules that typically occur in pairs ("dumbbells") but may occur also singly (Fig. 5-10). Because they are so small, calcium carbonate crystals represent part of the amorphous material seen in normal alkaline urine specimens.

Abnormal urinary crystals

Normal crystals of urine may be reported on the basis of microscopic examination alone. Abnormal crystals should not be reported without confirmatory chemical tests. The following description of abnormal crystals is superficial. If the occurrence of such crystals is suspected, a more detailed text must be consulted for microscopic appearance and confirmatory chemical procedures.

Cystine

Cystine crystals are colorless, refractive, hexagonal plates (Fig. 5-11). Although extremely rare, they may be seen in the urine of persons with a hereditary condition in which cystine seems to

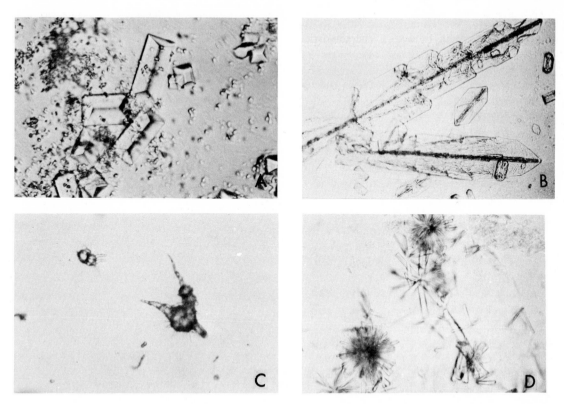

Fig. 5-10. Normal crystals in urinary sediment of an alkaline pH. A. Typical coffin-lid form of triple phosphate, with amorphous phosphates in background. B. Triple phosphate crystals going into solution; smaller, more typical forms are also present. C. Ammonium biurate. D. Calcium phosphate; most typical form. Low-power objective: B; high-dry objective: A, C, D.

replace uric acid in the urine. This is a serious situation that has kidney and liver involvement.

usually appear together and are associated with severe liver disease.

Tyrosine

Tyrosine crystals are fine needles arranged in sheaves and are usually black (Fig. 5-11).

Leucine

Leucine crystals are yellow, oily-looking spheres with radial and concentric striations. They are extremely rare. Leucine and tyrosine crystals

Cholesterol

Cholesterol crystals are said to be large, flat, hexagonal plates with one or more corners notched out. They are extremely rare—we have never seen such crystals in urine. Crystals of x-ray dye media (such as Renografin) are fairly commonly found associated with a very high specific gravity and a falsely positive delayed protein precipitation test; they should not be mistaken for cholesterol.

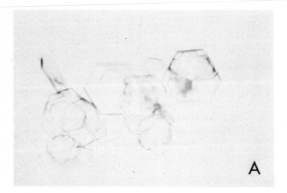
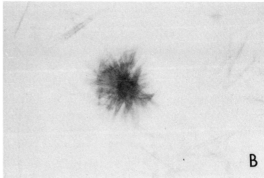
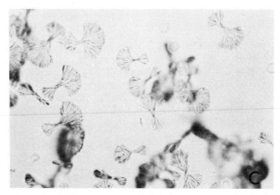

Fig. 5-11. Abnormal (pathological) crystals in urinary sediment. A. Cystine. B. Tyrosine. C. Sulfadiazine; red cells are also present. Photomicrographs taken using the high-dry objective.

Hippuric acid

Hippuric acid crystals are brownish needles or prisms. They are both extremely rare and of little clinical significance.

Sulfonamides

Sulfonamide crystals have various forms depending on the form of the drug. They are most insoluble at an acid pH. They include the following (Fig. 5-11):

1. Sulfanilamide is rarely seen. It occurs as large, colorless needles, frequently in sheaves or rosettes.
2. Sulfapyridine occurs as colorless arrowheads or whetstones, also as brown needles in large conglomerate masses or rosettes.
3. Sulfathiazole occurs as brownish shocks of wheat with central binding or rosettes with radial striations, also as colorless diamond and hexagonal plates, sometimes in rosettes.
4. Sulfadiazine is the most dangerous form of the drug in urine. It occurs as colorless to greenish brown shocks of wheat with eccentric binding and rosettes with radial striations, sometimes covered with needlelike processes.
5. Sulfaguanidine appears as colorless needles grouped as shocks of wheat with eccentric binding, also as rectangular plates with slight bulging in the long axis.
6. Sulfamethylthiazole occurs as colorless to

greenish brown needles clumped in the shape of a fan.

Sulfonamides are rarely found in urine, as more soluble forms of the drugs are available and the pH of the urine is kept alkaline to prevent precipitation. If present they represent a most serious situation, for their precipitation in the renal tubules will result in mechanical destruction of the tubules, which may lead to renal failure or shutdown. Sulfonamide crystals are therefore associated with blood in the urine as a result of bleeding in the renal tubules.

Ampicillin

Ampicillin crystals appear as long thin colorless needles in acid urine. They are seen only rarely as the result of large doses of the drug such as may be necessary for treatment of bacterial meningitis.

X-ray media

Crystals of compounds such as meglumine diatrizoate (Renografin) used for diagnostic x-ray procedures may be precipitated in the urine as flat, four-sided plates, or long thin rectangles (Fig. 5-12). They are not abnormal crystals in the sense of the others described in this section, since they are not metabolic products nor do they harm the patient. Rather, they may be regarded as a contaminant in the urine, and do not require chemical confirmation. However, these crystals should not be mistaken for cholesterol. When they are present the urine specimen is cloudy, has a high specific gravity (over 1.035), and may show a delayed falsely positive precipitation test for protein.

Contaminants and artifacts

Many objects and structures in the urinary sediment are contaminants or artifacts, and distract the attention of the observer from the important urinary constituents. These are the objects that students tend to see first when a microscopic examination of the urine is attempted. It seems to be a general rule that if an object is easy to see, it is unimportant.

Contaminating substances and artifacts that are often present in the urinary sediment include *cotton threads, hair, wool fibers,* and *wood fibers.* These are fairly common and easy to recognize. When wooden applicator sticks are used to mix the urinary sediment, wood fibers are common contaminants. These are *not* casts. *Scratches* on the cover glass are often mistaken for casts by the inexperienced observer. Their regular, highly refractive appearance is characteristic. *Bubbles* are also refractive and structureless and soon accepted as something to be overlooked. *Oil droplets* from lubricants or dirty collection containers may be confused with red blood cells. They are highly refractive and structureless, however (Fig. 5-12). Contaminating oil must be distinguished from fat globules that occur in lipuria, usually in conjunction with fatty casts and oval fat bodies. The use of polarizing filters is helpful in making this distinction. Granules of *starch* are also common contaminants. They may be introduced from surgical gloves. Starch granules, along with other common contaminants, also pose a problem in that they are doubly refractive, showing a Maltese cross pattern when examined with polarized light. In this case, observation with bright-field illumination clearly differentiates starch from fat globules containing esters of cholesterol (Fig. 5-12). Crystals of talc are also common urinary contaminants and should be recognized as such and then ignored.

Laboratory procedure: Microscopic examination of the urinary sediment

1. Pour exactly 10 ml of well-mixed urine into a graduated centrifuge tube, and centrifuge at 2000 r/min for 5 minutes.

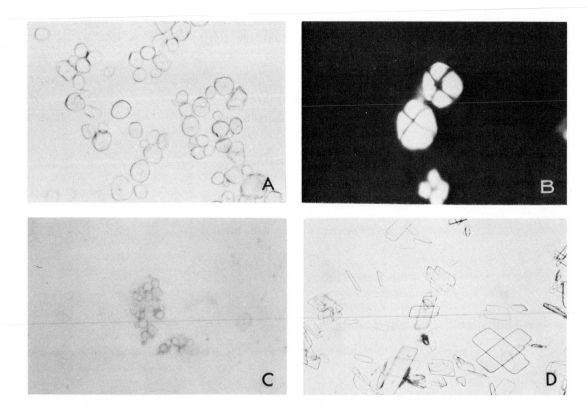

Fig. 5-12. Contaminants in the urinary sediment. A. Starch granules (compare with fat globules); bright field, unstained. B. Starch granules viewed with polarized light showing Maltese cross. C. Fat globules; bright field, unstained. D. X-ray dye medium (Renografin); bright field, unstained. Photomicrographs taken using the high-dry objective.

2. Decant 9 ml of clear supernatant urine, leaving exactly 1 ml (±0.1 ml) to ensure consistency in grading results. Use a disposable pipet to bring the volume of sediment to exactly 1 ml with the clear supernatant urine. Removal of more than 9 ml and readjustment to 1 ml is preferable to removal of less than 9 ml. A disposable system is commercially available for the collection, centrifugation, and concentration of urinary sediment. This system employs a 1:12 concentration and makes use of a disposable transfer pipet with a built-in plastic disk to facillitate easy discard of supernatant urine while retaining 1 ml of sediment (KOVA System, ICL Scientific, Fountain Valley, Calif.).

3. Resuspend the sediment for examination by mixing thoroughly.

4. Transfer a drop or two of well-mixed sediment to a clean, labeled glass slide with a disposable pipet or wooden applicator stick. The size of the drop is important. The fluid should completely fill the area under the cover glass but without overflowing the area or causing the cover glass to float. Some workers prefer to examine the sediment in a counting chamber to ensure even depth. This presents problems of proper disinfection and is not recommended, especially because of the prevalence of hepatitis virus in the clinical laboratory. Disposable, optically clear microscope slides with four individual covered

examination chambers of a uniform area and depth are also commercially available (KOVA Slide, ICL Scientific).

5. Carefully place a cover glass over the sediment, taking care that no bubbles appear. If bubbles appear, a new preparation must be made on a clean slide. Bubbles are confusing and make grading impossible, since they prevent random distribution of the substances to be graded.

6. Examine two preparations for each urinary sediment. After removing a sufficient portion of the unstained sediment (usually enough for only one preparation) add a drop or two of stain (e.g., Sedi-Stain) to the remaining portion of sediment and mix thoroughly. Alternatively, the sediment may be stained directly on the microscope slide before covering by adding a small portion of stain with the tip of a disposable glass pipet or wooden applicator to the drop of sediment on the slide. This method leaves an adequate amount of unstained sediment for further examination.

7. Place the preparation, either stained or unstained, on the microscope stage, and focus and adjust the light, using the low-power objective. Adjust the light by careful positioning of the condenser and iris diaphragm. The tendency is to have too much light, but the light must not be overly reduced. Be sure the sediment itself is brought into focus, rather than the cover glass. It is easier to achieve focus with specimens that are stained. Finally, vary the fine adjustment continuously to maintain focus.

8. Be systematic in the examination. Begin by looking around the four sides of the cover glass. Do not examine the preparation for more than 3 minutes, or drying will occur and the identifications will be inaccurate. First, look for the substances that are identified and graded under low power. Then change to high power, refocus and readjust the light, and search for the substances that are graded and identified under high power. All gradings are based on the average number of structures seen in a minimum of 10 microscopic fields. To ensure accurate results,

prepare two separate portions of sediment, and count the structures seen in five microscopic fields in each preparation (the first portion should be prepared and observed before the second is prepared). To obtain a meaningful average, observe and count structures in the four quadrants and center of each preparation. Describe separately the structures searched for under low and high power. Casts and cells are most important; look for these most carefully, observing the less important crystals and miscellaneous structures almost in retrospect.

a. With the low-power objective ($\times 100$), search for the following:

(1) Casts. Since they tend to roll to the edges of the cover glass, look for them around all four edges of the preparation, and then in the center. When a cast is discovered, change to high power to identify it. Grade casts as negative, occasional, 1+, 2+, 3+, or 4+ on the basis of the average number seen in a minimum of 10 low-power fields (Table 5-3). If more than one type of cast is found in a single specimen, identify and grade each type separately.

(2) Crystals and amorphous material. Look for these structures in the same way as for casts. Report normal crystals as a few or many per low-power field. Confirm abnormal crystals by a chemical test, and then grade them on the average number seen in a minimum of 10 low-power fields (Table 5-3). Some amorphous material and crystals can be found only under high power.

(3) Miscellaneous structures. Various miscellaneous structures such as larger crystals can be seen and are reported as a few or many per low-power field. They should be noted while casts are searched for.

b. With the high-power objective ($\times 440$), search for the following:

Table 5-3. Grading system for the urinary sediment[a]

Constituent	Negative	Occasional	1+	2+	3+	4+
Red cells/hpf[b]	0	Fewer than 4	4–8	8–30	More than 30, fewer than packed	Packed field
Leukocytes and epithelial cells other than squamous/hpf	0	Fewer than 5	5–20	20–50	More than 50, fewer than packed	Packed field
Casts/lpf[c]	0	Fewer than 1	1–5	5–10	10–30	More than 30
Abnormal crystals/lpf	0	Fewer than 1	1–5	5–10	10–30	More than 30

[a]This grading system applies to a microscope field viewed with the usual ×10 eyepiece and the ×10 and ×44 objective lenses. The approximate diameters of such a field under low and high power are 1.5 and 0.35 mm, respectively. A correction should be applied when a microscope with a different-sized field is used in order to maintain consistency in the reporting of results.

[b]hpf = high-power field.

[c]lpf = low-power field.

(1) Red blood cells. Grade them as negative, occasional, 1+, 2+, 3+, or 4+ on the basis of the average number seen in a minimum of 10 high-power fields (Table 5-3).

(2) Leukocytes and epithelial cells. Grade as negative, occasional, 1+, 2+, 3+, or 4+ on the basis of the average number seen in a minimum of 10 high-power fields (Table 5-3).

(3) Identify casts and search for smaller crystals and amorphous material.

(4) Miscellaneous structures. These include yeast, bacteria, squamous epithelium, and small crystals. Identify and report these structures as a few or many.

ADDIS COUNT

Although the routine microscopic examination of the urinary sediment that has just been described gives qualitative or semiquantitative results, a more quantitative evaluation may be desirable. An *Addis count* is such a quantitative enumeration of red cells, combined leukocytes and epithelial cells, and casts in a 12-hour collection of urine.[69,70] The Addis count is valuable in detecting or following renal disease.

Specimen requirements

Since a 12-hour collection of urine is required for this procedure, attention must be given to the factors that will ensure preservation of the elements to be counted. This presents problems, as some of the most important structures are the most difficult to preserve. For casts, a concentrated specimen of low pH is desirable. This is most easily obtained by collecting the specimen overnight, while the patient is not normally eating or drinking. Intake of fluids should be restricted or not permitted during the collection period, as the patient's condition permits. Formalin is the preservative of choice for the preservation of cells and casts and also inhibits the growth of microorganisms. Commercial Formalin tablets are available. Sufficient Formalin may be introduced by rinsing the collection bottle with it and discarding the excess; no more Formalin than this should be used. It is advisable to keep the specimen at room temperature during and after collection to prevent precipitation of dissolved materials, which may obscure the cells and casts and make counting more difficult. The specimen should be examined as soon as possible after the collection, however.

Principle

The total volume of the 12-hour collection of urine is thoroughly mixed and carefully measured. An aliquot of urine is then concentrated (usually 10:1) and the sediment remaining after centrifugation is placed in a counting chamber. The number of red cells, combined leukocytes and epithelial cells, and casts are counted and the numbers of cells and casts excreted in 12 hours are calculated. The amount of protein excreted in the same period and the specific gravity can also be measured and are of value in the eventual diagnosis or treatment of the patient.

The usual qualitative examination of the urinary sediment is most valuable for the general diagnosis of renal disease, while the Addis count is helpful in evaluating the course of a particular disease. It is not a routine procedure and it does not replace the usual examination, as the two have entirely different functions. In addition, the Addis count is cumbersome and time-consuming for both the patient and the laboratory. There is great room for error in the calculations, and a slight error in the number of cells or casts counted can make a difference of several million

in the calculated numbers excreted because of the large dilution factors.

Procedure

1. Mix the specimen for 5 minutes and measure the volume carefully.
2. Make a routine microscopic examination of the urinary sediment with 10:1 concentration of the sediment. From these results determine the volume in which to resuspend the sediment, as described below.
3. Transfer 10 ml of urine to a special Addis graduated centrifuge tube.
4. Centrifuge for 5 minutes at 2000 r/min.
5. Pour off the supernatant urine and save it for a protein determination. Adjust the volume of the remainder to 1 ml. When the amount of sediment is large, adjust the volume to 2-5 ml. Alter the calculations appropriately.
6. Mix well to resuspend the sediment.
7. With a capillary pipet, mount the resuspended sediment on both sides of two Levy-Hausser counting chambers with improved Neubauer rulings.
8. With the low-power objective, count the number of casts in the four largest ruled areas on the two sides of the two counting chambers $(4 \times 9 = 36 \text{ mm}^2)$.
9. With the high-power objective, count the red cells and the combined leukocytes and epithelial cells in 4 mm^2 (count 1 mm^2 in each side of the chamber). Do not count squamous epithelial cells.

Calculations

The numbers of cells and casts excreted in 12 hours are reported separately. They are determined as follows:

$$\text{No. counted/mm}^2 \times \tfrac{1}{10} = \text{no./mm}^2$$
(corrected for 10:1 concentration)

$$\text{No./mm}^2 \times \frac{1}{0.1 \text{ mm}} = \text{no./mm}^3$$

$$\text{No./mm}^3 \times 1000 = \text{no./ml}$$

$$\text{No./ml} \times \text{12-hr volume (ml)} = \text{no. excreted in 12 hours}$$

Normal values

For red blood cells:
  $0\text{-}5 \times 10^5$ in 12 hours
For leukocytes and epithelial cells:
  $0\text{-}1 \times 10^6$ in 12 hours
For casts:
  $0\text{-}5 \times 10^3$ hyalin casts in 12 hours

QUALITY CONTROL IN URINALYSIS

The urinalysis laboratory, like all departments of the clinical laboratory, requires a quality control program to ensure that results are meaningful for the physician and the patient. The popular use of commercial products such as multiple-reagent strips has changed practices in the urinalysis laboratory. They generally ensure rapid and reliable screening of all specimens for a far greater range of abnormal constituents than was possible with the former, more time-consuming chemical procedures. However, the principle of each test and its limitations and possible sources of interference and error must be understood. It is necessary to know which tests can be used only to screen for the presence or absence of a substance and which tests yield qualitative (semiquantitative) results. For tests that are useful merely to screen specimens, adequate confirmatory methods must be understood and employed. Tests must be performed in a technically correct manner and the reagent strips must be kept properly so that they react as they are designed to. The latter is ensured by the use of control specimens, which may be either commercial preparations or solutions prepared by the laboratory.

Control solutions must be used each day. Their use is becoming routine as a means of meeting the accreditation standards of a growing number of regulatory agencies. Both the Joint Commission of Accreditation of Hospitals and the College of American Pathologists have called for the regular use of urinalysis controls. They are particularly necessary because the least trained and most inexperienced personnel continue to be placed in this important division.

Several quality control products are commercially available and suitable for use in the laboratory. Most are obtained in lyophilized form (freeze-dried human urine) and require reconstitution before use. Positive and negative controls are available, and both should be used in the routine testing program. The products are assayed for expected results with commonly used reagent strips and methods. The assayed values that are available for a product will be a factor in determining which product is used by a laboratory.

Urinalysis controls may be used both as a check on the urinalysis reagents and procedures, and as a means of evaluating the ability of the laboratory personnel to correctly perform and interpret the tests. New bottles of reagent strips and tablets should be tested when they are first opened. All previously opened bottles of reagent strips and tablets should be tested each morning. Controls should be included whenever new reagents are used. Control solutions should be employed that check for both falsely negative and falsely positive results, the relative sensitivity at different concentrations, and the stability of the reagents. Results should be recorded in such a way as to ensure that the laboratory remains in control. The notation system used will vary from laboratory to laboratory; control results may be tabulated on daily and weekly graphs similar to those used for clinical chemistry analyses.

One system describing when control specimens should be tested is the following:

1. Test all opened bottles each morning.
2. Test each new bottle on opening.
3. Record data on the record sheet daily.

All bottles should be covered tightly when not in use. Directions given by the manufacturer for storage should be carefully followed. If any discoloration appears on the reagent strips or tablets, discard the bottle immediately. Note the expiration date and do not use any product after that date.

Urinometers and/or refractometers should also be checked daily for accuracy and the data should be recorded in an acceptable manner. The method of checking urinometers and refractometers has been described under Specific Gravity (and Refractive Index) in this chapter.

Of course, the best quality control system will be useless if the urine specimen is not collected and handled in an acceptable manner, before and after reaching the urinalysis laboratory, or if it is mislabled. Such mistakes remain the most frequent cause of error in routine urinalysis. One method of at least partial control of handling or specimen errors is to include blind controls or blind duplicates in the daily collection of urine specimens to be analyzed.

Probably the oldest and still most useful tool in quality control of urinalysis is a final inspection of all the results that make up the urinalysis before they are reported to the physician or placed on the patient's laboratory record. Correlation of expected findings has been discussed throughout this section whenever applicable. To correctly inspect the laboratory record for correlated results, the worker must know the limitations of the tests and the reason for their use. Physical properties, chemical test results, and constituents seen in the urinary sediment should be correlated. Some of the expected results, from a visual inspection of the report form, are listed below.

1. Physical appearance: red or a variation of red (smoky, pink, orange, brown, or black)
   Suspect: red blood cells, hemoglobin, myoglobin
   pH: acid or alkaline
   Protein: positive or negative
   Blood: positive (unless there is ascorbic acid interference)
   Sediment: red blood cells if caused by blood, red cell casts (or a variation such as granular casts) if caused by glomerular disease
2. Physical appearance: dark amber (concentrated urine) with fluffy pink precipitate (brick dust)
   pH: acid
   Specific gravity: relatively high
   Chemical tests: variable
   Sediment: amorphous urates, uric acid
3. Physical appearance: cloudy, white because of presence of x-ray medium
   Specific gravity: greater than 1.035
   Protein: delayed positive protein precipitation test
   Sediment: unusual crystals of x-ray media
4. Physical appearance: cloudy, white
   Suspect: normal alkaline urine, lower urinary tract infection, or upper urinary tract infection
   pH: alkaline
   Specific gravity: may be low (variable)
   Protein: positive or negative
   Blood: positive or negative
   Nitrites: positive or negative
   Sediment: amorphous phosphates (most often), bacteria, leukocytes (neutrophils), epithelial cells (renal to squamous), casts (cellular, granular, waxy, hyalin)
5. Physical appearance: pale, foamy
   Suspect: nephrotic syndrome
   Specific gravity: low
   Protein: very high (4+)
   Sediment: oval fat bodies, fatty casts, free fat
6. Physical appearance: pale, greenish
   Suspect: diabetes mellitus
   pH: acid

Specific gravity: high
Protein: positive or negative
Glucose: positive
Ketones: positive
Sediment: yeast may be present

7. Physical appearance: vivid yellow-brown (beer-brown) or orange-red

Suspect: jaundice
Bilirubin: positive
Urobilinogen: positive
Sediment: may show bile-stained casts or cells

8. Whenever protein is present, the sediment should be carefully inspected for the presence of casts.

AUTOMATION IN URINALYSIS

Although multiple-reagent strips in themselves may be thought of as automation (in a nonmechanical sense), true automation has come to the urinalysis laboratory. Instruments are available that measure the intensity of color formation in the various areas of the multiple-reagent strips by means of an electrooptical reflectance system. These instruments are produced and distributed by the reagent strip manufacturers. The electronic interpretation of results is intended to eliminate human error. There are both completely automatic systems, which allow processing of several specimens with a minimum of operator attention, and portable instruments, which electronically measure the color formation of individual strips. The more automated systems are useful in large institutions that perform a

large number of urinalyses per day. In addition to more conventional recording systems, the instruments are computer-compatible and can be connected with a data transmission system.

The use of automated screening systems should provide time for other parts of the urinalysis, leaving valuable time for careful microscopic analysis of the urinary sediment. Care must be taken with standardization and controls, and the instrument must not be misused. The operator must still be aware of the principles and limitations of the tests. A gross examination of the urine specimen must not be omitted, and the instrumental results must be checked against the gross appearance and correlated with findings in the urinary sediment before final results are reported.

REFERENCES

1. Stanley S. Raphael et al., "Lynch's Medical Laboratory Technology" 3d ed., vol. 1, pp. 10 and 146, W. B. Saunders Company, Philadelphia, 1976.
2. *Ibid.*, pp. 144–148.
3. Israel Davidsohn and John Bernard Henry (eds), "Clinical Diagnosis by Laboratory Methods," 15th ed., p. 108, W. B. Saunders Company, Philadelphia, 1974.
4. W. D. Foster, "A Short History of Clinical Pathology," E. & S. Livingstone, Ltd., London, 1961.
5. Davidsohn and Henry, *op. cit.*, p. 17.
6. Robert M. Kark, James R. Lawrence, Victor E. Pollak, Conrad L. Pirani, Robert C. Muehrcke, and Homera Silva, "A Primer of Urinalysis," 2d ed., p. 10, Hoeber Medical Division, Harper & Row, New York, 1963.
7. Davidsohn and Henry, *op. cit.*, p. 45.
8. "Modern Urinalysis: A Guide to the Diagnosis of Urinary Tract Diseases and Metabolic Disorders," p. 19, Ames Company, division of Miles Laboratories, Inc., Elkhart, Ind., 1973.
9. H. E. Goldberg, "Principles of Refractometry," Instrument Division, American Optical Company, Buffalo, N.Y., 1964.
10. "Instructions for Use and Care of the AO TS

Meter (a Goldberg Refractometer)," Instrument Division, American Optical Company, Buffalo, N.Y., 1964.

11. Philip B. Hawk, Bernard L. Oser, and William H. Summerson, "Practical Physiological Chemistry," 13th ed., McGraw-Hill Book Company, New York, 1954.

12. C. J. Watson and Ellis S. Benson, "Outlines of Internal Medicine," 10th ed., pt. V, p. 568, William C. Brown Company, Dubuque, Iowa, 1962.

13. Kark et al., *op. cit.,* pp. 36–38.

14. M. H. Cook and A. H. Free, The Quantitation of Sugar in Urine, *Am. J. Med. Technol.,* vol. 24, pp. 305–311, 1958.

15. M. M. Belmonte, E. Sarkozy, and E. R. Harpur, Urine Sugar Determination by the Two-Drop Clinitest Method, *Diabetes,* vol. 16, pp. 557–559, 1967.

16. A. H. Free, E. C. Adams, M. L. Kercher, H. M. Free, and M. H. Cook, Simple Specific Test for Urine Glucose, *Clin Chem.,* vol. 3, p. 163, 1957.

17. J. P. Comer, Semiquantitative Specific Test Paper for Glucose in Urine, *Anal. Chem.,* vol. 28, p. 1748, 1956.

18. Kark et al., *op. cit.,* pp. 38–40.

19. Lot B. Page and Perry J. Culver, "A Syllabus of Laboratory Examinations in Clinical Diagnosis," rev. ed., pp. 306–307, Harvard University Press, Cambridge, Mass., 1960.

20. J. M. Court, H. E. Davies, and R. Ferguson, Diastix and Keto-Diastix, a New Semiquantitative Test for Glucose in Urine, *Med. J. Aust.,* vol. 1, p. 525, 1972.

21. Kark et al., *op. cit.,* pp. 20–21.

22. *Ibid.,* p. 23.

23. Richard W. Lippman, "Urine and the Urinary Sediment," 2d ed., pp. 8–9 Charles C Thomas, Springfield, Ill., 1957.

24. Watson and Benson, *op. cit.,* p. 566.

25. Richard J. Henry, Donald C. Cannon, and James W. Winkelman, "Clinical Chemistry, Principles and Techniques, 2d ed., pp. 434–435, Harper & Row, Hagerstown, Md., 1974.

26. A. H. Free, C. O. Rupe, and I. Metzler, Studies with a New Colorimetric Test for Proteinuria, *Clin. Chem.,* vol. 3, p. 716, 1957.

27. G. Clough and T. G. Reah, A Protein Error, *Lancet,* vol. 1, p. 1248, 1964.

28. I. D. Rennie and H. Keen, Evaluation of Clinical Methods for Detecting Proteinuria, *Lancet,* vol. 2, p. 489, 1967.

29. Page and Culver, *op. cit.,* p. 309.

30. A. H. Free and H. M. Free, Nature of Nitroprusside Reactive Material in Urine in Ketosis, *Am. J. Clin. Pathol.,* vol. 30, p. 7, 1958.

31. H. M. Free, R. R. Smeby, M. H. Cook, and A. H. Free, A Comparative Study of Qualitative Tests for Ketones in Urine and Serum, *Clin. Chem.,* vol. 4, p. 323, 1958.

32. M. M. Chertack and J. C. Shernick, Evaluation of a Nitroprusside Dip Test for Ketone Bodies, *J. Am. Med. Assoc.* vol. 167, p. 1621, 1958.

33. Watson and Benson, *op. cit.,* p. 570.

34. M. Z. Barakat, S. K. Shehab, and M. M. El-Sadr, New Tests for Bile and Detection of Bile in Serum and Urine, *Clin. Chem.,* vol. 3, p. 135, 1957.

35. A. H. Free and H. M. Free, A Simple Test for Urine Bilirubin, *Gastroenterology,* vol. 24, p. 414, 1953.

36. H. Sobotka, A. V. Luisada-Opper, and M. Reiner, A New Test for Bilirubin in Urine, *Am. J. Clin. Pathol.,* vol. 23, p. 607, 1953.

37. J. A. Tallack and S. Sherlock, A New Tablet Test for Bilirubin in Urine, *Br. Med. J.,* vol. 2, p. 212, 1954.

38. S. Schwartz, M. H. Berg, I. Bossenmaier, and H. Dinsmore, Determination of Porphyrins in Biological Materials, *Methods Biochem. Anal.,* vol. 8, pp. 221–293, 1960.

39. S. Schwartz, M. Keprios, and R. Schmid, Experimental Porphyria. II. Type Produced by Lead, Phenylhydrazine, and Light, *Proc. Soc. Exp. Biol. Med.,* vol. 79, p. 463, 1952.

40. Watson and Benson, *op. cit.,* p. 578.

41. C. J. Watson, I. Bossenmaier, and R. Cardinal, Acute Intermittent Porphyria, *J. Am. Med. Assoc.* vol. 175, p. 1087, 1961.

42. C. J. Watson and S. Schwartz, A Simple Test for Urinary Porphobilinogen, *Proc. Soc. Exp. Biol. Med.,* vol. 47, p. 393, 1941.

43. D. S. Young, L. C. Pestaner, and Val Gibberman, Effects of Drugs on Clinical Laboratory Tests, *Clin. Chem.,* vol. 21, p. 386D, 1975.

44. C. B. Hager and A. H. Free, Urine Urobilino-gen as a Component of Routine Urinalysis, *Am. J. Med. Technol.,* vol. 36, pp. 227–233, 1970.

45. D. Kutter, A. P. M. Van Oudheusden, K. Eisenberg, A. Hennecke, A. R. Helbing, and E. W. Busch, Usefulness of a New Test Strip for Detecting Urobilinogen in Urine, *Dtsch. Med. Wochenschr.,* vol. 98, pp. 112–114, 1973.

46. Young et al., *loc. cit.*

47. Watson and Benson, *op. cit.,* p. 574.

48. "Modern Urinalysis: A Guide to the Diagnosis of Urinary Tract Diseases and Metabolic Disorders," pp. 45–46, Ames Company, division of Miles Laboratories, Inc., Elkhart, Ind., 1973.

49. Alfred H. Free and Helen M. Free, "Urodynamics, Concepts Relating to Urinalysis," pp. 50–55, Ames Company, division of Miles Laboratories, Inc., Elkhart, Ind., 1974.

50. J. R. Leonards, Simple Test for Hematuria Compared with Established Tests, *J. Am. Med. Assoc.* vol. 179, p. 807, 1962.

51. D. Kutter, A. Van Oudheusden, A. Hilvers, K. Nechvile, T. Van Buul, and P. Koller, The Usefulness of a New Test Strip for the Detection of Erythrocytes and Hemoglobin in Urine, *Dtsch. Med. Wochenschr.,* vol. 99, p. 2332, 1974.

52. J. Braun and W. Straube, A New Rapid Test for Diagnosing Microhaematuria Compared with Results of Microscopic Examination, *Dtsch. Med. Wochenschr.,* vol. 100, p. 87, 1975.

53. Free and Free, "Urodynamics, Concepts Relating to Urinalysis," *op. cit.,* p. 51.

54. P. Griess, Bemerkungen zu der Abhandlung des H. H. Weselsky und Benedikt über einige Aza Verbindungen, *Ber. Dtsch. Ophthalmol. Ges.,* vol. 12, p. 426, 1879.

55. R. Sternheimer and B. Malbin, Clinical Recognition of Pyelonephritis with a New Stain for Urinary Sediments, *Am. J. Med.* vol. 11, p. 312, 1951.

56. Davidsohn and Henry, *op. cit.,* p. 36.

57. *Ibid.,* pp. 23 and 36.

58. *Ibid.,* p. 35.

59. Meryl H. Haber, "Urine Casts, Their Microscopy and Clinical Significance," p. 67, Division of Educational Media Services, American Society of Clinical Pathologists, Chicago, 1975.

60. Lippman, *op. cit.,* p. 11.

61. Lippman, *op. cit.*

62. Haber, *op. cit.,* p. 11.

63. *Ibid.,* p. 5.

64. Lippman, *op. cit.,* p. 20.

65. Haber, *op. cit.,* p. 11.

66. George E. Schreiner, "Urinary Sediments," Medical Communications, Inc., New York, 1969.

67. Haber, *op. cit.,* p. 40.

68. *Ibid.,* p. 58.

69. T. Addis, "Glomerular Nephritis," pp. 10–16, Macmillan, New York, 1948.

70. Lippman, *op. cit.,* pp. 103–106.

BIBLIOGRAPHY

Campbell, M. R. and J. H. Harrison: "Urology," 4th ed., vol. 1, W. B. Saunders Company, Philadelphia, 1970.

Davidsohn, Israel and John Bernard Henry (eds), "Clinical Diagnosis by Laboratory Methods," 15th ed., W. B. Saunders Company, Philadelphia, 1974.

Free, Alfred H. and Helen M. Free: "Urodynamics, Concepts Relating to Urinalysis," Ames Company, division of Miles Laboratories, Inc., Elkhart, Ind., 1974.

Freeman, James A. and Myrton F. Beeler: "Laboratory Medicine—Clinical Microscopy," Lea & Febiger, Philadelphia, 1974.

Haber, Meryl H.: "Urine Casts, Their Microscopy and Clinical Significance," Division of Educational Media Services, American Society of Clinical Pathologists, Chicago, 1975.

Kark, Robert M., James R. Lawrence, Victor E. Pollak, Conard L. Pirani, Robert C. Muehrcke, and Homera Silva: "A Primer of Urinalysis," 2d ed., Hoeber Medical Division, Harper & Row, New York, 1963.

Lippman, Richard W.: "Urine and the Urinary

Sediment," 2d ed., Charles C Thomas, Springfield, Ill., 1957.

"Modern Urinalysis: A Guide to the Diagnosis of Urinary Tract Diseases and Metabolic Disorders," Ames Company, division of Miles Laboratories, Inc., Elkhart, Ind., 1973.

Raphael, Stanley S. et al.: "Lynch's Medical Laboratory Technology," 3d ed., vol. I, W. B. Saunders Company, Philadelphia, 1976.

Strauss, Maurice B. and Louis G. Welt: "Diseases of the Kidney," 2d ed., Little, Brown and Company, Waltham, Mass., 1971.

"Urine Under the Microscope," Rocom Press, division of Hoffmann-LaRoche, Inc., Nutley, N.J., 1973.

Young, D. S., L. C. Pestaner, and Val Gibberman: Effects of Drugs on Clinical Laboratory Tests, *Clin. Chem.,* vol. 21, 1975.

SIX
EXAMINATION OF MISCELLANEOUS EXTRAVASCULAR FLUIDS

Extravascular fluids (body fluids other than blood or urine) are examined in various departments of the clinical laboratory, depending on the nature of the test requested. Cell counts are routinely done on most body fluids, and for this reason the specimen is often sent directly to the hematology laboratory after collection (see under Collection, Preservation, and Preparation of Laboratory Specimens in Chap. 1 for more information on specimen collection). The extravascular fluids are termed pleural (around the lungs), pericardial (around the heart), peritoneal (around the abdominal and pelvic cavities), synovial (around the joints), and cerebrospinal (around the brain and spinal cord). Each of these fluids is handled in special ways. Analyses of synovial fluid and cerebrospinal fluid will be discussed separately. The examination of the other body fluids (serous fluids) will be discussed in general terms.

Several general observations are made for all body fluids. Cell counts and specific gravities are usually determined. Smears are made and, after staining with Wright's stain, are examined microscopically. Protein is measured and a mucin or clotting test is done. For other tests ordered, the specimen is sent to a particular department; for instance, glucose, protein, or chloride tests would be done in the chemistry department.

SEROUS FLUIDS (PLEURAL, PERICARDIAL, AND PERITONEAL)

Collection of serous fluids

Normally, there is about 1–10 ml of pleural fluid moistening the pleural surfaces. It surrounds the lungs and lines the walls of the thoracic cavity. If inflammation occurs, the plasma protein level drops, congestive heart failure is present, or there is decreased lymphatic drainage, there can be an abnormal accumulation of pleural fluid. A term used to describe such an abnormal accumulation is pleural effusion. Pleural fluid should be collected in three sterile tubes [anticoagulated with heparin or ethylenediaminetetraacetic acid (EDTA)] that are labeled sequentially. The first tube is used for culture and Gram stain and the others for cell counts, Wright's stain, total protein, glucose, cytology, and other studies as indicated. If a mucin test is to be done, a portion of the pleural fluid should be placed in a plain tube without anticoagulant.

The pericardial space enclosing the heart normally contains about 20-50 ml of a clear, straw-colored ultrafiltrate of plasma, called pericardial fluid. This fluid forms continually and is reabsorbed by the nearby lymph vessels (lymphatics), leaving a small but constant volume. When an abnormal accumulation of pericardial fluid occurs, it fills up the space around the heart and can mechanically inhibit the normal action of the heart. In this case, immediate aspiration of the excess fluid is indicated. This is a major procedure and must be done by a physician. At least three tubes of pericardial fluid should be obtained: an EDTA tube for gross and microscopic examination, a sterile plain or heparinized tube for microbiological studies, and a heparinized tube for chemical analyses.

Like pleural and pericardial fluids, peritoneal fluid is a plasma ultrafiltrate. Normally less than 100 ml of the clear, straw-colored fluid is present in the peritoneal cavity (the abdominal and pelvic cavities). An abnormal accumulation of the fluid is indicated by severe abdominal pain and may be caused by a ruptured abdominal organ, hemorrhage resulting from trauma, postoperative complications, or an unknown cause. If this occurs, the excess fluid is aspirated. The presence of such an accumulation must always be considered in the light of other findings. For the collection of peritoneal fluid, three collection tubes should be used. For cell counts, gross observations, and Wright's stained smears, an EDTA tube should be used. A sterile plain or heparinized tube can be used for microbiological examination, and a heparinized tube for chemistry determinations.

Serous effusions have been classified as transudates and exudates on the basis of the amount of protein present and the specific gravity. Body fluids with a total protein content under 3 g/dl are considered transudates; those with a total protein content over 3 g/dl are considered exudates.[1] Exudates result from conditions where the capillary permeability is increased, or there is some interference with the lymphatic drainage of the body spaces, especially the pleural spaces.

Routine examination of body fluids (serous fluids)

Gross appearance

Normal serous fluid is pale and straw-colored. This is the color seen in a transudate. Turbidity increases as the amount of cells and debris increases. An abnormally colored fluid may appear milky white (chylous or pseudochylous), cloudy, or bloody on gross observation. A cloudy serous fluid is often associated with an inflammatory reaction, either bacterial or viral. Blood-tinged fluid can be seen as a result of a traumatic tap, and grossly bloody fluid can be seen when an organ such as the spleen or liver or a blood vessel has ruptured. Bloody fluids are also seen in malignant disease states, after myocardial infarction, in tuberculosis, in rheumatoid arthritis, and in systemic lupus erythematosus.

Clotting

To observe the ability of the serous fluid to clot, the specimen must be collected in a plain tube with no anticoagulant. Ability of the fluid to clot indicates a substantial inflammatory reaction.

Red and white blood cell count

Cell counts are done on well-mixed serous fluid that has been mounted on a counting chamber, in much the same way as for blood. In many serous fluids the cell count is very low, so a drop of undiluted specimen may be mounted on the counting chamber; this is especially true when the fluid appears clear or almost clear. To count red cells, the specimen is mounted directly with a drop from a capillary pipet. To count white cells, the pipet is first rinsed with acetic acid and then the specimen is drawn into the pipet, filling it. After shaking and mounting the specimen, the white cell count is made in the same way as for blood. If the body fluids appear turbid and high in protein, they may be diluted with saline, using a regular blood-diluting pipet. The dilution factor must be used in the final calculations. When protein is present, acetic acid cannot be used to destroy the red cells (for the white cell count) because it precipitates protein, which would obscure the field.

A 10-mm^2 area is counted, using the high-dry objective of the microscope. The cells are classified as red or white and the number seen per microliter is reported. Red and white cells are counted at the same time but recorded separately. Leukocyte counts over 500 cells/μl are usually clinically significant. If there is a predominance of neutrophils (polymorphonuclear cells), bacterial inflammation is suggested. A predominance of lymphocytes suggests viral infection, tuberculosis, lymphoma, or carcinoma.

Specific gravity

To determine the specific gravity of the body fluid, a refractometer may be used. In another, somewhat outdated method a well-mixed drop of the fluid is dropped from a pipet into a series of copper sulfate solutions ranging in specific gravity from 1.008 to 1.075, and the falling drop is observed. If the specific gravity of the fluid is lower than that of the copper sulfate solution, the drop will float; if it is higher, the drop will sink.

Smears of the body fluid

Fluid preserved with EDTA is centrifuged for 5 minutes at 1500 r/min. The usual amount centrifuged is 5–10 ml. The supernatant is discarded or used for the protein test. The tube is then inverted and a drop of the sediment is removed with a bacteriologic loop and placed on a cover glass. A second cover glass is used to spread the drop of fluid, as is done with peripheral blood smears, and the smear is air-dried rapidly. It is then stained with Wright's stain and microscopically examined. In the examination a leukocyte differential is done; the white cells resemble those seen in peripheral blood smears. Generally 300 cells are counted and classified as neutrophils, lymphocytes, eosinophils, and other cells. If any malignant tumor cells are seen, or appear to be present, the smear must be checked by a pathologist or qualified medical technologist.

Smears or cell counts cannot be done on a clotted specimen. Smears for tumor cells are stained with Wright's or Giemsa stain, or by using the Papanicolaou method. Only unclotted body fluid is suitable for tumor cell studies.

Protein test by the Esbach method

The protein test is done on the supernatant (cell-free) body fluid. In Esbach's method (a now rarely used procedure), the supernatant is added to a special Esbach tube to the mark labeled 1 and diluted with deionized water to the mark labeled 10. Esbach reagent is added to the mark labeled R. The contents of the tube are mixed and allowed to stand at room temperature for 24 hours. If protein is present, it is precipitated by Esbach reagent. At the end of the 24 hours, the volume of the precipitate is read from the Esbach tube in grams per liter and then corrected for the dilution. In normal serous fluid, very little protein is present. Albumin passes through the membranes into the fluid first and then the larger protein molecules. With fibrinogen entering the effusion, clotting will occur.

Most protein tests are now done using electrophoresis.

Other chemistry tests

In bacterial infections, body fluids have lower concentrations of glucose than does the blood, and their glucose levels may be determined in the chemistry department. If a glucose determination is ordered on serous fluid, a blood sample must be collected simultaneously and both specimens must be collected in sodium fluoride tubes. Protein tests using electrophoresis and sometimes chloride tests may also be done.

Microbiological examination

This will include Gram stains and cultures on all body fluid effusions of unknown etiology (see under Chap. 10).

CEREBROSPINAL FLUID

The usual examination of the cerebrospinal fluid (CSF) specimen includes several observations, many of which can be made in the hematology laboratory. Abnormal color, the presence of turbidity, or clot formation is noted. The examination includes cell counts, smears, chemistries, and cultures.

Cerebrospinal (or spinal) fluid is a clear, lymph-like, sterile, extravascular fluid that circulates in the ventricles of the brain, the subarachnoid spaces, and the spinal cord. The normal adult has 125–150 ml of spinal fluid, and the newborn has about 5 ml. Spinal fluid has four main functions: it is a mechanical buffer that prevents trauma, it regulates the volume of the intracranial contents, it is a nutrient medium of the central nervous system, and it is an excretory channel for metabolic products of the central nervous system.

When a spinal tap is ordered, it is done for serious reasons. It can be ordered when meningeal irritation is present (as in meningitis or hemorrhage), in involvement of the central nervous system (as in paralysis or when abnormal reflexes are observed), when there is increased intracranial pressure (as in severe headache, convulsions, and coma), for drainage (as in subdural hematoma), and to introduce x-ray contrast media or drugs.

Cerebrospinal fluid differs from serous and synovial fluids because of the selective permeability of the membranes and adjacent tissues containing it. Some drugs, such as penicillin and streptomycin, do not enter the spinal fluid from the blood. Electrolytes such as sodium, magnesium, and chloride are more concentrated in spinal fluid than in plasma or plasma ultrafiltrates, while bicarbonate, glucose, and urea are less concentrated in spinal fluid. Protein enters the spinal fluid in very small amounts. Very few cells are found in normal spinal fluid.

Collection of spinal fluid

There is a certain risk to the patient in the procedure for obtaining a specimen of spinal fluid, hence such specimens must be handled with the utmost care. In practice, three sterile tubes containing about 5 ml each are collected during the spinal tap. These tubes are numbered in sequence of collection and immediately brought to the laboratory. It is important that any cell count or glucose determinations be done as soon as possible after collection to prevent deterioration of cells and glucose.

The glucose level in spinal fluid is about 20 mg/dl less than that in blood, but the amounts may vary, and both levels should be measured simultaneously. Bacteria and cells utilize glucose. The glucose level in spinal fluid is especially reduced in bacterial meningitis, but *not* in viral meningitis, primary brain tumor, or vascular accidents. It is low in metastatic tumor and insulin shock, and elevated in diabetic coma.

Routine examination of cerebrospinal fluid

Gross appearance

Normal spinal fluid is crystal-clear. Color should be noted by holding the sample beside a tube of distilled water and a clean white paper.[2] Slight haziness in the specimen indicates a white cell count of 200–500 cells/μl, and turbidity indicates a higher white cell count (over 500 cells/μl). Turbidity may be observed by holding newspaper behind the tube of specimen and observing the print.

Bloody fluid can result from a traumatic tap. If blood in a specimen results from this, the successive collection tubes will show less bloody fluid, eventually becoming clear. If blood in a specimen is caused by a subarachnoid hemorrhage, the color of the fluid will look the same in all the collection tubes. When the hemorrhage is old, the supernatant fluid, or fluid from which the cells have settled, will be yellow (xanthochromic). The yellow color is caused by bilirubin, formed from hemoglobin from the lysed red blood cells, and it appears about 12 hours after a bleeding episode. When the protein level is elevated, a yellow color in the fluid is observed because bilirubin is ordinarily carried in the albumin fraction.

Turbidity in spinal fluid may result from the presence of large numbers of leukocytes, as previously discussed, or from bacteria. In addition to the gross observations of turbidity and color, the spinal fluid should be examined for clotting. Clotting may occur with a traumatic tap or with a moderate or marked protein elevation.

Red and white blood cell counts

If the spinal fluid appears clear, cell counts may be performed in a hemocytometer counting chamber without using diluting fluid. All spinal fluids are considered contaminated and should be handled carefully. The use of rubber gloves is recommended. All disposable supplies and equipment used in handling the specimen or doing the laboratory tests should be discarded in the proper receptacles for contaminated materials. Proper disinfectants should be used to eliminate possible contamination. Contagious meningitis may be transmitted to the worker if the spinal fluids are not handled properly. Cell counts should be done as soon as possible after the

specimen is obtained because cells lyse on prolonged standing and the counts become invalid. Counts should be done within 30 minutes.

To count *red cells*, mount the well-mixed specimen with a clean, dry Pasteur pipet directly onto both sides of the counting chamber. Count the red cells in 10 mm^2, using the low-power objective ($\times$10). Count 9 mm^2 on one side of the chamber and the middle 1 mm^2 on the other side of the chamber. Red cells can be distinguished from white cells by changing to the high-dry ($\times$45) objective, when necessary. The red cells are small, round, yellow, and occasionally crenate. The percentage of crenate cells is reported, in addition to the total number of red cells per microliter. Every red cell is included in the count, crenate or not. If the spinal fluid is grossly bloody, the specimen must be diluted by using a red or white cell diluting pipet and Hayem's solution or saline. Usually a 1:10 or 1:20 dilution with a white cell diluting pipet (Thoma type) is adequate. Normally there are no red cells in spinal fluid.

To count *white cells*, rinse a disposable Pasteur pipet with glacial acetic acid, drain it carefully, wipe the outside completely dry with gauze, and touch the tip of the pipet to the gauze to remove any excess acid. It is very important that no glacial acetic acid is left on the outside of the pipet because it would contaminate the spinal fluid specimen when the pipet is placed in it. This rinsed pipet is used to mount a drop of well-mixed spinal fluid on a counting chamber. The acid will destroy the red cells and darken or intensify the nuclei of the white cells. Both sides of the counting chamber should be used. After mounting the specimen, it may be necessary to wait about 3–5 minutes for the complete destruction of the red cells. No bubbles can be present in the counting chamber; if they are, the specimen must be remounted.

The white cells are counted in 10 mm^2, using the low-power objective. When a white cell is seen, switch to the high-dry objective and classify the cell as polymorphonuclear or mononuclear. If the white cell count is high, it is probably better to do the entire count and the white cell differential with the high-power objective. When the white cell count is above 10 cells/μl, the cell differential is reported as a percentage, and when the count is below 10 cells/μl, the number counted is reported rather than a percentage. In enumerating the white cells in spinal fluid, the classification as polymorphonuclear or mononuclear is important to the physician for the diagnosis. A predominance of polymorphonuclear cells usually indicates a bacterial infection, while the presence of many mononuclear cells indicates a viral infection. The normal white cell count in spinal fluid is 0–8 cells/μl; more than 10 cells/μl is considered abnormal.

Smears of spinal fluid for the white cell differential

When the count is over 50 white cells/μl, a differential study is done on smears made from centrifuged spinal fluid sediment. The spinal fluid is centrifuged for 5 minutes at 3000 r/min and the supernatant is saved for chemistry determinations. The sediment is used to prepare smears on glass slides, and the smears are dried rapidly and stained with Wright's stain. Exactly 100 white cells are counted and classified as polymorphonuclear or mononuclear; the percentage of each is reported. If any tumor cells are seen, the sediment should be placed in Formalin and sent to the pathologist for further study.

Chemistry tests

Several chemistry determinations can be done with spinal fluid. The tests for glucose, protein, chloride, and bilirubin are the most common ones. For a glucose determination, the glucose in the specimen must be preserved by adding sodium fluoride to the sample tube immediately to prevent glycolysis. The determination should be done as soon as possible. As mentioned previously, simultaneous blood and spinal fluid glucose determinations must be done, as it is the difference between these values that is clinically significant.

Protein tests and protein electrophoresis are often done, and tests for bilirubin and chloride are less commonly done. The chloride level in spinal fluid is normally higher than that in blood; normal values are 122–132 meq/L for spinal fluid and 98–109 meq/L for serum or plasma.[3] Blood chloride concentrations are usually measured along with the spinal fluid chloride concentration, as the ratio of these values is normally maintained. Spinal fluid chloride levels fall in meningitis and become closer to the blood chloride levels. Spinal fluid levels of other electrolytes that are normally lower than blood levels rise during inflammation and become closer to the levels in the blood.

The normal protein content of spinal fluid is usually given as 45 mg/dl, but higher normal values are obtained with newer techniques for protein determination. Electrophoresis has replaced the colloidal gold test for the evaluation of spinal fluid protein fractions.

Microbiological examination

Gram stains and culturing are done in the microbiology department. Spinal fluid specimens are normally sterile. Gram stains are most useful in the diagnosis of acute bacterial meningitis, as the organisms can actually be seen in the stained specimen when observed microscopically (see under Chap. 10).

Serology tests

The Venereal Disease Research Laboratory (VDRL) test is a well-known serological test for syphilis that is done on spinal fluid (see under Chap. 8).

SYNOVIAL FLUID

Synovial fluid is found around the joints. Synovial membranes line the joints, bursas, and tendon sheaths. In composition, normal synovial fluid resembles plasma ultrafiltrate with the addition of hyaluronic acid. The presence of hyaluronic acid differentiates synovial fluid from other serous fluids and spinal fluid. Hyaluronic acid is excreted by synovial cells and possibly fibroblasts, which are found in the synovial membrane, and it gives synovial fluid its normal viscosity. Normal synovial fluid is straw-colored and viscous, resembling uncooked egg white, and does not clot. About 1 ml is present in each large joint, such as the knee, ankle, hip, elbow, wrist, or shoulder. Indications for aspiration of synovial fluid include arthritis of unknown etiology, manifested by effusion (abnormal accumulation); possible infectious arthritis; effusions of unknown etiology; and pain or decreased mobility. Effusion of synovial fluid is usually clinically observed before aspiration, and it is usually possible to aspirate 10-20 ml of the fluid for laboratory examination.

In the management of joint disorders, a differential diagnosis is essential so that the right kind of treatment can be used. One of the simple techniques in such a diagnosis is the examination of synovial fluid. The analysis of synovial fluid can give an immediate diagnosis in some disorders, and provides valuable information concerning other diseases of the joints.

In normal synovial fluid the white cell count is very low—about 50 cells/μl—and the majority of the white cells seen are mononuclear. The glucose concentration of synovial fluid is usually about 90 percent that of plasma or serum, and the protein content is low, about 1.7 g/dl.[4]

The differential diagnosis of diseased synovial fluid usually classifies the fluid as noninflammatory, inflammatory, or infected. *Noninflammatory* synovial fluid suggests the presence of traumatic acute arthritis, osteoarthritis, or frequently systemic lupus erythematosis. It is usually clear and viscous and has 200-2000 white cells/μl, less than 25 percent of which are polymorphonuclear. The glucose and protein contents are approximately the same as in normal synovial fluid. *Inflammatory* fluid is characteristic of rheumatoid arthritis, gout, pseudogout, and rheumatic fever. This fluid is cloudy yellow, has low viscosity, and has a moderately high white cell count (10 000-20 000 cells/μl), with 60-70 percent polymorphonuclear. The glucose content is normal and the protein content high. *Infected* fluid usually suggests a bacterial infection. It is generally cloudy and has low viscosity. The white cell count is over 50 000 cells/μl, and the proportion of polymorphonuclear cells is greater than 70 percent. The glucose content is characteristically very low—often as much as 10 mg/dl lower than normal.[5]

Collection of synovial fluid

The volume collected is divided according to the laboratory tests needed. One suggested division is as follows: one plain tube for viscosity, clot formation, and gross appearance; one EDTA tube for cell counts, cell differential, and crystal studies; one sterile plain or heparinized tube for microbiological cultures and Gram smears; one fluoride tube for glucose determination (for this test the specimen should be collected from a patient who is fasting); and appropriate additional tubes for serology or other chemistry determinations. When a test for glucose is to be done on synovial fluid, a blood sample is drawn simultaneously for analysis.

Routine examination of synovial fluid

Gross appearance

The first step in the analysis of synovial fluid is to observe the specimen for color and clarity.

The noninflammatory fluid is usually clear. To test for clarity, read newspaper print through a test tube containing the specimen. As the cell and protein content increases, the turbidity increases, and the print becomes more difficult to read.

In a traumatic tap of the joint, blood will be seen in the collection tubes in an uneven distribution; also, the blood may clot, and it diminishes as the aspiration continues. A truly bloody synovial fluid is uniform in color, the blood does not clot, and the sample gives a xanthochromic supernatant when centrifuged. Bloody effusions are seen with hemophilia, tumors, and trauma.

String test

The string test evaluates the viscosity of the synovial fluid. It can be done by "stringing" the fluid between the thumb and index finger. The use of rubber gloves is recommended. A drop of normal synovial fluid will form a string several inches long because of its viscosity. Inflammatory fluids contain enzymes that break down hyaluronic acid. Anything that decreases the hyaluronic acid content of synovial fluid lowers its viscosity.

Mucin clot test

This also tests for viscosity and is based on the polymerization of hyaluronic acid. To perform the mucin clot test, synovial fluid is added drop by drop to dilute acetic acid.[6] The resulting clot may fragment easily, indicating inflammatory fluid, or may remain firm, indicating noninflammatory fluid. Clots are graded as good, fair, poor, and very poor. Good clots do not break up easily when they are agitated, and they are surrounded by clear solution. A soft clot in turbid solution is graded as fair. A poor clot breaks up easily when agitated, ending up in small pieces, and is surrounded by a cloudy solution. If no clot forms and there are only flakes in a cloudy suspension, this is graded as very poor.[7]

Red and white blood cell count

The appearance of a drop of synovial fluid under an ordinary light microscope can be helpful in estimating the cell counts initially and in demonstrating the presence of crystals. The presence of only a few white cells per high-power field ($\times 45$) suggests a noninflammatory disorder. A large number of white cells would indicate inflammatory or infected synovial fluid. The total white blood cell count and differential count are very important in diagnosis. When cells are counted in other fluids, such as blood, the usual diluting fluid is dilute acetic acid. This cannot be used with synovial fluid because it may cause mucin clotting. Instead, a solution of saline containing methylene blue is used. The synovial fluid is diluted 1:20 with a white cell diluting pipet. The diluted cells are mounted in a counting chamber. Counts below 200 white cells/μl with less than 25 percent polymorphonuclear cells and no red cells are normally observed in synovial fluid. Monocytes, lymphocytes, and macrophages are seen. A low white cell count (200–2000 cells/μl) with predominantly mononuclear cells suggests a noninflammatory joint fluid, while a high white cell count suggests inflammation and a very high white cell count with a high proportion of polymorphonuclear cells strongly suggests infection.

Smears for white blood cell differential

Smears are made as for peripheral blood; they should be thin, as hyaluronic acid will distort the cells. The films may be prepared from fresh fluid at the time of aspiration, or from sediment centrifuged from the fluid collected in EDTA tubes. Centrifuged sediment gives a more concentrated preparation and is easier to examine. Smears are air-dried and stained with Wright's stain.

Lupus erythematosus (LE) cells are frequently found in stained synovial fluid from patients with systemic lupus erythematosus and occasionally in fluid from patients with rheumatoid arthritis (see under Lupus Erythematosus Cell Test in Chap. 3). The *in vivo* formation of LE cells in synovial fluid probably results from trauma to the white cells.

Microscopic examination for crystals

A drop of unclotted synovial fluid (generally preserved with EDTA) is examined with an ordinary light microscope. The drop is placed on a slide and cover-slipped. Needle-shaped, intracellular urate crystals (sodium acid urate) seen in a simple wet preparation of synovial fluid are characteristic of gouty arthritis (Fig. 6-1). Pseudogout, a crystal-deposition disease distinct from gout, is demonstrated by the presence of rhomboid calcium pyrophosphate. Cholesterol crystals are seen in synovial fluid from persons with rheumatoid arthritis and not in normal synovial fluid. They are flat, clear, rhombic crystals with one corner punched out.

Use of polarized light

More definitive microscopic identification of crystals in synovial fluid can be made with the use of polarized light. To set up the microscope, a polarizing filter is placed between the light source and the condenser, and another polarizing filter is placed between the eyepiece and the objective. These filters can be added to an ordinary microscope. When the filter between the eyepiece and the objective is rotated and the field is thereby darkened, urate crystals will appear birefringent and needle- or rod-shaped; calcium pyrophosphate crystals will appear birefringent and rhomboid. Calcium pyrophosphate crystals are diagnostic of pseudogout, which has symptoms that mimic those of gout, rheumatoid arthritis, or osteoarthritis. Urate crystals are

Fig. 6-1. Sodium acid urate crystal in neutrophil, characteristic of gouty arthritis. The picture at the left shows an intracellular crystal with bright-field illumination; the same crystal is shown at the right with polarized light. Photomicrographs were taken with the high-dry objective.

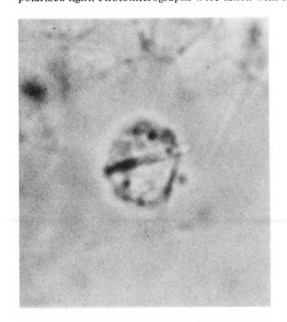 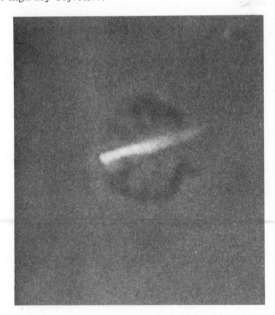

found in almost 100 percent of acute gouty joints and in 75 percent of chronic gouty arthritis.

Birefringent bodies have two or three different refractive indexes. Crystals that are birefringent appear differently colored in polarized light, depending on their orientation to the direction of a full-wave retardation plate, or first-order red filter. The filter is not actually red, but when it is placed over the bottom polarizer on the microscope and rotated to a certain position the field will appear red. A urate crystal at right angles to polarized light passing through the red plate appears blue, but the same crystal parallel to the light appears yellow. A calcium pyrophosphate crystal reacts in the opposite way, appearing yellow when it is perpendicular to the light passing through the plate and blue when it is parallel. In positive birefringence the refractive index for light vibrating parallel to the axis of the crystal is greater than that for light vibrating perpendicular to it; crystals perpendicular to the plane of slow vibration of light are yellow, and those parallel are blue.

Microbiological examination

Pathogenic organisms can be identified by use of the Gram stain and by culturing the synovial fluid. Cultures for suspected bacteria or mycobacterial or fungal infections are an essential part of the synovial fluid analysis. Immediate bedside inoculation of the sample onto chocolate agar

and the use of special media for the propagation of gonococcal organisms are suggested. Gonococcal arthritis is a joint disease that is sometimes difficult to diagnose unless special techniques and care are used.

Chemistry tests

The determination of glucose in the synovial fluid is valuable when infectious diseases are suspected. For example, when the glucose level is significantly lower in synovial fluid than in serum or plasma, infection of the joint is suggested. Samples of the patient's synovial fluid and blood must be obtained at the same time for a comparison of the two values to be valid. With inflammatory joint disease (e.g., rheumatoid arthritis), the total protein level of synovial fluid approaches that of plasma. Normally, the total protein level of synovial fluid is under 2 g/dl, and that of plasma is 4–7 g/dl. Other chemistry determinations on synovial fluid include certain enzyme studies.

Immunology tests

A rheumatoid factor has been reported in the synovial fluid as well as in the serum of patients with rheumatoid arthritis. The presence of the rheumatoid factor in the synovial fluid but not in the serum can be helpful in the diagnosis of this disease.

NASAL SMEARS FOR EOSINOPHILS

Persons with an allergic reaction show a distinct increase in the number of eosinophilic cells in a differential count on a smear of the nasal discharge. Smears may be made directly from the nostril by using a swab or from material blown into waxed paper or oiled silk by the patient. The nasal material is spread as thinly as possible on a glass slide and air-dried, and the slide is

stained with Wright's stain or Hansel's stain. The eosinophils contain bright red granules and are easily recognized under the oil-immersion objective. An increase in the number of eosinophils normally indicates that the patient may be in an allergic state rather than having an infection of some kind.

The exact role of eosinophils in allergic im-

munologic reactions has not been determined.[8] It is possible that antigen-antibody complexes or histamine, which are involved in such reactions, may attract eosinophils chemotactically. The eosinophils in the nasal discharge come from the blood. Many allergic conditions are characterized by eosinophilia. In this state, eosinophils are found in peripheral blood, marrow, sputum (in bronchial asthma), nasal and conjunctival discharges (in hay fever), and lesions (in some skin diseases).

The nasal smear examination is simple and useful. It can tell the physician whether a patient's upper respiratory tract involvement is caused by an allergy or a nasal infection. Proper treatment can then be started. Cytological studies are an indispensable aid in differentiating allergic and infectious factors.

Procedure for staining nasal smears with Hansel's stain

1. After the smear has been air-dried, it is covered with Hansel's stain for 30 seconds (Hansel's stain is available from Lide Laboratories, Inc., St. Louis, Mo.). The time may be increased for thick mucus secretions.

2. Distilled water is added to take up the stain and the mixture is allowed to remain on the smear for another 30 seconds.

3. The slide is then tilted to pour off the stain. Any excess is removed by flooding with distilled water.

4. With the slide tilted, 95% ethyl alcohol or 75% methyl alcohol is dropped over the stained smear to decolorize it. Care should be taken to not use too much alcohol, for the cytoplasm of the neutrophils may be excessively decolorized and will appear pink. This could cause confusion in looking for eosinophils.

5. The slide is carefully dried by fanning it in the air.

6. Alternatively, Wright's stain may be used for staining nasal smears.

Interpretation of the nasal smear

The stained smear is examined first under low power and then with the oil-immersion objective. Eosinophils may be recognized by their red cytoplasm and large, deep red granules. The nucleus is stained blue. Normally, the nasal smear contains mucus with scattered neutrophils, mononuclear cells, and occasional epithelial cells. If neutrophilia is pronounced, infection is probably present, especially if bacteria are present in large numbers. Eosinophilia is now accepted as positive evidence of nasal allergy. However, there can be a mixture of infection and allergy.

One method of evaluating the nasal smear is based on enumerating the eosinophils seen in four representative fields. If 10 percent or more eosinophils are seen in any of the four fields, nasal allergy is presumed to be present.

REFERENCES

1. Israel Davidsohn and John Bernard Henry (eds.), "Clinical Diagnosis by Laboratory Methods," 15th ed., p. 1273, W. B. Saunders Company, Philadelphia, 1974.
2. *Ibid.*, p. 1258.
3. Richard J. Henry, Donald C. Cannon, and James W. Winkelman, "Clinical Chemistry, Principles and Techniques," 2d ed., p. 720, Harper & Row, Hagerstown, Md., 1974.
4. Bernard F. Germain, "Synovial Fluid Analysis in the Diagnosis of Diseases of the Joints," p. 5, A Scope Publication, The Upjohn Company, March 1976.
5. *Ibid.*
6. *Ibid.*, p. 6.
7. Davidsohn and Henry, *op. cit.*, p. 1266.
8. M. Litt, Eosinophils and Antigen-Antibody Reactions, *Ann. N.Y. Acad. Sci.*, vol. 116, p. 964, 1964.

BIBLIOGRAPHY

Davidsohn, Israel and John Bernard Henry (eds.): "Clinical Diagnosis in Laboratory Methods," 15th ed., W. B. Saunders Company, Philadelphia, 1974.

Germain, Bernard F.: "Synovial Fluid Analysis in the Diagnosis of Diseases of the Joints," A Scope Publication, The Upjohn Company, March 1976.

Raphael, Stanley S. et al.: "Lynch's Medical Laboratory Technology," 3d ed., vol. II, W. B. Saunders Company, Philadelphia, 1976.

SEVEN
EXAMINATION OF THE FECES

Several useful diagnostic laboratory procedures are performed on fecal or stool specimens. The specimens are tested in various departments of the clinical laboratory, depending on the nature of the substance being tested for. Most of the determinations are usually performed in the urinalysis laboratory (more recently called the clinical microscopy laboratory).

After an initial physical examination, the substances most often looked for in an examination of the feces include blood, fat and fibers, and ova and parasites. A microbiological examination for *Salmonella* and *Shigella* sp. and Gram staining for staphylococcal overgrowth are also done. Large amounts of fat may be found to be excreted (*steatorrhea*) through microscopic analysis for fat and fibers. In such cases, tests are required to differentiate diseases of the pancreas from other causes of steatorrhea. Tests for blood are used primarily to detect gastrointestinal bleeding. It must be determined whether occult blood is caused by carcinoma, ulcer, or some other nonmalignant process. A routine examination for ova and parasites may be done in some parts of the country, where they are common, but not in others, where they are extremely rare. In general, when ova are to be looked for, the feces must be concentrated by a method such as zinc sulfate flotation. Certain parasites, especially pinworms, are commonly found by a cellophane tape method. The identification of ova and parasites is not discussed in this book. Physical examination of the feces, tests for occult blood, and the microscopic examination for fat are included in this chapter.

COLLECTION

Specimens should be collected in clean containers made of plastic-covered cardboard or in glass jars (approximately 2 ounce) with a screw cover. The specimen must be collected without being contaminated by urine, and the amount depends on the test to be done. The container should be properly labeled, including the time of collection (e.g., 24-hour collection or random specimen) and the laboratory test desired (a request slip should accompany all specimens sent to the laboratory). The patient must be properly instructed about the manner in which the specimen

is to be collected or incredible situations will occur. This instruction is usually the responsibility of the physician or nursing staff, but it may sometimes be the responsibility of the laboratory. At any rate, the basic guidelines should be stated by the laboratory.

GROSS EXAMINATION FOR PHYSICAL CHARACTERISTICS

Normal findings

A soft but formed stool specimen is normally seen. The amount varies greatly, depending on the individual and eating habits. Persons on strictly vegetarian diets normally excrete greater amounts of feces than those on diets with a high meat content. With this in mind, the amounts excreted are normally about 100–250 g/day.

The normal color of the stool specimen is brown. This color is caused by stercobilin, a pigment derived from bilirubin after conversion to urobilin. The formation of the normal color requires bacterial oxidation to take place in the colon. Without bacteria (a situation that may occur when patients are on antibiotic therapy) the stool loses its normal brown color. The normal color is also influenced by diet.

The newborn infant passes *meconium*, a viscid, elastic, greenish black material composed of amniotic fluid, biliary and intestinal secretions, and epithelial cells. In the first days after birth (neonatal period) the stool is normally soft and yellow because of the presence of unchanged bilirubin. As the child becomes older, the stools become brown and formed as solid foods are introduced and milk is decreased in the diet.

Abnormal or pathological findings

Yellow to yellow-green color

This color is seen in diarrhea, or when the normal bacterial flora is not present in the bowel, as in antibiotic therapy.

Tan, clay color, or putty color

Such specimens are seen when stercobilin is absent and there is some increase in fat. This is the very characteristic *acholic* stool seen with jaundice resulting from biliary obstruction.

Fat (gray)

The excretion of abnormally large amounts of fat in the feces is called steatorrhea. The specimens are bulky, frothy, foul-smelling, and greasy in appearance. They are associated with cystic fibrosis and with malabsorption syndromes such as celiac disease.

Black, tarry

Unusually dark specimens may be seen after the ingestion of iron or charcoal. However, bleeding from the upper gastrointestinal tract characteristically produces the dark, tarry stools of frank *melena*. The intensity of the color depends on the rate of passage through the gastrointestinal tract. Therefore, massive bleeding from the upper gastrointestinal tract may occasionally be associated with brown or reddish stools.

Blood streaks

Streaks of obvious blood on the exterior of the specimen are associated with diseases of the lower rectum and anus.

Mucus and pus

These may be seen macroscopically in strings or sometimes in balls. Mucus in the feces is seen in

inflammatory conditions such as colitis, as are blood and pus. They may also indicate a bowel tumor. Pus is seen in diseases such as ulcerative colitis and bacillary dysentery.

Gray color

This may be seen after a barium enema or a barium meal, which is used for diagnostic x-ray procedures.

Parasites

Adult roundworms or segments of tapeworms may be seen macroscopically in the feces.

HEMOGLOBIN IN FECES (OCCULT BLOOD)

Principles of tests and significance

Tests for hemoglobin in fecal specimens are often referred to as tests for *occult blood.* This is because hemoglobin may be present in the feces, as evidenced by positive chemical tests for blood, and yet not be detected by the naked eye. In other words, occult blood is hidden blood and requires a chemical test for its detection. Occasionally there will be enough blood in the feces to produce a tarry black or even bloody specimen. However, even bloody specimens should be tested chemically for occult blood. In such cases the outer portion is avoided and the central portion of the formed stool is sampled. The detection of occult blood in the feces is important in determining the cause of hypochromic anemias resulting from chronic loss of blood and in detecting ulcerative or neoplastic diseases of the gastrointestinal system. Blood in the feces may result from bleeding anywhere along the gastrointestinal tract, from the mouth to the anus.

Numerous tests have been described for the detection of hemoglobin (or blood) in both urine and feces. Most of these tests are based on the same general principles and reaction. They all make use of peroxidase activity in the heme portion of the hemoglobin molecule. The reagents most commonly used as color indicators are gum guaiac, benzidine, *o*-tolidine, and *o*-dianisidine. Benzidine is no longer recommended for tests as it is a carcinogenic reagent.

o-Tolidine may also be carcinogenic. All of the tests described require the presence of hydrogen peroxide or a suitable precursor. The peroxidase activity of the hemoglobin molecule results in the liberation of oxygen from hydrogen peroxide (H_2O_2), and the released oxygen oxidizes gum guaiac, benzidine, or *o*-tolidine to colored oxidation products, which are usually blue or green. These reactions are summarized below:

$$\text{Hemoglobin} + H_2O_2 \xrightarrow{\text{peroxidase}} \text{oxygen}$$

$$\text{Oxygen} + \text{reduced form of chromogen} \longrightarrow$$

$$\text{blue or green oxidation products}$$

The reagents that are commonly used in testing for hemoglobin vary in sensitivity. *o*-Tolidine is generally reported to be the most sensitive, benzidine is less sensitive, and gum guaiac is the least sensitive. However, there are significant discrepancies in these reports. In addition, the sensitivity of each test can be varied by changing the concentrations of the reagents and the relative amounts of the reagents and the stool specimen. The manner in which the specimen is sampled and mixed before testing also probably affects the results.

Interfering substances that may give falsely positive results include those of dietary origin with peroxidase activity, such as iron, meat, and fat, as well as copper, bismuth, bromides, iodides, Formalin, and white cells and bacteria with peroxidase activity. In general, the more sensitive a test is to hemoglobin, the less reliable it is, since it will be more likely to detect interfering substances. For this reason, gum guaiac has been considered the most reliable indicator and o-tolidine the least reliable. The gum guaiac test is the one most often used as a screening test for occult blood in feces.

Bleeding at any point in the gastrointestinal system representing as little as 2 ml of blood lost daily may be detected by the tests for occult blood. However, falsely negative results occur for unknown reasons, possibly because of inhibitors in the feces. Various systems are used in the routine examination of the feces for occult blood. In some systems, the feces must be examined on three successive days before a test may be considered negative. There is still a considerable chance that the results may be misleading, and the clinical history, physical examination, and radiological findings are necessary for the final diagnosis.

If the screening of specimens with gum guaiac gives a positive result for a person on a normal diet, certain follow-up studies must be made. They will depend on other physical and clinical findings. Often the follow-up will require collecting stool specimens after the patient has been on a diet free from red meat for at least 3 days. The patient must also exclude tooth brushing and ingestion of drugs such as aspirin, which may cause bleeding. Another follow-up that is reliable and of minimal trouble for the patient involves the use of chromium-labeled red blood cells. In this procedure, red cells are separated from the patient's blood, labeled with chromium-51, and reinjected. Stool and blood specimens are collected and assayed for radioactivity. This is an accurate way to detect bleeding in the gastrointestinal tract, although it is not a routine procedure.

Various commercial tests have been developed to test for the presence of hemoglobin in both the feces and the blood. Hematest and Occultest (Ames Co., Elkhart, Ind.) use o-tolidine as the color reagent. They have been adjusted so as not to give the falsely positive reactions typical of o-tolidine tests, although they still seem to do so. Hemoccult (Smith Kline Diagnostics, Sunnyvale, Calif.) utilizes a filter paper impregnated with gum guaiac. It seems to be a good screening test, especially because patients can easily collect and mail specimens for testing. When any of the commercial products are used, the manufacturer's directions should be followed and the literature consulted for possible reactions with interfering substances.

Gum guaiac filter paper test

Reagents

1. Glacial acetic acid.
2. Hydrogen peroxide (3 ml/dl). Dilute 10 ml of 30 ml/dl H_2O_2 to 100 ml with deionized water. Store in the refrigerator for up to 1 month.
3. Gum guaiac (3 g/dl) in 95% ethanol. Dilute 3 g of gum guaiac to 100 ml with 95% ethanol. Store in the refrigerator for up to 1 month.
4. Working reagent. Combine 1 part of gum guaiac and 1 part of hydrogen peroxide. Prepare fresh daily.

Procedure

1. Be sure the hands, equipment, and working area are clean and free from traces of blood.
2. Mix the specimen as thoroughly as possible.
3. Spread a small amount of feces on a filter paper.
4. Add two drops of glacial acetic acid.
5. Add four drops of the working guaiac-peroxide reagent.
6. Observe, grade, and report results as follows: negative, no blue color; small, faint blue color forming slowly; moderate, clear blue color appearing almost immediately but never intense; and large, intense blue color forming immediately.

Note: This procedure is usually performed using a fume hood.

Sensitivity

The gum guaiac test detects 10 mg hemoglobin per deciliter of aqueous solution.

Controls

Since there are several causes of both falsely positive and falsely negative reactions in the tests for occult blood, it is essential that both positive and negative controls be included. *Positive* controls consist of the reagents normally employed, plus blood. Whole blood is substituted for feces, and the procedure is performed as usual. If the test works, the reaction should be equivalent to a large amount of blood in the feces. If not, new working reagents should be prepared and the control retested. The positive control is used to check the reagents for falsely negative reactions. *Negative* controls consist of the reagents normally employed, without any specimen. In this case the result should be negative. If not, make new working reagents or use different filter paper. The negative control is used to check both the reagents and the filter paper for falsely positive results.

Hemoccult

Hemoccult is available as either a slide or tape dispenser that contains filter paper uniformly impregnated with guaiac. A developing solution containing a stabilized mixture of hydrogen peroxide and denatured alcohol is also supplied with the test. When a stool specimen containing occult blood is applied to the guaiac-impregnated paper, peroxidase in the specimen comes in contact with the guaiac. When the developing solution is then applied to the test paper, a reaction be-

tween the guaiac and peroxidase results in a blue or bluish green color.

The reaction requires that the blood cells be hemolyzed for proper release of peroxidase. This usually takes place when blood is present in the stool, probably because of water in the intestinal tract. However, if whole undiluted blood is applied to the test paper, the blood cells may not be hemolyzed and the reaction may be weak or atypical. A drop of water applied to the test paper to hemolyze the blood before the developing solution will alleviate this problem. A certain percentage of initially positive specimens may become negative on storage of the slides. This loss of sensitivity is a function of both the amount of blood present and the length of storage. The loss is greater at low levels of blood. Rehydration of the slide with either tap or distilled water reverses this loss of sensitivity. Therefore, a drop of water should be applied to the slide before application of the developing solution.

The test will detect *in vitro* dilutions of blood as high as 1:5000. In clinical studies where specimens were applied to the test paper and allowed to dry, as little as 2 ml of blood was detected in 100 g of feces. In tests on fresh specimens developed immediately after application of the specimen, as little as 4 ml of blood was detected in 100 g of feces. Therefore, the test is significantly more sensitive to the presence of occult blood if the specimens are allowed to dry on the slide before the developing solution is applied.

Because the reagent-impregnated paper is dry, the test paper is stable for prolonged periods when stored under normal conditions. However, it will lose sensitivity and may discolor if exposed to sunlight or another ultraviolet light source, or to extreme heat. Reagent paper that has turned blue or blue-green before use should be discarded. The developer solution evaporates if it is left uncapped. It is flammable and should not be exposed to extreme heat. Contact with the skin should be avoided.

Procedure—Slide method

Only a very small specimen, thinly applied, is necessary for the test. The test may be done by the physician during a rectal examination, by the patient after careful instruction, or in the laboratory. The reaction is more sensitive if the specimen is allowed to dry before application of the developing solution. To increase the probability of detecting occult blood in each stool, it is recommended that slides be prepared from two different parts of the stool, or that the specimen be well mixed if the test is done in the laboratory.

1. Open the perforated window in back of the slide.
2. Apply one drop of water (tap or distilled). Allow it to penetrate the specimen.
3. Apply two drops of developing solution.
4. Record the results after 30 seconds. Any trace of blue is positive for occult blood.

FECAL FAT (MICROSCOPIC EXAMINATION)

The appearance of fecal specimens with steatorrhea has already been described. The microscopic examination of a random stool specimen for the presence of increased amounts of fat can be used as a screening procedure for the detection of steatorrhea. In such an examination the specimen is observed microscopically after being treated with Sudan dyes. Fecal fat is composed of neutral fats, fatty acids, and soaps, each of which takes on a characteristic appearance when stained with Sudan dyes. Since fats are normally present in the feces, the observations should be interpreted with caution.

Reagents

1. Ethanol (95% by volume).
2. Saturated solution of Sudan III in ethanol.
3. Glacial acetic acid (36% by volume).

Neutral fat (triglycerides)

Procedure

1. Place a small amount of thoroughly mixed feces on a glass slide.
2. Add two or three drops of water to the sample and mix thoroughly with an applicator stick. If the specimen is liquid, omit the water.
3. Add two drops of 95% ethanol and mix thoroughly.
4. Add about three drops of Sudan III reagent.
5. Mix with the edge of a cover glass.
6. Apply a cover glass to the preparation and let stand for 5 minutes.
7. Examine for yellow-orange to red refractive globules of fat under the microscope, using the high-power objective (×450). Globules of fat tend to collect at the edge of the cover glass.

Discussion

Fatty acids are lightly staining flakes or needle-like crystals, which do not stain and may be missed. Soaps do not stain but appear as well-defined amorphous flakes or rounded masses of coarse crystals. Neutral fats appear as large yellow, orange, or red droplets. A few neutral fat globules are found in a normal specimen. The presence of a large amount of neutral fat may indicate that the patient has had mineral or castor oil, or used rectal suppositories.

Stools from some patients with *pancreatic disease* show a marked increase in neutral fat because of the absence of pancreatic lipase, which is necessary to digest the fat. This is often seen in children with cystic fibrosis and is confirmed with a sweat chloride test. Excess fat may also appear in feces with lipase when there is a rapid transit time through the intestine, as with some diseases of the small intestine or surgical removal of part of the intestine.

Normally, fewer than 50 droplets ranging from 1 to 4 μm in diameter are seen in each high-power field. This is approximately equivalent to 6 g of fat in 24 hours.

Total fat (as fatty acids)

Soaps and other fat combinations including triglycerides are dissociated as free fatty acids by the addition of 36% glacial acetic acid and heat. This converts the neutral fats and soaps to fatty acids and melts the fatty acids, causing them to form droplets, which stain strongly with Sudan III. The slide is examined while it is warm. After acidification and heat, up to 100 stained droplets of fat ranging from 1 to 4 μm in diameter may

normally be seen per high-power field. Patients with steatorrhea caused by a disease of the small intestine, such as celiac disease or sprue, are likely to show increases in fatty acids and soaps. This results from lack of absorption of these substances and may also be seen in acute diarrhea or after surgical removal of portions of the intestine. An increase in total fat (as fatty acid) is seen in cases of steatorrhea caused by pancreatic and liver disease where there is a lack of bile salts, and in small intestine disease.

The feces are also examined for fibers. However, undigested food particles are commonly seen, and their presence depends on many factors such as the extent of cooking of the food and the transit time through the gastrointestinal tract. The presence of fibers is therefore difficult to interpret. In adults, large numbers of undigested meat fibers are excreted when there is pancreatic disease or carcinoma of the head of the pancreas. In children, such fibers may accompany diarrhea or steatorrhea.

BIBLIOGRAPHY

Bradley, G. M.: Basic Laboratory Medicine Syllabus, University of Minnesota Medical School 1977–1978 curriculum (unpublished).

Davidsohn, Israel and John Bernard Henry (eds.): "Clinical Diagnosis by Laboratory Methods," 15th ed., W. B. Saunders Company, Philadelphia, 1974.

Drummey, G. D., J. A. Benson, Jr., and C. M. Jones: Microscopic Examination of the Stool for Steatorrhea, *N. Engl. J. Med.*, vol. 264, p. 85, 1961.

Freeman, James A. and Myrton F. Beeler: "Laboratory Medicine–Clinical Microscopy," Lea & Febiger, Philadelphia, 1974.

Hemoccult Test for Occult Blood, Smith Kline Diagnostics, Sunnyvale, Calif. (product information).

Hepler, O. E., P. Wong, and H. D. Pihl: Comparison of Tests for Occult Blood in Feces, *Am. J. Clin. Pathol.*, vol. 23, p. 1263, 1953.

Mendeloff, A. I.: Selection of a Screening Procedure for Detecting Occult Blood in Feces, *J. Am. Med. Assoc.*, vol. 152, p. 789, 1953.

Page, Lot B. and Perry J. Culver: "A Syllabus of Laboratory Examinations in Clinical Diagnosis," rev. ed., Harvard University Press, Cambridge, Mass., 1960.

EIGHT
SEROLOGY

In the department of serology reactions between antigens and antibodies are used to determine the presence of disease. The body has a unique defense system against foreign substances known as the immunologic response. Foreign substances, or antigens, are recognized by lymphoid and plasma cells. Each type of antigen stimulates the production of equally specific antibodies by various body tissues. Several methods are used in the laboratory measurement of the immune response. The techniques used in these serological determinations include precipitation, agglutination, complement fixation, cytolysis, neutralization, flocculation, and fluorescent antibody studies. Determinations of blood groups and Rh factors for persons donating or receiving blood utilize serological methods (see Chap. 9).

Generally, *antigens* are large molecules with molecular weights over 10 000; they are usually proteins. An antigen is generally described as a substance that, when injected into an animal, is recognized as foreign and—provided immunologically active cells are present—provokes an immune reaction. The immune reaction is the production of *antibodies*—substances that protect the body against the antigens. There are times, however, when antibodies are not protective, as in the case of antibody-antigen reactions that cause hay fever, rash, or anaphylactic shock. Antigenicity is not confined to proteins. Certain nonantigenic, nonprotein substances known as *haptens* may bind themselves to protein, and the resulting hapten-protein complex is antigenic.

Some antibodies occur in humans naturally as a result of exposure throughout life to bacteria and plant material, in the form of food and through inhalation and ingestion. Antibodies can also be produced in response to natural infections, as with pneumonia and typhoid fever organisms, and their production can be artificially stimulated by the injection of antigens in vaccine form. Natural and artificial infections stimulate the production of immune, or protective, antibodies.

Humans are equipped with two strong lines of defense against the invasion of foreign substances. One is a nonspecific resistance to certain diseases that comes about through physiological and anatomic attributes. The other is the formation of antibodies. Together, these systems work effectively to protect humans throughout life.

If an antibody has been formed against a foreign substance, one good way to identify the infecting organism is to identify the antibody produced in response to it. This is the basis for serological determinations. Many years ago researchers in the field of immunology showed that if a known antigen, such as a certain bacteria, is exposed in a test tube to a patient's serum containing antibodies against that antigen, a reaction (*serological reaction*) will be observed. If the specific antibody is not present in the patient's serum, no reaction will be observed.

Antibodies that have been produced in response to a specific antigenic stimulus can be identified easily in the serum. The serological reaction produces an observable change in the mixture in the form of agglutination, pre-cipitation, fluorescence capability, lysis, or complement fixation, for example. The reaction takes different forms because of variations in the condition of the antigen, the presence of saline, and the temperature.

SEROLOGICAL REACTIONS

Agglutination

Agglutination means clumping. In this type of observable serological reaction, the combination of specific antigens and antibodies results in the formation of visible clumps, which settle out of the solution. Antibodies that form clumps are called *agglutinins* and the associated antigens are called *agglutinogens.* Agglutination occurs only if the antigen is in the form of particles, such as bacteria, red blood cells, latex particles, white blood cells, or any substance that appears cloudy when suspended in saline.

Agglutination reactions are involved in immunohematologic typing procedures (see Chap. 9). Another example of agglutination is seen in the Widal test, which is used to detect agglutinins in patients with typhoid fever. In this test the titer of serum antibodies against known suspensions of organisms is measured. During the course of this disease, the antibody titer of the causative organism (*Salmonella*) rises slowly at first, increases to a maximum level, and then gradually falls to an undetectable level. The Widal reaction has usually been observed in a tube, but more recently a slide method has been introduced. Other agglutination tests are available for syphilis, rheumatoid factor, C-reactive protein, infectious mononucleosis, pregnancy testing, and cold agglutinins.

Precipitation

Precipitation may be defined as the visible result of an antigen-antibody reaction between a soluble antigen and its antiserum (serum containing antibodies). Electrolytes are also needed to bring the process to its desired conclusions, along with the proper pH and temperature of the mixture. Antibodies that react to form precipitates are called *precipitins.*

Precipitin tests are widely used in the identification of bacteria. In Lancefield's grouping method, hemolytic streptococci are classified in groups A through K by using commercial antisera. Abnormal globulins produced as a result of certain inflammatory diseases can also be identified by precipitin techniques. Certain diseases alter the quantities of some proteins found in the serum, such as immunoglobulin, haptoglobulin, and complement. These increases or decreases are valuable diagnostic tools.

If the amount of antigen is gradually decreased while the antibody concentration remains constant, a point is reached where large amounts of agglutinate or precipitate appear rapidly. Conversely, when increasing amounts of antigen are added, a point is reached where no agglutinate or precipitate is observed. An excess of antibody is known as the *prozone phenomenon.*

Fluorescent antibody studies

Antibody against insoluble or particulate antigen, such as bacteria or cellular materials, may also be detected by the *fluorescent antibody* testing method (see under Fluorescence Microscopy in Chap. 10). When this technique is employed, the insoluble antigen is fixed to a clean glass slide and the patient's serum is added. If the corresponding antibody is present in the serum, an antigen-antibody complex is formed that is invisible. To assist in observing the presence of antibody, a form of anti-gamma globulin is added that contains the dye fluorescein.[1] Anti-gamma globulin with fluorescein will attach to specific antibody because the antibody is a globulin, and it will show up as whole cells stained with fluorescein. The dye fluoresces apple green when viewed through a fluorescence microscope. If antibody is absent, the anti-gamma globulin will be removed in the washing procedure and no fluorescence will be seen. Fluorescence methods are used to detect syphilis antibodies and certain bacteria such as streptococci.

Lysis

Some serological reactions cause the destruction of red blood cells containing antigens. Such reactions are used in blood bank procedures. *Lysis*, or hemolysis of the red cells, is a positive indication that a specific antigen-antibody reaction has taken place. The lysing antibody that causes the reaction is known as a *lysin.* One form

of *Streptococcus* produces streptolysin, an antigen that can destroy human or rabbit red blood cells.

Complement fixation

A valuable but time-consuming and difficult way to detect and quantitate soluble antibody is by *complement fixation* tests. These tests detect soluble antigen by virtue of the availability of complement. Complement is a group of serum proteins that, when present or combined with antigen-antibody complexes, lyse antigen if it consists of bacteria or other cellular material. The antigen-antibody complex binds the complement present, and thus it is no longer available to promote additional antigen-antibody reactions. In the hemolysis of red cells, for example, and in the destruction of bacteria (called bacteriolysis), three elements must be present for the reaction to be observed: antigen, antibody, and complement.

Complement fixation tests involve two stages of reactions (Fig. 8-1). The first is a serological

Fig. 8-1. Complement fixation test. Antigen and antibody are incubated with complement. The indicator system, consisting of red cells coated with antibody, is added. (A) Positive reaction. When antigen and antibody are present in the test system they fix or bind the available complement and none remains to lyse the added indicator cells. (B) Negative reaction. When antigen or antibody is lacking in the test system, complement is available to lyse the sensitized indicator cells.

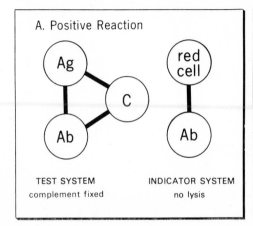

A. Positive Reaction

TEST SYSTEM
complement fixed

INDICATOR SYSTEM
no lysis

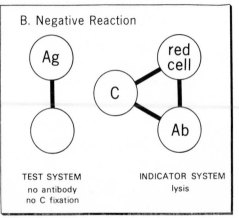

B. Negative Reaction

TEST SYSTEM
no antibody
no C fixation

INDICATOR SYSTEM
lysis

reaction between a test serum and antigen, where complement is adsorbed or bound by the antigen-antibody complex, but no visible lysis occurs. The second occurs when red cells coated with anti-red cell serum are added to the suspension. Failure to observe hemolysis is caused by the fixation of complement in the first step of the reaction. It is primarily the availability of complement in the system that determines whether lysis occurs, and the test thus indicates indirectly the presence or absence of specific antibody.

Complement fixation tests are used to identify some infectious disorders. A well-known example is the Wassermann complement fixation test for syphilis, which is now generally outdated.

SPECIMENS FOR SEROLOGY

Collection

Blood specimens should be collected before a meal to avoid the presence of chyle, an emulsion of fat globules that often appears in serum during digestion. Blood should be collected by venipuncture, using sterile needles and clean, plain collecting tubes (no anticoagulant). If syringes and needles are used, care must be taken to allow the blood to run gently into the tube to avoid rupturing cells. Capillary blood may be drawn into a plain capillary tube and allowed to clot. Care should be taken to avoid lysis of red cells since this might render the serum unstable. The specimen should stand undisturbed at room temperature for at least 30 minutes to allow for complete clotting and separation of cellular elements. Spinal fluid and other body fluids can also be used for serological testing. Occasionally, tests will require plasma or whole blood.

Preparation of serum

After the clot has completely formed (30 minutes to 1 hour is usually sufficient), the serum should be separated from the cells as quickly as possible by centrifugation. Care should be taken to transfer the serum to a fresh, clean container. Until the testing is done, serum specimens should be refrigerated (4-6°C). Specimens must not be hemolyzed and they must be free from particulate matter. Contamination with alkali or acid must be avoided as these substances have a denaturing effect on serum proteins and make the specimens useless for serological testing. Excessive heat and bacterial contamination are also to be avoided. Heat coagulates the proteins and bacterial growth alters protein molecules.[2]

Serum specimens can be stored in a refrigerator for up to 72 hours. If a longer storage period is necessary, the serum should be frozen. Specimens to be frozen must be properly sealed and labeled.

Specimens for cold agglutinin testing must be drawn into warmed syringes and *not* stored in the refrigerator.

The complement in serum must be inactivated for most serological testing. To inactivate complement, the tubes of serum are placed in a hot-water bath at 56°C for 30 minutes. If the protein complement is not inactivated it will promote lysis of the red cells and other types of cells and can therefore produce invalid results.

COMMON SEROLOGICAL TESTS

Serological tests are commonly done to assist in the diagnosis and treatment of many diseases and disorders. Among the more important and generally interesting reactions that are studied are those for syphilis, infectious mononucleosis (heterophil antibodies), C-reactive protein, cold agglutinins, febrile disease antibodies, pregnancy tests, lupus erythematosus cell factor, influenza antibodies, antibodies in thyroid disorders, and rheumatoid factors. Some of these will be discussed in the following sections.

The principles of serological testing are employed in tissue typing for organ transplantation. The immune mechanism is becoming recognized as an important factor in many disease states; it is a rapidly expanding avenue of research.

Syphilis serology

Serological tests are among the most important diagnostic procedures for syphilis. The laboratory results, together with clinical signs and the patient's history, aid the physician in deciding whether the patient has had a syphilitic condition. Syphilis tests were some of the first serological determinations done. They were introduced by Wassermann in 1906, when syphilis was a great threat to humans and many researchers had devoted years to the problem of finding a laboratory diagnosis for syphilis. To many, the terms syphilis and serology have become synonymous.

Syphilis is still a great medical problem. In the United States more than 3000 people a year die of syphilis; more than 26 000 are currently in mental hospitals as a result of syphilitic infections; an estimated 1 200 000 need treatment for syphilis; and of syphilitic cases, 1 in 200 will become blind, 1 in 50 will become insane, 1 in 25 will be crippled or incapacitated in some way, and 1 in 15 will become a syphilitic heart victim.[3] Early detection of and treatment of syphilis are of critical importance to prevent the infection from spreading and doing further harm to the patient.

Adequate diagnosis and treatment are important in all three stages of syphilis. The first stage extends from the initial inoculation with the

bacterium, a spirochete called *Treponema pallidum*, by direct contact (usually sexual) with an infectious lesion, to the formation of the chancre at the initial port of entry. The chancre is a primary lesion that appears 3-4 weeks after the initial inoculation. In this first stage, both the blood and the local lesion are infective. The sores often heal by themselves. In the second stage, a rash of the skin and mucous membranes appears. Exudates from the lesion are full of the syphilitic spirochetes. The patient is still highly contagious. Specific antibodies to the spirochete begin to appear about 4-6 weeks after the initial inoculation or 1-3 weeks after the appearance of the primary sore or chancre. In the third, or latent, stage of the disease, no clinical signs or symptoms are seen; it is recognized only by serological tests. If the disease goes untreated, severe complications can occur, as evidenced by the sad statistics given above.

In addition to specific antibodies to *T. pallidum*, patients with syphilitic infection respond immunologically by producing a nonspecific reagin antibody.

Tests for syphilis

The purpose of all tests for syphilis is to detect either reagin or true specific antibodies to *T. pallidum* in the blood of patients with the disease. Tests are of two types: nontreponemal tests, which use either cardiolipin or lipoid extracts as antigens and detect reagin, and treponemal tests, which use treponemal antigens and pick up specific antibodies.

Several treponemal tests for syphilis are designed to detect specific antibodies to *T. pallidum*. Live or dead (preserved) *T. pallidum* or extracts of the organism are used as antigens. One test—the fluorescent treponemal antibody absorption test (FTA-ABS)—is a reliable method of confirming syphilis (see under Fluorescent Antibody Studies).

Nontreponemal tests for syphilis are also of two main types: flocculation (using test tube or slide methods) or complement fixation. The flocculation tests include the VDRL (Venereal Disease Research Laboratory), Kahn, Kline, Hinton, RPR (rapid plasma reagin), and Mazzini tests. The Kolmer complement fixation test is the one used most commonly. The VDRL and RPR tests will be described in this section.

Venereal Disease Research Laboratory (VDRL) flocculation test

This test is the one most widely used today. It is done with cardiolipin-lecithin-cholesterol antigen and heat-inactivated serum from the patient, or with spinal fluid. It is a tube or a slide test, commonly the latter. Quality control measures must be employed to ensure reproducible and reliable results from laboratory to laboratory. Technique must be strictly adhered to and standardized reagents must be used to ensure good results. Positive and negative control sera of predetermined reactivity indicate when corrective action should be taken. Since this tests for nonspecific reagin, antibodies other than those of syphilis may react with the antigen. The test is therefore not 100 percent specific for syphilis, but it is practical, inexpensive, and reproducible.

The reagents necessary for the VDRL flocculation test include buffered saline solution and a stock antigen solution consisting of an alcoholic solution of cardiolipin, lecithin, and cholesterol. This stock antigen is available commercially in sealed ampules and is made into the working solution by adding buffered saline. The manufacturer's directions must be followed exactly. Some laboratories still prepare their own reagents, and formulas for them can be found in serology textbooks.[4] Positive and negative control sera are available commercially.

The special glass slides that are used contain 12 paraffin or ceramic rings in which the suspensions of specimen and reagents are placed and mixed. A hypodermic needle capable of delivering 60 drops per milliliter is attached to a syringe for delivering the antigen suspension. The patient's serum is delivered onto the glass slide from a 0.1- to 0.2-ml pipet calibrated in 0.01-ml divisions, or from a 0.05-ml disposable pipet. A 56°C water bath is used to inactivate the protein complement in the serum. A special machine is employed to rotate the mixture on the glass slide before reading the results. This serological rotator is set to revolve at 180 r/min. It facilitates complete and consistent mixing of sample and antigen.

Procedure[5]

1. Pipet 0.05 ml of the heat-inactivated serum from the patient into one ring of a slide. Pipet control sera in the same manner.
2. Add one drop ($\frac{1}{60}$ ml) of antigen emulsion onto each sample of serum.
3. Rotate slides for 4 minutes at 180 r/min on the rotator.
4. Read tests under the microscope immediately after rotation, using the ×10 objective. The antigen particles appear as short rods at this magnification.
5. Report as follows: nonreactive, no clumping or slight roughness; weakly reactive, small clumps; and reactive, medium to large clumps.

Rapid plasma reagin (RPR) test

RPR tests were developed as screening procedures for use in "field" situations, where equipment may be limited.[6] These tests are available commercially in kits that contain all the necessary reagents. A positive reaction with the RPR method must be followed up with a VDRL test, as RPR tests are more sensitive and less specific than the VDRL test. In one RPR test a special card with depressions on it is used. Three drops of blood from a finger puncture are allowed to fall into the depression on the card that contains an anticoagulant and a lectin (which causes agglutination of the red and white blood cells). After the plasma and cells have separated, 0.03 ml of the plasma is collected in a special capillary tube, placed onto an area of another plastic-coated card, and one drop ($\frac{1}{70}$ ml) of antigen suspension containing charcoal is added, using a special needle and dispensing bottle. The card is tilted for 4 minutes and read for agglutination, which appears on the card as black clumps against a white background. The manufacturer's instructions for the RPR test should be followed carefully.

C-reactive protein

C-reactive protein (CRP) was first recognized in 1930 as a constituent of the serum of patients with acute pneumonia that formed a precipitate with the C polysaccharide of the pneumococcus. This protein is found in the serum of persons suffering from acute phases of infections other than pneumonia and noninfectious inflammatory conditions. It is the basis for a capillary tube precipitation test and a rapid latex agglutination slide test that aid in the diagnosis of rheumatic fever and other inflammatory conditions. CRP is not found in clinically significant amounts in normal serum, and it disappears when the inflammatory condition has subsided.

As CRP is found in many infections and in noninfectious diseases, it is nonspecific, and its presence in the blood is a sensitive but nonspecific indicator of infection, inflammation, or tissue damage. The presence of CRP is clinically important even when it cannot be associated with a specific disease. It is consistently found in bacterial infections (particularly the colon-typhoid group), active rheumatic fever, acute myocardial infarction, and widespread malignant diseases, and is commonly found in active rheumatoid arthritis, viral infections, and tuberculosis.[7]

Test for C-reactive protein (capillary tube precipitation test)

The original method devised by Anderson and McCarty or a modification of it is used.[8] The method consists of observing and measuring the precipitate formed when CRP antiserum and patient's serum are mixed in a capillary tube. After a period of incubation, the degree of precipitation is observed and recorded for a positive test. A control serum should be included with the test serum.

Procedure[9]

1. Collect a fasting specimen of blood, allow it to clot, and separate the cells from the serum.

2. Draw up the CRP antiserum about 1.0–1.5 cm into the capillary tube. Wipe off the outside of the tube to remove excess antiserum.

3. Place the capillary tube into the patient's serum and draw up a volume equal to the volume of CRP antiserum in the previous step. The patient's serum must be in contact with the antiserum. Air pockets between the patient's serum and the test serum should be avoided.

4. Slowly invert the tube several times and allow the liquid contents to flow back and forth. Thorough mixing is important.

5. Place the tube in a Plasticine block or rack with the large air space toward the bottom. The meniscus of the tube should be above the Plasticine.

6. Leave the tube in an incubator at 37°C for 2 hours, followed by overnight incubation at 4°C.

7. Make a qualitative reading after the 2-hour incubation period by holding the tube between a light source and the eye. The presence of CRP is indicated by a white precipitate in the tube.

8. Make a semiquantitative reading after the overnight incubation by measuring the height of precipitate in the tube in millimeters. Read the amount of precipitation as follows: no precipitation, negative; slight precipitation, trace; 1 mm, 1+; 2 mm, 2+; 3 mm, 3+; and 4 mm or more, 4+.

9. Interpret these results as follows: absence of precipitation, no CRP present; and precipitation, CRP present.

Cold agglutinins

In the early 1940s, agglutinins were discovered in the serum of patients with primary atypical pneumonia, which agglutinated red blood cells of all blood groups at 0°C. Because these antibodies reacted only at low temperatures (0–10°C), they were called cold agglutinins (CA). They did not agglutinate the same red cells at 37°C. CAs are beta or gamma globulins that react in saline. They are nonspecific in their reactions because they react well with all red cell types. Red cell walls contain lipoid material that acts as an antigen or reactive site for CAs.

Normal persons can have CA titers up to 1:28, but more often a normal titer is approximately 1:8. CAs are found regularly in the blood of persons with diseases such as primary atypical pneumonia, tonsillitis, African trypanosomiasis, and staphylococcemia. High CA titers are often found in patients who are pregnant or who have cirrhosis of the liver, emboli of the veins or pulmonary system, influenza, or other acute respiratory infections.

Special precautions should be taken when drawing the blood specimen for CA tests. The syringes and needles, as well as the collecting tubes, should be warmed at 37°C before use in the venipuncture. The specimen should be kept warm in a container of some sort while it is delivered to the laboratory. In testing for cold agglutinins, the blood sample must be kept warm, preferably near 37°C, in a water bath. After the clot has completely retracted, the serum and cells are separated by centrifugation. The serum is removed and used in the test. If the test cannot be done within 2 days, the serum may be frozen.

A serial tube dilution procedure of Horstmann and Tatlock is generally used, with fresh human group O red cells as the antigen.[10] The tubes are incubated overnight in the refrigerator, and the presence of agglutination is determined before the cells are warmed. All positive tubes are then incubated at 37°C for 30 minutes. If the agglu-tination is caused by cold agglutinins, it will disappear or disperse on heating, whereas other antibody-mediated agglutination will not. To interpret the results, the titer is observed after incubation in the refrigerator. The titer is the highest serum dilution exhibiting 1+ or greater agglutination (1+ is the least amount of visible clumping). A titer of 1:32 to 1:64 in a single specimen from a convalescing patient is significant.

Antistreptococcic antibodies (ASO)

When humans are infected with group A streptococci (Lancefield's classification), enzymes are produced by the organism. One of the many enzymes produced by group A streptococci is called *streptolysin O*. This enzyme is capable of lysing red blood cells. When the organisms that produce streptolysin O are grown in a special broth culture and the broth is filtered after growth, the filtrates contain streptolysin O. Infection with group A streptococci results in the production of streptolysin O in the body. This acts as an antigen, stimulating the immune mechanism to develop antistreptolysin O (ASO) antibody. Observation of a high titer indicates that the organism is present and is causing disease.

When found in large amounts, ASO antibody is useful in diagnosing rheumatic fever, erythema nodosum, and acute glomerulonephritis, which are all diseases resulting from group A streptococci. Thus, ASO levels in serum have become widely used as evidence of a recent streptococcal infection.

The ASO antibody is a globulin, occurring mostly in the gamma globulin fraction of the serum. It can combine with and fix streptolysin O, neutralizing it *in vitro* and making it incapable of lysing red cells. The serological test used for the detection of ASO relies on several principles: (1) ASO can be specifically fixed with the antigen streptolysin O, inhibiting its hemolytic activity; (2) the amount of ASO can be estimated by serial dilution of the patient's serum in the presence of constant volumes of streptolysin O to the point where there is still complete prevention of hemolysis; and (3) the presence of ASO in the serum is directly related to the production of streptolysin O by the streptococcal bacteria in the infected patient. If no bacteria are present, or if they are eliminated, the ASO titer soon decreases. It is possible to find significant levels of ASO antibodies in healthy persons. Titers also vary with age, school-age children commonly having higher titers because of their continual exposure to streptococcal organisms. No normal ASO titer has been established, as there are so many variables. Consequently, the results of ASO titer determinations must be interpreted with caution.

Specimens for the ASO titer test should be collected aseptically, if possible, and the serum stored in a refrigerator until it is tested. If a specimen looks cloudy (contaminated), chylous (fatty), or red-tinged (hemolyzed), it should not be used for this test, as erroneous results will be obtained. Fresh-frozen or inactivated sera may be used for the ASO test.

The method that has been used routinely for years to measure the ASO titer involves a serial tube dilution technique.[11] Antigen for the procedure is obtained from the broth of an 18-hour culture of group A streptococci mixed with serial dilutions of the patient's serum and buffer. These mixtures are incubated at 37°C for 15 minutes, and a 5 percent suspension of human group O or rabbit red blood cells is then added. The tubes are reincubated at 37°C for 45 minutes, centrifuged for 1 minute at 1500 r/min, and read for hemolysis in the supernatant fluid. The end point, or titer, is the highest serum dilution that gives no hemolysis (that is, in which all the streptolysin O has been inactivated by combination with the ASO). The titer is reported in Todd units. The value in Todd units for each dilution is the reciprocal of that dilution.

Most healthy persons have ASO titers of up to 200 Todd units. Titers of over 200 Todd units

are considered abnormal, and titers of 300 or more Todd units may indicate active rheumatic fever or acute glomerulonephritis.[12]

Patients with complications of streptococcal infections that do not produce or discharge pus (nonsuppurative), such as rheumatic fever and acute glomerulonephritis, usually have a higher incidence of elevated ASO titers and higher numerical titers than patients with uncomplicated streptococcal infections.

Febrile disease antibodies

The etiology or cause of an infectious disease is usually determined by isolating and confirming the pathogen. An indirect method is sometimes needed, however, especially when the patient is observed late in the disease (particularly if antimicrobial therapy has partly suppressed the invading organism), when culture methods do not permit growth from very small numbers of bacteria, or when special growth requirements of certain bacteria have not been fulfilled. When these conditions exist, it is important to have a means of determining whether antibodies produced during the infection are present in the patient's serum. Detection of antibodies in the serum can also be used to confirm the pathogen already isolated.

Probably even more valuable than the detection of antibodies in the patient's serum is the titer of the serum. The titer is the highest dilution of the serum that will cause agglutination, or some other observable serological reaction, in the presence of the specific antigen. Blood should be tested during the acute phase of the disease and again several weeks later (usually after about 2 weeks). Many antibodies can be detected during infectious diseases; some arise in direct response to the invading pathogen, and others appear to have no direct relation to the causative organism.

Establishing the titer of the patient's serum antibody by agglutination with suspensions of known bacterial cells or antigens is a valuable diagnostic tool in fevers of unknown origin. These tests determine the greatest dilution of the patient's serum that will cause agglutination of a known bacterial antigen. The term *febrile* is associated with fever and fever-producing infections. Diseases causing febrile symptoms include brucellosis, salmonellosis, typhoid fever, paratyphoid fever, and certain rickettsial infections such as typhus fevers. The organisms causing these diseases are the antigens in febrile agglutination tests.

In all febrile agglutination tests, a positive reaction (agglutination) occurs when the test antigen is added to undiluted serum containing a specific antibody. To determine how much antibody is present in a patient's serum, the serum is diluted and each dilution is treated with the same test antigen. The process of agglutination usually takes place in two stages: the primary stage is when the antibody is adsorbed onto the surface of the test antigen, and the secondary stage is when the antibody-coated antigen particles agglutinate. The secondary stage depends on the presence of an electrolyte, usually saline.

The Widal reaction (already described under Agglutination) is used for the diagnosis of typhoid and paratyphoid infections. The Weil-Felix reaction is used in the diagnosis of rickettsial diseases such as typhus fever.

Pregnancy tests

Serological tests are done frequently in the laboratory to detect pregnancy in the early stages. Laboratory tests for pregnancy are based on the fact that during pregnancy, the placenta produces a hormone called chorionic gonadotropin. This hormone rapidly disappears after delivery. Human chorionic gonadotropin (HCG) is also produced in other conditions, as in the presence of a hydatidiform mole, choriocarcinoma, and in malignant teratomas of the ovaries and testes. In pregnancy, HCG is produced by the Langhans' cells of the developing placenta. It

is a glycoprotein with a molecular weight of about 30 000.

At about the eighth week of gestation, peak production of HCG is attained, and it is then present in the plasma at a concentration of about 25 000 international units (IU) per liter; the 24-hour urinary excretion amounts to about 30 000 IU.[13] (The international unit is defined as the specific gonadotropic activity of 0.1 mg of dried standard kept at the National Institutes of Health, London.[14]) After the eighth week of gestation HCG production sharply declines, until by the twelfth week the plasma level is about 7000 IU per liter and the daily urinary excretion is about 7000 IU. These lower values are then maintained for the remainder of pregnancy until the time of delivery, after which they disappear within 72 hours.

The presence of HCG is usually measured in the urine because a urine sample is so easy to obtain. Laboratory tests for pregnancy are generally used to detect HCG no earlier than 10 days after the last missed menstrual period and are used through the first trimester, or to about the twelfth week of pregnancy. After the first trimester, the levels of HCG may be undetectable by routine laboratory methods.

Early methods for the determination of pregnancy were biological ones that involved the use of animals. These tests were costly and very time-consuming. Test results were not available for several days, and often the animals had to be sacrificed to carry out the determination. Early biological tests employing animals, usually frogs, toads, rabbits, or rats, were the Aschheim-Zondek test and the Friedman test. The accuracy, economy, and convenience of immunologic tests for pregnancy have made animal tests a thing of the past in most laboratories.

Immunologic pregnancy tests are done in one of two ways. They differ in the carrier for the external source of HCG, which is either latex particles or red blood cells. Rapid slide agglutination or test tube agglutination methods are usually used. A variety of commercial kits are available for either method. The kits also include positive and negative controls, sensitized particles, and antiserum.

Most of the available commercial tests are slide tests and are based on the inhibition of latex particle agglutination. They are generally two-stage procedures. The accuracy of the commercial immunologic pregnancy tests depends on several factors. The manufacturer's directions must be followed carefully, the reagents must be properly shipped and stored, and the specimens must be properly collected and delivered promptly to the laboratory for testing. Other important factors are the stage of pregnancy, whether the pregnancy is normal or abnormal, the presence of interfering substances in the urine (including drugs, proteins, and red cells), the sensitivity and specificity of the assay procedure, and the use of quality control programs.

The two main types of pregnancy tests involve latex particle agglutination or hemagglutination inhibition. In the first of these methods, the HCG in the patient's urine specimen is treated with anti-HCG during the first stage of the procedure. Anti-HCG is manufactured by injecting purified HCG into animals (rabbits); the animal produces the specific antibody to HCG in its serum. If the patient's urine contains HCG (because of pregnancy or for one of the other reasons mentioned earlier), an antigen-antibody reaction occurs. In the second stage of the procedure, HCG-coated latex particles are added. If the antigen-antibody reaction occurred in the first stage, no agglutination will be observed because there is no more antibody to react with the coated latex particles. Therefore, a negative agglutination reaction is positive for pregnancy. If agglutination does occur, the result is negative for pregnancy. This method is usually carried out on a slide.

The second main type of pregnancy test is a hemagglutination inhibition method. This is also a two-stage method and can be carried out in a small test tube. The HCG in the patient's urine will neutralize anti-HCG antiserum that is added to the sample (again, an antigen-antibody reaction occurs if HCG is present in the specimen). Red cells coated with HCG are next added to the tube, and the tube is observed for agglutination. If the HCG in the patient's urine has reacted with the anti-HCG in the first stage, no agglutination will be observed in the second stage when the coated red cells are added. Unagglutinated red cells settle in a ring in the bottom of the tube. Agglutinated red cells settle in a button. A positive test for pregnancy is therefore reported when no agglutination is observed in the second stage of the test. A negative test is reported when agglutination occurs in the second stage. This test may be used with both urine and serum samples. For quantitation of HCG, a 24-hour urine specimen is required.

Since detergents may interfere with results, the specimen should be collected in a disposable urine container if possible. If these are not available, the patient must be instructed to use a clean rinsed container that does not contain traces of detergent or other substances that might interfere with the test. For all HCG tests an early morning urine sample is best. The specific gravity of the specimen should be at least 1.010. HCG is lost during storage, so the test should be done as soon as possible; otherwise the specimen may be preserved by freezing. The urine should be fresh and clear. The presence of hematuria or proteinuria may cause falsely positive results. Phenothiazine or promethazine drugs may also cause falsely positive results.

The stage of pregnancy has a marked influence on the test results, especially on the incidence of falsely negative results. Between the seventh or eighth and twelfth weeks of gestation, even a relatively insensitive assay will be almost 100 percent positive. If the assays are made before the sixth week of gestation, even the most sensitive assay may show an appreciable number of false negatives. Since the levels of HCG fall after the first trimester, falsely negative results may occur in the obviously pregnant individual.

A minimum quality control program for HCG assays requires that each assay be done in duplicate, that known negative and positive samples be assayed to check the system, and that tests be done regularly with samples of different, known HCG levels to check the low and high sensitivity of the system.

The most common reason for a positive test is pregnancy, but greatly increased levels of HCG may be seen in other instances. An increase in the level of HCG after the removal of a hydatidiform mole, for example, would indicate either that the mole was not completely removed, or that it was malignant and is redeveloping. The test for HCG is therefore a valuable tool for purposes other than the confirmation of pregnancy.

Heterophil antibodies in infectious mononucleosis

Infectious mononucleosis is an important acute infectious disease, probably viral in origin, that is represented by a relatively well-defined hematologic picture (see under Examination of the Blood Film in Chap. 3). Three distinct groups of antibodies are found in infectious mononucleosis: heterophil antibodies, Epstein-Barr virus (EBV) antibodies, and multiple autoantibodies, isoantibodies, and heteroantibodies. Heterophil antibodies are antibodies that react with an antigen entirely different from and phylogenetically unrelated to the antigen responsible for their production.[15] They are agglutinins that react particularly to sheep and horse red cells and are mainly class G immunoglobulins (IgG). Heterophil antibodies are detected by the Paul-Bunnell test.

Infectious mononucleosis is now thought to be caused by the EBV, a member of the herpes group of viruses. Antibodies to this virus are produced early in the disease and can be detected by complement fixation tests and im-

munofluorescence techniques. Demonstration of EBV antibodies is a complicated process and is beyond the scope of most routine laboratories. Heterophil antibodies are much more easily detected, and for this reason routine tests for the presence of heterophil antibodies are used for the diagnosis of infectious mononucleosis, along with hematologic findings.

Heterophil antibodies are present in low titer in the serum of normal persons and are known as Forssman antibodies. They resemble the antibodies found in infectious mononucleosis in that they agglutinate sheep red cells, but differ from them in that they are absorbed by an emulsion of guinea pig kidney, which is rich in Forssman antigen, and are not absorbed by beef cells, which are poor in Forssman antigen. In cases of serum sickness, or sensitization to animal (usually horse) serum, a further type of sheep red cell agglutination antibody is found and may be present in high titer. However, this is again distinguished from the antibody of infectious mononucleosis by being absorbed by guinea pig kidney, and from Forssman antibodies by being absorbed by beef red cells.[16] This is summarized in Table 8-1. This comparison was devised by Davidsohn in 1935 to 1937 and is used today as the basis for presumptive and differential tests.

The sheep cell agglutinins of infectious mononucleosis can be distinguished from those of serum sickness and other conditions by means of a differential test, using absorption with guinea

TABLE 8-1. Comparison of Forssman, serum sickness, and infectious mononucleosis antibodies

	Absorbed by	
Antibody	Guinea pig kidney	Beef red blood cells
Forssman	Yes	No
Serum sickness	Yes	Yes
Infectious mononucleosis	No	Yes

pig kidney and beef red cell antigens. The antibody that can be removed by absorption with guinea pig kidney is known as the Forssman antibody, and the guinea pig kidney as the Forssman antigen. The classical sheep red cell agglutination test is carried out in two steps: the presumptive test of Paul and Bunnell, and the differential test of Paul, Bunnell, and Davidsohn. These are the reference tests from which the rapid testing procedures have evolved. Modifications of these classical procedures utilize horse red cells instead of sheep red cells.

Under normal circumstances, rapid screening tests for infectious mononucleosis are done for the presence of heterophil antibodies. Horse red cells are usually used rather than sheep red cells, as they are more sensitive to heterophil antibodies. Persons suffering from infectious mononucleosis begin developing heterophil antibodies shortly after the appearance of the symptoms, usually during the first 2 weeks. Highest titers are found during the second and third weeks of the illness. The titer bears no relationship, however, to the severity of the illness. As a rule, heterophil sheep cell agglutinins appear in only 50–80 percent of cases of infectious mononucleosis, so negative results can be obtained when the disease is present. Negative tests therefore do not rule out the possibility of the disease.

The test for heterophil antibodies is of confirmatory diagnostic importance in cases of infectious mononucleosis with typical clinical and hematologic findings. It is of a deciding diagnostic importance early in the disease when there are unusual clinical findings and hematologic signs, some of which may be caused by complicating factors.

Recently, faster and easier screening tests have been introduced commercially and have replaced the laborious presumptive and differential tests in many laboratories. One such test is the spot test of Lee et al.[17] These rapid slide screening tests are based on the following principles: (1) the use of horse red cells instead of sheep red cells makes the test more sensitive and thus is espe-

cially valuable for low-titer serum found in the early stages of the disease; (2) the unwashed preserved horse red cells remain in a usable condition for at least 3 months and give stronger and quicker agglutination with infectious mononucleosis serum than do horse red cells preserved with Formalin; (3) some noninfectious mononucleosis serum also has a high horse agglutinin titer, and therefore serological tests cannot depend on titers alone; and (4) fine suspensions of guinea pig kidney and of beef red cell stromata give satisfactory instant absorption of antibodies and a clear-cut differentiation between infectious and noninfectious mononucleosis serum.[18]

These tests are done on a slide. The serum from the patient is mixed thoroughly with guinea pig kidney on one spot of the slide and with beef red cell stromata on another spot. The unwashed horse red cells (preserved) are added immediately to both spots. These reagents are available commercially in the form of test kits. Directions must be followed carefully. Agglutination is observed on both spots of the slide 1 minute after the final mixing. If agglutination is stronger on the spot where the guinea pig kidney suspension was mixed with the patient's serum, the test is positive. If it is stronger on the spot where the beef red cells were mixed with the patient's serum, the test is considered negative. If the agglutination is equal on both spots, the test is negative. If no agglutination appears on either spot, the test is negative. One commercially available test kit·utilizing this principle is called Mono-Spot and is manufactured by Ortho Diagnostics, Raritan, N.J.

The glass slides used for these rapid screening tests must be carefully cleaned under running water. Use of detergent could cause errors in the results. Most of the widely used immunologic assays for infectious mononucleosis are highly sensitive. It is still necessary, however, to use adequate and proper control programs as the only dependable method of detecting sources of technical errors. When the results are not clear-cut, it is always important to repeat them and to conduct additional dependable serological tests. Several tests are available. Repeating tests at a later date is also helpful.

REFERENCES

1. Leila, J. Walker and Howard Taub, "Fundamental Skills in Serology," p. 6, Charles C Thomas, Springfield, Ill., 1976.
2. Clois W. Bennett, "Clinical Serology," 7th printing, pp. 234–235, Charles C Thomas, Springfield, Ill., 1975.
3. *Ibid.*, p. 34.
4. *Ibid.*, pp. 56–58.
5. *Ibid.*, pp. 58–59.
6. Israel Davidsohn and John Bernard Henry (eds.), "Clinical Diagnosis by Laboratory Methods," 15th ed., p. 1221, W. B. Saunders Company, Philadelphia, 1974.
7. Bennett, *op. cit.*, p. 119.
8. H. C. Anderson and M. McCarty, Determination of the C-Reactive Protein in the Blood as a Measure of the Disease Process in Acute Rheumatic Fever, *Am. J. Med.*, vol. 8, p. 455, 1950.
9. Bennett, *op. cit.*, pp. 122–123.
10. D. M. Horstmann and H. Tatlock, Cold Agglutinin—A Diagnostic Aid in Certain Types of Primary Atypical Pneumonia, *J. Am. Med. Assoc.*, vol. 122, pp. 369–370, 1943.
11. L. A. Rantz and Randall, A Modification of the Technique for the Determination of the Antistreptolysin O Titer, *Proc. Soc. Exp. Biol. Med.*, vol. 59, p. 22, 1945.
12. Bennett, *op. cit.*, p. 141.
13. Stanley S. Raphael et al., "Lynch's Medical Laboratory Technology," 3d ed., vol. I, p. 527, W. B. Saunders Company, Philadelphia, 1976.
14. Davidsohn and Henry, *op. cit.*, p. 1281.
15. Bennett, *op. cit.*, p. 171.
16. Raphael et al., *op. cit.*, vol. II, p. 1102.
17. C. L. Lee, I. Davidsohn, and O. Panczyszyn, Horse Agglutinins in Infectious Mononucleosis. II. The Spot Test. *Am. J. Clin. Pathol.*, vol. 49, p. 12, 1968.
18. Davidsohn and Henry, *op. cit.*, pp. 264–265.

BIBLIOGRAPHY

Bennett, Clois W.: "Clinical Serology," 7th printing, Charles C Thomas, Springfield, Ill., 1975.

Carpenter, Philip L.: "Immunology and Serology," 3d ed., W. B. Saunders Company, Philadelphia, 1975.

Davidsohn, Israel and John Bernard Henry (eds.): "Clinical Diagnosis by Laboratory Methods," 15th ed., W. B. Saunders Company, Philadelphia, 1974.

Davidsohn, I., K. Stern, and C. Kashuiagi: The Differential Test for Infectious Mononucleosis, *Am. J. Clin. Pathol.*, vol. 21, p. 1101, 1951.

Galloway, E.: Comparison of Three Slide Tests for Infectious Mononucleosis with Davidsohn's Presumptive and Differential Heterophil Test, *Can. J. Med. Technol.*, vol. 31, p. 197, 1969.

Hyun, Bong Hak, John K. Ashton, and Kathleen Dolan: "Practical Hematology," W. B. Saunders Company, Philadelphia, 1975.

Raphael, Stanley S. et al.: "Lynch's Medical Laboratory Technology," 3d ed., vols. I and II, W. B. Saunders Company, Philadelphia, 1976.

Roitt, Ivan M.: "Essential Immunology," 3d ed., Blackwell Scientific Publications, Oxford, 1977.

Rose, Noel R. and Herman Friedman (eds.): "Manual of Clinical Immunology," American Society for Microbiology, Washington, D.C., 1976.

Walker, Leila J. and Howard Taub: "Fundamental Skills in Serology," Charles C Thomas, Springfield, Ill., 1976.

Wittman, Karl S. and John C. Thomas: "Medical Laboratory Skills," McGraw-Hill Book Company, New York, 1977.

NINE
IMMUNOHEMATOLOGY
(BLOOD BANKING)

The field of immunohematology has advanced rapidly in recent years, and all indications point to further advancement as techniques in laboratory medicine continue to change. Since 1951, new discoveries have been made at a rapid pace and the nature of the immunologic response to different antigens has been shown to be vastly more complicated than was at first supposed. Before 1951, nine independent blood group systems had been discovered. These important systems and their approximate dates of discovery are ABO (1900), MN (1927), P (1927), Rh (from rhesus) (1939), Lutheran (1945), Kell (1946), Lewis (1946), Duffy (1950), and Kidd (1951). The complexity of the red cell and its antigenic polymorphism seems almost endless, and it is expected that as methodology for studying the red cell antigen-antibody reactions improves, the boundaries of knowledge will continue to expand.

A study of the immunologic reactions of blood cells is critical when therapeutic replacement of blood is necessary. The many possible antigen-antibody reactions that can occur must be anticipated and tested for by the laboratory procedures available in the immunohematology laboratory. In many diseases and health problems, therapeutic administration of blood is indicated. Severe illness and death are closely associated with loss of blood, which impairs the ability of the circulatory system to deliver adequate amounts of oxygen to the body cells and critically upsets the delicate homeostatic water and acid-base balance of body fluids. Blood loss may be caused by hemorrhage, excessive destruction of red cells, or the body's inability to replenish its own blood supply. In specific instances, administration of whole blood or its components is indicated. Whole blood or plasma, for example, may be given in cases

of shock resulting from hemorrhage. Packed red cells are given in chronic anemia or carbon monoxide poisoning. Serum albumin is given in hypoproteinemia. The technique of replacing whole blood and its components is known as blood *transfusion*. The procedures involved in collecting, storing, processing, and distributing blood are called *blood banking*. The techniques and procedures involving the study of the immunologic responses of blood cells are called *immunohematology*.

Immunohematology and blood banking are unlike other fields of clinical laboratory investigation. Although accuracy is always important in the laboratory, it is absolutely essential in blood banking. Even the smallest error can directly result in the death of a patient from a hemolytic transfusion reaction. As R. R. Race says, "Blood group tests are different from most laboratory tests used in medicine in a vital way—the reported result must be correct, for the wisest physician cannot protect his patient from the consequences of a blood grouping error."[1]

This chapter is meant only as a very general introduction to the subject of blood banking. It is definitely not sufficient preparation for work in blood banking laboratories. Specific blood banking procedures will not be presented; only principles will be discussed. Several excellent texts are available in the field of blood banking; however, most of them seem complex (even unintelligible) to the person who has no background in this area. Probably the best single reference, in a practical sense, is the American Association of Blood Banks manual.[2] This indispensable reference will be found in any licensed blood bank and should be consulted by the regular blood bank staff.

To carry out blood banking procedures a thorough knowledge of the principles involved, recognition of the many difficulties that may be encountered, and exactness of technique are essential. Shortcuts must never be taken. Everyone working in a particular blood bank must use exactly the same technique. Also, an elaborate system of safeguards must be established and thoroughly understood by all personnel. These safeguards and checks may seem repetitive but are essential. When an incompatible transfusion reaction occurs, it is usually caused by a breakdown of, and/or failure to observe, the established system.

Complete, permanent, legible records must be kept of every sequence of the many steps involved in administering a unit of blood. This is because blood banking is an area in which medicolegal problems are apt to occur. Results and observations are always entered directly on the permanent record and never recopied, as recopying will invariably result in error at some time.

GENERAL INFORMATION

Blood

Whole human blood consists of two major portions: solid and liquid. The solid portion consists primarily of the formed elements—red blood cells, white blood cells, and platelets—and makes up about 45 percent of the total blood volume. The liquid portion consists of the plasma, which makes up about 55 percent of the total volume. The blood volume of normal adults is approximately 5-6 L, or 10-12 pt. In blood banking a *unit* of blood is often referred to; for practical purposes it may be considered 1 pt.

Infused blood, or blood that is administered by transfusion, must be anticoagulated. However, the portion of blood that is used for blood bank procedures such as typing and cross matching must be clotted blood. If anticoagulated blood is used, there is a chance that small fibrin clots may be present in the plasma and may be incorrectly interpreted as a positive result. Therefore, laboratory blood bank tests employ red cells and serum (the liquid remaining after blood has been allowed to clot), not red cells and plasma. Another important reason for using serum rather than plasma in laboratory testing is that complement activation is usually prevented by anticoagulant. Most anticoagulants bind calcium, which is necessary for complement integrity. Persons doing blood banking procedures are repeatedly reminded that complement activity occurs in laboratory tests only when serum is used. In the body, plasma does not have the added anticoagulant, and therefore the complement integrity is not lost. Therefore, complement activation occurs as readily in plasma in the laboratory as it does in serum in the body.

Historical interest in transfusions

The importance of blood must have been realized from the earliest times. Early humans must have observed that loss of blood could lead to death.

In addition, some primitive groups had rituals in which the blood of one person was given to another; it was thought that in this way various characteristics of the donor could be given to the recipient. The discovery of the circulation of blood by Harvey in 1616 did much to advance interest in blood transfusion. In one early transfusion, attempted by Denis in 1667, lamb's blood was transfused into a man. At first this seemed to benefit the man, who was given a total of three such transfusions. However, after the third transfusion of lamb's blood the man suffered a reaction and died. It was found that it is impossible to transfuse the blood of one species of animal into another, whether from animal to human, human to animal, or animal of one species to animal of another species. Transfusions were also attempted within the same species of animal, from human to human and from one animal to another of the same species. These transfusions seemed to work about half the time, but far too often the result was death.

Introduction to blood groups

It is now known that the incompatibility of many transfusions was caused by the presence of certain factors on red cells. Each species of animal, humans included, has a certain factor that is unique to that species and is present on the red cells of all members of that species. If the red cells of sheep, for example, are transfused into a human, an anti-sheep substance will be produced in the blood of the human. The anti-sheep substance will destroy any sheep red cells that are subsequently introduced. This cell destruction is what is meant by an incompatible transfusion reaction, and it results in the death of the recipient.

It is also known that certain factors are common to some, but not all, members of a particular species. If blood containing such a factor is transfused into a recipient whose red cells do not contain that factor, the recipient will form an anti-factor that will result in an incompatible transfusion reaction.

So far, this seems rather simple. Why all the difficulty in blood banking? All that is necessary is to find the factor present on the red cell and transfuse only blood containing that factor. The principle is correct, but a great number of factors may be present on one person's red cells. The factors that are known have been grouped into units referred to as *blood group systems.* Approximately 300 blood group systems have been described. A partial list includes

ABO	Kidd	Lutheran	Kell
Rh	P	I	Xg
Lewis	Diego	MNSs	Duffy

More systems are being discovered all the time. The factor or factors that exist on a person's red cells within a particular blood group system represent that person's type for that system. The number of possible types within one system varies. In the ABO system there are six main types, plus additional types determined by less frequent subgroups. The more complex Rh-Hr system has 110 possible types. Taking all systems and type combinations into account, over 500 billion different types of blood are possible. In essence, each person has a unique blood type.

At this point it would seem that blood transfusion is impossible, since no two persons should have exactly the same type of blood. Fortunately, only certain factors are likely to give problems in transfusion (i.e., incompatible transfusion reactions), although there is always the possibility that an unknown or untested-for factor may occur that will result in such a reaction. The factors most likely to cause reactions are located within the ABO and Rh-Hr systems and must be tested for whenever blood is administered. Other factors are routinely tested for indirectly through cross matching and antibody screening techniques.

Thus far, only the terms *factor* and *anti-factor* have been used. These are not scientific terms. What has been called a factor is actually an *antigen*, and an anti-factor is an *antibody*. People who are given an antigen not present on their red cells produce an antibody in their plasma that will react with the foreign antigen. This is evidenced by the destruction of the red cell containing the foreign antigen.

Inheritance of blood groups

All the factors or antigens present on a person's red cells are inherited. Each antigen is controlled by a *gene*, which is the unit of inheritance. In other words, antigens are inherited as genes. If the gene for a particular antigen is present, that antigen will be found on all the red cells.

Each cell (except for mature red cells) consists of cytoplasm and a nucleus. If the nucleus is observed under the microscope at approximately the time of cell division, several long, threadlike structures will be visible. These structures are referred to as *chromosomes*. Each species has a specific number of chromosomes, and the chromosomes occur in pairs. Humans have 46 chromosomes and 23 chromosome pairs. The paired chromosomes are similar in size and shape and have their own distinct functions. A complete set of 23 chromosomes is inherited from each parent. Chromosomes occur in pairs in all cells of the body, except the sex cells (sperm and ovum), which contain 23 single chromosomes.

Since the gene is the unit of inheritance, it must also be located within the nucleus. Genes are exceedingly small particles that, when associated in linear form, make up the chromosome. They are too small to see under the microscope but together are visible as the chromosome. Genes are now thought to be made up of deoxyribonucleic acid (DNA). Each trait that is inherited is controlled by the presence of a specific gene. The genes responsible for a particular trait always occur at exactly the same point or position on a particular chromosome—this position is referred to as the *locus* of the gene. Research in the field of genetics is continually

revealing new information about the location of genes on the chromosome and about diseases that are genetically inherited or environmentally induced. Most of what is generally known concerns genes that are located on the sex chromosomes. However, if genes for different inherited traits are known to be carried on the same chromosome, they are said to be *syntenic*. This term is useful in referring to genes on a single chromosome that are too far apart to display absolute linkage in inheritance. Genes that are located on the same chromosome and are normally inherited together are known as *linked* genes. The closer the loci of the genes, the closer the linkage is said to be.

Inherited traits are somewhat variable within a species. For example, eye color varies and it is known to be inherited. Therefore, each possible eye color must be the result of a gene for that color. Variants of a gene for a particular trait are referred to as *alleles* for that trait. Since we have only two genes (one pair) for any given trait, our cells will have only two alleles. However, the number of possible alleles for a trait varies. A person who has identical alleles for a trait is said to be *homozygous* for that trait. For example, a person with blue eyes carries two blue-eye genes and is homozygous for blue eyes. A person who has two different alleles for a trait is *heterozygous* for that trait—for example, having a blue-eye gene in addition to a brown-eye gene.

In general, certain alleles may be stronger than, or may mask the presence of, other alleles. In the case of eye color, brown-eye genes mask the presence of blue-eye genes, and are said to be *dominant* over blue-eye genes. People who have one brown-eye and one blue-eye gene have eyes that appear brown. Blue-eye genes are then said to be *recessive* in relation to brown-eye genes. One must have two blue-eye genes in order to have blue eyes. However, in blood banking, the various alleles for a particular blood group system are equally dominant, or *codominant*. If the gene is present (and there is a suitable testing solution available), it will be detected.

Two other genetic terms that are often used in blood banking are *phenotype* and *genotype*. The phenotype is the blood type determined by tests made directly on the blood, even though other factors may be present. The genotype refers to the actual total genetic pattern for any system. It is usually impossible to determine the complete genotype in the laboratory; this usually requires additional studies, especially family studies.

Antibodies and antigens

All blood banking is based on a knowledge of antigens and antibodies. Unfortunately, they cannot be defined simply. They have been discussed in terms of factor and anti-factor. In general, an antigen may be thought of as a foreign substance—foreign in the sense that if it is introduced into the body of a person who does not already have the antigen, an anti-substance called an antibody will be produced. The antibody is found in the plasma and other body fluids. It reacts with the foreign antigen in some observable way, and it is specific for the antigen against which it is formed—that is, it reacts with only its corresponding antigen and no other antigen.

The significance of antigens and antibodies is not limited to blood banking. They are the basis of immunity. Various bacteria have antigenic properties. Therefore, when introduced into a host, they elicit antibody formation. The antibody formed in response to the foreign antigen (in this case bacteria) protects the person from subsequent infections by that particular bacterium. For example, a person who has had chicken pox is immune to the disease in the future. The immunity is a function of antibody production by the host. However, immunity is not immediate, as can be seen from the fact that on first infection the person is ill or incapacitated by the disease. Antibodies require about 2 weeks to develop sufficiently, after which subsequent exposure to the antigen will elicit an effective antigen-antibody reaction and therefore protective immunity.

In blood banking, antibody formation does not result in protective immunity. The blood antigens are present on the red cells, and the antibody is found in the plasma or serum. The antigen-antibody reaction results in the destruction of the antigen-carrying red cell by antibody in the serum of the foreign host. Clinically, the result of this red cell destruction is the hemolytic transfusion reaction. The reaction varies from patient to patient, but generally the immediate reaction is characterized by chills, high temperature, pain in the lower back, nausea, vomiting, and shock as indicated by decreased blood pressure and rapid pulse. These first effects of the reaction are rarely fatal; however, the by-products of red cell destruction pose many problems, primarily severe renal involvement. The patient may eventually die from kidney failure.

Chemically, antigens are usually proteins, although polysaccharides, polypeptides, or polynucleotides may also be antigenic. They are usually large molecules with a molecular weight of 10 000 or more. The cause of the specificity of antigens is not known. It may be the shape or spatial configuration of the molecule, the presence and arrangement of amino acids and carbohydrates, or other chemical properties.[3] However, not all antigens are equally antigenic. Some are extremely effective in their ability to cause antibody production, while others are relatively weak and not as likely to result in antibodies. If this were not true, blood could never be transfused.

The same blood antigens are found not only on the red cells but also in other body fluids such as urine, saliva, plasma, and gastric juice.

Depending largely on the type of antigen involved, the antigenic material stimulates a response in either the cellular immune system or the humoral immune system. On some occasions both systems are involved and there are interactions between the two systems. It is now known that the immune response to a particular antigen may also result in an increase in the numbers of specifically reactive lymphocytes. There are two groups of these specifically reactive lymphocytes: T lymphocytes; which are responsible for mediating specific cellular immunity, and B lymphocytes, which are the cells' response to antigen in the formation of antibody immunoglobulins. The T cells develop under the influence of the thymus in the human, and the B cells, at least in the chicken (where much of the research concerning this has been done), develop under the influence of the bursa of Fabricius. There is a "bursal equivalent" in humans, but its exact location is not known. In immunohematology the products of B cells, the circulating antibodies present in the serum, are studied almost to the total exclusion of other aspects of the immune response.[4]

Antibodies are produced in response to foreign antigenic stimuli. For example, persons whose red cells contain group A antigen are unable to form anti-A antibody. However, several factors influence the amount of antibody that will be formed after foreign antigen stimulation. First, the stronger the antigen, the greater the antibody response. In blood banking the ABO and D antigens are very strong, whereas such antigens as Lutheran and Kidd are relatively weak. The number of foreign antigens that are introduced at a particular time also influences the amount of antibody production. In general, exposure to only one antigen elicits a stronger antibody response than simultaneous exposure to more than one antigen. The number of exposures to foreign antigen also plays a role in antibody response. Repeated exposures result in greater antibody formation.

The interval between exposures to a foreign antigen also has a role in antibody formation. A number of exposures repeated rapidly are less likely to result in antibody formation than the same number of exposures spaced over a longer period of time. The quantity of antigen introduced has some effect; however, the number of

exposures and interval between them are more important in terms of antibody production.

There is apparently a threshold amount of antigen related to antibody production. If more than this threshold amount of antigen is introduced, the amount of antibody produced is relatively small in proportion to the quantity of antigen. In addition, a large excess of antigen may completely inhibit an antibody response. This is important in blood banking, for a relatively small amount of incompatible blood produces as much antibody as a relatively large amount. The transfusion of any incompatible blood may result in serious sensitization of the patient.

Finally, there are individual and age differences in antibody formation. Some persons are more prone to form antibodies than others. Newborn infants do not form antibodies but receive them passively from the mother across the placenta. They begin forming gamma globulin and therefore antibody at about 3 months and usually have a normal gamma globulin level by 6 months. This is important when newborn infants are typed for antibodies in the ABO system.

Antibodies are proteins. It is believed that they are synthesized by B lymphocytes or plasma cells from gamma globulin. When a foreign antigen is first introduced, the antibody cannot be detected immediately in the serum or plasma. It is observed about 10–14 days after antigenic stimulation, and the titer (concentration) is greatest at about 20 days, after which it gradually decreases.

A second exposure to the same antigen, however, rapidly results in detectable amounts of antibody in the plasma or serum. There appears to be some sort of memory phenomenon that results in an immediate antibody response on the second or subsequent exposures. This secondary antibody response also produces a higher and longer-lasting titer of antibody. In addition, the antibody is more effective in its reaction with antigen or has better combining properties.

Antibodies have also been classified in terms of

physical types.[5] The major classes are slightly different forms of gamma globulin and are called IgG (γG), IgM (γM), and IgA (γA). There are also IgD (γD) and IgE (γE), about which less is known. Of the first three, IgG is the smallest, with a molecular weight of about 150 000, and IgM is the largest, molecular weight about 900 000, as seen in Fig. 9-1. IgA ranges in size, with a molecular weight from about 150 000 to 350 000. IgG and IgM are probably the most important blood group antibodies. IgM is the type of antibody that results from primary exposure to foreign antigen. Secondary exposure results in IgG formation. Repeated stimulation results in IgG antibody formation.

IgM is the first type of antibody that the newborn infant is able to form, and it is effectively synthesized at about 9 months. IgG is effectively synthesized at about 3–4 years, whereas IgA is not produced until adolescence. IgG is the only type of antibody that is able to cross the placenta. This is important in respect to hemolytic disease of the newborn (HDN).

A different antibody classification includes *natural* and *immune* antibodies. The natural antibody appears to exist without antigenic stimulus, whereas the immune antibody is the result of stimulation by specific blood group antigens. An example of natural antibodies in blood are the anti-A and anti-B antibodies found in the ABO blood group system. In this system, if the red cell lacks the A antigen, anti-A antibody will be found in the serum. If the red cell lacks the B antigen, anti-B antibody will be found in the serum. Hence the name natural antibody. Substances very similar to blood group antigens A and B are so widely distributed in nature that the antibody will develop in anyone if the antigen is not present. Certain bacteria and foods may have A- or B-like antigens. The natural anti-A and anti-B antibodies are routinely used in testing for the ABO blood group. (They are saline solution-active and of the IgM type.) There are several other natural IgM blood group antibodies.

Immune antibodies are also referred to as *un-*

Fig. 9-1. Examples of antibody molecular structure. Two antibody molecules shown to have blood group activity are IgG and IgM. IgG is a simple monomer composed of two heavy chains and two light chains connected by disulfide bonds or bridges. IgM is in the form of a pentamer. Each has reactive sites capable of combining with corresponding antigens.

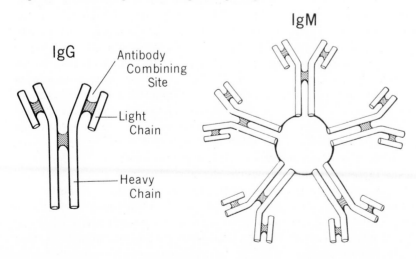

IgM

IgG

Antibody Combining Site

Light Chain

Heavy Chain

expected antibodies. They are usually the result of specific antigenic stimulation, and they result from immunization by way of *pregnancy, transfusion,* or *injection of red cells.* Once immunization exists, it is permanent. Immune antibodies are of the IgG, IgA, or IgM type.

Means of detecting antigen-antibody reactions in blood banking

Two terms that are used in discussing biological reactions are *in vivo* and *in vitro. In vivo* means in the living body, and *in vitro* means in glass (or in a laboratory setting). A biological reaction that normally occurs in the body (*in vivo*) may be demonstrated *in vitro,* or under laboratory conditions. Blood banking reactions that are used in determining blood groups and compatibility are *in vitro* reactions.

To determine a person's blood type, some sort of substance must be available to show what antigens are present on the red cell. The substance used for this purpose is referred to as an *antiserum.* An antiserum is a prepared and highly purified solution of antibody. It is named on the basis of the antibody it contains. For example, a solution of anti-A antibodies is called *anti-A antiserum.*

Most of the antisera that are used in blood banking are prepared commercially and purchased by the blood bank. In general, antiserum is prepared in one of two ways: (1) animals are deliberately inoculated with antigen and the resulting serum, which contains antibody, is purified and standardized for use as an antiserum, or (2) serum is collected from humans who have been sensitized to an antigen through transfusion, pregnancy, or intramuscular injection. Antiserum must meet certain requirements to be acceptable for use. It must be specific for the antigen to be detected—that is, specific under the manufacturer's recommended test conditions. It must have a sufficient titer to detect antigen. It must have a certain avidity for, or strength of reaction

with, corresponding red cells. It must also be sterile, clear, provided in a good container with a dropper, and stable. It should be marked with an expiration date and must never be used after this date. In addition, it must be stored at $4°C$ when not in use. Exact requirements for antiserum are defined by the Food and Drug Administration. When commercial antiserum is used, the manufacturer's directions must be followed carefully.

When antiserum is mixed with red cells, an antigen-antibody reaction may or may not occur. If a reaction does occur, the corresponding antigen must be present on the red cell, and the result is a positive reaction. If a reaction does not occur, the antigen is absent, and the result is negative. A positive reaction with anti-A antiserum demonstrates the presence of A antigen on the red cell, and so on.

In the original definition of antibody, it was stated that antibody resulting from antigenic stimulation will react with the antigen in an observable manner. In blood banking, two types of observable reactions may occur: *agglutination* and *hemolysis.*

Agglutination is clumping, or close association, of red cells caused by a specific antibody for antigen present on the cells. A positive antigen-antibody reaction results in an immediate combination of antibody and antigen on the red cell, followed by the visible agglutination, which takes longer to form. The IgG antibody, for example, is thought to be a somewhat Y-shaped structure with a reactive site at the end of each arm of the Y (Fig. 9-1). Each reactive site is capable of combining with corresponding antigen. Agglutination is thought to be the result of bridging of the red cells by antibody reacting with antigen sites on adjacent red cells. This bridging causes the red cells to stick together. Several such bridges result in visible clumping. The degree of agglutination varies. Very strong agglutination forms a large mass of cells that can be easily seen macroscopically. Less strong agglutination results in correspondingly smaller clumps of cells that can also be seen macroscopically, and finally in clumps of cells that can be seen only microscopically. The ability to observe all degrees of agglutination requires great care and experience. It is not a simple task, yet it is imperative that the degree of agglutination be detected.

Hemolysis is the result of lysis, or destruction, of the red cell by a specific antibody. It is probably the third stage in an antigen-antibody reaction and does not occur in all cases. The antibody causes rupture of the cell membrane with release of hemoglobin. The result is a crystal-clear red solution, with no cloudiness since no cells are present. Whenever hemolysis occurs, it is a positive antigen-antibody reaction. However, it is often overlooked and reported as negative, since agglutination is much more common and hemolysis looks much like a negative reaction with no agglutination. In the case of a negative reaction, however, the cells remain in a smooth, cloudy suspension. Misinterpretation of hemolysis is a cause of falsely negative results in the blood bank and may end in disaster for the patient.

For hemolysis to occur, a substance called *complement* must be present in the serum. Complement is a complex substance with at least nine components. It is important in blood banking because some antigen-antibody reactions require the presence of complement to be demonstrated *in vitro*, and although almost all normal sera contain complement when fresh, complement is destroyed by heat. Therefore, to have complement activity, sera must be either fresh or stored correctly. Complement will remain active if stored for 24-48 hours at 4°C or for 2 months at −50°C. If an antibody is to be detected that utilizes complement, it must be provided in the test medium.

In summary, the detection of antigen on red cells requires the demonstration of a positive reaction of the cells with a specific solution of antibodies (antiserum). The technique by which the red cell and antiserum are brought together varies widely, depending on a number of factors. The most important factor is the manner of action of the particular antigen-antibody system being tested for; in other words, knowledge of the antibodies of the blood group system involved is necessary.

In general, blood group tests are performed either on microscope slides or in test tubes. When test tubes are used, they are 10 by 75 or 12 by 75 mm. Other factors are adequate serum, storage of red cells, the concentration of cell suspensions, the testing medium (isotonic saline solution, albumin, or enzymes), the temperature of incubation, the incubation period, centrifugation, reading and interpretation of agglutination reactions, the use of reagents, and the glassware. The correct conditions are essential for reliable tests. Development of correct techniques requires thorough knowledge of all these considerations as well as of the blood groups. The technique will also depend on the brand of antiserum that is used and the manufacturer's directions, which must be followed for accurate results.

THE ABO BLOOD GROUP SYSTEM

The ABO blood group system was first discovered and described in 1900 and 1901 by Karl Landsteiner. By taking the blood of six of his colleagues, separating serum and cells, and mixing each cell suspension with each serum, Landsteiner was able to divide the blood into three groups: A, B, and O. In 1902 the fourth group, AB, was discovered by von Decastello and Struli, two of Landsteiner's pupils.[6]

The ABO system is now thought to consist of blood groups, or phenotypes, A, B, AB, and O. These four groups may be explained by the presence of two antigens (or factors) on the red cell surface, the A antigen and the B antigen. If a person belongs to group A, the A antigen is present on the red cell. Group B persons have B antigen on their cells. Group AB individuals have both A and B, while group O people have neither A nor B.

The antigen present on the red cell is determined by genes on the chromosomes. Three allelic genes can be inherited in the ABO system: the A, B, and O genes. Since each person has two genes for any trait, one from each parent, the following combinations of alleles are possible: AA, AO, AB, BB, BO, and OO. These combinations represent the possible genotypes in the ABO system.

If the A gene is present on the chromosome, A antigen will be present on the red cell. The presence of B gene results in B antigen on the red cell. The presence of O gene results in neither antigen on the red cell.

ABO typing procedures

In testing blood for the ABO group, a suspension of red cells in saline solution is prepared. This suspension is tested by mixing one portion with a solution of known anti-A antiserum (anti-A antibodies). A second portion is mixed with known anti-B antiserum (anti-B antibodies). The mixtures are then observed for a reaction. A positive reaction is the occurrence of agglutination or hemolysis. A negative reaction is the absence of agglutination or hemolysis. Results may be grouped as follows:

Group A blood—positive reaction of cells with anti-A antiserum

Group B blood—positive reaction of cells with anti-B antiserum

Group O blood—negative reaction of cells with both anti-A and anti-B antiserum

Group AB blood—positive reaction of cells with both anti-A and anti-B antiserum

In these typing reactions, the blood is merely tested for the presence or absence of A and B antigens. No direct test is made for the presence

or absence of the O gene. This is phenotyping, or typing by means of tests made directly on the blood. Since blood is tested only for the A and B antigens, genotypes AA and AO will both type as blood group A. Genotypes BB and BO both contain B antigen and will type as blood group B. Genotype AB will type as group AB, since both antigens are present to react with the appropriate antisera. All blood that types as group O must belong to the genotype OO, since the blood will not react with either anti-A or anti-B antiserum.

As is the case with any blood group system, corresponding antigens and antibodies cannot normally coexist in the same person's blood. In other words, persons who are blood group A cannot form anti-A antibodies and will not have anti-A antibodies in their serum. However, in the ABO system, unlike other blood group systems, if the A or B antigen is lacking on the red cell, the corresponding antibody will be found in the serum. These are the so-called natural antibodies discussed previously. Adults lacking group A antigen will be found to have anti-A antibody in their sera. The sera of adults with red cells lacking B antigen have anti-B antibody.

These naturally occurring anti-A and anti-B antibodies are important for several reasons, especially for ABO blood grouping in the laboratory. It is essential to avoid giving a blood transfusion to a person whose serum contains an antibody for an antigen present on the transfused red cells. If this occurred, there would be an immediate and severe hemolytic transfusion reaction. It is absolutely essential that the correct ABO blood type be transfused, or a severe reaction and death might result. For these reasons, the occurrence of natural anti-A and anti-B antibodies is made use of in the ABO typing procedure. In addition to testing red cells with known antibody, as described, the serum is tested with known group A_1 * and group B red

* A_1 is a subgroup of A antigen that will be defined later. For the present it may be considered synonymous with A antigen.

cells to determine what antibodies are present. In these tests, serum from the undetermined blood is separated from the cells. One portion of the serum is mixed with red cells known to contain group A_1 antigen. A second portion of serum is mixed with cells known to contain group B antigen. The mixtures are then observed for a positive or negative reaction as evidenced by agglutination or hemolysis. If there is a positive reaction with known group A_1 cells, the serum contains anti-A antibodies. If there is a positive reaction with known group B cells, the serum contains anti-B antibodies. If the serum reacts with both A_1 and B cells, both anti-A and anti-B antibodies are present. If no reaction occurs with either cell type, both antibodies are lacking. Remembering that in the ABO system the serum contains the corresponding antibody for the A or B antigen lacking from the red cell, the results may be grouped as follows:

Group A blood—positive reaction of serum with group B cells

Group B blood—positive reaction of serum with group A cells

Group O blood—positive reaction of serum with both A and B cells

Group AB blood—no reaction with either A or B cells

Typing reactions that employ undetermined red cells and known antibody or antiserum are referred to as *antigen*, *cell*, *direct*, or *front-typing* reactions. Typing reactions that employ undetermined serum and known red cells are referred to as *antibody*, *serum*, *indirect*, or *back-typing* reactions. These reactions are summarized in Table 9-1.

When the ABO group is to be determined, both the cells and the serum should be typed as described. The antigen- and antibody-typing results should then be compared to be sure that mistakes have not occurred and that the results are consistent. This is an excellent way to guard against mistakes in ABO grouping. However, in certain instances the antigen- and antibody-typing results show discrepancies.

Natural antibodies of the ABO system

One cause of cell and serum discrepancies involves the natural antibodies, which are expected

Table 9-1. ABO typing reactions

Blood group	Antigen on red cells	Antibody in serum	Antigen, front, or direct typing		Antibody, back, or indirect typing		Possible genotype
			Reaction of undetermined cells with anti-A antiserum	Reaction of undetermined cells with anti-B antiserum	Reaction of undetermined serum with A_1 cells	Reaction of undetermined serum with B cells	
A	A	Anti-B	+	−	−	+	*AA* *AO*
B	B	Anti-A	−	+	+	−	*BB* *BO*
AB	A and B	Neither	+	+	−	−	*AB*
O	Neither	Anti-A and anti-B	−	−	+	+	*OO*

to occur in most adults. They cannot be expected to exist in newborn infants, since infants do not normally begin to produce antibodies until they are 3-6 months of age. The titer of natural antibodies normally increases gradually through adolescence and then decreases gradually. For this reason, serum-grouping results may also show discrepancies in very elderly patients.

It should also be mentioned that there is a variation of the antibody titer in the population. In general, the anti-A titer seems to be higher than the anti-B titer. In the laboratory the antibody titer of serum will only rarely approach the antibody titer of commercially prepared antiserum. For this reason, reactions with cell-grouping tests are generally stronger and easier to read than serum-grouping reactions.

The occurrence of subgroups of group A or group B antigen might also result in discrepancies between cell- and serum-grouping reactions. The classification of blood in the ABO system into groups A, B, AB, and O is an oversimplification. Both group A and group B may be further classified into subgroups. The most important subdivision is that of group A into A_1 and A_2. Practically, these subgroups are of little clinical importance. They are not tested for routinely but should be kept in mind when there is difficulty in ABO grouping or compatibility testing. The concept of an *H substance* as a precursor material from which A and B antigens are produced is involved in the various subgroups (called ABH substances). These subjects will not be discussed further here. The student should consult a more detailed text such as "Blood Groups in Man"[7] or "Technical Manual of the American Association of Blood Banks."[8] It is because of the existence of subgroups that A_1 test cells must be used in ABO serum grouping. Subgrouping tests will involve the use, for example, of anti-AB serum, absorbed anti-A serum, and lectins.

It must be stressed that if discrepancies between the results of cell and serum grouping occur, they must be resolved. These problems should be referred to a person with sufficient training and experience in the area of blood banking.

Immune antibodies of the ABO system

Thus far, only natural anti-A and anti-B antibodies have been discussed. However, anti-A and anti-B antibodies may also be of the immune type. Serum may contain immune antibodies in addition to the natural ones. Natural antibodies are normally found in the serum of adults if the red cell lacks the corresponding antigen, and they probably arise from the inevitable stimulation by ABH substances widely distributed in nature. Immune anti-A or anti-B antibodies result from specific antigenic stimulation. This stimulation may occur through incompatible transfusion, pregnancy, or injection of ABH substances or substances having ABH activity.

Immune and natural antibodies differ in physical and chemical properties and in their serological behavior. In addition, natural ABO antibodies react best if the red cells are suspended in saline solution and the test is carried out at room temperature or $4°C$. Immune antibodies differ in that they react better if cells are suspended in albumin or serum and incubated at $37°C$. There are other differences in mode of reaction in the laboratory, and they must be taken into account when the occurrence of an immune-type anti-A or anti-B antibody is suspected or possible—for example, in cases of HDN with ABO incompatibility and in screening blood for low titers of anti-A and anti-B.

The natural antibody is a large molecule with a molecular weight of about 900 000, whereas the immune antibody has a molecular weight of about 150 000. Probably because of this size difference, natural antibodies are unable to cross the placental barrier, whereas immune antibodies may cross it. This is important in hemolytic disease of the newborn. Natural antibodies are of the IgM (γM) type, whereas immune antibodies are of the IgG (γG) type.

Universal donors and recipients

One concept that must be discussed in conjunction with the ABO system is that of "universal donors" and "universal recipients." These are terms familiar to most people, yet to the blood banker the concept is somewhat oversimplified. It is used only in cases of extreme emergency.

When blood is to be transfused, there are two questions that must be kept in mind: (1) Does the patient's serum contain an antibody against an antigen on the transfused red cell? and (2) Does the serum to be transfused contain an antibody against an antigen on the patient's red cells? The first situation is the more serious one. It can result in a major reaction and in the death of the patient. This is because all the transfused blood will be destroyed by antibody in the patient's circulatory system, resulting in accumulation of toxic waste products and probably in severe renal failure and death.

The second situation, in which the donor serum contains antibody against the patient's red cells, is not as serious. A minor reaction would occur, because only a small amount of blood compared to the patient's total blood volume is infused. As a result, only a small proportion of the patient's red cells are actually destroyed by donor serum, and this is offset by the benefits of the donor red cells that remain intact and viable.

These transfusion situations are made use of in the concepts of universal donor and recipient. Universal donor blood is group O blood. It is felt that group O blood can be safely transfused into a person with any ABO blood type, because patient's serum cannot contain an antibody to group O cells. In other words, a major reaction cannot occur. However, group O blood does contain anti-A and anti-B antibodies. Therefore, if it is given to group A persons, a minor

reaction can occur with anti-A antibodies. In case of group B persons, there can be a minor reaction with anti-B antibodies, while the AB person can have a minor reaction with both anti-A and anti-B.

Because these minor reactions can occur, it is preferable that group O blood that is to be used as universal donor blood have most of the plasma removed. If this is not possible, the donor blood must be screened with certain additional tests.[8] There is no universally accepted method of screening for "safe" blood for such use. An additional problem is the possible presence of immune anti-A or anti-B antibodies in addition to the natural forms.

In the case of the group AB patient, it is even more dangerous to transfuse group O blood, since both anti-A and anti-B antibodies are present to react with the patient's red cells. For this reason, if group AB blood cannot be secured for transfusion it is preferable to use either group A or group B blood, rather than group O. If group A blood is to be used, the anti-B titer should be determined; if group B blood, the anti-A titer. The so-called universal recipients are those with group AB blood, since they may be infused with group A, B, or O blood in emergency situations.

In summary, it should be stressed that ABO type-specific blood should be used whenever possible. Whenever group O blood is used for the A, B, or AB patient and A or B blood for the AB patient, a certain risk does exist. Although screening methods are available to test the titer of anti-A and/or anti-B, these methods are not perfect, and a severe transfusion reaction may still take place. However, a blood bank should always have some tested low-titer blood on hand for use in emergencies. These include situations where group-specific blood is not available and blood must be transfused, where there may not be enough time to type the patient's blood and test for compatibility, or where the patient's blood group cannot be accurately determined. In cases of ABO hemolytic disease of the newborn, group O blood may be necessary. Finally, there may be such unusual circumstances as disasters or military situations where blood cannot be typed for use.[9] Group O was routinely used on the battlefield in Korea and Vietnam.

THE Rh-Hr BLOOD GROUP SYSTEM

Definition of Rh factors and inheritance

The Rh blood group system is considerably more complex than the ABO system. Basically, it consists of six related blood group factors, or antigens, C, D, E, c, d, and e, and the corresponding antibodies anti-C, anti-D, anti-E, anti-c, and anti-e ("anti-d" antibody does not exist). Because of the lack of an anti-d antibody, the existence of d as an antigen is disputed. For this reason, the so-called presence of d should be thought of as the absence of D antigen.

More than one system of nomenclature is used to define the antigens of the Rh-Hr system. There are the Rh system of Wiener,[10] the CDE system of Fisher and Race,[11] and the numerical system of Rosenfield et al.[12] These systems are compared in Table 9-2. Because neither the CDE nor the Rh system is universally accepted, all commercial antiserum labels and direction sheets are required by the Food and Drug Administration, Bureau of Biologics, to include both the Rh and the CDE terms. The Rh term is given first and is followed by the CDE term in parentheses. For example, anti-Rh_0 (anti-D).

The six antigens that have been defined are not the only antigens in the Rh system, for

variants have been described. To date there are at least 35 related factors in the system.[13] However, C, D, E, c, and e are the most important factors.

The Rh factors that have been discovered on red cells are inherited traits, as are the antigens of the ABO system. However, in the ABO system only three allelic genes could be inherited. In the Rh system, D, C, E, d, c, and e are not all alleles for the same position. Rather, C and c are alleles for the same trait, while D and d are alleles for another chromosome position, as are E and e. The factors are inherited in groups of three, so that a particular chromosome will have one position for the Dd alleles, a second position for the Cc alleles, and a third position for the Ee alleles. In other words, each chromosome carrying the Rh determinants has three closely linked loci for the three related Rh alleles. Everyone has loci for six Rh genes.

Thus, there are three pairs of Rh-Hr factors that are genetically related. Everyone must have at least one of or both of the paired alleles Cc, Dd, and Ee. Since D and d are alleles for the same trait, if D is absent, d must be present, and if d is absent, D must be present.[11] This means that there are three possible combinations of genes for the Dd alleles. A person may possess two D genes, DD, and be homozygous for D. Or a person may possess a D gene and a d gene, Dd, and be heterozygous for D. Finally, the person may possess two d genes, dd, and be homozygous for d. This is also true of the Cc and the Ee alleles: persons may be homozygous or heterozygous for Ee and Cc.

Since the Rh alleles are inherited in groups of three paired factors, and each person has two chromosomes for the Rh factors, each person has

Table 9-2. Comparative nomenclature of the Rh-Hr antigens

CDE system (Fisher-Race)		Rh system (Wiener)		Numerical system (Rosenfield et al.)	
D	d	Rh_0	Hr_0	Rh1	
C	c	rh′	hr′	Rh2	Rh4
E	e	rh″	hr″	Rh3	Rh5

a total of six Rh factors. This means that there are eight possible combinations of three factors that can be carried on a particular chromosome. These possible combinations of factors in CDE notation and the corresponding Rh notation, and their approximate frequency are given in Table 9-3.

One of the eight possible Rh-Hr gene combinations is inherited from each parent, so that the total Rh-Hr genotype for a person would be denoted as *CDE/cde* or *CDe/cDe*, and so on. In Wiener's Rh-Hr notation corresponding to the CDE system, the capital letter R refers to the presence of D (Rh_0) antigen, while r refers to the presence of d (Hr_0). The superscript in Wiener's notation refers to the antigens C, c, E, and e.

Thus far, only one theory of Rh-Hr inheritance has been presented here—the theory of Fisher and Race.[11] In this theory the three genes on each chromosome carrying the Rh-Hr determinants are felt to be so closely linked that, in effect, they are inherited as a unit. In other words, the unit of inheritance is considered to be the chromosome rather than the gene in this case. This theory recognizes the existence of six genes, each gene controlling the identical factor in the blood. There is no difference between the gene and the factor.

The other theory of Rh-Hr inheritance is that proposed by Wiener.[10] Weiner differentiated between the genes and the factors that are found in the blood. Wiener felt that there is a single gene on each Rh-Hr chromosome that determines the presence of three factors in the blood. Since there are eight possible combinations of Rh-Hr factors, this theory recognizes eight possible genes. In other words, inheritance of the R^1 gene will result in the presence of C (rh'), D (Rh_0), and e (hr'') antigens on the red cells. A person inheriting an R^1 gene from one parent and an R^z gene from the other would be of genotype R^1/R^z (or *CDe/CDE*), and that person's red cells will contain C (rh'), D (Rh_0), E (rh''), and e (hr'') antigens. Wiener supported his theory of

Table 9-3. Rh chromosomes and approximate frequency

CDE notation (Fisher-Race)	Rh-Hr notation (Wiener)	Approximate frequency in white population[a]
CDe	R^1	Common
cDE	R^2	Common
CDE	R^z	Rare
cDe	R^O	2%
Cde	r'	1%
cdE	r''	1%
CdE	r^y	Very rare
cde	r	Common

[a]F. Stratton and P. H. Renton, "Practical Blood Grouping," p. 154, Charles C Thomas, Springfield, Ill., 1958.

inheritance with the fact that examples of crossovers (mutations resulting from paired chromosomes breaking and recombining) have not been found. In virtually every other case of closely linked inherited traits, crossovers have been found.

In any case, the net effect is the same. People will always have six Rh-Hr factors in their blood. The only real difficulty is that the two theories of inheritance have resulted in more than one system of nomenclature that must be learned by the student.

Historical background

The discovery of the Rh system was based on work by Landsteiner and Wiener in 1940 and by Levine and Stetson in 1939.[11] A woman who delivered a stillborn fetus was studied by Levine and Stetson. The woman had never received a blood transfusion; however, after delivery she was transfused with her husband's blood. Both the woman and her husband were blood group O. Following transfusion, the woman experienced a severe hemolytic reaction.

Similar transfusion reactions had previously been known to occur following the first transfusion after childbirth, and they did not seem to be associated with the ABO system. Levine and Stetson developed an explanation of their patient's transfusion reaction that has been proved to be correct. They explained the reaction by proposing that the woman's red cells did not contain a "new" antigen. However, the child inherited this new antigen from the father, and the fetal cells containing it found their way into the mother's circulatory system. This resulted in the formation of antibody to the new antigen. Therefore, when the woman was transfused with her husband's blood, her serum contained an antibody to the new antigen contained on her husband's red cells. It was also found that the woman's serum agglutinated not only her husband's red cells but the red cells of 80 of 104 ABO-compatible bloods. Levine and Stetson did not name this new antigen.

The naming of this new factor eventually resulted from studies by Landsteiner and Wiener in 1940.[11] They inoculated rabbits and guinea pigs with the red cells of rhesus monkeys, and found that the resulting rabbit antibody agglutinated the red cells of all rhesus monkeys and, more importantly, the red cells of about 85 percent of samples of the white population of New York City. The 85 percent of the cells that were agglutinated by the anti-rhesus serum were called *Rh-positive*, and the remaining 15 percent not agglutinated were called *Rh-negative*. Later it was shown that an antibody found in the serum of certain patients who had hemolytic reactions after transfusion of ABO-compatible blood was apparently the same as the antibody in the anti-rhesus serum. It was also found that the antibody contained within the serum of the women studied by Levine and Stetson in 1939 was similar to the antibody in the anti-rhesus serum.

Rh-positive and Rh-negative

It is now known that the new antigen described by Levine and Stetson is the D (or Rh_0) antigen.

Persons whose red cells contain D antigen either as *D/D* or *D/d* are now termed Rh-positive. They represent approximately 85 percent of the population. In other words, the antibody responsible for several transfusion reactions is the anti-D (anti-Rh_0) antibody. Persons whose red cells lack the D (Rh_0) antigen are termed Rh-negative. Rh-negative persons are then *d/d*. They represent about 15 percent of the population. (The great majority of Rh-negative persons are *cde/cde*. This genotype is what is meant by a truly Rh-negative person. Other very rare genotypes that are *d/d* must be considered Rh-negative as blood recipients.)

Characteristics of the Rh-Hr antigens

The factors C, D, E, c, and e are all antigenic. This means that they are capable of stimulating the production of antibodies if introduced into the body of a person whose red cells completely lack them. The Rh antigens are permanent inherited characteristics that remain constant throughout life. However, not all the Rh antigens are equally antigenic. The D (Rh_0) antigen is the strongest and will result in immunization if introduced into a foreign host. For this reason the term Rh-positive merely refers to the presence of D antigen without respect to the other Rh factors. The antigenic strength of D also makes it imperative that blood be tested for Rh type before transfusion. Rh-negative persons must never be transfused with Rh-positive (D-positive) blood, for they will certainly develop anti-D antibodies. This would not be lethal at the time of the first transfusion; however, subsequent transfusion with D-positive blood would result in a hemolytic reaction. In the case of the woman who was sensitized by an Rh-positive fetus, transfusion with D-positive blood resulted in a hemolytic reaction with the first transfusion.

While D is the most antigenic of the Rh antigens, the other factors (except d) are also antigenic. If strength is considered in terms of antibody frequency, anti-c is most common, followed by anti-E, anti-C, and finally anti-e. Combinations of antibodies in the same blood are also seen.

Characteristics of the Rh-Hr antibodies

Like all antibodies, the Rh antibodies are made from the gamma globulin portion of the blood plasma. They are specific for the antigen against which they were formed. Unlike the ABO antibodies, all Rh antibodies are immune or unexpected antibodies. There are *no* naturally occurring Rh antibodies. They all result from specific antigenic stimulation, whether by transfusion, pregnancy, or injection of antigen. The lack of natural antibodies in the Rh system is important for several reasons. Practically, it means that antibody typing is impossible in the Rh system. All typing methods in this system depend upon antigen-typing or cell-typing procedures involving unknown antigen and known antiserum.

Rh-typing procedures

Commercial antiserum is available for the C, D, E, c, and e factors. There is no way of testing for the d factor, since no anti-d antibody has been found. Two types of Rh antibodies are available commercially. One type is active in saline solution, while the other is of the so-called incomplete type and does not react in saline solution. This is extremely important in the laboratory if results are to be accurate.

Antibody of the saline solution-active type is labeled "for saline tube tests." When this preparation is used, reactions must be carried out on saline suspensions of red cells and the test must be performed in a test tube. Slide tests cannot be performed. The first Rh antibodies discovered were active in saline solution.

It was eventually found that some of the Rh antibodies, although not detectable in saline suspensions of red cells, could be demonstrated if a slightly different technique was used. Rather than saline solution, the cells were suspended in serum or a medium containing sufficient protein. The antibodies that were detectable only when suspended in protein were termed incomplete, or albumin-active, antibodies, as opposed to the complete, or saline solution-active, antibodies. Later, another class of antibody was found to be demonstrable only by means of anti-human globulin, or Coombs' reagent. This type of antibody was termed incomplete univalent. It is now known that all antibodies have more than one valence (i.e., reactive site), although some are detectable in saline suspension, others require sufficient protein, and still others are demonstrable only by means of the anti-human globulin test.

The differences in reactivity have been found to depend on the length of the antibody molecule. The molecules that are reactive in saline suspensions of cells are of the larger IgM (γM) type. Their length is sufficient to cause bridging of adjacent cells in suspension (agglutination). However, red cells in suspension are known to carry an electrical charge, the *zeta potential*, which causes them to repel each other. The IgM-type antibody molecules are so long that they extend beyond the range of the zeta potential and can react with antigenic sites on adjacent cells. Molecules of the smaller IgG (γG) type are so short that they do not extend beyond the zeta potential and cannot react with adjacent cells. To demonstrate the existence of IgG molecules by means of agglutination, the repulsion caused by the zeta potential must be overcome or reduced. It can be reduced by suspending the cells in a sufficiently high-protein medium (either their own serum or a commercial protein preparation, or both). Other techniques for the demonstration of IgG include high-speed centrifugation and enzyme methods.

Commercial Rh antisera may be of either the

saline solution-active or albumin-active variety. The type of preparation is stated on the manufacturer's label. If the preparation is of the saline solution-active variety, the cells must be suspended in saline solution, since the presence of protein may block the reaction, resulting in falsely negative results. In general, saline solution-active antibodies require a test tube method and incubation at 37°C. Slide methods are not adequate. The proper antiserum is labeled "for saline tube tests."

Commercial antisera of the albumin-active, high-protein, variety contain IgG-type antibodies. In general, the albumin-active antisera are more avid preparations, and for this reason many of them may be used with either a slide or the test tube technique. In addition, the reaction takes place in less time than with saline solution-active antibody, and the incubation time is shortened. The tube methods with albumin-active antiserum may not even require incubation at 37°C but may produce a reaction at room temperature. In general, Rh antibodies will not react unless the preparation is warmed to (or incubated at) 37°C. Antisera of the incomplete, or albumin-active, variety are labeled "for slide or rapid tube test (or modified tube test)." Again, it is essential to follow the manufacturer's directions.

When blood is to be transfused, the patient must be tested for the presence or absence of the D (Rh$_0$) antigen. This is because the D factor is so antigenic that most persons who are D-negative (Rh$_0$-negative) or d/d may produce an anti-D antibody if transfused with D-positive blood. All persons who are D-negative (d/d) must be transfused with Rh-negative or d/d blood. Conversely, since d (Hr$_0$) has never been shown to be antigenic, Rh-positive persons may be safely transfused with Rh-negative (d/d) blood.

Since the D (Rh$_0$) factor is the most antigenic of the Rh factors, many laboratories test only for the presence or absence of this factor and transfuse Rh-positive or Rh-negative blood accordingly. In most cases this is sufficient, since other Rh antibodies are comparatively rare and

are tested for indirectly by compatibility testing or antibody screening techniques. If only the D factor is to be tested for, the incomplete, albumin-active, anti-Rh$_0$ (anti-D) antiserum is usually used. Anti-D antiserum is available commercially in both a saline solution-active and an albumin-active form. However, there are certain weaker forms of the D antigen (high- and low-grade D^u) that are not detectable with saline solution-active anti-D antiserum. For this reason, if only one test is to be performed, the incomplete, albumin-active form of anti-D must be used. Blood that is negative with this test may be further tested for the presence of the D^u variant by means of the anti-human globulin (Coombs) reaction.

Although blood must be tested for only the presence or absence of D antigen and transfused accordingly, tests for other Rh factors may be performed. Antisera are available for the C, c, D, E, and e factors. Often blood is tested routinely for C, c, D, and E. Although anti-e is available, it is so rare that the antiserum is too expensive to be used routinely. There are several reasons for performing tests for C, c, D, and E routinely: in cases of multiple transfusions over extended periods of time, blood that is specific for all these types may be given, for the patient may have developed another Rh antibody.

By performing additional Rh tests, either the complete Rh genotype may be determined positively, or the most probable genotype may be determined by consulting the frequency charts that are available from these typing reactions. This is especially important in determining the probability of occurrence of hemolytic disease of the newborn (HDN) in mothers negative for a factor that the father is positive for. In this case, both the mother and father are typed and the most probable genotypes are determined to predict the possibility of HDN in their children. Finally, the results of tests with these other Rh-typing sera may be used to check the laboratory results by consulting frequency charts. The occurrence of a very infrequent typing reaction will often point to an error in the typing procedure itself.

The anti-C, anti-E, and the anti-D (anti-Rh$_0$) antisera are available in both complete, saline solution-active form and incomplete, albumin-active form. Blood is often routinely tested for D antigen with both these antisera as a means of checking the accuracy of the test for D antigen. Since all Rh antibodies are immune ones and it is impossible to antibody-type, it is useful to have a means of checking results for the D antigen. The saline and albumin forms of anti-D antiserum should give the same result. The use of albumin-active anti-D allows for the detection of D antigen in a shorter period of time than with saline anti-D. In the case of the D^u variants of the D antigen, only the incomplete form of anti-D antiserum will give positive results. For a more complete explanation of D^u testing, the American Association of Blood Banks (AABB) technical manual should be consulted.

Anti-C and anti-E antisera (in addition to anti-D) are normally available in a saline solution-active form. Antisera of this type will be labeled "for saline tube tests," and the tests must be performed in test tubes. In general, equal amounts of antiserum and 2–4% suspensions of red cells (one or two drops of each) are mixed in 10- by 75- or 12- by 75-mm test tubes and incubated at 37°C for about 1 hour. After incubation, the tubes may be centrifuged. Most blood banking laboratories use a special centrifuge called the Serofuge (manufactured by the Clay-Adams Co., Parsipanny, N.J.). This centrifuge is set to run at a constant speed and is used to spin serum-cell mixtures before reading. It rotates rapidly: 15 seconds at 1000 g in a Serofuge is comparable to 60 seconds at 135 g in a conventional centrifuge.[14] By using this type of centrifuge, time can be saved and the results of typing tests determined quickly. The results are very carefully read macroscopically by resuspending the cells and tipping the tubes. Negative results are often confirmed by observation under the microscope. The exact technique will vary with different brands of antiserum, and the manufacturer's directions must be followed.

Anti-c (anti-hr') antiserum is normally available in an incomplete, albumin-active form labeled "for slide or rapid tube test (or modified tube test)." In the slide technique, a suspension of cells in their own serum is added to antiserum on a warmed microscope slide and observed for agglutination. Alternatively, the cells may be suspended either in serum or saline solution and added to antiserum in a test tube. The tube is usually incubated at 37°C for 15 or 30 minutes (less than with saline solution-active antiserum). Again the manufacturer's directions must be followed, and the technique will vary somewhat with different brands of antiserum.

Conclusion

In summary, the Rh system is considerably more complex than the ABO system. Everyone has six Rh blood group factors but only two ABO blood group factors. One may be either homozygous or heterozygous for the three paired Rh factors, as for the A, B, and O factors. The ABO system has both natural and immune antibodies, while the Rh system has only immune antibodies. In transfusions ABO type-specific blood should always be given. With the Rh system, blood may be tested for only the presence or absence of D antigen and transfused accordingly. However, it is sometimes necessary to give blood that is type-specific for the Rh factors.

Commercial Rh antiserum may be of either the saline solution-active or albumin-active type. The procedure used depends on the form of antiserum employed. Techniques vary with different brands of antiserum.

Experience is invaluable when testing for the Rh factors. Techniques must be mastered and performed with great care. Shortcuts must never be taken, and the methods and reasons for them must be thoroughly understood.

THE ANTIGLOBULIN REACTION (COOMBS' TEST)

Under Rh-typing Procedures we discussed different types of antibodies and their laboratory reactions. Antibodies were classified as complete or incomplete depending on their ability to react in saline suspensions of red cells or the requirement for additional techniques, such as the addition of protein to the test medium. This was related to the size of the antibody molecule and its ability to overcome electrical charges on red cells in suspension (the zeta potential). In general IgM antibodies are large enough to extend beyond the zeta potential and agglutinate red cells in saline suspensions. However, many IgG antibodies are unable to bring about agglutination unless the zeta potential is reduced by such means as adding protein to the red cell suspension. Even after the addition of protein, some IgG antibody molecules will not bring about agglutination. Antibodies that are unable to cause agglutination in any of the laboratory techniques mentioned thus far are detectable by means of the antiglobulin, or Coombs, technique. They have been described in the past as incomplete

univalent antibodies; however, they are now known to be bivalent in action, although this can only be demonstrated by the antiglobulin technique.

The antibodies that are detectable by the antiglobulin technique react with red cells. However, the reaction is not observable in terms of agglutination. The antibodies coat the red cells by reacting with antigenic sites on the cell surfaces. The other arm of the antibody molecule is not able to react with antigen on a second red cell, with resultant bridging and agglutination. To demonstrate the coating of red cells by this incomplete antibody, some sort of reagent must be available to show that the cells have reacted with antibody, as seen in the example in Fig. 9-2. It must be remembered that these incomplete antibodies are fully capable of reacting in the body and, if present, will result in severe transfusion reactions.

In developing a reagent to demonstrate the coating of incomplete antibody on red cells, use is made of the fact that all antibodies are some

Fig. 9-2. Coombs' reaction (anti-human globulin reaction). Rabbit IgG with anti-human IgG specificity is shown combining or reacting with human IgG on human red blood cells.

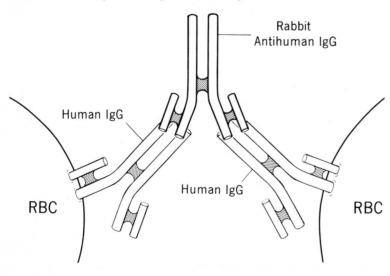

Rabbit
Antihuman IgG

Human IgG

Human IgG

RBC

RBC

form of human globulin. The reagent need only be an antibody to human globulin. This is the basis of the antiglobulin, or Coombs, test. The reagent is an antibody to human globulin, or anti-human globulin antibody. This antiglobulin antibody will react with any antibody coating a red cell. Since it is sufficiently long (it is actually an IgM-type antibody), it will react with antibody coating adjacent red cells, and bridging or agglutination of the red cells results.

Anti-human globulin (Coombs') reagent is produced commercially by the companies that produce blood group antisera. The anti-human globulin reagent is prepared by inoculating laboratory animals with human serum or the globulin fraction of human serum. The laboratory animals produce an antibody to the human globulin, or anti-human globulin antibody. The laboratory animal is bled and the serum collected. This serum is purified by various techniques until it is specific for human globulin. The anti-human serum is often prepared in such a way that it reacts with both gamma globulin and complement. The antiglobulin portion of the serum is actually anti-IgG globulin. However, antibodies other than those of the IgG type must be detected by the antiglobulin test, and it has been found that some of these other antibodies utilize complement in their reaction—they are said to *fix* complement. Anti-human globulin reagent that reacts with both IgG-type antibodies and complement is called *broad-spectrum* antiglobulin reagent.[15]

Antiglobulin test procedures (direct and indirect tests)

There are two ways in which the antiglobulin test is performed. These are the direct and indirect methods.[15,16]

The *direct antiglobulin (Coombs) test* is performed on red cells that are suspected of being coated with antibody. The cells are first washed

meticulously with saline solution to remove all traces of serum (hence human globulin) from the test medium. Any serum remaining will react with the antiglobulin reagent, causing falsely negative results.

The test is performed in test tubes measuring 10 by 75 or 12 by 75 mm. The cells are washed by completely filling the test tube with a forceful stream of saline solution, resulting in a homogeneous suspension of cells in saline solution. The tube is then centrifuged, and the cells are packed at the bottom of the tube. After centrifuging, the tube is inverted and all the saline solution is decanted in one motion, shaking the tube to remove all saline solution. The tube is then turned upright and shaken to resuspend the cells. The tube must never be covered with the finger or palm of the hand at any stage of mixing, for protein from the skin can inactivate or neutralize the antiglobulin reagent.

The cells are washed with saline solution in this manner at least three times. More washing may be necessary if periodic evaluation of the washing technique shows that three times is not adequate. An alternative way to wash and centrifuge the cells is to use one of the cell-washing centrifuges that are now available. These centrifuges can be preset to the desired number of washes and are extremely useful for antiglobulin tests. After the final washing, the saline solution is decanted as completely as possible. The cells are shaken to facilitate resuspension and the antiglobulin reagent is added. The test tube is then incubated and centrifuged as the manufacturer's directions specify, and the results are read macroscopically and microscopically for the presence or absence of agglutination. The direct antiglobulin test is used in the diagnosis of HDN and autoimmune hemolytic anemia, and in the investigation of transfusion reactions.

The *indirect antiglobulin (Coombs) test* begins a step before the direct method, although it eventually requires the same washing technique and reaction with antiglobulin reagent. The indirect test begins with a serum suspected of containing antibodies. The serum is mixed with red cells that contain antigen for the suspected antibody in the serum. The test cells are suspended in saline solution, albumin, or serum (depending on the antibody), mixed with the suspected serum, and incubated for a sufficient period of time for a reaction to occur. Incubation is usually for 15-30 minutes at 37°C, but this varies with the antigen-antibody system involved. If the serum contains an antibody for an antigen on the test cells, there will be a reaction—a coating of antibody on the test cells. To demonstrate the reaction, the cells must be washed with saline solution and treated in the same way as in the direct antiglobulin test.

The indirect antiglobulin test has several uses. It is used in cross matching blood to detect incompatibility before transfusion, to test the serum of pregnant women when HDN could occur, to test donor serum for unexpected antibodies, and to demonstrate certain blood group antigens (such as low-grade D^u antigen). Finally,

various investigative studies require the use of this technique.

Neither the indirect nor the direct antiglobulin test is specific for any one antibody. They give the same reaction with any antibody contained in human serum. To determine the identity of the antibody responsible for a positive reaction, the antigens present on the red cells must be known. This is done by a process of elimination, using various commercial red cell preparations containing known antigens.

The antiglobulin test is not simple. The reagent is a particularly unstable preparation and must be stored with great care. It is inactivated in several different ways. The AABB manual lists 12 causes of falsely negative and 10 causes of falsely positive results.[17] All these must be understood before the antiglobulin test can be performed with reliability. Because of these numerous sources of error, positive and negative controls must be included when the antiglobulin test is performed.

HEMOLYTIC DISEASE OF THE NEWBORN (ERYTHROBLASTOSIS FETALIS)

Hemolytic disease of the newborn, also called erythroblastosis fetalis, occurs when a child inherits an antigen for which its mother is negative. The disease most commonly involves factors of the Rh and ABO blood group systems, although it may result from incompatibilities in virtually any blood group system. For this disease to occur, however, the child must be positive for an antigen for which the mother is negative.

This condition develops while the fetus is in the uterus. The mechanism involves sensitization or immunization of the mother to foreign antigen present on her child's red cells. Although the circulatory systems of a mother and her child are separate, and only small molecules such as nutrients can cross the placenta, there can be some seepage of fetal red cells into the mother's

circulatory system. This is most likely to occur very late in pregnancy or at the time of birth. If any incompatible fetal red cells do find their way into the mother's circulatory system, she develops an antibody to the antigen on them. Once such immunization occurs, it is permanent. The antibody formed by the mother is of the IgG type and it can cross the placenta into the circulatory system of the fetus, where it reacts with corresponding antigen on the red cells of the fetus, with resultant destruction of the cells. HDN is the condition that exists when maternal antibody crosses the placenta and reacts with antigen on fetal red cells. This was the cause of death of the child delivered by the woman studied by Levine and Stetson in 1939, which led to the discovery of the Rh blood group system.

Rh factors

HDN most commonly involves the Rh blood group system. It most often involves the D antigen, the mother being negative for D (*d/d*) and the father positive for D. The child inherits this factor from the father and is D-positive (*D/d*). If any of the D-positive red cells of the fetus cross into the mother's circulatory system, she develops an immune anti-D antibody. This antibody, of the IgG type, crosses the placenta and reacts with the red cells of the fetus. Fortunately, sensitization usually occurs only very late in pregnancy or at the time of delivery, so the first child is rarely affected by HDN. Further, any child who is D-negative cannot be affected by anti-D antibody in the mother's circulatory system. For this reason, genotyping parents in possible cases of HDN is very useful in predicting the chance of occurrence of the disease. For example, if the husband is heterozygous for the D antigen (*D/d*) and the mother is D-negative (*d/d*), chances are that only half the children will inherit the D antigen (Fig. 9-3). On the other hand, if the father is homozygous for D (*D/D*), all the children will inherit the D antigen and there is a 100 percent chance of HDN (Fig. 9-3). (Only children who are D-positive can be affected by the disease, since only they are positive for a factor that the mother is negative for.)

It has been mentioned that the first child is rarely affected by HDN. In fact, fewer than 20 percent of Rh-negative women actually become immunized during pregnancy.[18] Although a woman can usually have one or two children who are both Rh-positive and encounter no difficulties, her immunization is permanent. Further, once the disease develops in one child, subsequent children positive for the antigen are likely to be affected at least as severely. More important, if a woman has been sensitized before pregnancy as a result of transfusion of incompatible blood or injection of antigenic material, even the first child can be severely affected [see under Prevention of Rh Immunization (use of Rh immune globulin)].

It has been mentioned that the anti-D antibody is the most common cause of HDN. Other antibodies causing this disease include anti-c, anti-K (Kell), anti-E, and even incompatibilities in the ABO system.

Prevention of Rh immunization (use of Rh immune globulin)

In the early 1960s a dramatic decrease in the incidence of HDN was seen following the introduction of Rh immune globulin (RhIG), which could prevent immunization to the D antigen during pregnancy. This was an extremely im-

Fig. 9-3. Chance of development of hemolytic disease of the newborn (HDN) based on genotypes for the D factor.

Father heterozygous for D (*D/d*)
Mother homozygous for d (*d/d*)
50% chance of hemolytic disease

	D	d
d	D/d	d/d
d	D/d	d/d

Father homozygous for D (*D/D*)
Mother homozygous for d (*d/d*)
100% chance of hemolytic disease

	D	D
d	D/d	D/d
d	D/d	D/d

portant advance, and the incidence of immunization by pregnancy to the Rh antigen D is very different now. Research at first was based on the theory that the Rh immune globulin would have to be given during pregnancy, since that was when primary immunization was believed to occur. These attempts were not entirely successful, however. Later research showed that if the Rh immune globulin was injected into Rh-negative women who had delivered Rh-positive babies within 72 hours of delivery, they were well protected against Rh problems in subsequent pregnancies.

At present, Rh immune globulin is injected intramuscularly within 72 hours of delivery in mothers who fulfill the following requirements: (1) they are D-negative and D^u-negative, (2) they have no detectable anti-D antibody, and (3) their newborn infants are D-positive or D^u-positive.[19]

Rh immune globulin has also been used, with some success, to prevent sensitization in D-negative individuals who have been transfused accidentally with D-positive blood. More research is being done in this area.

RhIG is supplied as a sterile, clear solution to be injected intramuscularly. It is a highly concentrated solution of IgG and anti-Rh_0(D), free of hepatitis virus, and derived from human plasma.[20] One commercially available RhIG is called RhoGAM (Ortho Diagnostics, Raritan, N.J.).

The anti-D antibody can be detected 12–60 hours after the administration of RhIG and is sometimes found for as long as 5 months. If it is detected 6 months after delivery, active immunization and failure of the RhIG can be assumed. Such failures are infrequent, but they can occur if RhIG is given too late or in too small a dose, or if Rh immunization has already occurred during the pregnancy. Most of the D-positive fetal cells enter the maternal circulation at the time of delivery. The amount of fetal blood present in the maternal circulation is important for the RhIG dosage. For example, a dose of RhIG that will prevent the formation of anti-D in a woman who has 10 ml of fetal blood in her circulation may be totally ineffective in a woman with 60 ml of fetal blood.[21] The amount of fetal bleeding into the maternal circulation is best determined by use of a quantitative Kleihauer-Betke stain or a modification of this method.[22]

Acid elution stain (modified Kleihauer-Betke method)

This stain is based on the fact that fetal hemoglobin is resistant to acid elution (separation of a substance by extraction) whereas adult hemoglobin is not. That is, when a thin blood smear is exposed to an acid buffer, the adult red cell loses its hemoglobin into the buffer, leaving only the red cell stroma, whereas the fetal red cell is unaffected and retains its hemoglobin. The smears are examined under the microscope after staining and the percentage of fetal cells in the maternal blood is used to calculate the approximate volume of fetal hemorrhage into the maternal circulation. Either clotted blood or anticoagulated blood may be used for this test.

ABO factors

HDN can also occur as a result of factors in the ABO system. In this case, the mother is usually blood group O and the child inherits the A or B antigen from its father. If this occurs and any fetal cells find their way into the mother's circulation, she develops an immune IgG antibody in addition to her natural IgM anti-A or anti-B antibody. If an immune IgG antibody is produced, it crosses the placenta and reacts with corresponding antigen on the red cells of the fetus. Fortunately, although ABO sensitization may occur fairly often, hemolytic disease caused by ABO incompatibility is less severe and the child may be only mildly affected and require little or no treatment.[23]

Treatment of hemolytic disease of the newborn

When HDN does occur, it varies considerably in severity. In its most severe form, the child is stillborn or aborts early in pregnancy. If the child is alive when born, it may be affected so mildly as to require little treatment, or it may be severely affected by the products of destruction of the red cells and by anemia. The cell destruction results in hemolytic anemia accompanied by abnormal levels of serum bilirubin with the clinical appearance of jaundice. The bilirubin will result in irreversible brain damage if present in sufficient concentration. If the child survives and is not treated adequately, the brain damage will result in severe mental retardation.

Treatment in severe cases of HDN includes blood transfusion. This is referred to as an *exchange transfusion*, for most of the child's blood is replaced with the transfused blood. The exchange transfusion will serve to correct the anemia and remove the abnormal levels of serum bilirubin, thus preventing brain damage.

The type of blood used for transfusion depends on the antibody responsible for the disease. The outstanding consideration is that the blood be negative for the factor against which the antibody has been formed. In other words, the child is given blood that is compatible with the mother. In the case of HDN caused by the formation of anti-D antibody in the mother's serum, the child is transfused with blood that is specific for its own ABO type but negative for the D antigen. This is because not all of the child's blood is replaced at the time of exchange, some maternal antibody is left. Therefore, blood is given that will not react with the remaining antibody yet will not harm the child. In cases of ABO incompatibility that require exchange, the mother is usually group O and the child group A or B. In such cases the child is transfused with low-titer group O blood of the child's Rh type.

Many laboratory tests are performed in cases of HDN, on the parents' (primarily the mother's) blood prior to birth and on the child's blood after birth. The first step is to type the mother and father for ABO and Rh during pregnancy to see if HDN can occur. In other words, is the father positive for any factor that the mother is negative for? Depending on the results of genotyping the mother and father, with reference to frequency charts and family studies, the probability of occurrence of the disease can be predicted. The mother's serum is usually screened by means of the indirect antiglobulin (Coombs) test to see if an antibody exists. If an antibody is found, it is identified and the titer is determined. This titer is rechecked throughout pregnancy as an indication of the possible severity of the disease.

After birth, several tests may be performed on the child's blood, in addition to further tests on the maternal serum. Initially, a sample of umbilical cord blood is tested for ABO group and Rh type, and a direct antiglobulin (Coombs) test is performed. Some other laboratory tests include hemoglobin determinations, blood smear examination and differential, reticulocyte count, and serum bilirubin determinations on the child's blood.

The decision to perform exchange transfusion will depend on a combination of laboratory results and on the clinical condition of the child. Preparation can and should be made before birth, so that the exchange can be done as soon as possible if necessary.

COMPATIBILITY TESTING OR CROSS MATCHING

Whenever blood is to be transfused, two considerations must be kept in mind. First, blood must be selected that will not be harmful to the patient or result in a transfusion reaction. Second, blood must be selected that will be of maximum benefit to the patient. For these reasons, whenever blood is to be transfused the *compatibility test* or *cross matching* must be performed.

When blood is selected for transfusion, the patient and the donor are tested for ABO type and for the presence or absence of the D (Rh_0) antigen. The ABO group is matched and the Rh type is selected with respect to the D factor. Patients whose cells contain the D antigen are given blood positive for the D factor (Rh-positive blood), while patients who are negative for the D antigen are always given blood that is negative for the D antigen (Rh-negative blood). The other antigens that collectively make up a person's complete blood type are not matched when blood is to be transfused.

In general, the cross match is used to help detect (1) unexpected antibodies in the patient's serum, (2) some ABO incompatibilities, and (3) some errors in labeling, recording, or identifying patients or donors.[24] Unfortunately, compatibility testing is not a perfect or foolproof method that guards against all problems that may arise. The most frequent causes of transfusion of incompatible blood are errors of an organizational, clerical, or technical nature. Although these errors may be detected by means of the cross match, this is not always the case. The laboratory must always work with great care to avoid mistakes of this nature. In addition, although ABO incompatibility may be detected in the cross match, not all such errors are found by this method. Correct typing remains absolutely necessary.

In addition, incompatibility will be discovered only if the patient's serum contains an unexpected antibody. Cross matching will not prevent immunization if the patient is transfused with foreign antigen. For example, an Rh-negative person who has never been exposed to Rh-positive antigenic material will not show incompatibility if cross-matched with Rh-positive blood, but the person may develop an anti-D antibody. Errors of Rh typing will be detected only if the recipient's serum contains an Rh

antibody. Furthermore, no single cross-matching procedure will detect all unexpected antibodies that may be present in the patient's serum. Finally, even if the blood is found to be compatible, the cross match will not ensure the normal survival of donor red cells.[24] Blood must be processed and stored correctly.

There are several different ways to perform the compatibility test. No method is perfect or can even be said to be preferable. In general, there are (1) the saline solution or serum cross match, (2) the high-protein cross match, (3) the antiglobulin (Coombs) cross match, and (4) enzyme cross matches. Each of these types may be performed as a *major* or a *minor* cross match.

The division into major and minor cross matches is related to the principles involved in considering group O persons as universal donors and group AB persons as universal recipients. The major cross match involves testing the donor's red cells with the patient's serum to detect any antibody in the patient's serum that will react with the donor's red cells. The presence of such antibody in the patient's serum would certainly result in a major transfusion reaction, for all the infused donor cells would be destroyed by the patient's antibodies. Of course, even if the patient's serum did contain an unexpected antibody, it would be detected only if the donor's cells contained the corresponding antigen. For this reason, the patients' serum is usually screened with a red cell preparation containing a great variety of antigens in order to detect a greater variety of unexpected antibodies than may be detected by means of a major cross match of prospective donors.[25]

The minor cross match is just the opposite—it tests the donor's serum with the patient's red cells to detect the presence of an antibody in the donor's serum that is specific for an antigen on the patient's red cells. Antibody in the donor's serum will be detected only if the patient's red cells contain the corresponding antigen. The minor cross match will not detect every antibody in the donor's serum. This test is referred to as the minor cross match because even if it were positive, the transfusion reaction would be minor, in the sense that the donor's antibody would be so diluted by infusion into the patient that only a few of the patient's red cells would be destroyed and the donor cells would remain intact and viable. This was the rationale for using group O blood as universal donor blood, and both cases have the same disadvantages. Although the major cross match is required whenever blood is to be transfused, the minor cross match may be optional. Since donor's serum must be adequately tested for unexpected antibody by an antibody-screening technique, the minor cross match is no longer commonly done.[26] However, no one technique is perfect, and many investigators feel that both antibody-screening techniques and minor cross matches should be performed routinely, since they detect different problems.[27]

Whether one or both cross matches are performed, different techniques may be used. No single technique will detect all unexpected antibodies. Usually a combination of techniques is used. However, the antiglobulin phase, or test, must be included.

Saline solution or serum cross match[28]

The various general types of cross matches will be discussed in the paragraphs that follow, although the exact procedures will not be given.

The saline solution or serum test involves mixing serum and a suspension of cells in serum or saline solution. This may be a major test, using patient serum and donor cells, or a minor test, using donor serum and patient cells. The test tube is first incubated at room temperature, centrifuged, and observed for the presence of agglutination or hemolysis. At this stage ABO incompatibility will be observable, as will incompatibility caused by antibodies of the P, MNSs, Lewis, Lutheran, or Wright systems.

If the test is negative at this point, the test tube is further incubated at 37°C for a sufficient period of time and observed once again. Saline solution-reacting antibodies of the Rh-Hr and Lewis systems will be detected, and antibodies of the P, MNSs, or Kell systems may sometimes react at this stage.

If the saline solution or serum cross match is still negative, it may be further tested by means of the antiglobulin cross match.

High-protein cross match[28]

The high-protein cross match involves mixing serum with a suspension of cells in their own serum and adding a commercial preparation of albumin. This may be a major test, using patient serum and donor cells, or a minor test, using donor serum and patient cells. The preparation is mixed, centrifuged, and observed. It is then incubated at 37°C for a sufficient length of time and observed again. The high-protein cross match will detect most Rh-Hr antibodies, including some that are not detected by the saline solution method. The preparation may also be further tested by the antiglobulin test.

Antiglobulin (Coombs) cross match[28]

The antiglobulin, or Coombs, cross match may be an extension of either the saline solution or the albumin cross match of the major and minor types. It is the one technique that must be included in any cross-matching procedure, since it is the best way to detect most of the IgG-type antibodies. After incubation of either the saline solution or high-protein preparation at 37°C, the cells are thoroughly washed with saline solution, as described for the direct and indirect antiglobulin tests. The antiglobulin serum is added and the test carried out as recommended by the manufacturer. This is an indirect antiglobulin (Coombs) test between a patient and a prospective blood donor. The antiglobulin cross match will detect almost all Rh-Hr antibodies. In addition, it may be the only means of detecting some antibodies, especially in the Duffy, Kidd, and Kell blood group systems.

Enzyme cross matches[28]

There are also cross-matching procedures that make use of enzyme preparations such as bromelin, ficin, papain, and trypsin. Although these may be useful as additional methods, they should not be used as the only means of compatibility testing and should not replace the antiglobulin test. They may detect some Rh-Hr antibodies not found by other methods, but may not detect some antibodies of the MNSs, Kell, and Duffy systems. This type of cross match is rarely done in the immunohematology laboratory today.

Summary

Some sort of compatibility testing regimen is required whenever blood is to be transfused. Unfortunately, there is no one ideal cross-matching method and no way to guarantee that all mistakes or incompatibilities have been discovered. Of course, if an incompatibility is discovered at any point, its cause must be determined. This determination is far beyond the scope of this brief outline of the cross-matching procedure. In addition, numerous technical problems that may be encountered have not been discussed here. Yet, if typing and cross matching have been performed with care according to the correct procedure used by the particular blood bank, transfusion of blood can be a relatively safe procedure of tremendous benefit to the patient.

BLOOD COMPONENTS FOR TRANSFUSION

Only human blood and its components are used for transfusion into humans. As stated previously, the therapeutic replacement of blood or its components is indicated in many instances. The use of component therapy gives the patient a better form of treatment and often permits considerable economy in the use of blood. In addition, the risk of immune reactions may be minimized. For example, when a patient needs a special fraction of the blood, the red blood cells may not be necessary. When red cells are not transfused, the production of antibodies to them is avoided.

The "United States Pharmacopeia" includes established standards for the clinical use of blood. Preparations for blood transfusion may consist of whole fresh blood, red blood cells only, plasma, serum albumin, platelet concentrates, leukocytes, leukocyte-poor blood, and other special factors that can be isolated and transfused (Table 9-4). Materials prepared from blood by mechanical methods, especially by cen-

trifugation, are called *components*, whereas those separated by more complex processes are called blood *derivatives* or *fractions.* Modern equipment, such as refrigerated centrifuges and plastic bags, has made blood component preparation within reach for most every blood bank laboratory. Blood fractionation is still a complex process and is done only in laboratories with the necessary equipment and trained technologists; many of these are commercial laboratories.

The use of plastic bags for blood containers has been the most important advance for component blood therapy. By using plastic instead of glass, several containers can be interconnected for sterilization as a unit. Blood drawn into the primary container bag can be easily separated into components, which are then transferred aseptically into one or more of the satellite container bags.[29] In this way, plasma and cells can be prepared, stored, and administered individually, without the potential for contamination that is always present when the blood container

Table 9-4. Some blood components and derivatives and their uses[a]

Blood component or derivative	Use
Fresh whole blood	Acute blood loss requiring massive replacement
Stored whole blood	Acute blood loss
Packed red blood cells	Therapy for anemia
Platelet concentrate	Functional or quantitative platelet defects
Leukocyte-poor blood	For individuals with leukocyte antibodies
Washed red blood cells	To circumvent reactions caused by plasma antigens
Freshly frozen plasma	Coagulation factor defects
Albumin	Burns, protein depletion, blood volume restorer
Gamma globulin	Hypogammaglobulinemia and therapeutic antibody uses
Factor II–VII–X–IX concentrate	Correction of vitamin K-dependent factor deficiencies

[a]Adapted from Stanley S. Raphael et al., "Lynch's Medical Laboratory Technology," 3d ed., vol. II, p. 1298, W. B. Saunders Company, Philadelphia, 1976.

is "entered" for transfusion into the recipient or patient.

Collection of blood

Blood for eventual transfusion must be collected and handled under strictly sterile conditions to prevent bacterial contamination. Skin cleansing is done differently by different blood banks. One method is to use a tincture of green soap and 70% alcohol first, followed by tincture of iodine to sterilize the puncture site. The venipuncture is made after applying a tourniquet in the proper manner.

Blood collected for transfusion must be treated with an anticoagulant. Plastic or glass containers may be used. They contain the proper amount of anticoagulant, usually a sterile citrate-phosphate-dextrose (CPD) solution, or acid citrate-dextrose (ACD) solution. The usual amount of blood drawn for one unit of whole blood is 450 ml. Proper labeling of the collecting container is of the utmost importance. The name of the product (i.e., whole blood), amount collected, kind and amount of anticoagulant, donor number, required storage temperature, expiration date, ABO blood group, and Rh type (once these tests are completed) should be shown on the label. When the proper amount of blood has been collected, a series of small tubes are filled with blood and are used for the blood bank studies in the laboratory. These samples used for blood processing must also be properly labeled.

Storage of blood

Blood bank blood must be stored in a refrigerator with a constant temperature of 1-6°C. Some sort of alarm must be available that will go off whenever the temperature is not within these limits. A thermometer for recording the temperature should also be installed. Whole blood, collected with citrate, can be stored for only 21 days. After 21 days, this blood is outdated and is removed. Stored whole blood is inspected daily for color, turbidity, appearance of clots, and presence of hemolysis. Blood is removed when it does not meet the appearance criteria established by the laboratory.

Common components and derivatives

Whole blood

Whole blood is made up of plasma and the formed elements. It is collected aseptically and must be free of transmissible diseases such as hepatitis. Clotting is prevented by use of ACD or CPD solution, the preparation usually being called *citrated whole human blood*. In cases of severe hemorrhage, whole blood is used to replace red cells and plasma. Whole blood can be stored for up to 21 days if refrigerated at 1-6°C.

Red blood cells

Blood component preparation begins with the separation of plasma from whole blood, leaving the red cells. Red cells for transfusion can be prepared by sedimentation or centrifugation. The technique used must maintain the sterility of both the plasma and the red cells. If the container is not entered when the red cells are prepared, the expiration date for the red cells remains the same as for the original whole blood. If the container is entered, the red cells are considered usable for only 24 hours.[30] Packed red cells are especially useful in treating certain anemic conditions.

Plasma

When the red cells are removed from whole blood, plasma remains. It is the liquid portion of blood that has been anticoagulated. Slightly more than half the volume of whole blood is plasma. Plasma can be used in clinical situations where bleeding has occurred, as in the case of shock, where liquid replacement is critical. Its use has become less common as other substances have been developed for fluid replacement therapy, however. Freshly frozen plasma is a good source of labile clotting factors and is used in the treatment of hemophilia, for example. At present, freshly frozen plasma is used for most plasma transfusions.

The clinical need for various blood fractions has resulted in increased commercial production of these fractions from blood plasma. Albumin can be used to treat extensive burns and pancreatitis. Gamma globulin is the antibody-containing portion of plasma that is separated and used therapeutically for its antibody content.

Platelet concentrates

Nearly all therapy for low platelet counts involves platelet concentrate transfusion. Platelet concentrates are prepared by differential centrifugation of whole blood shortly after donation. Regulations state that platelets must be processed within 4 hours after blood is drawn from the donor. In current practice platelet concentrates to be used for thrombocytopenia therapy are stored at room temperature for as short a time as possible, usually 24 hours or less.[31]

CONCLUSION

This chapter has been only a brief introduction to the complex field of immunohematology and blood banking. Specific blood-grouping and cross-matching methods have been omitted. The current edition of the "Technical Manual of the American Association of Blood Banks" is useful for these procedures. Also, it is extremely important to *always* follow the manufacturer's instructions when using any specific blood-grouping or -typing antisera. Complete instructions are always included with the reputable commercial products. Other topics that have not been covered completely in this chapter but must be understood before the student can work in the blood bank include causes of error, cleaning of glassware, organization of the blood bank, selection of blood donors, labeling of blood, and record-keeping protocol. Excellent discussions of these subjects have been published in standard blood bank texts. In addition, knowledge may be gained from firsthand experience in a licensed blood bank.

In the field of blood banking there are numerous situations that may result in error. In general, these may be organizational, clerical, or technical errors.[1] Organizational and clerical errors may be made by the blood bank staff or by personnel in other services involved in the transfusion of blood. These errors often involve incorrect identification of the patient or of the blood removed from the patient and sent to the laboratory for testing.

Transfusion involves a series of tests that are performed by several persons. Included are clerical manipulations where even a mistake on the part of a typist in transcribing a laboratory report could result in fatal errors if adequate checks did not exist. Because of the number of persons and tests involved in blood transfusion, a blood bank has elaborate organizational procedures that must be followed exactly to ensure that the correct blood be transfused into the correct patient. The American Association of Blood Banks has definite requirements and recommendations. Organizational systems involve such items and procedures as request forms, methods of labeling tubes of blood from the patient, manner of recording results in the laboratory, labeling and numbering of donor blood, selection of blood donors, and storage of blood.

Technical errors are the direct responsibility of the blood banking laboratory and its staff. They may be personal errors, where the technician is directly responsible, or impersonal errors resulting from various factors that enter into the laboratory technique. In any blood-grouping or compatibility testing method, impersonal technical factors can result in falsely positive or falsely negative results. Some may happen in all tests, and some are peculiar to a specific method. These sources of error are beyond the scope of this discussion but they must be understood by the blood bank technician if the results are to be reliable and accurate.

It is hoped that this brief outline of blood banking will serve as a useful introduction to the student. Work in this area will require much additional knowledge and study.

REFERENCES

1. R. R. Race, in I. Dunsford and C. C. Bowley (eds.), "Techniques in Blood Grouping," Oliver and Boyd, Ltd., Edinburgh and London, 1955.
2. "Technical Manual of the American Association of Blood Banks," American Association of Blood Banks, Washington, D.C., 1977.
3. Nancy J. Bigley, "Immunologic Fundamentals," pp. 13–17, Year Book Medical Publishers, Inc., Chicago, 1975.
4. Peter D. Issitt and Charla H. Issitt, "Applied Blood Group Serology," 2d ed., pp. 3–4, Spectra Biologicals, division of Becton, Dickinson & Company, Oxnard, Calif., 1975.
5. Bigley, *op. cit.*, p. 39.
6. R. R. Race and R. Sanger, "Blood Groups in Man," 6th ed., p. 8, Blackwell Scientific Publications, Oxford, 1975.
7. Race and Sanger, *op. cit.*
8. "Technical Manual of the American Association of Blood Banks," *op. cit.*, pp. 188–197.
9. *Ibid.*, p. 196.
10. A. S. Wiener and I. B. Wexler, "Heredity of the Blood Groups," chap. 5, Grune & Stratton, New York, 1958.
11. Race and Sanger, *op. cit.*, chap. 5.
12. R. E. Rosenfield, F. H. Aleen, Jr., S. N. Swisher, and S. Kochwa, A Review of the Rh Serology and Presentation of a New Technology, *Transfusion*, vol. 2, p. 287, 1962.
13. Issitt and Issitt, *op. cit.*, p. 117.
14. Stanley S. Raphael et al., "Lynch's Medical Laboratory Technology," 3d ed., vol. II, p. 1323, W. B. Saunders Company, Philadelphia, 1976.
15. "Technical Manual of the American Association of Blood Banks," *op. cit.*, pp. 156–158.
16. Douglas W. Huestis, Joseph R. Bove, and Shirley Busch, "Practical Blood Transfusion," 2d ed., pp. 111–115, Little, Brown and Company, Boston, 1976.
17. "Technical Manual of the American Association of Blood Banks," *op. cit.*, pp. 163–164.
18. *Ibid.*, p. 219.

19. *Ibid.*, p. 226.
20. *Ibid.*
21. Issitt and Issitt, *op. cit.*, p. 335.
22. E. M. Clayton, Jr., E. B. Foster, and E. P. Clayton, New Stain for Fetal Erythrocytes in Peripheral Blood Smears, *Obstet. Gynecol.*, vol. 35, p. 642, 1970.
23. "Blood Group Antigens and Antibodies as Applied to Hemolytic Disease of the Newborn," p. 27, Ortho Diagnostics, Raritan, N.J., 1968.
24. "Technical Manual of the American Association of Blood Banks," *op. cit.*, p. 188.

25. Huestis et al., *op. cit.*, p. 211.
26. "Technical Manual of the American Association of Blood Banks," *op. cit.*, p. 188.
27. "Blood Group Antigens and Antibodies as Applied to Compatibility Testing," pp. 12–13, Diagnostic Division, Ortho Pharmaceutical Corporation, Raritan, N.J., 1967.
28. N. J. Bryant, "An Introduction to Immunohematology," pp. 179–182, W. B. Saunders Company, Philadelphia, 1976.
29. Huestis et al., *op. cit.*, p. 285.
30. *Ibid.*, p. 286.
31. *Ibid.*, pp. 298–302.

BIBLIOGRAPHY

Bigley, Nancy J.: "Immunologic Fundamentals," Year Book Medical Publishers, Inc., Chicago, 1975.

Bryant, N. J.: "An Introduction to Immunohematology," W. B. Saunders Company, Philadelphia, 1976.

Davidsohn, Israel and John Bernard Henry (eds.): "Clinical Diagnosis by Laboratory Methods," 15th ed., W. B. Saunders Company, Philadelphia, 1974.

Dusford, I. and C. C. Bowley: "Techniques in Blood Grouping," Oliver and Boyd, Ltd., Edinburgh and London, 1955.

Erskine, Addine G.: "Principles and Practices of Blood Grouping," C. V. Mosby Company, St. Louis, 1973.

Greendyke, Robert M. and Jane Corner Banzhaf: "Introduction to Blood Banking," 2d ed., Medical Examination Publishing Company, Inc., Flushing, N.J., 1974.

Huestis, Douglas W., Joseph R. Bove, and Shirley Busch: "Practical Blood Transfusion," 2d ed., Little, Brown and Company, Boston, 1976.

Issitt, Peter D. and Charla H. Issitt: "Applied Blood Group Serology," 2d ed., Spectra Biologicals, division of Becton, Dickinson & Company, Oxnard, Calif., 1975.

Mollison, P. L.: "Blood Transfusion in Clinical Medicine," 5th ed., Blackwell Scientific Publications, Oxford, 1972.

Race, R. R. and R. Sanger: "Blood Groups in Man," 6th ed., Blackwell Scientific Publications, Oxford, 1975.

Raphael, Stanley S. et al.: "Lynch's Medical Laboratory Technology," 3d ed., vol. II, W. B. Saunders Company, Philadelphia, 1976.

"Standards for Blood Banks and Transfusion Services," 8th ed., American Association of Blood Banks, Washington, D.C., 1976.

Stratton, F. and P. H. Renton: "Practical Blood Grouping," Charles C Thomas, Springfield, Ill., 1958.

"Technical Manual of the American Association of Blood Banks," American Association of Blood Banks, Washington, D.C., 1977.

Wiener, Alexander S.: "Advances in Blood Grouping," Grune & Stratton, New York, 1961.

Wiener, A. S. and I. B. Wexler: "Heredity of the Blood Groups," Grune & Stratton, New York, 1958.

Wittman, Karl S. and John C. Thomas: "Medical Laboratory Skills," McGraw-Hill Book Company, New York, 1977.

TEN
MICROBIOLOGY

Microbiology involves the study of organisms so small that they cannot be seen with the naked eye. They can be observed only with a microscope. For most routine studies the bright-field microscope is used, and the organism appears dark against a bright background. Other optical systems that are sometimes used in microbiology are the dark-field, phase-contrast, ultraviolet, fluorescent, and electron microscopes.

Microorganisms, or microbes, are distributed throughout nature and interact in human and other life cycles. For example, certain bacteria are normal constituents of the human intestinal tract. These microorganisms benefit from this association, for they derive essential food materials from the host. The host also benefits, for the microorganisms synthesize and aid in the digestion of vitamins that are essential for human life. The life cycle in general involves the bacterial breakdown of dead plants and animals into simpler substances, which can be utilized by green plants to make foodstuffs that are utilized by higher animals. Some plant microorganisms that inhabit the digestive tracts of ruminants, such as cows, are essential for the digestion of cellulose, which is the major foodstuff of these animals.

Although microorganisms are generally beneficial and essential for life, some are harmful to their hosts. These are disease-producing, or *pathogenic*, microorganisms. The discussion in this chapter will be concerned with the less numerous, pathogenic microorganisms.

The pathogenic microorganisms include living organisms of both the plant and animal kingdoms. The only true microbes of the animal kingdom are the *protozoa*, which are single-celled animals. Most of the protozoa are harmless, but some may be pathogenic. The protozoa are further subdivided into amebas, ciliates, flagellates, and sporozoa. An example of a disease resulting from protozoa is amebic dysentery, which is caused by a specific protozoan ameba.

Certain pathogenic worms are often included in the field of microbiology, although they are not microorganisms. Examples of worms that cause disease are the tapeworm *Taenia solium*, the fluke *Fasciolopsis buski*, and the roundworm *Strongyloides stercoralis*. An even higher class of animals, the arthropods, are included in microbiology in some instances. These organisms themselves rarely cause disease; however, they serve as vectors in certain microbial infections. Some insects are essential in one stage of the life cycle of true microorganisms that cause malaria. Also, some ticks are bloodsucking parasites themselves.

Several different groups of microorganisms are studied in the microbiology laboratory, including bacteria, viruses, rickettsiae, fungi, protozoa, and algae. Organisms in each of these groups can cause disease. Medical microbiology is concerned with identifying pathogens and developing effective ways to eliminate or control them.

The field of medical microbiology is generally divided into areas of specialization, depending on the type of microorganism being studied. For example, the study of bacteria is called *bacteriology*, the study of viruses *virology*, the study of fungi *mycology*, the study of protozoa *protozoology*, the study of rickettsiae *rickettsiology*, and the study of algae *phycology*. In addition, certain parasites are also studied in many microbiology departments; the study of parasites is called *parasitology*.

In this chapter the discussion deals more with bacteriology than any other area of microbiology. However, it is possible to apply the skills learned in dealing with bacteria to the other areas. As in other divisions of the medical laboratory, if the basic skills are understood and learned well, many other specific tests and procedures can easily be done. The routine procedures, such as initial media inoculation, preparation of media, and staining of slides, are extremely important for the final identification process. Techniques involved in the growth (culture) and identification of various pathogenic bacteria will also be discussed in this chapter.

CLASSIFICATION OF MICROORGANISMS

In discussing microorganisms, it is necessary to touch on the method by which living things are classified. By using biological classification methods, it is possible for the laboratory microbiologist to systematically identify microbes. This classification system provides a relatively simple method for placing microbes into categories according to their morphological and biochemical properties.

In the terminology of biological classification, the word *species* is frequently used. It is the basic unit of the biological world. The species category is based on reproduction: members of the same species are able to mate successfully and produce others of their kind. The *genus* is the next largest classification. The microbes studied in the medical laboratory will have two Latin names, the genus name (often abbreviated) and the species name. These Latin names are printed in italics. The same genus can include several different species, all of which are somewhat different from each other. For example, the genus *Hemophilus* includes several species. Depending on the species, the organisms cause different diseases in humans. *Hemophilus influenzae* is a pathogen that causes acute respiratory tract infections, and *Hemophilus aegyptius* is responsible for

Fig. 10-1. Biological classification system.

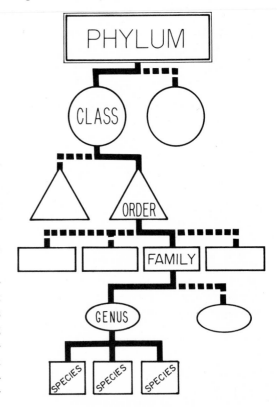

conjunctivitis (pinkeye).[1] At least four other species of this genus can cause human disease.

Continuing up the classification system, microbes that have common characteristics are grouped into successively larger categories. Similar genera are grouped into *families*, related families are classified as an *order*, related orders make up a *class*, and classes with common characteristics comprise a *phylum* (Fig. 10-1).

The majority of pathogenic microorganisms belong to the plant kingdom, which includes the fungi and simpler organisms. The systematic classification of these organisms is quite complex. Fungi are simple colorless plants that are further subdivided into the molds, yeasts, and bacteria. Microorganisms simpler than bacteria include pleuropneumonia and pleuropneumonia-like organisms, rickettsiae, and viruses.

TYPES AND COLLECTION OF SPECIMENS FOR MICROBIOLOGICAL EXAMINATION

When a patient has certain disease symptoms, the physician will often want to identify the causative agent if a microbiological infection is suspected. Positive identification of the causative agent is important in the correct treatment of the patient. Therefore, the physician will send appropriate specimens to the laboratory. In the case of a possible kidney or urinary tract infection, a urine specimen will be collected for bacterial analysis. If the patient has a sore throat, the throat will be swabbed with a cotton-tipped applicator, and this will be submitted for analysis. Possible dysentery will require the examination of stool specimens, while the examination of infected wounds will require swabs or appropriate material from the area of infection. Other sites of infection from which swabs or material is submitted to the laboratory for culture and identification include the blood; various body fluids; cervix; urethra; vagina; ear; endometrium; eye; spinal, ventricular, or subdural fluid; bronchi or trachea (sputum material); and various tissues.

General types of microbiology specimens collected

Sputum

When a specimen of sputum is collected, the patient must cooperate fully to ensure that a proper specimen is obtained. Sputum is usually collected in the morning, and it should be sent to the laboratory and processed immediately. Deep coughing will usually bring up a good sputum specimen. It is necessary to avoid collecting nasal or salivary fluids. A wide-mouthed sterile container is best used for collecting this type of specimen.

Urine

The collection of urine for microbiological studies also requires the cooperation of the patient. A midstream sample, usually the first morning specimen, is suitable for culture, provided care has been taken to clean the urethral area before the collection (see also under Collection, Preservation, and Preparation of Laboratory Specimens in Chap. 1). A sterile container must be used for the collection. When a patient is too ill or cannot void properly, a specimen is obtained by catheterization. This is not done unless necessary, however. The specimen should be sent to the laboratory for immediate processing.

Blood

A blood sample for culture is extremely useful, as normal blood is sterile and should not contain any microorganisms. Special blood-collecting equipment is used. Sterile collecting bottles containing the proper nutrient broth media, blood-collecting sets with needles and tubing that allows the blood to flow into the collecting bottle, as well as the proper skin cleansing equipment, are necessary to ensure a properly collected blood specimen for culture. Special care must be taken to clean the venipuncture site carefully before puncture to avoid possible contamination of the blood sample.

Cerebrospinal fluid

Spinal fluid is collected only by a physician. Rapid handling of spinal fluid samples in the laboratory is extremely important, since some of the organisms associated with meningitis quickly "self-destruct" after collection. Spinal fluid is collected by lumbar puncture into tubes. The tubes are sent to the laboratory immediately for various studies.

Swabs of various fluids

Swabs are used to collect cultures from various openings of the body, such as the nose, throat, mouth, vagina, anus, and wounds. These swabs must be collected carefully and placed in the proper transport media before they are taken to the laboratory for processing. It has been found that certain organisms survive longer when polyester rather than cotton swabs are used.

Feces

Feces normally contain large numbers of bacteria, and a specimen of feces is usually cultured to isolate certain types of pathogenic organisms. Feces are usually collected early in the day and should be cultured immediately. Swabs of the rectal area are also commonly used.

Culturing considerations for specimens

There are certain possible sources of infection of each area from which material may be submitted for examination. The microbiologist must be aware of the types of infective agents that may be responsible for a disease and test for these accordingly. Likewise, for each source of infected material there is a certain set of tests that must be performed to discover the cause of infection.

When material is submitted to the microbiology laboratory for culture and identification, certain procedures are the responsibility of the people actually collecting the specimen. This is rarely done by the laboratory personnel. However, it is the responsibility of the laboratory to inform the hospital staff of correct procedures for collecting microbiological specimens and to provide suitable containers for this purpose. The following are general considerations for the collection of specimens.

The treatment of a disease or infection often involves the use of antibiotics or other agents that destroy various pathogens. The antibiotics are often administered before the causative agent is identified, since such identification takes 1 day or more while the patient requires immediate treatment. However, culture of the causative agent will often be impossible once antibiotics have been administered. Therefore, the appropriate specimen should be obtained before antibiotics are administered.

It is important to remember that material should be collected for culture from the location where the suspected organism is most likely to be found. An example of this is the culture of specimens from draining lesions containing coagulase-positive staphylococci. This type of specimen should also be collected with as little external contamination as possible.

Another factor that contributes to the successful isolation of the causative agent is the stage of the disease during which the specimen is collected. Enteric pathogens are found in much greater numbers in the acute stage of certain diarrheal intestinal infections, and are therefore more likely to be isolated from specimens obtained at this stage. Viruses causing meningitis are isolated from cerebrospinal fluid with greater frequency when the fluid is obtained at the onset of the disease. It is important that the physician understand the necessity of collecting microbiological specimens at the correct time, as well as in the proper manner.

Specimen containers

Correct identification of a causative agent requires isolation and growth of a *pure culture* of that organism in the laboratory. To do this, the original specimen must be collected in a sterile container and not contaminated at any stage in its subsequent transfer to or isolation in the laboratory. The microbiology laboratory should provide sterile containers to the nursing station or physician with specific information about the type of container to be used for various types of specimens and about the manner of collection. It is also important, for the protection of the laboratory personnel and anyone else handling the specimen, that the specimen be placed entirely within the appropriate container and not allowed to contaminate the outside. Microbiology specimens often contain dangerous pathogens that could infect anyone coming in contact with the infected material.

The container holding the specimen should neither contribute its own microbial flora nor increase or decrease the original flora contained in the specimen. A variety of containers have been manufactured for collecting microbiology specimens. Some are reused after proper cleaning and sterilization, and some are disposable. One of the most useful pieces of collecting equipment is a wooden applicator stick tipped with cotton, calcium alginate, or polyester. Applicator sticks tipped with the appropriate fiber, packaged in a capped sterile tube, are available commercially. These sticks may be used for the collection of material from the throat, nose, eye, or ear; from wounds and sites of operation; from urogenital orifices; and from the rectum. In many instances, another tube containing sterile broth is included

with these units, and when the specimen has been collected on the swab it is immediately placed in the broth tube to prevent drying out. The whole outfit is properly labeled and promptly sent to the laboratory.

Recently, many innovations have been made in sterile, disposable culture units of various types. To prolong the survival of microorganisms that have been collected, transport media can be used. This is especially desirable when a significant delay occurs between collection and culturing. Swabs of infectious material can be prevented from drying out by immersion in broth or another holding medium until culture is done. If the suspected organism is an anaerobe, conventional transport tubes should not be used. The crucial factor in the successful final culturing of anaerobic (oxygen-sensitive) organisms is the transport of the original specimen. Atmospheric oxygen, which kills such organisms, must be kept out until the specimen has been processed anaerobically by the laboratory. Special double-stoppered collection tubes containing oxygen-free carbon dioxide or nitrogen can be used. The specimen is injected through the rubber stopper, avoiding the introduction of air. If only a swab can be obtained, the swab should be one that has been prepared in a special "gassed-out" tube and then transported to the laboratory in a rubber-stoppered tube partially filled with an anaerobic medium (see under Oxygen).

Initial laboratory handling of specimens

Most pathogenic organisms are not greatly affected by small changes in temperature, but they are generally susceptible to drying out. Certain bacteria, however, such as meningococci in cerebrospinal fluid, are quite susceptible to low temperatures and require immediate culturing. Most pathogenic organisms are preserved by refrigeration if immediate culturing cannot be done. Refrigeration will also prevent overgrowth of other organisms that are present, which could make the isolation of the significant microbe more difficult. Refrigeration is particularly effective for specimens of urine, feces, sputum, and material on swabs from a variety of sources. It is not effective for anaerobic organisms from wound cultures; these specimens should be kept at room temperature until cultured. Still other specimens require freezing to preserve the organism. It is important that those working in the microbiology laboratory understand thoroughly the factors that affect the survival of the organisms being handled. Only when the specimens are properly collected and properly handled initially by the laboratory will the final results of the culturing methods be valid.

Once the specimen has been placed in the appropriate container, it should be delivered to the laboratory immediately and not allowed to stand at the nursing station. Although many organisms remain alive for long periods after collection, some are extremely fastidious outside the host and require rapid inoculation into a suitable culture medium in order to be detected. In fact, some organisms are so fragile that arrangements must be made to take a special culture medium to the patient so that the material can be placed directly on it. Some pathogens will be obscured by the rapid and overwhelming growth of other organisms that are normally present in the material to be cultured. For example, fecal samples normally contain several types of bacteria that will obscure the detection of such pathogens as *Shigella* if the specimen is not delivered to the laboratory and plated onto a suitable medium soon after collection.

When the specimen reaches the laboratory, it is not always possible to inoculate the correct culture medium immediately. Most specimens may be stored under refrigeration at 4-6°C until the culture medium can be inoculated. With certain microorganisms, however, the medium must be inoculated immediately, and it is the responsibility of the laboratory personnel to know which organisms require immediate inoculation.

Finally, the physician should inform the laboratory of the source of the material to be examined and of the tentative diagnosis. This information will help to ensure that the correct medium is inoculated with the specimen and will aid in the correct identification of the pathogen.

PROTECTION OF LABORATORY PERSONNEL AND STERILIZATION OF MATERIALS

Since the material to be examined in the microbiology laboratory may contain dangerous pathogens, it is necessary to protect the microbiologist. All microbiology laboratories have rules that must be followed for the protection of the workers.

First, nothing should ever be put into the mouth in the laboratory. Smoking, eating, or drinking in the laboratory is absolutely prohibited, as these are ideal modes of infection. Personal objects should not be placed on the work area, as they may become contaminated with pathogens.

The work area should be cleaned with an agent such as Pheneen, 5% phenol, or bleach before and after use each day. A mild disinfectant such as Pheneen or diluted solution of bleach is used primarily for cleaning. It is also important to keep the laboratory free of dust, for this can be the cause of infection by dangerous pathogens. If the work area is actually contaminated, a potent disinfectant such as 5% phenol must be used. For example, if a culture is dropped or spilled, 5% phenol should be poured over the contaminated area, covered with paper towels, and let stand for at least 15 minutes. Then the contaminated material must be removed and placed in an appropriate container to be autoclaved.

The hands should be washed thoroughly with soap before leaving the microbiology laboratory. They must also be washed in case of contamination. The microbiologist should not work with uncovered open cuts or broken skin. These should be covered with a bandage or some suitable material.

Since open flames are routinely used in the laboratory to sterilize the inoculating "loops" and needles and to flame the lips of test tubes before inoculation, there is a constant fire hazard in the microbiology laboratory. This may be minimized by turning off burners whenever they are not in use. In addition, burners should be kept away from lamps and cotton plugs or other material that is flammable.

These are only a few general rules for working in the microbiology laboratory. Specific laboratories will have additional rules, which are established for the safety of the personnel.

Sterilization techniques

Since microorganisms are so widely distributed in nature, it is essential that sterile media be used to grow pure cultures of bacteria. In general, all equipment and glassware and all media used in the microbiology laboratory must be absolutely sterile to ensure the preparation of pure cultures of microorganisms. Equipment in which microorganisms have been cultured or anything contaminated by infected material must be sterilized. It must also be sterilized before it is discarded in order to prevent infection of those responsible for its removal. If equipment is to be reused, it must be sterilized before a new microorganism can be isolated and identified.

Sterilization refers to the killing or destruction of all forms of life. There are various ways in which it may be achieved. In general, physical means such as heat or filtration and chemical means such as oxidation are involved.

Use of heat

The effect of heat on organisms is generally known, and heat is the most widely used and efficient physical means of sterilization. Heat may be employed in the form of *dry heat* or *moist heat*. Dry heat destroys bacteria by oxidation, while moist heat works through the coagulation of protein.[2] Except for burning or incineration, sterilization by moist heat is generally more rapid. However, the type of sterilization method that is used will depend on the nature of the material being sterilized, since many materials are destroyed by burning and many are harmed by the application of moist heat. Sterilization by dry heat includes burning and the use of hot air. Sterilization by moist heat includes the use of boiling water, "live" steam (steam at atmospheric pressure), and steam under pressure.

Burning is an especially useful means of sterilization in various steps in the culture and identification of microorganisms. Infected material from the original specimen, material from isolated colonies, and material from liquid cultures are usually manipulated by means of a transfer needle or inoculating loop. These needles and loops are made of inert metals such as platinum or suitable alloys such as Nichrome. They are unharmed when held in a Bunsen or alcohol flame and are sterilized in this manner. Therefore, when material is to be transferred, the inoculating loop or wire is flamed until it glows in a Bunsen or alcohol flame, cooled to room temperature by waiting approximately 30 seconds, and then reflamed after use to sterilize it. The Bunsen or alcohol flame is also used to flame the lip of test tubes containing culture media before and after microorganisms are introduced. The tops of certain culture media in Petri plates are also flamed when the plates are "poured," or the medium is prepared.

Use of dry air

Sterilization by dry heat is achieved by use of a *dry-air* chamber that is similar to an oven.[2] The material must be kept at a temperature between 150 and 160°C for at least 1 hour. To be sterilized in this time the material must be a good heat conductor. This method is most useful for materials that are destroyed by moist heat. Sterilization by dry heat is often used for pipets and other glassware in the microbiology laboratory.

Use of moist heat

Moist-heat sterilization by *boiling water* is convenient because it requires little special equipment. Boiling in water for 5 minutes is sufficient to kill all vegetative forms of bacteria. Unfortunately, certain species of bacteria of the genus *Bacillus* have the ability to form spores under unfavorable conditions, but return to normal when favorable conditions return. Since spores are highly resistant forms of bacteria, they pose a great problem in sterilization. To kill spores by boiling in water generally requires 1-2 hours, although certain spores have been known to survive 16 hours of boiling. For this reason, certain chemicals may be added to the water to achieve more rapid sterilization by boiling. For example, 1 g/dl sodium carbonate makes the destruction of spores more rapid and also prevents rusting of certain metals sterilized in this manner. To achieve more rapid sterilization, 2-5% carbolic acid (phenol) may be used; this will usually kill anthrax spores in 10-15 minutes.[2]

For sterilization by *live steam*, or steam at atmospheric pressure, an Arnold sterilizer is usually employed, although makeshift apparatus may be devised from kitchen equipment. A modification of sterilization by live steam that is sometimes required in the microbiology laboratory is fractional sterilization, or tyndallization. This method is required for materials or media that cannot tolerate high temperature and high pressure. However, live steam does not kill spores. To achieve the destruction of spores, the material to be sterilized is exposed to live steam for 15-30 minutes on three successive days. The vegetative cells that are present are killed by the first exposure to steam, and the exposed material is then incubated until the next day. During this time, spores develop into vegetative cells, which are killed by the next exposure to steam. The third exposure ensures sterility. This method, however, can be used only if the material to be sterilized is conducive to bacterial growth. It is especially useful for sterilizing culture media, but is not effective for such material as glassware.

Use of steam under pressure (the autoclave)

The most effective means of sterilization with moist heat involves the use of *steam under pressure*, and a special device called an *autoclave*. It is the method of choice for any material that can fit in the apparatus and is not injured by moisture, high temperature, and high pressure. Most media prepared in the microbiology laboratory are sterilized in the autoclave before use. Most equipment is sterilized in this manner, as are infected materials that are to be discarded.

Several types of autoclaves are available. Basically, the device is a heavy metal chamber with a door or lid that can be fastened to withstand the internal steam pressure, a pressure gauge, a safety valve, and a temperature gauge. The steam may be supplied by boiling water in the chamber or from heating pipes. Whatever type of autoclave is used, it is essential that *all* the air be displaced from the chamber by steam before the system is sealed. If this is not done, the chamber will contain unsaturated steam, which is a mixture of dry heat and moist heat and is significantly less efficient in achieving complete sterilization.

The exact details of operation of the autoclave may be found in the operating instructions provided with the autoclave. The material is exposed to pure steam in the autoclave at 121°C for 15-20 minutes. This temperature is achieved by applying pressure. Generally, 15 lb above atmospheric pressure is required to reach 121°C. This time and temperature will kill all forms of bacterial life, including spores. The temperature of steam in an autoclave at 15 lb gauge pressure at sea level is 121.3°C.[3]

It is strongly recommended that the efficiency of the autoclave be checked regularly. This may be conveniently done by one of several methods, using biological or chemical indicators. Commercial test kits provide sealed glass ampules containing a standardized spore suspension of *Bacillus stearothermophilus*, culture medium, and indicator. The ampule is autoclaved and exposed, incubated, and read. An unheated ampule is included as a positive control. The spores of *B. stearothermophilus* are destroyed when exposed to 121°C for 15 minutes.[4] Alternatively, the efficiency of the autoclave can be checked by using a chemical indicator in the form of an adhesive tape on which the word *sterile* is printed invisibly. The word becomes visible if the

autoclaving is sufficient. The tape may be placed on anything to be autoclaved and may be employed routinely.

Use of filtration and chemicals

In the preparation of certain media that are used in microbiology, none of the preceding methods of sterilization is applicable, since they result in deterioration of the media. In these cases, some other means such as filtration through sintered Pyrex (unglazed porcelain), infusorial earth, compressed asbestos, or membranes may be necessary. In some cases, chemical methods of sterilization such as the addition of thymol may be employed.

Not all methods of complete or partial sterilization or disinfection have been covered in this section. Sterilization or disinfection by chemical means has been largely omitted from this discussion, although it is routinely employed in microbiology. In addition, other physical means, such as radiation, may be used.

GENERAL OBSERVATIONS CONCERNING MICROORGANISMS

For the microbiologist to correctly identify the causative agent of an infection, several tests must be carried out. These tests involve a general knowledge of microorganisms and their mode of action. The field of microbiology is too extensive to be covered here. Many students using this book will already have taken a general microbiology course. Others will be given more information through lecture material or additional texts. This section deals only with the laboratory aspects of the subject.

Morphology of bacteria

Bacteria are a form of fungus. Fungi are the colorless plants—that is, plants that do not con-

tain chlorophyll. More specifically, bacteria are fungi belonging to the class Schizomycetes, which also includes related forms of the group Protophyta, the primitive plants.

Each species of bacteria has a characteristic shape, which is one of three basic shapes. Spherical or round bacteria are *cocci,* straight rod-shaped ones are *bacilli,* and spiral rod-shaped ones are *spirilla.* Most bacteria are either cocci or bacilli, the bacilli being the most numerous.

There are certain variations of the three basic shapes, such as club-shaped bacilli and bacilli with square ends. The particular species may be further classified according to whether the cells normally occur singly, in diploids or pairs, in chains, or in clusters. The prefix *diplo-* describes bacteria that occur as pairs of cells, *strepto-*

describes bacteria occurring as chains of cells, and *staphylo-* refers to irregular clumps or clusters of bacterial cells.

Although bacteria can be seen under the ordinary compound light microscope, they are extremely small structures. They are normally observed under oil immersion with an ×95–97 objective, giving a total magnification of ×950–970 when the ×10 ocular is used. Bacteria are measured in micrometers (1 μm $= \frac{1}{1000}$ millimeter or about $\frac{1}{25\,000}$ in). There is a good deal of variation in size among bacteria. Cocci may range from 0.15 to 2 μm in diameter, although most pathogens measure 0.8–1.2 μm. The bacilli show an even greater size variation. *H. influenzae* is a very small rod, about 0.5 μm long by 0.2 μm wide. *Bacillus anthracis* is a relatively large rod, 5–10 μm long and 1–3 μm wide.[5] For comparison, a red blood cell is approximately 7 μm in diameter.

If bacteria are placed on a glass slide and observed under the microscope, they appear as transparent, colorless structures and may be homogeneous or granular. They have a refractive index close to that of water, and therefore should be stained to be made more visible. Various staining procedures may be used, depending on the information desired. To observe gross morphological features, a simple stain such as crystal violet, fuchsin, methylene blue, or safranine may be used. However, the most widely used stain in the bacteriology laboratory is the Gram stain, which differentiates bacteria as gram-positive or gram-negative, besides showing gross morphological features. Other stains include acid-fast stain, capsule stains, flagella stains, stains for metachromatic granules, spore stains, relief stains, and stains for spirochetes, rickettsiae, yeast, and fungi. Some specific staining procedures and the preparation of slides are described later in this section.

Each bacterium has four distinct morphological parts: the protoplasm, cytoplasmic membrane, cell wall, and capsule. Different stains may be used to accentuate these parts. Other morpho-logical structures have been discovered by means of the electron microscope.

The morphological character of a bacterium is useful for identifying it. One should determine its general shape (sphere, straight rod, or spiral rod), its Gram-staining reaction, and its association with other bacterial cells (single, in chains, or in clusters). However, these and other morphological characteristics only rarely lead to the final identification of the bacterium. For the final identification it is necessary to know the cultural characteristics of the bacterium. This is discussed later in this section.

Each bacterium is a single cell and, like most cells, it possesses cytoplasm surrounded by a cell membrane, which in turn is surrounded by a cell wall. Some bacteria also have other external structures, such as flagella or capsules. Some typical organelles found within a single bacterium are the nucleus, ribosomes, vacuoles, and granules. Another important organelle contained within the cytoplasm is the spore. Bacteria can manufacture a slimy gelatinous layer around the cell wall, and this layer of slime often becomes an integral part of the bacterial cell structure called a capsule. If special staining techniques are used, the capsule may be seen more easily. The presence or absence of a capsule is used clinically to help identify the microorganism.

The most significant external structures of bacteria are flagella—long, threadlike structures anchored within the cell wall and cell membrane. The whiplike motion of the flagella enables the bacterial cell to move. Flagella vary in their number and position on the bacteria, and this pattern is also helpful in identifying the species.

The cytoplasm of bacteria contains a variety of granules, many of which can be identified by special staining procedures. Some bacteria have spores, or endospores, in their cytoplasm. Spores are able to survive under extremely unfavorable conditions, even when the active or vegetative bacterial cell dies. Thus, spore-forming bacteria can survive conditions that would kill non-spore-forming bacteria.

Laboratory procedures—Microscopic examination

Biological staining is the microscopic procedure most commonly used in microbiology to identify a particular bacterial species. Stains are chemical substances that contain colored dyes. Certain bacterial structures have affinities for particular dyes. Therefore special stains are useful for showing the morphology of bacteria and specific structures such as capsules, flagella, spores, and granules. *Simple* stains such as methylene blue or more complex *differential* stains are used to show special cellular details. One commonly used differential stain is the *Gram* stain. The way bacteria react to this stain depends on the chemical composition of the cell wall. Staining techniques are discussed further later in this chapter.

Cultural requirements of bacteria

Many (but not all) microorganisms may be grown in the laboratory away from their natural habitat. However, to grow microorganisms artificially it is necessary to provide the proper nutrients and growth conditions. The growth of microorganisms on artificial material is referred to as *culture* of the microorganism, and the mixture of nutrients on which the microorganism is grown is the *culture medium.*

Growth of a pure culture

Specimens for microbiological analysis must be collected in sterile containers because the identification of microorganisms generally requires isolation and growth of a pure culture of bacteria. A bacterium placed on a suitable culture medium will multiply until an isolated colony of bacteria is formed. It is assumed that each colony of bacteria originates from a single cell. In culturing bacteria in the laboratory, the infected material is treated in such a way that single bacterial cells are separated on the culture medium and allowed to grow into isolated colonies. Material from a single isolated colony is then further inoculated onto additional media, so that several colonies will appear, all arising from a single bacterium. The growth of several colonies originating from a single colony, and hence a single cell, is what is meant by a *pure culture.*

Laboratory procedures—Culture studies

Bacteria may be grown in or on specially prepared culture media. By studying the cultural characteristics of a particular bacterium, certain growth patterns may be seen and the species identification may be narrowed down. The types of culture media vary greatly. They may be prepared in liquid or solid form. A solid medium may be prepared in a flat, circular dish called a *Petri* dish or plate (see under Culture Media). When the specimen is placed on the medium in the plate, it is said to be *inoculated.* A tube of solid medium can be prepared as a *stab* or a *slant.* In a slant culture the surface of the medium is inclined at an angle (Fig. 10-2), and

Fig. 10-2. Examples of types of culture media in tubes: (a) stab culture tube, (b) slant culture tube, and (c) liquid broth culture tube.

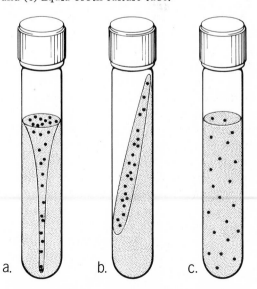

an inoculating loop or needle containing the specimen is placed on the surface of the medium. A tube of medium can also be inoculated by stabbing or passing through the medium with an inoculating needle, thus leaving the specimen behind in the medium. A tube prepared in this way is referred to as a stab tube. In a stab culture the surface of the medium is perpendicular to the sides of the test tube (Fig. 10-2). Tubes containing liquid broth media can also be inoculated with bacteria by using an inoculating loop (Fig. 10-2). (See under Special Equipment and Techniques for Microbiology Studies.)

Laboratory procedures—Biochemical tests

Many bacteria cannot be identified on the basis of microscopic or cultural studies alone. The biochemical properties and reactions of bacteria form the basis for an important series of identification procedures. Biochemical identification has been used increasingly in recent years and is an important function of the microbiology laboratory. Biochemical tests rely on bacterial physiology and the end products produced in reactions of bacterial cells.[6] The most important biochemical reactions involve fermentation, starch hydrolysis, hydrogen sulfide production, urea hydrolysis, and tryptophan hydrolysis. In each biochemical procedure, the unknown bacterium causes a change of some type in the medium, to which a specific test substance has been added. The change may be indicated by the formation of gas (carbon dioxide), which is collected in special tubes (Fig. 10-3), or by the formation of color. In some media a pH indicator is used—for instance, when an acid is produced during fermentation. Some bacteria can break down starch in the medium, and iodine is used to test for the presence or absence of starch. Metabolism of the amino acid tryptophan can produce *indole*, which can be detected by a color change in another indicator. Biochemical tests may be done individually, or they may be incorporated into culture media.

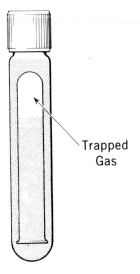

Fig. 10-3. Tube used to collect gas.

Colonial characteristics of bacteria

When inoculated onto suitable semisolid or solid nutrient media with the proper temperature and moisture, bacteria rapidly multiply and form macroscopic colonies. Under ideal conditions, the growth of a microbial cell is a geometric progression with time. For example, a single bacterium such as *Escherichia coli*, having a generation time of 20 minutes, would produce 2.2×10^{43} cells in 48 hours.[7] Certain limiting factors come into play that ultimately terminate growth, however. A culture that is a closed system will eventually stop growing as a result of exhaustion of essential nutrients, accumulation of toxic products, or development of an unfavorable pH.

The type of culture medium used—liquid or solid—can affect the appearance or growth of the colonies. In liquid media bacterial growth does not have a characteristic appearance, and organisms cannot be separated from "mixed cultures." By contrast, on solid media the appearance of a culture is extremely useful in initially differentiating the colony type and pure cultures can be isolated.

Bacteria multiply by binary fission, or division into two equal parts. Macroscopic bacterial colonies form in 24-48 hours. The colonies originate from individual cells, although each colony is a mass of individual cells, each of which functions independently. Different species of bacteria form colonies that differ in appearance; therefore, colony appearance is useful in identifying the species of bacterium. Colony characteristics that are observed for the purpose of identification include the following:

1. Bacteria without slime capsules produce colonies that appear dry and rough.
2. Bacteria with slime capsules produce colonies that appear smooth and shiny.

3. Bacteria may possess a pigment that gives a characteristic color (e.g., white, red, yellow, or orange) to the colony.
4. Bacteria may spread from the original colony, which indicates that they are motile. Nonmotile bacteria remain in discrete colonies.

Therefore, bacterial colonies should be observed for their relative size, shape, elevation, texture, marginal appearance, and color. This information, in addition to morphological appearance under the microscope and various staining reactions such as with Gram stain, helps in the eventual identification of a particular species of bacterium.

CULTURE MEDIA

The media used in clinical microbiology are generally prepared from precisely measured quantities of known substances that are formulated to give highly repeatable cultural results. Media of this type are produced synthetically and consist of the specific amino acids, sugars, salts, vitamins, and minerals needed to ensure the proper growth of certain bacterial species. They may be produced commercially or prepared by the individual laboratory and used for diagnostic purposes. Commercially prepared media in disposable culture plates or tubes are generally replacing media prepared in the individual laboratory. Broths are also used as culture media. They are less well chemically defined and are used mainly to maintain bacterial growth. They are generally not used for identification of bacterial species. Broths are meat extracts of protein materials—either peptone, an intermediate product of protein digestion, or digested protein.

A culture medium may be prepared as a solid, liquid, or semisolid, depending on the bacteriological studies to be done. Liquid media are well suited for studying the production of a gas, odor, or change in pH. Media in a semisolid or solid form are most useful for the observation of colony size, shape, and color.

Agar is used extensively in the preparation of solid media. It is a seaweed extract that is liquid when heated and solid when cooled. It does not affect bacterial growth and is an excellent base for nutrient media. Agar can be melted and poured into tubes or plates, where it will solidify when cool. The more agar used, the more solid the final medium will become. Plates, slants, and stabs are all prepared with agar as the base.

Culture medium requirements

Bacteria, like all living things, have specific requirements to sustain life and to reproduce. The culture requirements for bacteria include a source of nutrients, the proper temperature, an adequate supply of oxygen (or in some cases the absence of oxygen), and the correct pH. Some of these requirements are described in a manual published by Difco Laboratories.[8]

Food

First, the *proper food elements* must be available. Different microorganisms differ in their food requirements. Some grow on media containing simple mixtures of inorganic salts, since they are able to synthesize their own organic compounds. Others, especially many pathogens, are very particular and may require complex mixtures of nutrients, including many of the B vitamins and certain amino acids. In general, the culture medium must be able to supply carbon, nitrogen, and inorganic salts. Peptone is used in a variety of culture media as it contains nitrogen in a form (amino acids and simple nitrogen compounds) that can be used by most microorganisms. Certain bacteria require media to which serum, blood, or ascitic fluid has been added. In some media it is advantageous to add carbohydrates, and in some instances salts of calcium, manganese, magnesium, sodium, and potassium are required by the microorganism for growth.

In addition to nutrient sources, dyes or indicators may be added to culture media as a means of detecting metabolic activity by the microorganism or of promoting the growth of some microorganisms by inhibiting the growth of others. Finally, certain microorganisms either require or are enhanced by the presence of growth-promoting vitamin-like substances in the media.

Oxygen

Another factor that must be considered in culturing microorganisms is the presence or absence of *oxygen.* Some microorganisms require an atmosphere containing oxygen for growth; they are called *aerobes* or *aerobic organisms.* Others are able to derive oxygen from their food sources and are actually inhibited by atmospheric oxygen. To culture these *anaerobes* or *anaerobic organisms*, atmospheric oxygen must be excluded. There are also organisms with oxygen requirements between those of the obligate aerobes and obligate anaerobes. *Facultative anaerobes* are able to grow under either aerobic or anaerobic conditions. *Microaerophilic organisms* grow best under conditions of low oxygen tension and are inhibited by high oxygen tension.

Anaerobic conditions may be produced in the laboratory in a number of ways, including displacement of air by carbon dioxide, use of special media such as thioglycolate broth, inoculation into the deeper layers of solid media, and addition of small amounts of agar to liquid media.

Moisture

All microorganisms require some moisture for growth. Bacteria in general require a high concentration of water in their environment for growth and multiplication. Formation of highly resistant spores by bacteria that are spore formers is stimulated by drying or lack of water. Water is required for the metabolic reactions that take place in the bacterial cell and is the means of supplying nutrients to and removing waste products from the cell. Water is an integral part of the organism's protoplasm and accounts for much of the weight of the bacterial cell.

The amount of moisture in culture media varies. A medium may be used as a liquid, solid, liquefiable solid, or semisolid. Liquid media, or *broths*, may be converted to solid media by adding whole egg, egg white, or blood serum and heating until the mixture coagulates. Alternatively, potatoes may be used as a solid medium.

Liquefiable solid media are prepared by adding gelatin, which is a protein with a low melting point, or agar-agar, which is a complex carbohydrate prepared by adding certain seaweeds to a liquid medium such as nutrient broth. Agar-agar is superior to gelatin for this type of medium. It melts just before boiling, solidifies just above body temperature, and is digested by only a few bacteria. Gelatin has a lower melting point than agar-agar, many organisms do not develop satisfactorily at temperatures below its melting point, and many organisms liquefy gelatin. When gelatin is added to a broth, the medium too is referred to as a *gelatin*. For example, a mixture of gelatin and nutrient broth is called *nutrient gelatin*. Similarly, a mixture of agar-agar and nutrient broth would be called *nutrient agar.*

Semisolid media are prepared in much the same way as the liquefiable solid media. However, a much smaller amount of agar-agar is added.

pH

Another factor affecting the growth or culture of microorganisms is the *pH* of the medium. Not only must a culture medium contain the proper nutrients in the correct concentrations, it must have the correct degree of acidity or alkalinity. Most microorganisms prefer culture media that are approximately neutral, although some require a medium that is acid. Most microorganisms grow within a pH range of 3.0–9.0. Although changes in pH may not actually prevent the growth of a particular organism, its metabolic activities may not be normal if the pH is not optimum.

The pH of media is controlled by use of buffers, or substances that resist changes in hydrogen ion concentration. Buffers are especially useful for microorganisms that produce acid as part of their metabolism. These microorganisms would kill themselves by their own acid production if a suitable buffer were not present. Conversely, some bacteria produce alkaline products such as ammonia, which must also be buffered or the culture would destroy itself. Blood, milk, and seawater are all solutions that are naturally buffered and are therefore useful as culture media. Synthetic media often contain phosphate buffer systems.

Temperature

All organisms have a minimum *temperature* below which development ceases, an optimum temperature at which growth is maximum or luxuriant, and a maximum temperature above which death occurs. The majority of bacteria grow within the temperature range 15–43°C. However, the pathogens generally have a narrow temperature range with optimum growth at 35°C, and for this reason most cultures are incubated at 35°C. Since the heat of an incubator would promote drying, the incubator should always be equipped with containers of water or some other suitable source of humidity. In addition, most microorganisms grow in the absence of light, and sunlight should be avoided.

Sterile conditions

To obtain a pure culture of a microorganism, the culture medium must be *sterile*. Not only is sterilization necessary for separation of the inoculated organism, but contamination by other forms may influence or prevent the growth of the desired microorganism. Most culture media are sterilized by use of the autoclave. Quantities of medium up to 1 L should be autoclaved for 15 minutes at 121°C, and larger volumes may require a longer period. The culture media should be prepared according to directions and then placed in test tubes or Erlenmeyer flasks. These are plugged with nonabsorbent cotton, or loosely capped, and placed in the autoclave. The test tubes should be autoclaved in racks or baskets, and the flasks should not be more than two-thirds full. Oversterilization or prolonged heating must be avoided, as it can change the composition of the medium; it may cause precipitation in agar media or an increase in acidity. Some culture media may be harmed by autoclaving and may have to be sterilized by tyndallization or filtration.

Storage

Finally, culture media must be protected from *external contamination*. Media and cultures in

Petri dishes are protected from external contamination by the design of the dish. Test tubes and flasks may be plugged with cotton or covered with screw caps or loosely fitting metal covers. The plug or cover must not be too tight or too loose, and it must protect the lip of the container from contamination by dust. Screw caps must be used with care, for they may result in anaerobic or partially anaerobic conditions. Cotton plugs are useful because they prevent the entrance of foreign microorganisms and debris while admitting sterile filtered air, which is necessary for the growth of aerobic microorganisms. Loosely fitting metal caps are becoming more popular, as they do not pose a fire hazard or tend to fall out of test tubes that have been entered repeatedly, both of which are problems with cotton plugs.

Although media should not be stored for prolonged periods, they are generally prepared in reasonably large batches. Usually these batches should be stored under refrigeration (4°C) to prevent deterioration and dehydration. Certain media require special storage, but such information will be provided with the directions for preparing the medium. In general, a medium should be allowed to warm up to room temperature before it is inoculated, or microorganisms may be destroyed.

Selective, differential, and enrichment media

Although cultural as well as morphological characteristics are invaluable in the identification of bacteria, additional determinations are often necessary. Culture media may be employed to give additional information, and in this context they are termed selective, differential, or enrichment media.

Selective media

Selective media are semisolid plating media prepared by adding dyes, antibiotics, or other chemical compounds to certain media. These substances selectively inhibit the growth of certain microorganisms and permit the growth of others. Selective media are used for fecal and sputum specimens, where many normally occurring bacteria could obscure the presence of the pathogenic material. The normally occurring bacteria are selectively inhibited so that the pathogens can be seen if they are present.

Enrichment media

Enrichment media are usually liquid. They permit one organism to grow rapidly while inhibiting the growth of other organisms. Enrichment media are especially useful in the isolation of *Salmonella* or *Shigella* from stool cultures, which contain several bacteria—the *normal intestinal flora*—that are so numerous that they would obscure the growth of the pathogens. Therefore, cultures of stool specimens for pathogens normally include an enrichment medium that inhibits the normal intestinal flora and promotes the growth of the pathogens that must be identified. Subculture to a solid plating medium from the enrichment broth must be made to obtain isolated colonies for final identification.

Differential media

Differential media contain dyes, indicators, or other constituents that give colonies of particular organisms distinctive and easily recognizable characteristics. The final identification of an organism often involves isolation on a suitable culture medium and then characteristic reaction or growth on a differential medium. Such a characteristic reaction constitutes a confirmatory test for the microorganism.

PREPARATION OF SMEARS AND STAINING TECHNIQUES

One necessary step in the identification of a particular species of bacterium involves morphological observation under the microscope. Since bacteria are so small and have refractive indexes approximately equal to that of glass, a stain must be used to accentuate the microorganisms.

There is some merit in studying unstained preparations of bacteria, as bacterial motility may be observed in this way. Most bacteria can be observed unstained with the ordinary light microscope. Spirochetes, however, are so feebly refractive that it is necessary to use dark-field illumination or phase-contrast microscopy.

To stain bacteria, the material to be examined is thinly spread on a glass microscope slide and allowed to dry. The film should be thin enough so that individual bacteria can be seen. If the material to be examined is a liquid, such as a broth culture, it may be transferred by means of a sterile, cooled inoculating loop and spread directly on the dry slide. If it is taken from an isolated colony on a Petri plate or other dry material, a drop of sterile water must first be placed on the slide and the material added and mixed by using the sterile, cooled inoculating loop or needle.

After the material has air-dried, it must be *fixed* to the slide—that is, killed, hardened, and preserved for microbiological study. The fixing process prevents many of the bacterial cells from washing off the slide in subsequent operations. Fixation is achieved by simply passing the back of the microscope slide through the burner flame two or three times. The film side of the slide must not be exposed to heat, and the bottom of the slide must not be so hot that it cannot be held against the back of the hand. This heating coagulates the bacterial protein, causing cells to adhere to the slide. However, the air-drying and fixation do not necessarily kill all the bacterial cells on the slide, and to prevent accidental infection the slides must be handled carefully and placed in containers to be autoclaved before they are discarded.

Simple staining procedures

Simple staining procedures employing crystal violet, fuchsin, methylene blue, or safranine have only limited use in the microbiology laboratory. These are termed *simple* stains because only one stain is used and all structures present are stained the same color. They accentuate the otherwise colorless bacterial cell, but that is about all. When a simple stain is used, organisms should be observed for size, shape, and uniformity of staining. The procedure for using one simple stain in microbiology, the methylene blue stain, is as follows.

Procedure using methylene blue

1. Spread a thin film of material on the clean microscope slide, air-dry it, and heat-fix it. Place the slide on the staining rack.
2. Flood the surface of the slide with methylene blue staining solution. Allow the stain to remain on the slide for 2 minutes.
3. Wash the slide gently with running water to remove excess stain.
4. Allow the slide to dry naturally.
5. Examine the smear with the oil-immersion microscope lens, noting the size, shape, and uniformity of staining of the microorganisms present.

Differential staining methods

Differential staining methods are very useful in microbiology, for in addition to showing gross morphological features, they serve to differentiate bacteria or divide them into useful groups. Two of the most widely used differential stains are the Gram stain and acid-fast stain.

The Gram stain

The Gram stain is particularly useful in bacteriology. There are several modifications of the method, but it generally involves the primary stain crystal violet; the addition of iodine, which serves as a mordant; decolorization with an alcohol-acetone solution; and counterstaining with a secondary stain such as safranine. (A mordant is a substance that combines with a particular dye, forming an insoluble complex, or "lake," and fixing the color in the substance dyed.) This staining method divides bacteria into two broad groups. Bacteria that stain *purple* as a result of retention of the crystal violet-iodine complex are termed *gram-positive.* Bacteria that stain *red* from the counterstain are termed *gram-negative.* Differentiation into these categories is particularly helpful in determining the subsequent tests and means of culture for eventual identification of the bacteria. It is also a guide to treatment of the patient, for certain antibiotics are generally effective against gram-positive bacteria, while gram-negative bacteria are not as susceptible to their action.

One method of Gram staining (basically the Hucker modification) is as follows.[9]

Reagents

1. Crystal violet stain.
   a. Stock crystal violet. Dissolve 20 g of crystal violet 85% dye in 100 ml of 95% ethanol.
   b. Stock oxalate solution. Dissolve 1 g of ammonium oxalate in 100 ml of distilled water.
   c. Working solution. Dilute the stock crystal violet solution 1:10 with distilled water.

Mix this with 4 volumes of stock oxalate solution. Store in a glass-stoppered bottle.
2. Gram iodine solution. Dissolve 1 g of iodine crystals and 2 g of potassium iodide in 5 ml of distilled water. Add to this 240 ml of distilled water and 60 ml of a 5% aqueous solution of sodium bicarbonate. Mix well and store in an amber glass bottle.
3. Alcohol-acetone decolorizer. Mix 250 ml of 95% ethanol with 250 ml of acetone. Store in a glass-stoppered bottle.
4. Safranine counterstain.
   a. Stock safranine. Dissolve 2.5 g of safranine stain in 100 ml of 95% ethanol.
   b. Working safranine. Dilute stock safranine 1:5 or 1:10 with distilled water. Store in a glass-stoppered bottle.

Procedure

1. Flood the heat-fixed slide with crystal violet stain and wait 10 seconds.
2. Pour off stain and rinse with iodine solution.
3. Cover with iodine solution and wait for 10 seconds.
4. Rinse with running water, shaking off the excess.
5. Decolorize quickly with the alcohol-acetone solution, or with 95% alcohol if the alcohol-acetone decolorization proves to be too rapid. Continue until no more color is extracted by the solvent. This usually takes 10–20 seconds, but take care not to decolorize the film too much.
6. Flood with safranine for 10 seconds.
7. Rinse with water, then allow to air-dry.

In the first step, all organisms present are stained violet by the primary stain, crystal violet. The iodine added in the second and third steps forms a crystal violet-iodine complex, which is fixed or retained in gram-positive but not in gram-negative organisms. The mechanism involved in the retention of this complex in gram-positive and not gram-negative organisms is not completely understood, but it reflects significant differences between the two groups.

The fifth step, decolorization with a mixture of acetone and alcohol, removes all color from gram-negative organisms but does not affect gram-positive ones, which remain purple. Since the gram-negative organisms are colorless after the fifth step, they are counterstained in the sixth step with the red secondary stain safranine so that they can be visualized under the microscope.

If a slide were observed under the microscope after each step of the Gram staining process, the following results would be noted. After steps 1, 2, and 3, all organisms would be colored purple. After step 5, gram-positive organisms would appear purple, and gram-negative organisms would be colorless. After step 6, all gram-positive organisms would appear purple and all gram-negative organisms red.

Acid-fast stain

Acid-fast stain is used mainly to detect organisms that cause tuberculosis and leprosy. These organisms are extremely difficult to stain by ordinary methods because of their highly resistant fatty (or lipid) cell membranes. Once stained, they retain the dye color and decolorization is difficult, even with an acid-alcohol solution—hence the term acid-fast bacteria. Other bacteria are easily decolorized by the acid-alcohol reagent.

The Ziehl-Neelsen acid-fast method uses carbol-fuchsin as the primary stain, heat as the mordant, a mixture of hydrochloric acid and alcohol as the decolorizer, and methylene blue as the counterstain. The Kinyoun acid-fast method uses a slightly different carbol-fuchsin preparation and Tergitol 7 as the mordant. After the first step, all bacteria present on the slide appear red. Following decolorization with acid-alcohol reagent, the acid-fast bacteria appear red and all other bacteria are colorless. After counterstaining with methylene blue, the acid-fast bacteria appear red and all other cells appear blue.

The Kinyoun carbol-fuchsin method may be performed as follows.[10]

Reagents

1. Kinyoun carbol-fuchsin stain. Dissolve 4 g of basic fuchsin in 20 ml of 95% ethanol. Add 100 ml of distilled water slowly while shaking the preparation. Melt phenol in a 56°C water bath. Add 8 ml of melted phenol to the stain, using a pipet with mechanical suction (do not pipet by mouth). To accelerate the staining procedure add 1 drop of Tergitol 7 to every 30–40 ml of the Kinyoun carbol-fuchsin stain.
2. Acid-alcohol reagent. Add 3 ml of concentrated hydrochloric acid to 97 ml of 95% ethanol.
3. Counterstain. Dissolve 0.3 g of methylene blue in 100 ml of distilled water.

Procedure

1. Flood the heat-fixed smear with Kinyoun's carbol-fuchsin stain containing Tergitol 7 for 1 minute.
2. Wash with water.
3. Decolorize by adding acid-alcohol reagent drop by drop with continual agitation until carbol-fuchsin no longer washes off. This requires approximately 2 minutes for smears of average thickness.
4. Wash with water.
5. Counterstain with methylene blue for 20–30 seconds.
6. Wash with water and air-dry.

SPECIAL EQUIPMENT AND TECHNIQUES FOR MICROBIOLOGY STUDIES

Microbiologists use special techniques and equipment to isolate and grow pure cultures of micro-organisms free of contamination by other micro-organisms that are present everywhere. Such techniques and equipment include the inoculating needle or loop, the Bunsen burner, tube cultures, the Petri dish, and artificial media.

Disposable plastic equipment

In the microbiology laboratory today, much of the equipment used is in the form of disposable plasticware or glassware. By far the most common types of plastic used are the polypropylenes and polystyrenes. This plastic material can be produced glass-clear and quite cheaply. It can be purchased presterilized in various forms, such as Petri dishes, test tubes, syringes, and precision pipets. Initial sterilization is not necessary and subsequent decontamination is simple.

Inoculating needle and loop

Probably the most important tool of the microbiologist is the inoculating needle or loop. These implements may be either a straight wire or a wire with a loop at one end inserted into a suitable holder. The wire is usually platinum or an alloy, such as Nichrome, that can be heated to glowing without being harmed and returned to room temperature fairly rapidly. An object that can be safely heated until it is red is sterilized almost instantaneously. The needle or loop is used to transfer microorganisms from one medium to another or from a culture to a microscope slide. Because it can be sterilized quickly, it can be used repeatedly for this purpose. When a transfer is to be made, the needle or loop is sterilized in a flame, used to perform the transfer, then resterilized before it is set aside. The procedure for sterilizing the inoculating loop by flaming is as follows (Fig. 10-4).

Procedure

1. Hold the inoculating loop between the thumb and index finger. This leaves the three

Fig. 10-4. Flaming of wet and dry inoculating loops.

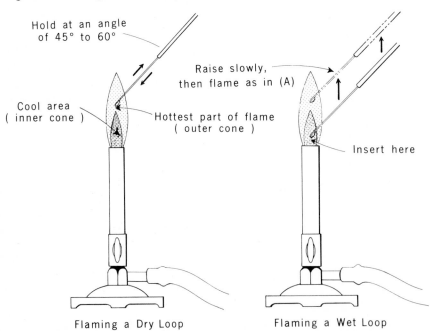

Hold at an angle
of 45° to 60°

Raise slowly,
then flame as in (A)

Cool area
(inner cone)

Hottest part of flame
(outer cone)

Insert here

Flaming a Dry Loop

Flaming a Wet Loop

outer fingers free—for example, to remove cotton plugs or tops from test tubes.

2. Push the loop into the upper flame of the Bunsen burner at an angle of about 45-60°. (Observe the special technique described below if the loop is wet.) Continue heating until the entire loop is red hot. Then briefly flame the hub of the loop holder.

3. Allow the loop to cool to room temperature before using. If used hot, it will kill the organism under study.

A flame normally has two parts: the outer part is the *outer cone*, and within this part, extending down to the base or origin of the flame, is the *inner cone.* The hottest part of the flame is the upper portion, above the top of the inner cone. The inner cone at the base of the flame is cool. If an inoculating needle or loop filled with bacteria is inserted into the hottest part of the flame, a small amount of steam will form. This will result in explosive sputtering of the material to the desk top, hands, and clothing of the worker. This is extremely dangerous, as the bacteria are often still viable when this occurs and can produce infection. To prevent this, an alternative method of flaming must be followed. If the needle or loop is wet, it must be first inserted into the cool inner cone at the base of the flame. It is then slowly raised through the inner cone and finally flamed in the hottest part of the flame. The needle or loop must always be flamed before it is set aside.

Tube cultures and tube culture transfers

Microorganisms are commonly grown and maintained in presterilized test tubes that contain a liquid or liquefiable solid medium and have been plugged with cotton or covered with loose-fitting metal caps or screw caps. In general, the cotton plug or cap is removed with and held in the outer three fingers of the hand holding the inoculating needle. The lip of the tube is flamed

before and after entry to prevent contamination of the culture. The transfer is performed with a sterilized inoculating needle.

Plate cultures and transfers

Petri dishes are often used for cultures. They are shallow glass or plastic plates with loose-fitting covers of the same material, shape, and depth as the dish but slightly larger in diameter. The deep cover prevents contamination of the dish. Petri dishes are used for liquefiable solid media. The medium is poured into the dish, allowed to harden, covered, and stored in an inverted position in order to prevent condensation on its surface. The plates are also stored in an inverted position after inoculation; they are labeled on the back of the portion of the plate in which the medium is contained. Plates of liquefiable solid media may be used as streak plates or as pour plates.

Streak plates are prepared by streaking material across the surface of the hardened medium contained in a Petri dish. Streaking is especially useful for isolating individual colonies originating from a single bacterial cell (Fig. 10-5). These isolated colonies may then be transferred to another medium. Thus, pure cultures may be prepared from mixtures of bacteria. Characteristics of isolated colonies may also be observed on streak plates.

Fig. 10-5. Preparation of a streak plate.

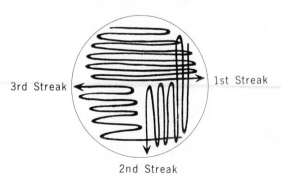

3rd Streak   1st Streak

2nd Streak

The technique of streaking a plate will vary from laboratory to laboratory and even within a particular laboratory, depending on the source of material and characteristics of the microorganism under investigation. It should be remembered that the streak plate is used primarily as a means of obtaining isolated colonies of microorganisms (see under Quantitative Urine Cultures and under Throat Cultures). The aim is therefore to inoculate successively smaller quantities of material onto the medium, so that at one point the organisms are plated thinly enough to allow the growth of individual isolated colonies.

If a swab is submitted for culture, it may be used to make the inoculation onto the medium, instead of an inoculating loop (see under Throat Cultures).

There are certain important things to remember when using the plate culture method. Plates should be perfectly dry before use, or the organism will tend to spread; this will hinder the formation of individual colonies. When a loop is used to inoculate the plate, it should be held lightly and not dug into the medium. One should always work near a Bunsen burner when inoculating, since the upward surge of air created by the flame tends to carry dust in the air away from the plate.[11]

In general, a small and sometimes measured amount of material is streaked onto the periphery at one side of the plate. Streaking is achieved by drawing the inoculating loop across the surface of the medium in a zigzag motion. The first streak is continued across approximately half the plate. The plate is then turned 90° and streaked again, beginning at the periphery, overlapping the previously inoculated area once or twice. The second streak is continued across half the plate. Finally, the plate is turned at 90° once again and streaked a third time, beginning at the periphery, drawing the loop through the second streak once, and continuing across the remaining quarter of the plate (Fig. 10-5). The isolated colonies will generally be found in the third area of streaking.

Sometimes the needle must be flamed between each streak as well as before and after inoculation. Sheep blood agar plates are often cut one or more times with the inoculating loop at the conclusion of streaking in the third and/or the first area of streaking in order to observe hemolysis reactions of certain bacteria. Some of these techniques are described under Media Used in Medical Bacteriology.

Pour plates represent another manner of inoculating culture media in Petri dishes. They are less commonly used than streak plates. Pour plates are generally used to determine the number of viable organisms in a liquid—particularly in testing such liquids as milk and water for bacterial contamination. In the medical microbiology laboratory, the pour plate may also be used for cultures of blood.

In using the pour plate, one generally first dilutes the specimen serially to achieve isolation of colonies. The diluted specimen is then inoculated into a liquefiable solid medium that is in the liquid state. The medium and inoculum may be mixed in a test tube or in the plate itself, depending on the technique being used. Thorough mixing must be achieved in any case. When the medium has been inoculated at the appropriate temperature for the desired length of time, it is allowed to harden. Plates are then observed for growth and the colonies are counted to obtain an estimate of the concentration of microorganisms in the original specimen. The use of pour plates rather than streak plates provides at least partially anaerobic conditions in the deeper layers of the plate, facilitating the culture of anaerobic microorganisms. As with streak plates, colonies may be observed on the pour plate itself or introduced into additional media in order to obtain pure cultures or observe growth on differential media.

Preparation of artificial culture media[12]

Preparing artificial culture media for the growth of microorganisms in the laboratory used to be a difficult task. The microbiologist had to concoct a medium having the various growth requirements (nutrients, oxygen, moisture, pH, temperature, and sterility). Today, with the availability of commercially prepared dehydrated culture media, the microbiologist no longer needs to completely assemble the media and cook them. Now the preparation of culture media is much like the preparation of any reagent in the laboratory. The medium is supplied in dry form. Basically, all that is necessary is rehydration. Of course, certain precautions must be observed that take into account microbial requirements. The medium is generally supplied in a labeled bottle that gives its exact chemical composition and instructions for preparation, in terms of quantity of dehydrated medium necessary per liter of reconstituted medium. The person preparing the culture medium must accurately weigh the required amount of dehydrated medium, dissolve it in freshly distilled water or freshly boiled distilled water that has been cooled to room temperature, and sterilize the reconstituted medium.

It is important to use freshly distilled water or distilled water that has been boiled and cooled to room temperature, because when distilled water is stored it absorbs gases from the atmosphere that alter the composition and pH of the medium. It is necessary to avoid contamination of the medium while it is being prepared, even though it is to be sterilized before use. It is absolutely essential that only chemically clean, sterile glassware be used for medium preparation. All traces of detergent must be removed from the glassware, as residual detergent inhibits the growth of bacteria.

If the medium is to be used in test tubes, it is

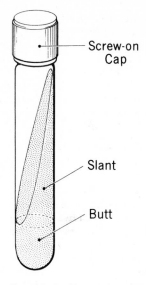

Fig. 10-6. Slant tube, showing slant and butt.

usually dispensed and autoclaved in the tubes. If liquefiable solid medium is to be used in slant tubes, it is dispensed in the liquid state into test tubes, autoclaved, and then allowed to harden while set at an angle (Fig. 10-6). If the medium is to be used in plates, it is generally autoclaved in an Erlenmeyer flask and dispensed into sterile plates under aseptic conditions.

It is also possible to purchase culture media that have been rehydrated, dispensed in sealed plates or tubes, and sterilized, and are therefore completely ready for use. Such commercially prepared media are now in general use.

In most laboratories cotton plugs for tubes and flasks have been replaced by plastic caps, screw caps, or metal closures of some type. Sterile, disposable Petri dishes or plates have also come into widespread use.

MEDIA USED IN MEDICAL BACTERIOLOGY

Since the eventual identification of a particular microorganism requires its culture on various media (selective, enrichment, or differential), some of the more commonly used media in the medical bacteriology laboratory[13,14,15] are discussed here. However, since there is no one system that is universally employed in the identification of pathogens, some routinely used media may well have been omitted.

After this study of media, the student should be able to recognize the common media by their appearance, know what change in the appearance of a medium constitutes a positive reaction, and be able to correlate a characteristic change in the medium with the ability of organisms to carry on certain chemical reactions. The students should be able to (1) recognize the reactions of various indicators at different pH values, (2) associate the ingredients of the medium with the purpose for using the medium, and (3) interpret a change in the indicator in terms of the metabolic product that caused the change. Because most media have rather cumbersome names, they are commonly known by certain abbreviations, with which the student should be familiar.

Since most commonly used media are contained in either test tubes or Petri dishes, the following material is divided in two sections, namely media in test tubes and media in Petri dishes.

Media in test tubes

Trypticase soy broth (tryp broth)

Contains:

Trypticase soy
Yeast extract
PABA (*p*-aminobenzoic acid)
Agar (0.15% to provide anaerobic conditions)

Tryp broth is a very good general purpose medium. Almost everything grows well in it. There are many similar broths with slightly different names. All contain dextrose, some type of peptone, inorganic salts, and water. Most cultures are inoculated into tryp broth to maintain the growth of *all* organisms in the specimen. A small amount of agar is added to the medium to make it thicker, but not enough to solidify it. This

permits the growth of some anaerobic organisms, since oxygen does not diffuse to the bottom of the medium if agar is added.

Thioglycolate broth (thio broth)

Contains:

Trypticase
Cystine
Dextrose
Sodium chloride
Sodium thioglycolate
Resazurin (an oxidation-reduction indicator)
Small amount of agar

Thio broth is used particularly for the cultivation of anaerobic organisms. It contains thioglycolic acid (sodium thioglycolate) and agar to encourage anaerobic growth. The medium is in a reduced state, and contains the indicator resazurin, which turns pink if the medium is oxidized. If more than one-third of the medium is pink, it contains too much oxygen for anaerobic growth. The oxygen can be driven off by heating the tube of medium. All cultures in which an anaerobic organism is suspected are inoculated into thio broth.

Sugar fermentation broths

Contains:

Beef extract
Peptone
Sodium chloride
Bromocresol purple
Sugar solution (1%)

Different bacteria ferment different sugars, producing either lactic acid or lactic acid and gas. The ability of microorganisms to ferment certain sugars often serves to identify them. Sugar tubes contain peptone broth in addition to a 1% solution of the sugar in question. The medium also contains a pH indicator, bromocresol purple, which is purple in alkaline solutions and yellow in acid solutions. The tube of medium contains a smaller tube, which is inverted into the larger tube (Fig. 10-3).

If a microorganism ferments the sugar into which it has been inoculated, it produces lactic acid from the sugar and therefore lowers the pH of the medium. This change of pH is indicated by a color change of the bromocresol purple indicator from purple to yellow. Hence, the formation of a yellow color indicates fermentation of the sugar, or a positive reaction. If gas is also produced by the inoculum, the smaller inverted tube is filled with carbon dioxide. Growth may occur in sugar tubes without the production of lactic acid (i.e., without fermentation). There will be no color change in this case. The three sugars used most in the identification of bacteria are dextrose, sucrose, and lactose. Maltose and mannitol fermentation studies are also occasionally desired. The sugar contained in the culture tubes must be indicated by the color of the cotton plug (or some other suitable system), since all sugar tubes look exactly alike.

Agar slants

Agar slants contain liquefiable solid media made by heating nutrient agar, placing it in a sterile tube, and cooling the tube at a slant (Fig. 10-6). An agar slant is usually used to preserve a pure culture of a microorganism, either to maintain the culture or to hold it for further chemical tests. Slants are inoculated by streaking the inoculum on the slant in a zigzag movement from bottom to top.

Simmons citrate agar

Contains:

Magnesium sulfate
Monoammonium phosphate
Dipotassium phosphate
Sodium citrate

Sodium chloride
Agar
Bromothymol blue

Simmons citrate is also an agar slant. It is not a nutrient agar, but contains simple inorganic salts. It is used to test the ability of the organism to utilize sodium citrate as its sole source of carbon and monoammonium phosphate as its sole source of nitrogen. The medium also contains the indicator bromothymol blue to indicate growth. Bromothymol blue is green (the color of the uninoculated medium) when the organism is not growing and turns blue when it is. Therefore, a positive reaction is observed as a change of the color of the medium from green to blue. This medium is important in separating different types of gram-negative rods.

Peptone water with tryptophan (indole medium)

This is the culture medium used for the *indole test*. Tryptophan is an amino acid. The ability of bacteria to split indole from the tryptophan molecule is highly diagnostic. If a microorganism growing in peptone water with tryptophan has produced indole, the addition of Kovac's reagent to the culture results in a red color. Therefore, a positive test for indole production is the production of a red color after addition of Kovac's reagent. The indole test is useful in the identification of gram-negative rods.

Clark-Lubs broth

Contains:

Peptone water
Dextrose (2%)

Clark-Lubs medium is important as the culture medium for two differential tests, the methyl red test and the Voges-Proskauer test, used in the identification of gram-negative rods.

Methyl red test

This is a test of hydronium ion concentration, or pH. The organism is inoculated into Clark-Lubs broth and incubated at 35°C for 48 hours. After incubation, four to five drops of methyl red indicator are added to the broth. The appearance of a reddish color indicates a pH below 4.4. A yellow color indicates a pH above 4.4.

Voges-Proskauer test

This tests the ability of the inoculum to produce acetylmethylcarbinol from glucose. In a positive test the addition of potassium hydroxide to the culture produces a red color as acetylmethylcarbinol is formed.

Triple sugar iron agar (TSI slants)

Contains:

Nutrient (peptone)
Sodium chloride
Lactose (1%)
Sucrose (1%)
Dextrose (0.1%)
Sodium thiosulfate
Phenol red indicator (yellow in acid pH and red in alkaline pH)
Ferrous ammonium sulfate (black in the presence of hydrogen sulfide)
Agar

TSI slants are slant tubes having a lump, or butt, of medium at the bottom and a slant above (Fig. 10-6). It is essential that the slants be inoculated with a pure culture. Therefore, a single, well-isolated colony should be used for the inoculum. The medium is inoculated by streaking the slant and then stabbing the butt with a straight inoculating needle.

The medium is especially useful as a first step in the identification of gram-negative rods. It is used to test the ability of gram-negative rods to ferment dextrose, sucrose, and lactose, and to produce hydrogen sulfide (H_2S). Fermentation of sugars is accompanied by acid production, which is indicated by a change in the color of the phenol red indicator from red to yellow. Production of hydrogen sulfide is indicated by the formation of a black color as hydrogen sulfide combines with ferrous ammonium sulfate. Splitting of the agar in the butt indicates gas production.

Since a variety of reactions occur in the TSI slants, there must be a scheme for observing and recording these reactions. Reactions in the slant and butt are recorded as acid (A) or alkaline (Alk) and the production of hydrogen sulfide (H_2S) and/or gas (G) is noted. An acid reaction is indicated by the presence of a yellow color, and an alkaline reaction by a red color. No reaction would be recorded as NR. Various observations and interpretations are shown in Table 10-1.

As indicated, failure of the organism to ferment any of the three sugars results in an Alk/Alk reaction (or no reaction), indicated by a red slant and butt. An Alk/A reaction (red slant and yellow butt) results when only dextrose is fermented. Organisms fermenting only dextrose will originally give an A/A reaction, or yellow slant and butt. However, the small amount of

Table 10-1. Observations of triple sugar iron agar (TSI) slants

Notation	Color change	Metabolic change
A/A	Yellow slant, yellow butt	Dextrose fermented, lactose or sucrose or both fermented
Alk/A	Red slant, yellow butt	Dextrose fermented, lactose and sucrose not fermented
Alk/Alk or NR	Red slant, red butt	None of the three sugars fermented, or no reaction
H_2S G	Black in butt Splitting of agar in butt	H_2S production Gas production

dextrose present is used up as the incubation continues. The slant is under aerobic conditions and reverts to alkaline (or red) in 18–24 hours. In the butt, however, anaerobic conditions exist, there is no reversion to alkaline pH, and the acid (or yellow) reaction remains.

An A/A reaction (yellow slant and butt) results when dextrose and lactose or sucrose or both are fermented. The medium contains 10 times more lactose and sucrose than dextrose. Therefore, organisms fermenting lactose or sucrose or both do not use up the sugars except after very prolonged incubation. Fermentation of sucrose and/or lactose is indicated by acid (yellow) conditions in both the slant and the butt. However, with prolonged incubation (48–72 hours), lactose and sucrose may also be used up, and formerly acid reactions may revert to alkaline. Therefore, the time of incubation is critical. The time recommended to obtain typical reactions is 18 hours.

There are other media that are similar to TSI. One such medium is Kligler's iron agar. This medium differs in that it tests fermentation of only dextrose and lactose. Sucrose is not included.

Cristianson's urea slant (with 1-in butt)

Contains:

Peptone
Urea
Glucose (0.1%)
Phenol red indicator
Buffer

This is an enrichment agar slant that is used to test the ability of a microorganism to utilize urea as its only source of nitrogen. To do this, the organism must produce the enzyme urease. Breakdown of urea by the action of urease results in the production of ammonia, which raises the pH of the medium, as indicated by a color change of the phenol red indicator to red. The organism is streaked onto the slant only.

The butt is *not* stabbed. Some organisms give a red color in only the slant; others color both the butt and the slant.

Tests for urease production may also be done on urea broth, which contains a buffered urea solution and phenol red indicator.

Selenite broth

Contains:

Sodium selenite (0.4%)
Lactose
Sodium phosphate
Peptone

This is an enrichment medium used for stool cultures. The medium inhibits the growth of gram-positive organisms and coliform bacilli (gram-negative organisms that are part of the normal intestinal flora), while favoring and therefore isolating *Shigella* and *Salmonella*, the causative agents of dysentery and typhoid fever, respectively. The medium suppresses growth of organisms other than *Shigella* and *Salmonella* for 12–18 hours. After this time coliforms and streptococci (enterococci) grow rapidly. Therefore, after 18 hours of incubation, cultures grown in selenite broth must be subcultured onto a MacConkey plate or other suitable differential medium. Selenite broth is most effective under reduced oxygen tension. Therefore, it is dispensed into tubes to a depth of 2 in. The broth should be inoculated heavily with fecal material—an amount about the size of a pea.

Motility indole-ornithine test medium (MIO)

Contains:

Decarboxylase medium
L-Ornithine hydrochloride
Peptone
Tryptone
Agar

This is a semisolid medium used to test bacteria for motility. The sterile medium is inoculated by stabbing through its center with a straight wire to no more than one-fourth the depth of the tube. Motility is indicated by growth of the organism away from the stab.

It is essential that this medium be at least 2 in deep in the tube to provide the anaerobic conditions necessary for the detection of ornithine decarboxylase activity. Production of ornithine decarboxylase is indicated by a purple color throughout the tube. With a negative ornithine decarboxylase reaction, the bottom of the tube will be bright yellow with a narrow rim of purple at the top. This test is valid only for organisms that ferment dextrose.

To detect the production of indole, a few drops of Kovac's reagent are added to the tube. A pink color indicates that indole was produced.

Loeffler's slant

Contains:

One part dextrose
Whole egg
Infusion broth
Three parts coagulated beef serum

This medium is used for detection of *Corynebacterium diphtheriae*, the causative agent of diphtheria. The medium is inoculated with swabs of material taken from the throat. After 24 hours of incubation the growth is placed on a clean glass microscope slide, stained with Loeffler's methylene blue, and examined for typical morphological features of the diphtheria bacterium.

Litmus milk

Contains:

Skim milk
Litmus

This medium is used to determine the action of bacteria on milk. Bacteria may ferment, coagulate, peptonize (i.e., convert to a clear fluid), or reduce milk. The litmus indicates acid (pink) and alkaline (blue) changes. It also indicates reduction, by turning colorless.

Media in Petri dishes

Sheep blood agar (SB or BA)

Contains:

Trypticase soy
Yeast extract
Sodium chloride
Agar
PABA
Fresh sterile sheep blood (5%)

This medium supports the growth of most ordinary bacteria. It is therefore used for primary plating and for subculturing. It is a good general medium for the growth of pathogens, since the blood adds many of the accessory substances that pathogens require. Most pathogens can be recognized on sheep blood. The medium is also useful in distinguishing different types of streptococci by their ability to hemolyze the red blood cells present in the medium. They are differentiated as follows:

Alpha streptococci—green hemolysis
Beta streptococci—clear hemolysis
Gamma streptococci—no hemolysis

Human blood can also be used in nutrient agar; however, false hemolysis is often observed. Horse blood works well. SB may inhibit the growth of *Hemophilus influenzae*, a common respiratory pathogen in children. Rabbit blood, however, promotes the growth of this organism.

Rabbit blood agar (RB)

This medium consists of 5% fresh sterile rabbit blood in nutrient agar. It is the primary medium for nose and throat cultures of material taken from pediatric patients or when *Hemophilus* infection is suspected. It is used for the isolation of *H. influenzae*, since it contains the X and V growth factors required by this organism. RB is rarely used for other cultures because it produces too diffuse hemolysis.

Chocolate agar (Choc)

Contains:

GC base medium (Difco Laboratories, Inc., Detroit, Mich.), a nutrient base medium that has a low concentration of agar (1%) and provides the higher moisture content required by some fastidious organisms

Supplement B (Difco) or Isovitalex (Baltimore Biological Laboratories, Cockeysville, Md.), which supplies glutamine, X factor, V factor, cocarboxylase, and other growth factors

Hemoglobin

Choc is prepared by adding blood to the base medium at 75–80°C. The heat denatures proteins in the blood, causing the blood to coagulate and turn brown. This gives a richer medium than ordinary blood agar and is used in the cultivation of the pathogenic *Neisseria* species. These organisms cause gonorrhea and meningitis and are difficult to grow. They require an atmosphere of 10% carbon dioxide in addition to the special medium. The medium also supplies the special growth requirements for *H. influenzae.*

Phenylethyl alcohol agar (PEA)

Contains:

Trypticase
Peptone
Sodium chloride
Agar
Phenylethyl alcohol (0.25%)
Fresh sterile sheep blood (5%)

This is essentially SB (sheep blood agar) with phenylethyl alcohol added. The medium inhibits the growth of gram-negative organisms except *Pseudomonas aeruginosa*. It allows growth of gram-positive organisms and permits their identification and separation, even when they are mixed with gram-negative organisms. If *P. aeruginosa* is present in a mixed culture and isolation of gram-positive organisms is desired, the culture is mixed with ether and then streaked onto the PEA plate, since ether destroys *Pseudomonas*. Hemolysis cannot be observed on the PEA plate.

Bordet-Gengou agar (BG)

Contains:

Potato agar base
Sodium chloride
Peptone
Fresh sterile rabbit or sheep blood (15%)
Glycerol (to conserve moisture) (1%)

This is a special plate used in the diagnosis of whooping cough, caused by *Bordetella pertussis*. Colonies of the organism have a special diagnostic appearance on this medium. Penicillin may also be added to the medium to inhibit growth of the normal bacterial flora. However, certain strains of *B. pertussis* are also inhibited by penicillin, so two BG plates should be inoculated, one with and one without penicillin.

Levine's eosin methylene blue agar (EMB)

Contains:

Eosin (0.2%), which gives a metallic sheen to *Escherichia coli*
Methylene blue (0.005%), which inhibits gram-positive organisms
Lactose (1%)
Peptone
Dipotassium phosphate
Agar

This medium promotes the growth of gram-negative organisms and inhibits that of gram-positive organisms. In addition, many gram-negative organisms have a characteristic appearance on EMB. Lactose fermenters produce acid, which precipitates the two dyes and gives colonies of the lactose-positive organisms a purple center. Urine cultures are inoculated onto EMB plates as well as sheep blood agar, since many urinary tract infections are caused by gram-negative rods. Mac-Conkey agar can be used in place of EMB.

MacConkey agar (Mac)

Contains:

Nutrients (peptone)
Bile salts (0.15%)
Sodium chloride
Lactose (1%)
Neutral red, an acid-base indicator (red indicates an acid reaction, yellow an alkaline reaction)
Crystal violet, which inhibits gram-positive organisms
Agar

Mac is a differential medium used in the primary plating of routine cultures (urine in particular). The medium should be lightly inoculated. Crystal violet is included to inhibit the growth of gram-positive organisms, and bile salts are present to inhibit nonpathogenic gram-negative organisms. The medium is used in the diagnosis of dysentery, typhoid, and paratyphoid bacteria, which do not ferment lactose. Colonies of organisms that do ferment lactose are red in this medium because the lactic acid that results from fermentation reacts with the bile salts, with subsequent absorption of neutral red. Therefore, the pathogens that do not ferment lactose are seen as yellow or colorless colonies on this medium.

Mac medium is sometimes used in place of EMB, since it tends to inhibit the spread of *Proteus* species more than EMB does.

Salmonella-Shigella agar (SS)

Contains:

Nutrients (beef extract and peptone)
Lactose (1%)
Bile salts (0.85%—a higher concentration than in Mac)
Sodium citrate, which inhibits coliforms
Sodium thiosulfate, which inhibits coliforms
Ferric citrate, an H_2S indicator
Neutral red, an acid-base indicator
Brilliant green, which inhibits gram-positive organisms

SS is a highly selective medium that is very inhibitory to coliforms and gram-positive organisms. It is used along with Mac in routine stool cultures. The medium should be heavily inoculated. It is designed to isolate the *Salmonella* and *Shigella* species in the presence of other gram-negative organisms. Colonies of lactose fermenters are red and those of nonfermenters are yellowish or colorless. Organisms that produce hydrogen sulfide show black centers on this medium.

Sabouraud agar with chloramphenicol

This medium promotes the growth of fungi while inhibiting bacterial growth. It has a low pH and high osmotic pressure. It should always be incubated at room temperature. Chloramphenicol is included to inhibit gram-positive and gram-negative organisms. Actinodine may be included to inhibit nonpathogenic fungi.

ROUTINE PROCEDURE FOR MICROBIOLOGY STUDIES

Since the isolation and identification of microorganisms require skills in several fundamental laboratory techniques, these skills must be practiced by everyone involved in microbiological determinations. The procedures used in the identification depend on the type of organism that is suspected. There is no specific set of tests that are done on all specimens sent to the laboratory. Three basic steps are involved in the identification of microorganisms. These are microscopic observation, culture studies, and biochemical tests.

Microscopic observation

Properly prepared and stained preparations of specimens may give excellent clues to the media to be inoculated or the further examinations to be done. Preliminary reports on the results of Gram staining of spinal fluid, urethral smears, and sputum, for example, can be of great value to the physician in the treatment of the patient.

When preparing a smear, it is essential to use only clean slides. The material is spread thinly but evenly over the appropriate area of the slide, using an inoculating loop. This material may be from a suspension of bacteria in a liquid medium, a colony on a solid medium, or a patient specimen. The smear is allowed to dry and then heat-fixed by passing it rapidly through a flame (see under Preparation of Smears and Staining Techniques).

Several staining procedures are used in the microbiology laboratory. Gram staining is most likely to yield valuable information and should be done in all cases when a staining procedure is indicated. Gram stains are also used routinely for the examination of cultures to determine purity and for identification. Special stains for spores, capsules, flagella, and spirochetes may also be used.

Fluorescence microscopy

It is important at this point to discuss the fluorescent antibody (FA) techniques used in many laboratories. These techniques will probably replace some of the older serological methods for the final identification of certain microorganisms. It is possible to pretreat certain antibodies with fluorescent dye and then react them with bacteria specific for the complementary antigen. The antibody-antigen complex is fluorescent and can be observed under the microscope. In fluorescence microscopy, the specimen is self-illuminating and a light image is observed against a dark background. A special dark-field fluorescence microscope is used (see under Types of Microscopes in Chap. 1). Group A streptococci may be identified on pure cultures isolated from throat swabs from patients with acute pharyngitis (strep throat), and there is a rapid method for detecting human influenza virus infection by utilizing nasal smears.[16] In some cases, FA techniques completely replace time-consuming cultural methods. In others, preliminary identification of microorganisms by FA methods may be followed by cultural confirmation.

Culture studies

This step in the identification of microorganisms requires growing and isolating the suspected organism. A pure culture of the organism taken from the patient specimen must be obtained. Bacteria from patient specimens are almost always isolated by streaking on the surface of a culture medium in a culture plate or Petri dish. A suitable medium will allow a single bacterial cell to grow into a colony. Various culturing methods enable the microbiologist to separate individual cells on the media and eventually allow them to grow into separate colonies.

It is important that the streaking be done properly to provide the best opportunity for isolation of the bacterial colonies. When isolated colonies are grown, a portion of the pure culture may be picked up for identification. There are several ways in which a plate may be streaked to ensure the appearance of isolated colonies on incubation. One method is illustrated in Fig.

10-5. Special streaking methods are used for certain types of specimens. We will discuss the methods for streaking urine specimens and throat swab cultures as examples.

Other culture studies include the use of agar slants for maintenance of cultures or for certain biochemical studies, semisolid media for motility or biochemical studies, and broth media for maintenance or biochemical studies.

Quantitative urine cultures

A streak plate method for quantitating the growth of microorganisms in the urine is commonly used in many hospital laboratories. A special standardized inoculating loop, holding 0.001 ml of urine or fluid, is used to transfer the specimen to the culture plate and to streak the plate. In common practice, a general medium such as SB and a selective medium such as Mac or EMB are streaked with the urine specimen. This is done in such a way that the drop of urine is spread as uniformly as possible on the plate (Fig. 10-7). After streaking and incubation, the number of colonies seen is multiplied by 1000 to give the number of colonies in 1 ml of urine. The blood agar plate gives a total colony count, as most common organisms grow on it. The selective medium indicates whether gram-negative rods (and some inhibited gram-positive organisms) are present. The EMB and Mac media also indicate whether the organisms are lactose-positive or -negative. *E. coli*, *Klebsiella* sp., and *Enterobacter* sp. are lactose fermenters that show pink col-

Fig. 10-7. Streak plate for quantitative urine culture.

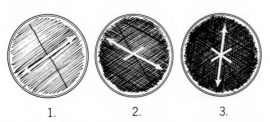

1.   2.   3.

onies, whereas *Proteus* sp. and *Pseudomonas* sp. are lactose-negative (do not ferment lactose) and show yellowish colonies. *Proteus* sp. may also be recognized on blood agar by its spreading growth. Gram-positive organisms such as staphylococci and streptococci grow well on blood agar but are inhibited on EMB or Mac medium.

In streaking the urine for a quantitative colony count, the urine must first be mixed well. The special loop is flamed, cooled, and dipped into the bubble-free surface of the specimen. The loopful of urine is streaked undiluted over the surface of the plates. After streaking the sheep blood plate, three or four small cuts are made in the agar to check for hemolysis. The culture plates should be incubated at 35-37°C in an inverted position for 18-24 hours. After incubation, the organisms growing on each plate are counted and the number multiplied by 1000. Normal urine is sterile. Plates that show no growth may be discarded and reported as no growth. Bacteriuria is considered clinically significant when laboratory findings show the presence of 100 000 (10^5) or more bacteria colonies per milliliter of urine specimen.

Throat cultures

Throat cultures are done by swabbing the rear pharyngeal wall and tonsillar area. Cultures are made by rolling the swab onto one edge of an SB plate, being certain to get as much of the specimen off onto the plate as possible. The inoculating loop is flamed and used to streak the plate out from the inoculated area, as shown in Fig. 10-8. The streaking is done so as to isolate the bacterial colonies as much as possible. Three or four cuts should then be made into the agar to check for hemolysis. After incubation, hemolysis can be observed. This phenomenon is useful in distinguishing different types of streptococci by their ability to hemolyze the red cells present in the medium. The hemolysis is differentiated as follows: alpha streptococci produce a green hemolysis reaction, beta streptococci produce a

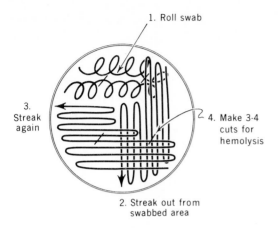

1. Roll swab

3. Streak again

4. Make 3-4 cuts for hemolysis

2. Streak out from swabbed area

Fig. 10-8. Streak plate for throat culture.

clear hemolysis reaction, and gamma streptococci do not produce hemolysis.

After 18-24 hours of incubation, throat culture plates should be examined for pathogens. If pathogens are present, appropriate subculturing is done for their final identification. Throat cultures are used primarily to detect the presence of beta hemolytic streptococci belonging to Lancefield's group A. This is the major throat pathogen, although other pathogens may sometimes be clinically significant. If pathogens are not present, the result should be reported as normal flora. Normal throat cultures show a predominance of alpha hemolytic streptococci and commensal *Neisseria* sp. Other organisms also constitute normal flora.

Anaerobic culture methods

Most of the common pathogenic bacteria are aerobic and grow well in the presence of oxygen. Some pathogenic organisms are incapable of growth in oxygen and are classified as anaerobic organisms. All specimens for anaerobic studies must be cultured as soon as possible after collection to avoid loss of viability. Special methods are required for the isolation and study of anaerobic bacteria.

The techniques for culturing anaerobic organisms are essentially of three types, involving the use of (1) media containing reducing substances that eliminate oxygen, (2) media and methods by which oxygen can be excluded, and (3) anaerobic jars, plates, and incubators from which oxygen can be removed and replaced by hydrogen or nitrogen.

One of the most useful media for growing anaerobic organisms is thio broth. It contains sodium thioglycolate, which absorbs oxygen from the medium. It can be used to study and identify anaerobes, but is generally not very satisfactory for the isolation of cultures. For isolation, it is desirable to streak plates of blood agar, infusion agar, or thioglycolate agar. When the plates have been streaked, they are placed in an anaerobic jar or other special container and the oxygen is removed.

Prereduced media are now commercially available. They appear to be very practical and reliable for the isolation of anaerobic bacteria.

Commercial dip culture products

Among the modern innovations being tested in some laboratories are commercial dip culture kits. In the case of urine culture, several commercial products are available. These products vary somewhat, but in general consist of a slide or paddle covered on both sides with combinations of culture media. The dip slide is dipped into a freshly voided urine specimen. If bacteria are present in the specimen, some of the organisms will adhere to the surfaces of the slide. The dip cultures are incubated for an appropriate length of time and checked for colony growth.

Nitrite tests have been incorporated into reagent strips used in many laboratories for routine urine analysis (see Chap. 5). Common organisms that cause urinary tract infections, such as species of *Enterobacter*, *Escherichia*, *Proteus*, *Klebsiella*, and *Pseudomonas*, contain enzymes that reduce nitrate in the urine to nitrite (see Chap. 5). One product, called Microstix (Ames Co., Elkhart, Ind.), which is also a dip test for nitrite, contains two types of media pads, one favoring growth of all bacterial types commonly found in urinary tract infections, and the other supporting growth of only gram-negative organisms. A special pouch for incubation is included.[17]

QUALITY CONTROL IN THE MICROBIOLOGY LABORATORY

Quality control is necessary in microbiology as in the other areas of the laboratory. The development of quality control for microbiology is recent, however.

Control of equipment

Equipment used in the microbiology laboratory can be easily controlled—for example, by monitoring the temperatures, daily or weekly, of incubators, refrigerators, water baths, freezers, and autoclaves. Also, every laboratory handling biological material must have a safety hood.

Control of media

Most media are now purchased ready-made from media companies. They are generally of high quality and provide good batch-to-batch consistency of results. If media are prepared by the laboratory, strict controls must be employed in the preparation. Directions for preparation must be followed exactly. The best way to control the quality of media is by *performance testing—*

checking the media with cultures of known stock microorganisms.

Control of reagents and antisera

New batches of reagents can be tested by using known positive and negative culture controls. Reagents should be dated when they are prepared, as are reagents in other areas of the laboratory. New reagents should be tested with known control cultures. Gram-staining reagents are best checked by staining and examining slides prepared with known suspensions of gram-negative and gram-positive organisms.

Control of specimens and specimen collection

If proper controls are not placed on the collection of patient specimens and on the procedures for handling these specimens in the laboratory, the identification of pathogens is not very meaningful. Strict controls of collection techniques must be enforced and repeat collections must be made if the circumstances demand it.

TESTS FOR SUSCEPTIBILITY OF BACTERIA TO ANTIBIOTICS

One of the main functions of the medical microbiology laboratory is to assist the physician in identifying and treating diseases caused by microbes. Therefore, a very important task of the laboratory is to test the isolated organisms for susceptibility to antimicrobial agents, or antibiotics. To a large extent, the laboratory report

showing susceptibility or resistance to a particular antibiotic determines whether the agent is used or withdrawn.

In doing tests for antibiotic sensitivity, the laboratory must maintain a high level of accuracy in the testing procedures, there must be a high degree of reproducibility of results, and there must be a good correlation between the results and the clinical response of the patient.[18]

Various methods are used to determine the susceptibility of a microorganism to an antibiotic. Some methods involve dilution tests, such as broth tube dilution or agar plate dilution. Another commonly used method is the agar diffusion test, employing antibiotic-impregnated disks. In this section we describe the method that is used most often and is the most economical—the high-potency disk-agar diffusion method.

It is important to remember that any *in vitro* test for antibiotic sensitivity is an artificial measurement and will give only an estimate of the effectiveness of the agent against the microorganism. The only absolute test of antibiotic sensitivity is the clinical response of the patient to the dosage of the antibiotic.

Disk-agar diffusion method for determination of antibiotic susceptibility (modified Bauer-Kirby procedure)[19]

This method is perhaps the most useful one for testing for antibiotic susceptibility. It is quick, economical, and can give reproducible results. The method was originally described by Bondi et al. in 1947.[20] Originally, filter paper disks were impregnated with antimicrobial agents in known concentrations and were carefully placed on an agar culture plate that had been inoculated with a culture of the bacterium being tested. Today, disks are commercially available, and a special disk dispenser is used to distribute the appropriate disks on the inoculated plate. The plate is incubated overnight and observed the following morning. There will be a zone of growth inhibition around the disk containing the agent to which the organism is *susceptible*, whereas the organism will grow up to and under the periphery of the disks containing agents to which it is *resistant*. Much work has been done to standard-

ize the disk procedure, and one modification used in many laboratories is that of Bauer and Kirby.[21]

The disk diffusion method is subject to Food and Drug Administration requirements, which cover standardization of media, formula, pH, agar depth, inoculum density, temperature, zone sizes, interpretative tables, and reference strains of bacteria for controls.

Selection of media for plating

For antibiotic sensitivity testing, the Mueller-Hinton (MH) agar plate is used. Mueller-Hinton agar can be prepared from commercial materials, following the manufacturer's instructions carefully. The plates should be stored in the refrigerator until used and should not be kept for more than 7 days, even under refrigeration, unless some method is used to prevent water loss by evaporation. Plates can be saved longer by wrapping them in polystyrene and keeping them refrigerated.

Handling and storage of disks

Disks for antibiotic susceptibility testing are usually supplied in separate containers with a suitable desiccant to prevent deterioration. Most antibiotic disks should be refrigerated until used, but some require freezing to maintain their potency. The manufacturer's instructions for storage and handling should be followed. All disks must be discarded on their expiration date.

Preparation of inoculum

A tube of tryp broth (5 ml) is inoculated with a pure culture of the organism to be tested and is incubated at 35°C for 4 hours or until the culture is visibly cloudy. This method is suitable only for fast-growing organisms. The turbidity of the test organism is compared with that of a barium sulfate standard, known as the McFarland standard. The standard must be vigorously mixed before use. The turbidity of the broth culture may be adjusted, if necessary, by diluting it with uninoculated broth in another tube. If the 4-hour broth tube does not have enough growth, it can be reincubated until adequate growth is observed. MH plates should be inoculated within 15 minutes of standardizing the broth.

Inoculation of the Mueller-Hinton agar plate

A sterile swab is dipped into the standardized broth culture (mixed well), and any excess fluid is removed from the swab by squeezing it on the side of the tube. The swab is streaked across the plate in much the same way as the quantitative urine culture plate (Fig. 10-7). While the MH plate is being streaked, the same swab is used to inoculate a sheep blood plate to check for purity. All organisms being tested should be inoculated onto their respective plates before any disks are applied. Plates should be labeled with the patient's name, type of specimen, organism, and date. They should be allowed to dry for at least 3 minutes before the disks are applied.

Application of disks

The appropriate disks are applied to all the plates, using a disk dispenser if one is available. Special disk dispensers are available with different combinations of antibiotic-impregnated disks. Each disk should be firmly pressed down onto the surface of the agar with a flamed and cooled

forceps to ensure complete contact with the agar. The disks should be distributed so that they are no closer than 15 mm to the edge of the Petri dish and so that no two disks are closer than 24 mm from center to center. Once a disk has been placed it should not be moved, as some diffusion of the antibiotic occurs almost immediately.

Incubation of plates

The plates are incubated at 35°C for 18 hours.

Reading of results

After incubation, the diameters of the zones of inhibition are measured with a caliper or a zone reader and recorded to the nearest whole millimeter. Susceptibility of the organism to the antibiotic is demonstrated by a clear zone of growth inhibition around the disk. Within the limitations of the test, the diameter of the inhibition zone is a measure of the relative susceptibility to a particular antibiotic. The diameters are compared with a sensitivity table for each antibiotic to see whether the organism is sensitive, intermediate, or resistant to that particular antibiotic. These results are reported to the physician. The term susceptible or sensitive implies that an infection caused by the strain tested may be expected to respond favorably to the particular antibiotic. Resistant strains, on the other hand, are not inhibited completely by the usual therapeutic concentration of the antibiotic.

REFERENCES

1. Karl S. Wittman and John C. Thomas, "Medical Laboratory Skills," p. 226, McGraw-Hill Book Company, New York, 1977.
2. David T. Smith, Norman F. Conant, et al., "Zinsser Microbiology," 12th ed., p. 102, Appleton-Century-Crofts, Inc., New York, 1960.
3. *Ibid.*, p. 104.
4. W. Robert Bailey and Elvyn G. Scott, "Diagnostic Microbiology," p. 5, 4th ed., C. V. Mosby Company, St. Louis, 1974.
5. Smith et al., *op. cit.*, pp. 13–14.
6. Wittman and Thomas, *op. cit.*, p. 239.
7. Stanley S. Raphael et al., "Lynch's Medical

Laboratory Technology," 3d ed., vol. I, p. 543, W. B. Saunders Company, Philadelphia, 1976.

8. "Difco Manual of Dehydrated Culture Media and Reagents for Microbiological and Clinical Laboratory Procedures," 9th ed., pp. 16–20, Difco Laboratories, Inc., Detroit, 1963.

9. Bailey and Scott, *op. cit.*, p. 392.

10. *Ibid.*, p. 389.

11. Raphael et al., *op. cit.*, p. 549.

12. "Difco Manual," *op. cit.*, pp. 21–22.

13. "Baltimore Biological Laboratories (BBL) Manual of Products and Laboratory Procedures," 5th ed., Baltimore Biological Laboratories, Cockeysville, Md., 1968.

14. Donna J. Blazevic, "Laboratory Procedures in Diagnostic Microbiology," pp. 127–149, Telestar Productions, Inc., St. Paul, Minn., 1976.

15. "Difco Manual," *op. cit.*

16. Israel Davidsohn and John Bernard Henry (eds.), "Clinical Diagnosis by Laboratory Methods," 15th ed., p. 933, W. B. Saunders Company, Philadelphia, 1974.

17. "Modern Urinalysis: A Guide to the Diagnosis of Urinary Tract Diseases and Metabolic Disorders," pp. 73–77, Ames Company, division of Miles Laboratories, Inc., Elkhart, Ind., 1973.

18. H. D. Isenberg, A Comparison of Nationwide Microbial Susceptibility Testing Using Standardized Discs, *Health Lab. Sci.*, vol. 1, pp. 185–256, 1964.

19. Blazevic, *op. cit.*, pp. 71–74.

20. A. Bondi, E. H. Spaulding, E. D. Smith, and C. C. Dietz, A Routine Method for the Rapid Determination of Susceptibility to Penicillin and Other Antibiotics, *Am. J. Med. Sci.*, vol. 214, pp. 221–225, 1947.

21. A. W. Bauer, W. W. M. Kirby, J. C. Sherris, and M. Turck, Antibiotic Susceptibility Testing by a Standardized Single Disc Method, *Am. J. Clin. Pathol.*, vol. 45, pp. 493–496, 1966.

BIBLIOGRAPHY

Bailey, W. Robert and Elvyn G. Scott: "Diagnostic Microbiology," 4th ed., C. V. Mosby Company, St. Louis, 1974.

"Baltimore Biological Laboratories (BBL) Manual of Products and Laboratory Procedures," 5th ed., Baltimore Biological Laboratories, Cockeysville, Md., 1968.

"Bergey's Manual of Determinative Bacteriology," 7th ed., Williams & Wilkins Company, Baltimore, 1957.

Blazevic, Donna J.: "Laboratory Procedures in Diagnostic Microbiology," Telestar Productions, Inc., St. Paul, Minn., 1976.

Cowan, S. T. and K. J. Steel: "Manual for the Identification of Medical Bacteria," 2d ed., Cambridge University Press, New York, 1974.

Davidsohn, Israel and John Bernard Henry (eds.): "Clinical Diagnosis by Laboratory Methods," 15th ed., W. B. Saunders Company, Philadelphia, 1974.

"Diagnostic Procedures and Reagents," 5th ed., American Public Health Association, Washington, D.C., 1970.

"Difco Manual of Dehydrated Culture Media and Reagents for Microbiological and Clinical Laboratory Procedures," 9th ed., Difco Laboratories, Inc., Detroit, 1963.

"Difco Supplementary Literature," Difco Laboratories, Inc., Detroit, 1968.

Kunin, Calvin M.: "Detection, Prevention, and Management of Urinary Tract Infections," Lea & Febiger, Philadelphia, 1972.

"Modern Urinalysis: A Guide to the Diagnosis of Urinary Tract Diseases and Metabolic Disorders," Ames Company, division of Miles Laboratories, Inc., Elkhart, Ind., 1973.

Raphael, Stanley S. et al.: "Lynch's Medical Laboratory Technology," 3d ed., vol. I, W. B. Saunders Company, Philadelphia, 1976.

Smith, Alice Lorraine: "Microbiology and Pathology," 9th ed., C. V. Mosby Company, St. Louis, 1968.

Wittman, Karl S. and John C. Thomas: "Medical Laboratory Skills," McGraw-Hill Book Company, New York, 1977.

INDEX